Medical Infrared Imaging

EDITED BY
Nicholas A. Diakides
Joseph D. Bronzino

CRC Press
Taylor & Francis Group
Boca Raton London New York

CRC Press is an imprint of the
Taylor & Francis Group, an **informa** business

This material was previously published in *Medical Devices and Systems* © 2006 by Taylor & Francis Group, LLC.

CRC Press
Taylor & Francis Group
6000 Broken Sound Parkway NW, Suite 300
Boca Raton, FL 33487-2742

© 2008 by Taylor & Francis Group, LLC
CRC Press is an imprint of Taylor & Francis Group, an Informa business

No claim to original U.S. Government works
Printed in the United States of America on acid-free paper
10 9 8 7 6 5 4 3 2 1

International Standard Book Number-13: 978-0-8493-9027-2 (Hardcover)

This book contains information obtained from authentic and highly regarded sources. Reprinted material is quoted with permission, and sources are indicated. A wide variety of references are listed. Reasonable efforts have been made to publish reliable data and information, but the author and the publisher cannot assume responsibility for the validity of all materials or for the consequences of their use.

No part of this book may be reprinted, reproduced, transmitted, or utilized in any form by any electronic, mechanical, or other means, now known or hereafter invented, including photocopying, microfilming, and recording, or in any information storage or retrieval system, without written permission from the publishers.

For permission to photocopy or use material electronically from this work, please access www.copyright.com (http://www.copyright.com/) or contact the Copyright Clearance Center, Inc. (CCC) 222 Rosewood Drive, Danvers, MA 01923, 978-750-8400. CCC is a not-for-profit organization that provides licenses and registration for a variety of users. For organizations that have been granted a photocopy license by the CCC, a separate system of payment has been arranged.

Trademark Notice: Product or corporate names may be trademarks or registered trademarks, and are used only for identification and explanation without intent to infringe.

Library of Congress Cataloging-in-Publication Data

Medical infrared imaging / editors, Nicholas A. Diakides and Joseph D. Bronzino.
    p. ; cm.
"A CRC title."
Includes bibliographical references and index.
ISBN-13: 978-0-8493-9027-2 (hardcover : alk. paper)
ISBN-10: 0-8493-9027-3 (hardcover : alk. paper)
    1. Infrared imaging--Diagnostic use. I. Diakides, Nicholas A. II. Bronzino, Joseph D., 1937-
    [DNLM: 1. Diagnostic Imaging--methods. 2. Infrared Rays--diagnostic use. 3. Thermography--methods. WN 180 M4903 2007]

RC78.7.D53M437 2007
616.07'54--dc22
                                                                 2007007402

Visit the Taylor & Francis Web site at
http://www.taylorandfrancis.com

and the CRC Press Web site at
http://www.crcpress.com

Preface

The evolution of technological advances in infrared sensor technology, image processing, "smart" algorithms, knowledge-based databases, and their overall system integration has resulted in new methods of research and use in medical infrared imaging. The development of infrared cameras with focal plane arrays not requiring cooling added a new dimension to this modality. New detector materials with improved thermal sensitivity are now available and production of high-density focal plane arrays (640 × 480) has been achieved. Advance read-out circuitry using on-chip signal processing is in common use. These breakthroughs permit low-cost and easy-to-use camera systems with thermal sensitivity less than 50 mK, as well as spatial resolution of 25–50 μm, given the appropriate optics. Another important factor is the emerging interest in the development of smart image processing algorithms to enhance the interpretation of thermal signatures. In the clinical area, new research addresses the key issues of diagnostic sensitivity and specificity of infrared imaging. Efforts are underway to achieve quantitative clinical data interpretation in standardized diagnostic procedures. For this purpose, clinical protocols are emphasized.

New concepts such as dynamic thermal imaging and thermal texture mapping (thermal tomography) and thermal multispectral imaging are being implemented in clinical environments. Other areas such as three-dimensional infrared are being investigated.

Some of these new ideas, concepts, and technologies are covered in this book. We have assembled a set of chapters that ranges in content from historical background, concepts, clinical applications, standards, and infrared technology.

Chapter 1 deals with worldwide advances in and a guide to thermal imaging systems for medical applications. Chapter 2 presents an historical perspective and the evolution of thermal imaging. Chapters 3–5 are comprehensive chapters on technology and hardware including detectors, detector materials, uncooled focal plane arrays, high performance systems, camera characterization, electronics for on-chip image processing, optics, and cost-reduction designs.

Chapter 6 deals with the physiological basis of the thermal signature and its interpretation in a medical setting. It discusses the physics of thermal radiation theory and the pathophysiology as related to infrared imaging. Chapters 7 and 8 cover innovative concepts such as dynamic thermal imaging and thermal tomography that enhance the clinical utility leading to improved diagnostic capability. Chapters 9 and 10 expose the fundamentals of infrared breast imaging, equipment considerations, early detection, and the use of infrared imaging in a multi-modality setting. Chapters 11 and 12 are on innovative image processing techniques for the early detection of breast cancer. Chapter 13 presents biometrics, a novel method for facial recognition. Today, this technology is of utmost importance in the area of homeland security and other applications. Chapter 14 deals with infrared monitoring of therapies using multispectral optical imaging in Kaposi's Sarcoma investigations at NIH. Chapters 15–20 deal with the use of infrared in various clinical applications: surgery, dental, skeletal and neuromuscular diseases, as well as the quantification of the TAU image technique in the relevance and stage of a disease. Chapter 21 is on infrared imaging in veterinary medicine. Chapter 22 discusses the complexities and importance of standardization, calibration, and protocols for effective and reproducible results. Chapter 23 deals with databases and primarily with the storage and retrieval of thermal images. Chapter 24 addresses the ethical obligations in infrared research and clinical practice.

This book will be of interest to both the medical and biomedical engineering communities. It could provide many opportunities for developing and conducting multidisciplinary research in many areas of medical infrared imaging. These range from clinical quantification to intelligent image processing for enhancement of the interpretation of images, and for further development of user-friendly high-resolution thermal cameras. These would enable the wide use of infrared imaging as a viable, noninvasive, low-cost, first-line detection modality.

Acknowledgments

I would like to acknowledge each and every author in this book for the excellent contributions. I am aware of their busy schedules and I appreciate the time they dedicated to this book.

Further recognition must be given to those who have continued to research and use infrared imaging in the medical field over many years and upon whose basis the present technological advancement in this field has emerged.

In addition, I would like to acknowledge the great contribution of the U.S. Department of Defense for successfully developing the infrared technology and for the continued strong support of the Army Research Office (ARO), Defense Advanced Research Project Agency (DARPA), and the Office of the Undersecretary of Defense (Science & Technology) toward the transfer of this technology to medicine.

Editors

Nicholas A. Diakides received his D.Sc. in electrical engineering (biomedical engineering, telecommunications and computer science) from George Washington University in 1979. He is president of Advanced Concepts Analysis, Inc. (1989–present), a corporation dealing with advanced biomedical technology and innovative defense research on sensors. He was involved in analysis and assessment of sensor systems, biomedical technology, medical imaging, and bioinformatics for the Office of the Secretary of Defense (OSD-S&T, DARPA, ARO, and ONR). In addition, since 1994 he has led the effort to establish internationally the use of advanced digital infrared imaging in medicine. Previously, he was the director of the Survivability Enhancement Division, U.S. Army Laboratory Command (1984–1989). From 1962 to 1983 he was program manager for various areas of infrared (IR) technology and electro-optics at the Army Night Vision and Electro-Optics Laboratory. Dr. Diakides' research interests include infrared imaging, "smart" image processing, computer-aided detection, knowledge-based databases, information technology, and telemedicine.

Dr. Diakides has been very active in IEEE-EMBS activities: publicity chair and member of the conference and technical program committees at the 16th annual international conference, Baltimore, Maryland, 1994; organizer and chair of all infrared imaging activities (tracks, sessions, workshops and mini-symposia) for IEEE-EMBS International Conferences (1994–2006). He is a IEEE-USA member of the following committees: R&D Policy (1994–present), Healthcare Engineering Policy (1989–1994), EMBS technical committee on imaging and image processing (2005–present). His editorial responsibilities include: guest editor, *IEEE EMB Magazine* special issues on medical infrared imaging (July/August 1999, May/June 2000, November/December 2002), co-editor *Medical Infrared Imaging* (CRC Press, 2007), section editor, "Infrared Imaging" in the *Biomedical Engineering Handbook* (3rd Edition, CRC Press, 2006). He has published more than 50 papers, as well as a book chapter (invited) on "Phosphor Screens" in the *Electronics Engineers' Handbook* (2nd Edition, McGraw-Hill Book Company, 1982).

Dr. Diakides is the inventor of the MedATR concept that led to the first IR-CAD for the early detection of breast abnormalities and other applications. He was the first to demonstrate the value of knowledge-based databases with standardized IR signatures validated by pathology and is a recipient of the Department of the Army R&D Achievement Award (1973). He is a fellow of the American Institute of Medical and Biological Engineering and a member of the executive committee of the American Academy of Thermology (1998–present).

Joseph D. Bronzino received the B.S.E.E. degree from Worcester Polytechnic Institute, Worcester, Massachusetts, in 1959, the M.S.E.E. degree from the Naval Postgraduate School, Monterey, California, in 1961, and the Ph.D. degree in electrical engineering from Worcester Polytechnic Institute in 1968. He is presently the Vernon Roosa Professor of Applied Science, an endowed chair at Trinity College, Hartford, Connecticut and president of the Biomedical Engineering Alliance and Consortium (BEACON), which is a nonprofit organization consisting of academic and medical institutions as well as corporations dedicated to the development and commercialization of new medical technologies (for details visit www.beaconalliance.org).

Dr. Bronzino is the author of over 200 articles and 11 books including the following: *Technology for Patient Care* (C.V. Mosby, 1977), *Computer Applications for Patient Care* (Addison-Wesley, 1982), *Biomedical Engineering: Basic Concepts and Instrumentation* (PWS Publishing Co., 1986), *Expert Systems: Basic Concepts* (Research Foundation of State University of New York, 1989), *Medical Technology and Society: An Interdisciplinary Perspective* (MIT Press and McGraw-Hill, 1990), *Management of Medical Technology* (Butterworth/Heinemann, 1992), *The Biomedical Engineering Handbook* (CRC Press, 1st ed., 1995; 2nd ed., 2000; Taylor & Francis, 3rd ed., 2005), *Introduction to Biomedical Engineering* (Academic Press, 1st ed., 1999; 2nd ed., 2005).

Dr. Bronzino is a fellow of IEEE and the American Institute of Medical and Biological Engineering (AIMBE), an honorary member of the Italian Society of Experimental Biology, past chairman of the Biomedical Engineering Division of the American Society for Engineering Education (ASEE), a charter member and presently vice president of the Connecticut Academy of Science and Engineering (CASE), a charter member of the American College of Clinical Engineering (ACCE) and the Association for the Advancement of Medical Instrumentation (AAMI), past president of the IEEE-Engineering in Medicine and Biology Society (EMBS), past chairman of the IEEE Health Care Engineering Policy Committee (HCEPC), past chairman of the IEEE Technical Policy Council in Washington, DC, and presently editor-in-chief of Elsevier's BME Book Series and Taylor & Francis' *Biomedical Engineering Handbook*.

Dr. Bronzino was also the recipient of the Millennium Award from IEEE/EMBS in 2000 and the Goddard Award from Worcester Polytechnic Institute for Professional Achievement in June 2004.

Contributors

P.D. Ahlgren
Ville Marie Medical and Women's Health Center
Montreal, Quebec, Canada

William C. Amalu
Pacific Chiropractic and Research Center
Redwood City, California, U.S.A.

Kurt Ammer
Ludwig Bolzman Research Institute for Physical Diagnostics and University of Glamorgan
Vienna, Austria

Michael Anbar
Department of Physiology and Biophysics
School of Medicine and Biomedical Science
University at Buffalo (SUNY)
Buffalo, New York, U.S.A.

Raymond Balcerak
Defense Advanced Research Projects Agency
Arlington, Virginia, U.S.A.

Normand Belliveau
Ville Marie Medical and Women's Health Center
Montreal, Quebec, Canada

Pradeep Buddharaju
Department of Computer Science
University of Houston
Houston, Texas, U.S.A.

Paul Campbell
Ninewells Hospital
Dundee, Scotland, U.K.

Victor Chernomordik
Laboratory of Integrative and Medical Biophysics
National Institute of Child Health and Human Development
Bethesda, Maryland, U.S.A.

Timothy D. Conwell
Colorado Infrared Imaging Center
Denver, Colorado, U.S.A.

Lois de Weerd
University Hospital of North Norway
Tromsø, Norway

Mary Diakides
Advanced Concept Analysis, Inc.
Falls Church, Virginia, U.S.A.

Nicholas A. Diakides
Advanced Concept Analysis, Inc.
Falls Church, Virginia, U.S.A.

C. Drews-Peszynski
Technical University of Lodz
Lodz, Poland

Ronald G. Driggers
Army CERDEC Night Vision and Electronic Sensors Directorate
Fort Belvoir, Virginia, U.S.A.

Robert L. Elliott
Elliott-Elliott-Head Breast Cancer Research and Treatment Center
Baton Rouge, Louisiana, U.S.A.

Amir H. Gandjbakhche
Laboratory of Integrative and Medical Biophysics
National Institute of Child Health and Human Development
Bethesda, Maryland, U.S.A.

Israel Gannot
Laboratory of Integrative and Medical Biophysics
National Institute of Child Health and Human Development
Bethesda, Maryland, U.S.A.

James Giordano
Center for Clinical Bioethics and Division of Palliative Medicine
Georgetown University Medical Center
Washington, DC, U.S.A.

Barton M. Gratt
School of Dentistry
University of Washington
Seattle, Washington, U.S.A.

Michael W. Grenn
Army CERDEC Night Vision and Electronic Sensors Directorate
Fort Belvoir, Virginia, U.S.A.

Steven J. Gulevich
Swedish Medical Center
Edgewood, Colorado, U.S.A.

Moinuddin Hassan
Laboratory of Integrative and Medical Biophysics
National Institute of Child Health and Human Development
Bethesda, Maryland, U.S.A.

David Hattery
Laboratory of Integrative and Medical Biophysics
National Institute of Child Health and Human Development
Bethesda, Maryland, U.S.A.

Jonathan F. Head
Elliott-Elliott-Head Breast Caner Research and Treatment Center
Baton Rouge, Louisiana, U.S.A.

William B. Hobbins
Women's Breast Health Center
Madison, Wisconsin, U.S.A.

Stuart B. Horn
Army CERDEC Night Vision and Electronic Sensors Directorate
Fort Belvoir, Virginia, U.S.A.

T. Jakubowska
Technical University of Lodz
Lodz, Poland

Bryan F. Jones
Medical Imaging Research Group
School of Computing
Glamorgan University
Pontypridd, Wales U.K.

John R. Keyserlingk
Ville Marie Medical and Women's Health Center
Montreal, Quebec, Canada

E.C. Klee
Nanyang Technological University
Singapore

Phani Teja Kuruganti
RF and Microwave Systems Group
Oak Ridge National Laboratory
Oak Ridge, Tennessee, U.S.A.

Richard F. Little
Laboratory of Integrative and Medical Biophysics
National Institute of Child Health and Human Development
Bethesda, Maryland, U.S.A.

Jasper C. Lupo
Applied Research Associates, Inc.
Alexandra, Virginia, U.S.A.

James B. Mercer
University of Tromsø
Tromsø, Norway

Arcangelo Merla
Department of Clinical Sciences and Bioimaging
University of G. d'Annunzio
and
Institute for Advanced Biomedical Technology
University Foundation "G. d'Annunzio"
and
Istituto Nazionale Fisica della Materia
Coordinated Group of Chieti
Chieti-Pescara, Italy

E.Y.K. Ng
School of Mechanical and Aerospace Engineering
College of Engineering
Nanyang Technological University
Singapore

Paul. R. Norton
Army CERDEC Night Vision and Electronic Sensors Directorate
Fort Belvoir, Virginia, U.S.A.

Antoni Nowakowski
Department of Biomedical Engineering
Gdansk University of Technology
Narutowicza, Gdansk, Poland

David D. Pascoe
Auburn University
Auburn, Alabama, U.S.A.

Jeffrey L. Paul
Defense Advanced Research Projects Agency
Arlington, Virginia, U.S.A.

Ioannis Pavlidis
Department of Computer Science
University of Houston
Houston, Texas, U.S.A.

Joseph G. Pellegrino
Army CERDEC Night Vision and Electronic Sensors Directorate
Fort Belvoir, Virginia, U.S.A.

Philip Perconti
Army CERDEC Night Vision and Electronic Sensors Directorate
Fort Belvoir, Virginia, U.S.A.

Ram C. Purohit
Auburn University
Auburn, Alabama, U.S.A.

Hairong Qi
ECE Department
University of Tennessee
Knoxville, Tennessee, U.S.A.

Francis E. Ring
Medical Imaging Research Group
School of Computing
Glamorgan University
Pontypridd, Wales U.K.

Gian Luca Romani
Department of Clinical Sciences and Bioimaging
University of G. d'Annunzio
and
Institute for Advanced Biomedical Technology
University Foundation "G. d'Annunzio"
and
Istituto Nazionale Fisica della Materia
Coordinated Group of Chieti
Chieti-Pescara, Italy

Gerald Schaefer
School of Engineering and Applied Science
Aston University
Birmingham, U.K.

Wesley E. Snyder
ECE Department
North Carolina State University
Raleigh, North Carolina, U.S.A.

M. Strzelecki
Technical University of Lodz
Lodz, Poland

Roderick Thomas
Faculty of Applied Design and Engineering
Swansea Institute of Technology
Swansea, U.K.

Tracy A. Turner
Private practice
Auburn, Alabama, U.S.A.

Jay Vizgaitis
Army CERDEC Night Vision and Electronic Sensors Directorate
Fort Belvoir, Virginia, U.S.A.

Abby Vogel
Laboratory of Integrative and Medical Biophysics
National Institute of Child Health and Human Development
Bethesda, Maryland, U.S.A.

Boguslaw Wiecek
Technical University of Lodz
Lodz, Poland

M. Wysocki
Technical University of Lodz
Lodz, Poland

Robert Yarchoan
HIV and AIDS Malignancy Branch
Center for Cancer Research
National Cancer Institute (NCI)
Bethesda, Maryland, U.S.A.

Mariam Yassa
Ville Marie Medical and Women's Health Center
Montreal, Quebec, Canada

E. Yu
Ville Marie Medical and Women's Health Center
Montreal, Quebec, Canada

Jason Zeibel
Army CERDEC Night Vision and Electronic Sensors Directorate
Fort Belvoir, Virginia, U.S.A.

Contents

1 Advances in Medical Infrared Imaging
  *Nicholas A. Diakides, Mary Diakides, Jasper C. Lupo, Jeffrey
  L. Paul, and Raymond Balcerak* **1**-1

2 The Historical Development of Thermometry and Thermal
  Imaging in Medicine
  Francis E. Ring and Bryan F. Jones **2**-1

3 Infrared Detectors and Detector Arrays
  *Paul R. Norton, Stuart B. Horn, Joseph G. Pellegrino, and
  Philip Perconti* **3**-1

4 Infrared Camera Characterization
  *Joseph G. Pellegrino, Jason Zeibel, Ronald G. Driggers, and
  Philip Perconti* **4**-1

5 Infrared Camera and Optics for Medical Applications
  *Michael W. Grenn, Jay Vizgaitis, Joseph G. Pellegrino, and
  Philip Perconti* **5**-1

6 Physiology of Thermal Signals
  David D. Pascoe, James B. Mercer, and Lois de Weerd **6**-1

7 Quantitative Active Dynamic Thermal IR-Imaging and
  Thermal Tomography in Medical Diagnostics
  Antoni Nowakowski **7**-1

8 Dynamic Thermal Assessment
  Michael Anbar **8**-1

9 Infrared Imaging of the Breast: A Review
  *William C. Amalu, William B. Hobbins, Jonathan F. Head,
  and Robert L. Elliot* **9**-1

10 Functional Infrared Imaging of the Breast: Historical Perspectives, Current Application, and Future Considerations
    John R. Keyserlingk, P.D. Ahlgren, E. Yu, Normand Belliveau, and Mariam Yassa 10-1

11 Detecting Breast Cancer from Thermal Infrared Images by Asymmetry Analysis
    Hairong Qi, Phani Teja Kuruganti, and Wesley E. Snyder 11-1

12 Advanced Thermal Image Processing
    Boguslaw Wiecek, M. Strzelecki, T. Jakubowska, M. Wysocki, and C. Drews-Peszynski 12-1

13 Physiology-Based Face Recognition in the Thermal Infrared Spectrum
    Pradeep Buddharaju and Ioannis Pavlidis 13-1

14 Infrared Imaging for Functional Monitoring of Disease Processes
    Moinuddin Hassan, Victor Chernomordik, Abby Vogel, David Hattery, Israel Gannot, Richard F. Little, Robert Yarchoan, and Amir H. Gandjbakhche 14-1

15 Biomedical Applications of Functional Infrared Imaging
    Arcangelo Merla and Gian Luca Romani 15-1

16 Fever Mass Screening Tool for Infectious Diseases Outbreak: Integrated Artificial Intelligence with Bio-Statistical Approach in Thermogram Analysis
    E.Y.K. Ng and E.C. Klee 16-1

17 Thermal Imaging in Diseases of the Skeletal and Neuromuscular Systems
    Francis E. Ring and Kurt Ammer 17-1

18 Functional Infrared Imaging in the Evaluation of Complex Regional Pain Syndrome, Type I: Current Pathophysiological Concepts, Methodology, Case Studies, Clinical Implications
    Timothy D. Conwell, James Giordano, and Steven J. Gulevich 18-1

19 Thermal Imaging in Surgery
    Paul Campbell and Roderick Thomas 19-1

20 Infrared Imaging Applied to Dentistry
    Barton M. Gratt 20-1

21 Use of Infrared Imaging in Veterinary Medicine
    Ram C. Purohit, Tracy A. Turner, and David D. Pascoe 21-1

22 Standard Procedures for Infrared Imaging in Medicine
   Kurt Ammer and Francis E. Ring **22**-1

23 Storage and Retrieval of Medical Thermograms
   Gerald Schaefer **23**-1

24 Ethical Obligations in Infrared Imaging Research and Practice
   James Giordano **24**-1

Index **I**-1

1
Advances in Medical Infrared Imaging

Nicholas A. Diakides
Mary Diakides
Advanced Concept Analysis, Inc.

Jasper C. Lupo
Applied Research Associates, Inc.

Jeffrey L. Paul
Raymond Balcerak
Defense Advanced Research Projects Agency

1.1 Introduction... 1-1
1.2 Worldwide Use of IR Imaging in Medicine 1-2
1.3 IR Imaging in Breast Cancer 1-5
    The Image Processing and Medical Applications • Website and Database • Sensor Technology for Medical Applications
1.4 Guide to Thermal Imaging Systems for Medical Applications.. 1-7
    Introduction • Background • Applications and Image Formats • Dynamic Range • Resolution and Sensitivity • Calibration • Single Band Imagers • Emerging and Future Camera Technology • Summary Specifications
1.5 Summary, Conclusions, and Recommendations 1-12
References 1-13

1.1 Introduction

Infrared (IR) imaging in medicine has been used in the past but without the advantage of twenty-first-century technology. In 1994, under the Department of Defense (DOD) grants jointly funded by the Office of the Secretary of Defense Science and Technology (S&T), the Defense Advanced Research Projects Agency (DARPA), and the Army Research Office (ARO), a concerted effort was initiated to revisit this subject. Specifically, it was to explore the potential of integrating advanced IR technology with "smart" image processing for use in medicine. The major challenges for acceptance of this modality by the medical community were investigated. It was found that the following issues were of prime importance:

1. Standardization and quantification of clinical data
2. Better understanding of the pathophysiological nature of thermal signatures
3. Wider publication and exposure of medical IR imaging in conferences and leading journals
4. Characterization of thermal signatures through an interactive web-based database
5. Training in both image acquisition and interpretation

In the past 10 years, significant progress has been made internationally by advancing a thrust for new initiatives worldwide for clinical quantification, international collaboration, and providing a forum for coordination, discussion, and publication through the following activities:

1. Medical IR imaging symposia, workshops, and tracks at IEEE/Engineering in Medicine and Biology Society (EMBS) conferences from 1994 to 2004

TABLE 1.1 Medical Applications and Methods

Applications	IR imaging methods
Oncology (breast, skin, etc.)	Static (classical)
Pain (management/control)	Dynamic (DAT, subtraction, etc.)
Vascular Disorders (diabetes, DVT)	Dynamic (active)
Arthritis/rheumatism	Multispectral/hyperspectral
Neurology	Multimodality
Surgery (open heart, transplant, etc.)	Sensor Fusion
Ophthalmic (cataract removal)	
Tissue viability (burns, etc.)	
Dermatological disorders	
Monitoring efficacy of drugs and therapies	
Thyroid	
Dentistry	
Respiratory (allergies, SARS)	
Sports and Rehabilitation Medicine	

2. Three Engineering in Medicine and Biology Magazines (EMBS), Special Issues dedicated to this topic [1–3]
3. The DOD "From Tanks to Tumors" Workshop [4]

The products of these efforts are documented in final government technical reports [5–8] and *IEEE/EMBS Conference Proceedings* (1994–2004).

Early IR-cameras used a small number of detector elements (1 to 180 individual detectors) that required cryogenic cooling in order to operate effectively without noise. The camera design incorporated a scanning mechanism with mirrors to form the image. Electrical contact was made to each individual detector— a very laborious and time-intensive task. The signal leads were brought out of the cryogenic envelope and each individual signal was combined. The processing was performed outside the focal plane array (FPA). This type of camera was heavy in weight, high in power consumption, and very expensive to manufacture. Hence, the technology focused on producing a more efficient, lower-cost system that ultimately led to the uncooled FPA-type cameras. In the FPA camera, the detectors are fabricated in large arrays, which eliminates the need for scanning. Electrical contact is made simultaneously to the detector array, thus reducing significantly the number of leads through vacuum. Furthermore, the uncooled FPA has the potential to accommodate on-chip processing, thus leading to faster operation and fewer leads.

Presently, IR imaging is used in many different medical applications. The most prominent of these are oncology (breast, skin, etc.), vascular disorders (diabetes Deep Venous Thrombosis (DVT), etc.), pain, surgery, tissue viability, monitoring the efficacy of drugs and therapies, and respiratory disorders (recently introduced for testing of Severe Acute Respiratory Syndrome (SARS)).

There are various methods used to acquire IR images: static, dynamic, passive, and active—dynamic area telethermometry (DAT), subtraction, and so forth [9]; thermal texture mapping (TTM); multi-spectral/hyperspectral; multimodality; and sensor fusion. A list of current applications and IR imaging methods are listed in Table 1.1. Figures 1.1 and 1.2 illustrate thermal signatures of breast screening and Kaposi sarcoma.

1.2 Worldwide Use of IR Imaging in Medicine

United States of America and Canada: IR imaging is beginning to be reconsidered in the Unites States, largely due to the new IR technology; advanced image processing; powerful, high-speed computers; and exposure of existing research. This is evidenced by the increased number of publications available in open literature and national databases such as "Index Medicus" and "Medline" (National Library of Medicine)

FIGURE 1.1 (See color insert at the back of the book.) An application of IR technique for breast screening: (a) healthy and (b) pathological breast. (Courtesy: Prof. Reinhold Berz, MD. Informatics Germany.)

FIGURE 1.2 (See color insert.) An application of IR technique for cancer research. (From Hassan, M., et al., 2004. *Technology in Cancer Research and Treatment*, 3, 451–457. With permission.)

on this modality. Currently, there are several academic institutions with research initiatives in IR imaging. Some of the most prominent are the following: The National Institutes of Health (NIH), Johns Hopkins University, University of Houston, University of Texas. NIH has several ongoing programs: vascular disorders (diabetes, deep venous thrombosis); monitoring angiogenesis activity—Kaposi sarcoma; pain-reflex sympathetic dystrophy; monitoring the efficacy of radiation therapy; organ transplant—perfusion; and multispectral imaging.

Johns Hopkins University does research in microcirculation; monitoring angiogenic activity in Kaposi sarcoma and breast screening; and laparoscopic IR images—renal disease.

University of Houston has recently created an IR imaging laboratory to investigate with IR the facial thermal characteristics for such applications as lie detection and other behavioral issues (fatigue, anxiety, fear, etc.).

There are multimodality medical centers specializing in breast cancer research and treatment that use IR routinely as part of their first-line detection system, which also includes mammography and clinical exam. Two of these are EHH Breast Cancer and Treatment Center, Baton Rouge, Los Angeles, and Ville Marie Oncology Research Center, Montreal, Canada. Their centers are fully equipped with all state-of-the-art imaging equipment. These centers are members of the coalition team for the development of a "knowledge-based" database of thermal signatures of the breast with "ground-truth" validation. There are also new research initiatives currently being conducted in leading medical centers.

China: China has a long-standing interest in IR imaging. More recently, the novel method TTM has added increased specificity to static imaging. It is known that this method is widely used in this country, but unfortunately there is no formal literature about this important work. This is urgently needed in order for TTM to be exposed and accepted as a viable, effective method by the international community. The clinical results obtained through this method should be published in open literature of medical journals and international conference proceedings. Despite the lack of the availability of this documentation, introduction of TTM has been made to NIH. They are now using this method and its camera successfully in detection and treatment in Kaposi sarcoma (associated with AIDS patients). After further discussions with them, interest has also been shown for its use in the area of breast cancer (detection of angiogenesis). There are further possibilities for high-level research for this method in the United States and abroad.

Japan: IR imaging is widely accepted in Japan by the government and the medical community. More than 1500 hospitals and clinics use IR imaging routinely. The government sets the standards and reimburses clinical tests. Their focus is in the following areas: blood perfusion, breast cancer, dermatology, pain, neurology, surgery (open-heart, orthopedic, dental, cosmetic), sports medicine, and oriental medicine. The main research is performed at the following universities: University of Tokyo (organ transplant); Tokyo Medical and Dental University (skin temperature characterization and thermal properties); Toho University (neurological operation); and Cancer Institute Hospital (breast cancer). In addition, about 40 other medical institutions are using IR for breast cancer screening.

Korea: Koreas began involvement in IR imaging during the early 1990s. More than 450 systems are being used in hospitals and medical centers. Primary clinical applications are neurology, back pain/treatment, surgery, and oriental medicine. Yonsei College of Medicine is one of the leading institutions in medical IR imaging research along with three others.

United Kingdom: The University of Glamorgan is the center of IR imaging; the School of Computing has a thermal physiology laboratory that focuses in the following areas: medical IR research, standardization, training (university diploma), and "SPORTI" Project funded by the European Union Organization. The objective of this effort is to develop a reference database of normal, thermal signatures from healthy subjects.

The Royal National Hospital of Rheumatic Diseases specializes in rheumatic disorders, occupational health (Raynaud's disease, carpal tunnel syndrome, and sports medicine).

The Royal Free University College Medical School Hospital specializes in vascular disorders (diabetes, DVT, etc.), optimization of IR imaging techniques, and Raynaud's phenomenon.

Germany: University of Leipzig uses IR for open-heart surgery, perfusion, and microcirculation. There are several private clinics and other hospitals that use IR imaging in various applications.

EvoBus-Daimler Chrysler uses IR imaging for screening all their employees for wellness/health assessment (occupational health).

InfraMedic, AG, conducts breast cancer screening of women from 20 to 85 years old for the government under a 2-year grant. IR is the sole modality used. Their screening method is called infrared regulation imaging (IRI) and it is listed in Figure 1.1.

Austria: Ludwig Bolzman Research Institute for Physical Diagnostics has done research in IR for many years and it publishes the *Thermology International* (a quarterly journal of IR clinical research and instrumentation). This journal contains papers from many thermology societies. A recent issue contains the results of a survey of 2003 international papers dedicated to thermology [10].

The General Hospital, University of Vienna, does research mainly in angiology (study of blood and lymph vessels) and diabetic foot (pedobarography).

Poland: There has been a more recent rapid increase in the use of IR imaging for medicine in Poland since the Polish market for IR-cameras was opened up. There are more than 50 cameras being used in the following medical centers: Warsaw University, Technical University of Gdansk, Poznan University, Lodz University, Katowice University, and the Military Clinical Hospital. The research activities are focused on the following areas: active IR imaging, open-heart surgery, quantitative assessment of skin burns, ophthalmology, dentistry, allergic diseases, neurological disorders, plastic surgery, thermal image database for healthy and pathological cases, and multispectral imaging (IR, visual, x-ray, ultrasound, etc.).

Advances in Medical Infrared Imaging

In 1986, the Eurotherm Committee was created by members of the European Community to promote cooperation in the thermal sciences by gathering scientist and engineers working in the area of thermology. This organization focuses on quantitative IR thermography and periodically holds conferences and seminars in this field [11].

Italy: Much of the clinical use of IR imaging is done under the public health system, besides private clinics. The ongoing clinical work is in the following areas: dermatology (melanoma), neurology, rheumatology, anesthesiology, reproductive medicine, and sports medicine. The University of G. d'Annunzio, Chieti, has an imaging laboratory purely for research on IR applications. It collaborates on these projects with other universities throughout Italy.

There are other countries, such as Australia, Norway, South America, Russia, and so forth, that have ongoing research as well.

1.3 IR Imaging in Breast Cancer

In the United States, breast cancer is a national concern. There are 192,000 cases a year; it is estimated that there are 1 million women with undetected breast cancer; presently, the figure of women affected is 1.8 million; 45,000 women die per year. The cost burden of the U.S. healthcare is estimated at $18 billion per year. The cost for early stage detection is $12,000 per patient and that for late detection is $345,000 per patient. Hence, early detection would potentially save $12 billion dollars annually—as well as many lives. As a result, the U.S. Congress created "The Congressionally Directed Medical Research Program for Breast Cancer." Clinical IR has not as yet been supported through this funding. Effort is being directed toward including IR. Since 1982, FDA has approved IR imaging (thermography) as an adjunct modality to mammography for breast cancer, as shown in Table 1.2.

Ideal characteristics for an early breast cancer detection method as defined by the Congressionally Directed Medical Research Programs on Breast Cancer are listed in Table 1.3. IR imaging meets these requirements with the exception of the detection of early lesions at 1000 to 10,000 cells that have not yet been fully determined.

TABLE 1.2 Imaging Modalities for Breast Cancer Detection Approved by FDA

Film-screen mammography
Full-field digital mammography
Computer-aided detection
Ultrasound
Magnetic resonance imaging (MRI)
Positron emission tomography (PET)
Thermography
Electrical impedance imaging

Source: Mammography and Beyond, Institute of Medicine, National Academy Press, 2001.

TABLE 1.3 Ideal Characteristics for an Early Breast Cancer Detection Method

Detects early lesions
Available to population (48 million U.S. women ages 40 to 70 years)
High sensitivity/High specificity (in all age groups)
Inexpensive
Noninvasive
Easily trainable and with high quality assurance
Decreases mortality
Infrared imaging meets all the above requirements

A program is underway in the United States to develop a prototype web-based database with a collection of approximately 2000 patient thermal signatures to be categorized into three categories: normal, equivocal, and suspicious for developing algorithms for screening and early detection of tumor development.

The origin of this program can be traced back to a 1994 multiagency DOD grant sponsored by the Director for Research in the Office of the Director, Defense Research and Engineering, the DARPA, and the ARO. This grant funded a study to determine the applicability of advanced military technology to the detection of breast cancer—particularly thermal imaging and automatic target recognition (ATR). The study produced two reports, one in 1995 and another in 1998; these studies identified technology, concepts, and ongoing activity that would have direct relevance to a rigorous application of IR. Rigor was the essential ingredient to further progress. The U.S. effort had been dormant since the 1970s because of the limitations imposed by poor sensors, simplistic imaging processing, lack of ATR, and inadequate computing power. This was complicated by the fact that the virtues of IR had been overstated by a few developers.

In 1999, the Director for Research in the Office of the Director, Defense Research and Engineering and the Deputy Assistant Secretary of the Army for Installations and Environment; Environmental Safety and Occupational Health formulated a technology transfer program that would facilitate the use of advanced military technology and processes in breast cancer screening. Funds were provided by the army and the project was funded through the Office of Naval Research (ONR).

A major milestone in the U.S. program was the Tanks to Tumors workshop held in Arlington, VA, December 4–5, 2001. The workshop was cosponsored by Office of the Director, Defense Research and Engineering, Space and Sensor Technology Directorate; the Deputy Assistant Secretary of the Army for Environment, Safety and Occupational Health; the DARPA; and the ARO. The purpose was to explore means for exploiting the technological opportunities in the integration of image processing, web-based database management and development, and IR sensor technology for the early detection of breast cancer. A second objective was to provide guidance to a program. The government speakers noted that significant military advances in thermal imaging and ATR coupled with medical understanding of abnormal vascularity (angiogenesis) offer the prospect of automated detection from 1 to 2 years earlier than other, more costly and invasive screening methods.

There were compelling reasons for both military and civilian researchers to attend:

1. Recognition of breast cancer as a major occupational health issue by key personnel such as Raymond Fatz, Deputy Assistant Secretary of the Army for Installations and Environment; Environmental Safety and Occupational Health
2. Growing use of thermal imaging in military and civilian medicine (especially abroad)
3. Maturation of military technology in ATR, ATR evaluation, and low-cost thermal imaging
4. Emerging transfer opportunities to and from the military

In particular, ATR assessment technology has developed image data management, dissemination, collaboration, and assessment tools for use by government and industrial developers of ATR software used to find military targets in thermal imagery. Such tools seem naturally suited for adaptation to the creation and use of a national database for IR breast cancer imagery and the evaluation of screening algorithms that would assist physicians in detecting the disease early. Finally, recent IR theories developed by civilian physicians indicate that the abnormal vascularity (angiogenesis) associated with the formation of breast tumors may be detected easily by IR-cameras from 1 to 5 years before any other technique. Early detection has been shown to be the key to high survival probability.

The workshop involved specialists and leaders from the military research and development (R&D), academic, and medical communities. Together they covered a multidisciplinary range of topics: military IR sensor technology, ATR, smart image processing, database management, interactive web-based data management, IR imaging for screening of breast cancer, and related medical topics. Three panels were formed to consider: (1) Image Processing and Medical Applications; (2) Website and Database; and (3) Sensor Technology for Medical Applications. A subject area expert led each. The deliberations of each group were presented in a briefing to the plenary session of the final day. Their outputs were quite general; they still apply to the current program and are discussed below for the benefit of all future U.S. efforts.

1.3.1 The Image Processing and Medical Applications

This group focused on the algorithms (ATR approaches) and how to evaluate and use them. It advised that the clinical methods of collection must be able to support the most common ATR approaches, for example, single frame, change detection, multilook, and anomaly detection. They also provided detailed draft guidelines for controlled problem sets for ATR evaluation. Although they thought a multisensor approach would pay dividends, they stressed the need to quantify algorithm performance in a methodical way, starting with approaches that work with single IR images.

1.3.2 Website and Database

This panel concerned itself with the collection and management of an IR image database for breast cancer. It looked particularly at issues of data standards and security. It concluded that the Office of the Secretary of Defense (OSD)-supported Virtual Distributed Laboratory (VDL), created within the OSD ATR Evaluation Program, is a very good model for the medical data repository to include collaborative software, image management software, evaluation concepts, data standards, security, bandwidth, and storage capacity. It also advised that camera calibration concepts and phantom targets be provided to help baseline performance and eliminate unknowns. It noted that privacy regulations would have to be dealt with in order to post the human data but suggested that this would complicate but not impede the formation of the database.

1.3.3 Sensor Technology for Medical Applications

The sensor panel started by pointing out that, if angiogenesis is a reliable early indicator of risk, then thermal imaging is ideally suited for detection at that stage. Current sensor performance is fully adequate. The group discussed calibration issues associated with hardware design and concluded that internal reference is desirable to ensure that temperature differences are being measured accurately. However, they questioned the need for absolute temperature measurement; the plenary group offered no counter to this. This group also looked at the economics of thermal imaging and concluded that recent military developments in uncooled thermal imaging systems at DARPA and the Army Night Vision and Electronic Sensing Division would allow the proliferation of IR-cameras costing at most a few thousand dollars each. They cited China's installation of more than 60 such cameras. The panel challenged ATR and algorithm developers to look at software methods to help simplify the sensor hardware, for example, frame-to-frame change detection to replace mechanical stabilization.

IR imaging for medical uses is a multidisciplinary technology and must include experts from different fields if its full potential is to be realized. The Tanks to Tumors workshop is a model for future U.S. efforts. It succeeded in bringing several different communities together—medical, military, academic, industrial, and engineering. These experts worked together to determine how the United States might adopt thermal imaging diagnostic technology in an orderly and demonstrable way for the early detection of breast cancer and other conditions. The panel recommendations will serve to guide the transition of military technology developments in ATR, the VDL, and IR sensors to the civilian medical community. The result will be a new tool in the war against breast cancer—a major benefit to the military and civilian population. Detailed proceedings of this workshop are available from ACA, Falls Church, VA.

1.4 Guide to Thermal Imaging Systems for Medical Applications

1.4.1 Introduction

The purpose of this section is to provide the physician with an overview of the key features of thermal imaging systems and a brief discussion of the marketplace. It assumes that the reader is somewhat familiar with thermal imaging theory and terminology as well as the fundamentals of digital imaging. It contains a brief, modestly technical guide to buying sensor hardware, and a short list of active websites that can introduce the buyer to the current marketplace. It is intended primarily to aid the newcomer; however, advanced workers may also find some of these websites useful in seeking custom or cutting edge capabilities in their quest to better understand the thermal phenomenology of breast cancer.

1.4.2 Background

As discussed elsewhere, the last decade has seen a resurgence of interest in thermal imaging for the early detection of breast cancer and other medical applications, both civilian and military. There was a brief period in the 1970s when thermal imaging became the subject of medical interest. That interest waned because of the combination of high prices and modest to marginal performance. Dramatic progress has been made in the intervening years; prices have dropped—thanks to burgeoning military, domestic, and industrial use; performance has improved significantly; and new technology has emerged from defense investments. Imaging electronics, digitization, image manipulation software, and automatic detection algorithms have emerged. Cameras can be had for prices that range from about $3000 onward. Cameras under $10,000 can provide a significant capability for screening and data collection. The camera field is highly competitive; it is possible to rent, lease, or buy cameras from numerous vendors and manufacturers.

1.4.3 Applications and Image Formats

Currently, thermal imaging is being used for R&D into the phenomenology of breast cancer detection, and for screening and cuing in the multimodal diagnosis and tracking of breast cancer in patients. The least stressful and most affordable is the latter. Here, two types of formats can be of general utility: uncalibrated still pictures and simple uncalibrated video. Such formats can be stored and archived for future viewing. Use of such imagery for rigorous R&D is not recommended. Furthermore, there may be legal issues associated with the recording and collection of such imagery unless it is applied merely as a screening aid to the doctor rather than as a primary diagnostic tool. In other words, such imagery would provide the doctor with anecdotal support in future review of a patient's record. In this mode, the thermal imagery has the same diagnostic relevance as a stethoscope or endoscope, neither of which is routinely recorded in the doctor's office. Imagery so obtained would not carry the same diagnostic weight as a mammogram. Still cameras and video imagers of this kind are quite affordable and compact. They can be kept in a drawer or cabinet and can be used for thermal viewing of many types of conditions including tumors, fractures, skin anomalies, circulation, and drug affects, to name a few. The marketplace is saturated with imagers under $10,000 that can provide adequate resolution and sensitivity for informal "eyeballing" the thermal features of interest. Virtually any image or video format is adequate for this kind of use.

For medical R&D, in which still imagery is to be archived, shared, and used for the testing of software and medical theories, or to explore phenomenology, it is important to collect calibrated still imagery in lossless archival formats (e.g., the so-called "raw" format that many digital cameras offer). It is thus desirable to purchase or rent a radiometric still camera with uncompressed standard formats or "raw" output that preserves the thermal calibration. This kind of imagery allows the medical center to put its collected thermal imagery into a standard format for distribution to the VDL and other interested medical centers. There are image manipulation software packages that can transform the imagery if need be. On the other hand, the data can be transmitted in any number of uncompressed formats and transformed by the data collection center. The use of standard formats is critical if medical research centers are to share common databases. There is no obvious need yet for video in R&D for breast cancer, although thermal video is being studied for many medical applications where dynamic phenomena are of interest.

1.4.4 Dynamic Range

The ability of a camera to preserve fine temperature detail in the presence of large scene temperature range is determined by its dynamic range. Dynamic range is determined by the camera's image digitization and

Advances in Medical Infrared Imaging

formation electronics. Take care to use a camera that allocates an adequate number of bits to the digitization of the images. Most commercially available cameras use 12 bits or more per pixel. This is quite adequate to preserve fine detail in images of the human body. However, when collecting images, make sure there is nothing in the field of view of the camera that is dramatically cooler or hotter than the subject; that is, avoid scene temperature differences of more than approximately 30°C (e.g., lamps, refrigerators or radiators in the background could cause trouble). This is analogous to trying to use a visible digital camera to capture a picture of a person standing next to headlights—electronic circuits may bloom or sacrifice detail of the scene near the bright lights. Although 12-bit digitization should preserve fine temperature differences at 30°C delta, large temperature differences generally stress the image formation circuitry, and undesired artifacts may appear. Nevertheless, it is relatively easy to design a collection environment with a modest temperature range. A simple way to do this is to simply fill the camera field of view with the human subject. Experiment with the imaging arrangement before collecting a large body of imagery for archiving.

1.4.5 Resolution and Sensitivity

The two most important parameters for a thermal sensor are its sensitivity and resolution. The sensitivity is measured in degree Celsius. Modest sensitivity is on the order of a tenth of a degree Celsius. Good sensitivity sensors can detect temperature differences up to four times lower or 0.025°. This sensitivity is deemed valuable for medical diagnosis, since local temperature variations caused by tumors and angiogenesis are usually higher than this. The temperature resolution is analogous to the number of colors in a computer display or color photograph. The better the resolution, the smoother will be the temperature transitions. If the subject has sudden temperature gradients, those will be attributable to the subject and not the camera.

The spatial resolution of the sensor is determined primarily by the size of the imaging chip or pixel count. This parameter is exactly analogous to the world of proliferating digital photography. Just as a four-megapixel digital camera can make sharper photos than a two-megapixel camera, pixel count is a key element in the design of a medical camera. There are quite economical thermal cameras on the market with 320 × 240 pixels, and the images from such cameras can be quite adequate for informal screening; imagery may appear to be grainy if magnified unless the viewing area or field of view is reduced. By way of example, if the image is of the full chest area, about 18 in., then a 320-pixel camera will provide the ability to resolve spatial features of about a 16th of an inch. If only the left breast is imaged, spatial features as low as 1/32 in. can be resolved. On the other hand, a 640 × 480 camera can cut these feature sizes in half. Good sensitivity and pixel count ensures that the medical images will contain useful thermal and spatial detail. In summary, although 320 × 240 imagery is quite adequate, larger pixel counts can provide more freedom for casual use, and are essential for R&D in medical centers. Although the military is developing megapixel arrays, they are not commercially available. Larger pixel counts have advantages for consumer digital photography and military applications, but there is no identified, clear need at this time for megapixel arrays in breast cancer detection. Avoid the quest for larger pixel counts unless there is a clear need. Temperature resolution should be a tenth of a degree or better.

1.4.6 Calibration

Another key feature is temperature calibration. Many thermal imaging systems are designed to detect temperature differences, not to map calibrated temperature. A camera that maps the actual surface temperature is a radiographic sensor. A reasonably good job of screening for tumors can be accomplished by only mapping local temperature differences. This application would amount to a third eye for the physician, aiding him in finding asymmetries and temperature anomalies—hot or cold spots. For example, checking circulation with thermal imaging amounts to looking for cold spots relative to the normally warm torso. However, if the physician intends to share his imagery with other doctors, or use the imagery for research, it is advisable to use a calibrated camera so that the meaning of the thermal differences can be quantified and separated from display settings and digital compression artifacts. For example, viewing the same image on two different computer displays may result in different assessments. But, if the imagery is calibrated so that each color or brightness is associated with a specific temperature, then doctors can be sure that they view relevant imagery and accurate temperatures, not image artifacts.

It is critical that the calibration be stable and accurate enough to match the temperature sensitivity of the camera. Here caution is advised. Many radiometric cameras on the market are designed for industrial applications where large temperature differences are expected and the temperature of the object is well over 100°C; for example, the temperature difference may be 5°C at 600°C. In breast cancer, the temperature differences of interest are about a tenth of a degree at about 37°C. Therefore, the calibration method must be relevant for those parameters. Since the dynamic range of the breast cancer application is very small, the calibration method is simplified. More important are the temporal stability, temperature resolution, and accuracy of the calibration. Useful calibration parameters are 0.1°C resolution at 37°C, stability of 0.1°C per hour (drift), and accuracy of ±0.3°C. This means that the camera can measure a temperature difference of 0.1°C with an accuracy of ±0.3°C at body temperature. For example, suppose the breast is at 36.5°C, the camera may read 36.7°C.

Two methods of calibration are available—internal and external. External calibration devices are available from numerous sources. They are traceable to the National Institute of Science and Technology (NIST) and meet the above requirements. Prices are under $3000 for compact, portable devices. The drawback with external calibration is that it involves a second piece of equipment and more complex procedure for use. The thermal camera must be calibrated just prior to use and calibration imagery recorded, or the calibration source must be placed in the image while data is collected. The latter method is more reliable but it complicates the collection geometry.

Internal calibration is preferable because it simplifies the entire data collection process. However, radiometric still cameras with the above specifications are more expensive than uncalibrated cameras by $3000 to $5000.

1.4.7 Single Band Imagers

Today there are thermal imaging sensors with suitable performance parameters. There are two distinct spectral bands that provide adequate thermal sensitivity for medical use: the medium-wave IR band (MWIR) covers the electromagnetic spectrum from 3 to 5 μm in wavelength, approximately; the long-wave IR band (LWIR) covers the wavelength spectrum from about 8 to 12 μm. There are advocates for both bands, and neither band offers a clear advantage over the other for medical applications, although the LWIR is rapidly becoming the most economical sensor technology. Some experimenters believe that there is merit in using both bands.

MWIR cameras are widely available and generally have more pixels, and hence higher resolution for the same price. Phenomenology in this band has been quite effective in detecting small tumors and temperature asymmetries. MWIR sensors must be cooled to cryogenic temperatures as low as 77K. Thermoelectric coolers are used for some MWIR sensors; they operate at 175 to 220K depending on the design of the imaging chip. MWIR sensors not only respond to emitted radiation from thermal sources but also sense radiation from broadband visible sources such as the sun. Images in this band can contain structure caused by reflected light rather than emitted radiation. Some care must be taken to minimize reflected light from broadband sources including incandescent light bulbs and sunlight. Unwanted light can cause shadows, reflections, and bright spots in the imagery. Care should be taken to avoid direct illumination of the subject by wideband artificial sources and sunlight. It is advisable to experiment with lighting geometries and sources before collecting data for the record. Moisturizing creams, sweat, and other skin surface coatings should also be avoided.

The cost of LWIR cameras has dropped dramatically since the advent of uncooled thermal imaging arrays. This is a dramatic difference between the current state-of-the-art and what was available in the 1970s. Now, LWIR cameras are being proliferated and can be competitive in price and performance to the thermoelectrically cooled MWIR. Uncooled thermal cameras are compact and have good resolution and sensitivity. Cameras with 320 × 240 pixels can be purchased for well under $10,000. This year, sensors with 640 × 480 pixels have hit the market. Sensors in this band are far less likely to be affected by shadows, lighting, and reflections. Nevertheless, it is advisable to experiment with viewing geometry, ambient lighting, and skin condition before collecting data for the record and for dissemination.

1.4.8 Emerging and Future Camera Technology

There are emerging developments that may soon provide for a richer set of observable phenomena in the thermography for breast cancer. Some researchers are already simultaneously collecting imagery in both the MWIR and LWIR bands. This is normally accomplished using two cameras at the same time. Dual band imagery arguably provides software and physicians with a richer set of observables. Developers of automatic screening algorithms are exploring schemes that compare the images in the two bands and emphasize the common elements of both to get greater confidence in detecting tumors. More sophisticated software (based on neural networks) learns what is important in both bands. New dual band technology has emerged from recent investments by the DARPA. Uncooled detector arrays have been demonstrated that operate in both bands simultaneously. It is likely that larger or well-endowed medical centers can order custom imagers with this capability this year. Contact the Materials Technology Office at DARPA for further information.

Spectroscopic (hyperspectral) imaging in the thermal bands is also an important research topic. Investigators are looking for phenomenology that manifests itself in fine spectral detail. Since flesh is a thermally absorptive and scattering medium, it may be possible to detect unique signatures that help detect tumors. Interested parties should ask vendors if such cameras are available for lease or purchase.

Some researchers are using multiple views and color to attempt to enhance tomographic imaging processes and to image to greater depths using physical models of the flesh and its thermal profiles at different wavelengths. Contact the principal investigators directly.

1.4.9 Summary Specifications

Table 1.4 summarizes the key parameters and their nominal values to use in shopping for a camera.

1.4.9.1 How to Begin

Those who are new to thermal phenomenology should carefully study the material in this handbook. Medical centers, researchers, and physicians seeking to purchase cameras and enter the field may wish to contact the authors or leading investigators mentioned in this handbook for advice before looking for sensor hardware. The participants in the Tanks to Tumors workshop and the MedATR program may already have the answers. If possible, compare advice from two or more of these experts before moving on; the experts do not agree on everything. They are currently using sensors and software suitable for building the VDL database. They may also be aware of public domain image screening software. Once advice has been collected, the potential buyer should begin shopping at one or more of the websites listed in this section. Do not rely on the website alone. Most vendors provide contact information so that the purchaser may discuss imaging needs with a consultant. Take advantage of these advisory services to shop around and survey the field. Researchers may also wish to contact government and university experts before deciding on a camera. Finally, many of the vendors below offer custom sensor design services. Some

TABLE 1.4 Summary of Key Camera Parameters

	Applications	
	Recording	Informal
Format	Digital stills	Video or stills
Compression	None	As provided by manufacturer
Digitization (dynamic range)	12 bits or more	12 bits nominal
Pixels (array size)	320 × 240 up to 640 × 480	320 × 240
Sensitivity	0.04°C, 0.1°C max	0.1°C
Calibration accuracy	±0.3°C	Not required
Calibration range	Room and body temperature	Not required
Calibration resolution	0.1°C	Not required
Spectral band	MWIR or LWIR	MWIR or LWIR

vendors may be willing to lease or loan equipment for evaluation. High-end, leading edge researchers may need to contact component developers at companies such as Raytheon, DRS, BAE, or SOFRADIR to see if the state-of-the-art supports their specific needs.

Supplier websites: The reader is advised that all references to brand names or specific manufacturers do not connote an endorsement of the vendor, producer, or its products. Likewise, the list is not a complete survey; we apologize for any omissions.

http://www.infrared-camera-rentals.com/
http://www.electrophysics.com/Browse/Brw_AllProductLineCategory.asp
http://www.cantronic.com/ir860.html
http://www.nationalinfrared.com/Medical_Imaging.php
http://www.flirthermography.com/cameras/all_cameras.asp
http://www.mikroninst.com/
http://www.baesystems.com/newsroom/2005/jan/310105news4.htm
http://www.indigosystems.com/product/rental.html
http://www.indigosystems.com/
http://www.raytheoninfrared.com/productcatalog/
http://x26.com/Night_Vision_Thermal_Links.html
http://www.infraredsolutions.com/
http://www.isgfire.com/
http://www.infrared.com/
http://www.sofradir.com/
http://www.infrared-detectors.com/
http://www.drs.com/products/index.cfm?gID=21&cID=39

1.5 Summary, Conclusions, and Recommendations

Today, medical IR is being backed by more clinical research worldwide where state-of-the-art equipment is being used. Focus must be placed on the quantification of clinical data, standardization, effective training with high quality assurance, collaborations, and more publications in leading peer-reviewed medical journals.

For an effective integration of twenty-first-century technologies for IR imaging, we need to focus on the following areas:

- IR-cameras and systems
- Advanced image processing
- Image analysis techniques
- High-speed computers
- Computer-aided detection (CAD)
- Knowledge-based databases
- Telemedicine

Other areas of importance are

- Effective clinical use
- Protocol-based image acquisition
- Image interpretation
- System operation and calibration
- Training
- Better understanding of the pathophysiological nature of thermal signatures
- Quantification of clinical data

In conclusion, this noninvasive, nonionizing imaging modality can provide added value to the present multi-imaging clinical setting. This functional image measures metabolic activity in the tissue and thus can noninvasively detect abnormalities very early. It is well known that early detection leads to enhanced survivability and great reduction in health care costs. With these becoming exorbitant, this would be of great value. Besides its usefulness at this stage, a second critical benefit is that it has the capability to noninvasively monitor the efficacy of therapies [12].

References

[1] Diakides, N.A. (Guest Editor), Special Issue on Medical Infrared Imaging, *IEEE/Engineering in Medicine and Biology*, 17, July/August 1998.

[2] Diakides, N.A. (Guest Editor), Special Issue on Medical Infrared Imaging, *IEEE/Engineering in Medicine and Biology*, 19, May/June 2000.

[3] Diakides, N.A. (Guest Editor), Special Issue on Medical Infrared Imaging, *IEEE/Engineering in Medicine and Biology*, 21, November/December 2002.

[4] Paul, J.L. and Lupo, J.C., From Tanks to Tumors: Applications of Infrared Imaging and Automatic Target Recognition Image Processing for Early Detection of Breast Cancer, Special Issue on Medical Infrared Imaging, *IEEE/Engineering in Medicine and Biology*, 21, 34–35, November/December 2002.

[5] Diakides, N.A., Medical Applications of IR Focal Plane Arrays, Final Progress Report, U.S. Army Research Office, Contract DAAH04-94-C-0020, March 1998.

[6] Diakides, N.A., Application of Army IR Technology to Medical IR Imaging, Technical Report, U.S. Army Research Office Contract DAAH04-96-C-0086 (TCN 97-143), August 1999.

[7] Diakides, N.A., Exploitation of Infrared Imaging for Medicine, Final Progress Report, U.S. Army Research Office, Contract DAAG55-98-0035, January 2001.

[8] Diakides, N.A., Medical IR Imaging and Image Processing, Final Report U.S. Army Research Office, Contract DAAH04-96-C-0086 (TNC 01041), October 2003.

[9] Anbar, M., *Quantitative Dynamic Telethermometry in Medical Diagnosis and Management*, CRC Press, Boca Raton, FL, 1994.

[10] Ammer, K. (Editor In Chief), *Journal of Thermology, International*, 14, January, 2004.

[11] Balageas, D., Busse, G., Carlomagno, C., and Wiecek, B. (Eds.), *Proceedings of Quantitative Infrared Thermography*, 4, Technical University of Lodz, 1998.

[12] Hassan, M., et al., Quantitative Assessment of Tumor Vasculature and Response to Therapy in Kaposi's Sarcoma Using Functional Noninvasive Imaging, *Technology in Cancer Research and Treatment*, 3, 451–457, Adenine Press, 2004.

2
The Historical Development of Thermometry and Thermal Imaging in Medicine

Francis E. Ring
Bryan F. Jones
Glamorgan University

References 2-4

Fever was the most frequently occurring condition in early medical observation. From the early days of Hippocrates, when it is said that wet mud was used on the skin to observe fast drying over a tumorous swelling, physicians have recognised the importance of a raised temperature. For centuries, this remained a subjective skill, and the concept of measuring temperature was not developed until the sixteenth century. Galileo made his famous thermoscope from a glass tube, which functioned as an unsealed thermometer. It was affected by atmospheric pressure as a result.

In modern terms we now describe heat transfer by three main modes. The first is conduction, requiring contact between the object and the sensor to enable the flow of thermal energy. The second mode of heat transfer is convection where the flow of a hot mass transfers thermal energy. The third is radiation. The latter two led to remote detection methods.

Thermometry developed slowly from Galileo's experiments. There were Florentine and Venetian glassblowers in Italy who made sealed glass containers of various shapes, which were tied onto the body surface. The temperature of an object was assessed by the rising or falling of small beads or seeds within the fluid inside the container. Huygens, Roemer, and Fahrenheit all proposed the need for a calibrated scale in the late seventeenth and early eighteenth century. Celsius did propose a centigrade scale based on ice and boiling water. He strangely suggested that boiling water should be zero, and melting ice 100 on his scale. It was the Danish biologist Linnaeus in 1750 who proposed the reversal of this scale, as it is known today. Although International Standards have given the term Celsius to the 0 to 100 scale today, strictly speaking it would be historically accurate to refer to degrees Linnaeus or centigrade [1].

The Clinical thermometer, which has been universally used in medicine for over 130 years, was developed by Dr. Carl Wunderlich in 1868. This is essentially a maximum thermometer with a limited scale around the normal internal body temperature of 37°C or 98.4°F. Wunderlich's treatise on body temperature in health and disease is a masterpiece of painstaking work over many years. He charted the progress of all his patients daily, and sometimes two or three times during the day. His thesis was written in German for Leipzig University and was also translated into English in the late nineteenth century [2]. The significance of body temperature lies in the fact that humans are homeotherms who are capable of maintaining a constant temperature that is different from that of the surroundings. This is essential to the preservation of a relatively constant environment within the body known as homeostasis. Changes in temperature of more than a few degrees either way is a clear indicator of a bodily dysfunction; temperature variations outside this range may disrupt the essential chemical processes in the body.

Today, there has been a move away from glass thermometers in many countries, giving rise to more disposable thermocouple systems for routine clinical use.

Liquid crystal sensors for temperature became available in usable form in the 1960s. Originally the crystalline substances were painted on the skin that had previously been coated with black paint. Three of four colours became visible if the paint was at the critical temperature range for the subject. Micro-encapsulation of these substances, that are primarily cholesteric esters, resulted in plastic sheet detectors. Later these sheets were mounted on a soft latex base to mould to the skin under air pressure using a cushion with a rigid clear window. Polaroid photography was then used to record the colour pattern while the sensor remained in contact. The system was re-usable and inexpensive. However, sensitivity declined over 1 to 2 years from the date of manufacture, and many different pictures were required to obtain a subjective pattern of skin temperature [3].

Convection currents of heat emitted by the human body have been imaged by a technique called Schlieren Photography. The change in refractive index with density in the warm air around the body is made visible by special illumination. This method has been used to monitor heat loss in experimental subjects, especially in the design of protective clothing for people working in extreme physical environments.

Heat transfer by radiation is of great value in medicine. The human body surface requires variable degrees of heat exchange with the environment as part of the normal thermo-regulatory process. Most of this heat transfer occurs in the infrared, which can be imaged by electronic thermal imaging [4]. Infrared radiation was discovered in 1800 when Sir William Herschel performed his famous experiment to measure heat beyond the visible spectrum. Nearly 200 years before, Italian observers had noted the presence of reflected heat. John Della Porta in 1698 observed that when a candle was lit and placed before a large silver bowl in church, that he could sense the heat on his face. When he altered the positions of the candle, bowl, and his face, the sensation of heat was lost.

William Herschel, in a series of careful experiments, showed that not only was there a "dark heat" present, but that heat itself behaved like light, it could be reflected and refracted under the right conditions. William's only son, John Herschel, repeated some experiments after his father's death, and successfully made an image using solar radiation. This he called a "thermogram," a term still in use today to describe an image made by thermal radiation. John Herschel's thermogram was made by focussing solar radiation with a lens onto to a suspension of carbon particles in alcohol. This process is known as evaporography [5].

A major development came in the early 1940s with the first electronic sensor for infrared radiation. Rudimentary night vision systems were produced towards the end of the Second World War for use by snipers. The electrons from near-infrared cathodes were directed onto visible phosphors which converted the infrared radiation to visible light. Sniperscope devices, based on this principle, were provided for soldiers in the Pacific in 1945, but found little use.

At about the same time, another device was made from indium antimonide; this was mounted at the base of a small Dewar vessel to allow cooling with liquid nitrogen. A cumbersome device such as this, which required a constant supply of liquid nitrogen, was clearly impractical for battlefield use but could be used with only minor inconvenience in a hospital. The first medical images taken with a British prototype system, the "Pyroscan," were made at The Middlesex Hospital in London and The Royal National Hospital for Rheumatic Diseases in Bath between 1959 and 1961. By modern standards, these thermograms were very crude.

In the meantime, the cascade image tube, that had been pioneered during World War II in Germany, had been developed by RCA into a multi-alkali photocathode tube whose performance exceeded expectations.

These strides in technology were motivated by military needs in Vietnam; they were classified and, therefore, unavailable to clinicians. However, a mark 2 Pyroscan was made for medical use in 1962, with improved images. The mechanical scanning was slow and each image needed from 2 to 5 min to record. The final picture was written line by line on electro-sensitive paper. In the seventies, the U.S. Military sponsored the development of a multi-element detector array that was to form the basis of a real-time framing imager. This led to the targeting and navigation system known as Forward Looking InfraRed (FLIR) systems which had the added advantage of being able to detect warm objects through smoke and fog.

During this time the potential for thermal imaging in medicine was being explored in an increasing number of centres. Earlier work by the American physiologist J. Hardy had shown that the human skin, regardless of colour, is a highly efficient radiator with an emissivity of 0.98 which is close to that of a perfect black body. Even so, the normal temperature of skin in the region of 20 to 30°C generated low intensities of infrared radiation at about 10 μm wavelength [6]. The detection of such low intensities at these wavelengths presented a considerable challenge to the technology of the day. Cancer detection was a high priority subject and hopes that this new technique would be a tool for screening breast cancer provided the motivation to develop detectors. Many centres across Europe, the United States, and Japan became involved. In the United Kingdom, a British surgeon, K. Lloyd Williams showed that many tumours are hot and the hotter the tumour, the worse the prognosis. By this time, the images were displayed on a cathode ray screen in black and white. Image processing by computer had not arrived, so much discussion was given to schemes to score the images subjectively, and to look for hot spots and asymmetry of temperature in the breast. This was confounded by changes in the breast through the menstrual cycle in younger women. The use of false colour thermograms was only possible by photography at this time. A series of bright isotherms were manually ranged across the temperature span of the image, each being exposed through a different colour filter, and superimposed on a single frame of film.

Improvements in infrared technology were forging ahead at the behest of the U.S. Military during the seventies. At Fort Belvoir, some of the first monolithic laser diode arrays were designed and produced with a capability of generating 500 W pulses at 15 kHz at room temperature. These lasers were able to image objects at distances of 3 km. Attention then turned to solid state, gas, and tunable lasers which were used in a wide range of applications.

By the mid-seventies, computer technology made a widespread impact with the introduction of smaller mini and microcomputers at affordable prices. The first "personal" computer systems had arrived. In Bath, a special system for nuclear medicine made in Sweden was adapted for thermal imaging. A colour screen was provided to display the digitised image. The processor was a PDP8, and the program was loaded every day from paper-tape. With computerisation many problems began to be resolved. The images were archived in digital form, standard regions of interest could be selected, and temperature measurements obtained from the images. Manufacturers of thermal imaging equipment slowly adapted to the call for quantification and some sold thermal radiation calibration sources to their customers to aid the standardisation of technique. Workshops that had started in the late 1960s became a regular feature, and the European Thermographic Association was formed with a major conference in Amsterdam in 1974. Apart from a range of physiological and medical applications groups were formed to formulate guidelines for good practice. This included the requirements for patient preparation, conditions for thermal imaging and criteria for the use of thermal imaging in medicine and pharmacology [7,8]. At the IEEE EMBS conference in Amsterdam some twenty years later in 1996, Dr. N. Diakides facilitated the production of a CD ROM of the early, seminal papers on infrared imaging in medicine that had been published in *ACTA Thermographica* and the *Journal of Thermology*. This CD was sponsored by the U.S. Office of Technology Applications, Ballistic Missile Defence Organisation and the U.S. National Technology Transfer Center Washington Operations and is available from the authors at the Medical Imaging Research Group at the University of Glamorgan, U.K. [9]. The archive of papers may also be search online at the Medical Imaging Group's web site [9].

A thermal index was devised in Bath to provide clinicians with a simplified measure of inflammation [10]. A normal range of values was established for ankles, elbows, hands, and knees, with raised values obtained in osteoarthritic joints and higher values still in Rheumatoid Arthritis. A series of clinical trials with non-steroid, anti-inflammatory, oral drugs, and steroid analogues for joint injection was published using the index to document the course of treatment [11].

Improvements in thermal imaging cameras have had a major impact, both on image quality and speed of image capture. Early single element detectors were dependent on optical mechanical scanning. Both spatial and thermal image resolutions were inversely dependent on scanning speed. The Bofors and some American imagers scanned at 1 to 4 frames per sec. AGA cameras were faster at 16 frames per sec, and used interlacing to smooth the image. Multi-element arrays were developed in the United Kingdom and were employed in cameras made by EMI and Rank. Alignment of the elements was critical, and a poorly aligned array produced characteristic banding in the image. Prof. Tom Elliott F.R.S. solved this problem when he designed and produced the first significant detector for faster high-resolution images that subsequently became known as the Signal PRocessing In The Element (Sprite) detector. Rank Taylor Hobson used the Sprite in the high-resolution system called Talytherm. This camera also had a high specification Infrared zoom lens, with a macro attachment. Superb images of sweat pore function, eyes with contact lenses, and skin pathology were recorded with this system.

With the end of the cold war, the greatly improved military technology was declassified and its use for medical applications was encouraged. As a result, the first focal plane array detectors came from the multi-element arrays, with increasing numbers of pixel/elements, yielding high resolution at video frame rates. Uncooled bolometer arrays have also been shown to be adequate for many medical applications. Without the need for electronic cooling systems these cameras are almost maintenance free. Good software with enhancement and analysis is now expected in thermal imaging. Many commercial systems use general imaging software, which is primarily designed for industrial users of the technique. A few dedicated medical software packages have been produced, which can even enhance the images from the older cameras. CTHERM is one such package that is a robust and almost universally usable programme for medical thermography [9]. As standardisation of image capture and analysis becomes more widely accepted, the ability to manage the images and, if necessary, to transmit them over an intranet or internet for communication becomes paramount. Future developments will enable the operator of thermal imaging to use reference images and reference data as a diagnostic aid. This, however, depends on the level of standardisation that can be provided by the manufacturers, and by the operators themselves in the performance of their technique [12].

Modern thermal imaging is already digital and quantifiable, and ready for the integration into anticipated hospital and clinical computer networks.

References

[1] Ring, E.F.J., *The History of Thermal Imaging in the Thermal Image in Medicine and Biology*, eds. Ammer, K. and Ring, E.F.J., pp. 13–20. Uhlen Verlag, Vienna, 1995.

[2] Wunderlich, C.A., *On the Temperature in Diseases, A Manual of Medical Thermometry*. Translated from the second German edition by Bathurst Woodman, W., The New Sydenham Society, London, 1871.

[3] Flesch, U., Thermographic techniques with liquid crystals in medicine, In *Recent Advances in Medical Thermology*, eds. Ring, E.F.J. and Phillips, B., pp. 283–299. Plenum Press, New York, London, 1984.

[4] Houdas, Y. and Ring, E.F.J., *Human Body Temperature, its Measurement and Regulation*, Plenum Press, New York, London, 1982.

[5] Ring, E.F.J., The discovery of infrared radiation in 1800. *Imaging Science Journal*, 48, 1–8, 2000.

[6] Jones, B.F., A Reappraisal of Infrared Thermal Image Analysis in Medicine. *IEEE Transactions on Medical Imaging*, 17, 1019–1027, 1998.

[7] Engel, J.M., Cosh, J.A., Ring, E.F.J. et al., Thermography in locomotor diseases: recommended procedure. *European Journal of Rheumatology and Inflammation*, 2, 299–306, 1979.

[8] Ring, E.F.J., Engel, J.M., and Page-Thomas, D.P., Thermological methods in clinical pharmacology. *International Journal of Clinical Pharmacology*, 22, 20–24, 1984.

[9] CTHERM website www.medimaging.org.
[10] Collins, A.J., Ring, E.J.F., Cash, J.A., and Brown, P.A., Quantification of thermography in arthritis using multi-isothermal analysis: I. The thermographic index. *Annals of the Rheumatic Diseases*, 33, 113–115, 1974.
[11] Bacon, P.A., Ring, E.F.J., and Collins, A.J., Thermography in the assessment of antirheumatic agents. In *Rheumatoid Arthritis*, eds. Gordon and Hazleman, pp. 105–110. Elsevier/North Holland Biochemical Press, Amsterdam, 1977.
[12] Ring, E.F.J. and Ammer, K., The technique of infrared imaging in medicine. *Thermology International*, 10, 7–14, 2000.

3

Infrared Detectors and Detector Arrays

3.1	Photon Detectors	3-1
	Photoconductive Detectors • Photovoltaic Detectors	
3.2	Thermal Detectors	3-6
3.3	Detector Materials	3-7
3.4	Detector Readouts	3-12
	Readouts for Photon Detectors • Thermal Detector Readouts • Readout Evolution	
3.5	Technical Challenges for Infrared Detectors	3-14
	Uncooled Infrared Detector Challenges • Electronics Challenges • Detector Readout Challenges • Optics Challenges • Challenges for Third-Generation Cooled Imagers	
3.6	Summary	3-24
References	....	3-25

Paul R. Norton
Stuart B. Horn
Joseph G. Pellegrino
Philip Perconti
U.S. Army CERDEC Night Vision and Electronic Sensors Directorate

There are two general classes of detectors: *photon* (or quantum) and *thermal* detectors [1,2]. Photon detectors convert absorbed photon energy into released electrons (from their bound states to conduction states). The material band gap describes the energy necessary to transition a charge carrier from the valence band to the conduction band. The change in charge carrier state changes the electrical properties of the material. These electrical property variations are measured to determine the amount of incident optical power. Thermal detectors absorb energy over a broad band of wavelengths. The energy absorbed by a detector causes the temperature of the material to increase. Thermal detectors have at least one inherent electrical property that changes with temperature. This temperature-related property is measured electrically to determine the power on the detector. Commercial infrared imaging systems suitable for medical applications use both types of detectors. We begin by describing the physical mechanism employed by these two detector types.

3.1 Photon Detectors

Infrared radiation consists of a flux of photons, the quantum-mechanical elements of all electromagnetic radiation. The energy of the photon is given by:

$$E_{ph} = h\nu = hc/\lambda = 1.986 \times 10^{-19}/\lambda \text{ J}/\mu\text{m} \tag{3.1}$$

FIGURE 3.1 Photoconductive detector geometery.

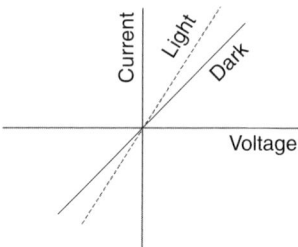

FIGURE 3.2 Current–voltage characteristics of a photoconductive detector.

where h is the Planck's constant, c is the speed of light, and λ is the wavelength of the infrared photon in micrometers (μm).

Photon detectors respond by elevating an bound electron in a material to a free or conductive state. Two types are photon detectors are produced for the commercial market:

- Photoconductive
- Photovoltaic

3.1.1 Photoconductive Detectors

The mechanism of photoconductive detectors is based upon the excitation of bound electrons to a mobile state where they can move freely through the material. The increase in the number of conductive electrons, n, created by the photon flux, Φ_0 allows more current to flow when the detective element is used in a bias circuit having an electric field E. The photoconductive detector element having dimensions of length L, width W, and thickness t is represented in Figure 3.1.

Figure 3.2 illustrates how the current–voltage characteristics of a photoconductor change with incident photon flux (Chapter 4).

The response of a photoconductive detector can be written as:

$$R = \frac{\eta q R E \tau (\mu_n + \mu_p)}{E_{ph} L} (V/W) \qquad (3.2)$$

where R is the response in volts per Watt, η is the quantum efficiency in electrons per photon, q is the charge of an electron, R is the resistance of the detector element, τ is the lifetime of a photoexcited electron, and μ_n and μ_p are the mobilities of the electrons and holes in the material in volts per square centimeter per second.

Noise in photoconductors is the square root averaged sum of terms from three sources:

- Johnson noise
- Thermal generation-recombination
- Photon generation-recombination

FIGURE 3.3 Photovoltaic detector structure example for mesa diodes.

Expressions for the total noise and each of the noise terms are given in Equations 3.3 to 3.6

$$V_{\text{noise}} = \sqrt{V_{\text{Johnson}}^2 + V_{\text{phg-r}}^2 + V_{\text{thg-r}}^2} \quad (3.3)$$

$$V_{\text{Johnson}} = \sqrt{4kTR} \quad (3.4)$$

$$V_{\text{ph g-r}} = \frac{\sqrt{\eta \phi (WL)} 2qRE\tau (\mu_n + \mu_p)}{L} \quad (3.5)$$

$$V_{\text{th g-r}} = \sqrt{\frac{np}{n+p} \tau \left(\frac{Wt}{L}\right)} 2qRE(\mu_n + \mu_p) \quad (3.6)$$

The figure of merit for infrared detectors is called D^*. The units of D^* are cm $(\text{Hz})^{1/2}/\text{W}$, but are most commonly referred to as Jones. D^* is the detector's signal-to-noise (SNR) ratio, normalized to an area of 1 cm^2, to a noise bandwidth of 1 Hz, and to a signal level of 1 W at the peak of the detectors response. The equation for D^* is:

$$D^*_{\text{peak}} = \frac{R}{V_{\text{noise}}} \sqrt{WL} \quad (\text{Jones}) \quad (3.7)$$

where W and L are defined in Figure 3.1.

A special condition of D^* for a photoconductor is noted when the noise is dominated by the photon noise term. This is a condition in which the D^* is maximum.

$$D^*_{\text{blip}} = \frac{\lambda}{2hc} \sqrt{\frac{\eta}{E_{\text{ph}}}} \quad (3.8)$$

where "blip" notes background-limited photodetector.

3.1.2 Photovoltaic Detectors

The mechanism of photovoltaic detectors is based on the collection of photoexcited carriers by a diode junction. Photovoltaic detectors are the most commonly used photon detectors for imaging arrays in current production. An example of the structure of detectors in such an array is illustrated in Figure 3.3 for a mesa photodiode. Photons are incident from the optically transparent detector substrate side and are absorbed in the n-type material layer. Absorbed photons create a pair of carriers, an electron and a hole. The hole diffuses to the p-type side of the junction creating a photocurrent. A contact on the p-type side of the junction is connected to an indium bump that mates to an amplifier in a readout circuit where the signal is stored and conveyed to a display during each display frame. A common contact is made to

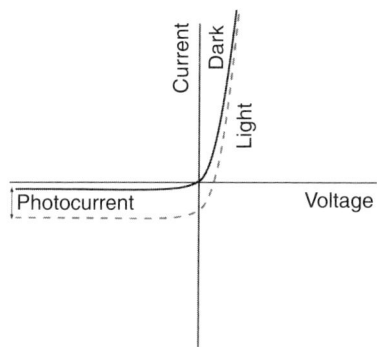

FIGURE 3.4 Current–voltage characteristics of a photovoltaic detector.

the n-type layer at the edge of the detector array. Adjacent diodes are isolated electrically from each other by a mesa etch cutting the p-type layer into islands.

Figure 3.4 illustrates how the current–voltage characteristics of a photodiode change with incident photon flux (Chapter 4).

The current of the photodiode can be expressed as:

$$I = I_0(e^{qV/kT} - 1) - I_{\text{photo}} \tag{3.9}$$

where I_0 is reverse-bias leakage current and I_{photo} is the photoinduced current. The photocurrent is given by:

$$I = I_0(e^{qV/kT} - 1) - I_{\text{photo}} \tag{3.10}$$

where Φ_0 is the photon flux in photons/cm^2/sec and A is the detector area.

Detector noise in a photodiode includes three terms: Johnson noise, thermal diffusion generation and recombination noise, and photon generation and recombination. The Johnson noise term, written in terms of the detector resistance $dI/dV = R_0$ at zero bias as:

$$i_{\text{Johnson}} = \sqrt{4kT/R_0} \tag{3.11}$$

where k is Boltzmann's constant and T is the detector temperature. The thermal diffusion current is given by:

$$i_{\text{diffusion noise}} = q\sqrt{2I_s\left[\exp\left(\frac{eV}{kT}\right) - 1\right]} \tag{3.12}$$

where the saturation current, I_s, is given by:

$$I_s = qn_i^2\left[\frac{1}{N_a}\sqrt{\frac{D_n}{\tau_{n0}}} + \frac{1}{N_d}\sqrt{\frac{D_p}{\tau_{p0}}}\right] \tag{3.13}$$

where N_a and N_d are the concentration of p- and n-type dopants on either side of the diode junction, τ_{n0} and τ_{p0} are the carrier lifetimes, and D_n and D_p are the diffusion constants on either side of the junction, respectively.

FIGURE 3.5 D^* as a function of the detector resistance-area product, R_0A. This condition applies when detector performance is limited by dark current.

The photon generation-recombination current noise is given by:

$$i_{\text{photon noise}} = q\sqrt{2\eta\Phi_0} \tag{3.14}$$

When the junction is at zero bias, the photodiode D^* is given by:

$$D^*_\lambda = \frac{\lambda}{hc}\eta e \frac{1}{\left[(4kT/R_0A) + 2e^2\eta\right]} \tag{3.15}$$

In the special case of a photodiode that is operated without sufficient cooling, the maximum D^* may be limited by the dark current or leakage current of the junction. The expression for D^* in this case, written in terms of the junction-resistance area product, R_0A, is given by:

$$D^*_\lambda = \frac{\lambda}{hc}\eta e\sqrt{\frac{R_0A}{4kT}} \tag{3.16}$$

Figure 3.5 illustrates how D^* is limited by the R_0A product for the case of dark-current limited detector conditions.

For the ideal case where the noise is dominated by the photon flux in the background scene, the peak D^* is given by:

$$D^*_\lambda = \frac{\lambda}{hc}\sqrt{\frac{\eta}{2E_{\text{ph}}}} \tag{3.17}$$

Comparing this limit with that for a photoconductive detector in Equation 3.8, we see that the background-limited D^* for a photodiode is higher by a factor of square root of 2 ($\sqrt{2}$).

3.2 Thermal Detectors

Thermal detectors operate by converting the incoming photon flux to heat [3]. The heat input causes the thermal detector's temperature to rise and this change in temperature is sensed by a bolometer. A bolometer element operates by changing its resistance as its temperature is changed. A bias circuit across the bolometer can be used to convert the changing current to a signal output.

The coefficient α is used to compare the sensitivity of different bolometer materials and is given by:

$$\alpha = \frac{1}{R_d} \frac{dR}{dT} \tag{3.18}$$

where R_d is the resistance of the bolometer element, and dR/dT is the change in resistance per unit change in temperature. Typical values of α are 2 to 3%.

Theoretically, the bolometer structure can be represented as illustrated in Figure 3.6. The rise in temperature due to a heat flux ϕ_e is given by:

$$\Delta T = \frac{\eta P_0}{G(1+\omega^2\tau^2)^{1/2}} \tag{3.19}$$

where P_0 is the radiant power of the signal in watts, G is the thermal conductance (K/W), h is the percentage of flux absorbed, and ω is the angular frequency of the signal. The bolometer time constant, τ, is determined by:

$$\tau = \frac{C}{G} \tag{3.20}$$

where C is the heat capacity of detector element.

The sensitivity or D^* of a thermal detector is limited by variations in the detector temperature caused by fluctuations in the absorption and radiation of heat between the detector element and the background. Sensitive thermal detectors must minimize competing mechanisms for heat loss by the element, namely, convection and conduction.

Convection by air is eliminated by isolating the detector in a vacuum. If the conductive heat losses were less than those due to radiation, then the limiting D^* would be given by:

$$D^*(T,f) = 2.8 \times 10^{16} \sqrt{\frac{\varepsilon}{T_2^5 + T_1^5}} \text{ Jone} \tag{3.21}$$

where T_1 is the detector temperature, T_2 the background temperature, and ε the value of the detector's emissivity and equally it's absorption. For the usual case of both the detector and background temperature at normal ambient, 300 K, the limiting D^* is 1.8×10^{10} Jones.

Bolometer operation is constrained by the requirement that the response time of the detector be compatible with the frame rate of the imaging system. Most bolometer cameras operate at a 30 Hz frame

FIGURE 3.6 Abstract bolometer detector structure, where C is the thermal capacitance, G is the thermal conductance, and ε is the emissivity of the surface. ϕ_e represents the energy flux in W/cm^2.

rate — 33 msec frame. Response times of the bolometer are usually designed to be on the order of 10 msec. This gives the element a fast enough response to follow scenes with rapidly varying temperatures without objectionable image smearing.

3.3 Detector Materials

The most popular commercial cameras for thermal imaging today use the following detector materials [4]:

- InSb for 5 μm medium wavelength infrared (MWIR) imaging
- $Hg_{1-x}Cd_xTe$ alloys for 5 and 10 μm long wavelength infrared (LWIR) imaging
- Quantum well detectors for 5 and 10 μm imaging
- Uncooled bolometers for 10 μm imaging

We will now review a few of the basic properties of these detector types.

Photovoltaic InSb remains a popular detector for the MWIR spectral band operating at a temperature of 80 K [5,6]. The detector's spectral response at 80 K is shown in Figure 3.7. The spectral response cutoff is about 5.5 μm at 80 K, a good match to the MWIR spectral transmission of the atmosphere. As the operating temperature of InSb is raised, the spectral response extends to longer wavelengths and the dark current increases accordingly. It is thus not normally used above about 100 K. At 80 K the $R_0 A$ product of InSb detectors is typically in the range of 10^5 to 10^6 Ω cm^2 — see Equation 3.16 and Figure 3.5 for reference.

Crystals of InSb are grown in bulk boules up to 3 in. in diameter. InSb materials is highly uniform and combined with a planar-implanted process in which the device geometry is precisely controlled, the resulting detector array responsivity is good to excellent. Devices are usually made with a p/n diode polarity using diffusion or ion implantation. Staring arrays of backside illuminated, direct hybrid InSb detectors in 256 × 256, 240 × 320, 480 × 640, 512 × 640, and 1024 × 1024 formats are available from a number of vendors.

HgCdTe detectors are commercially available to cover the spectral range from 1 to 12 μm [7–13]. Figure 3.8 illustrates representative spectral response from photovoltaic devices, the most commonly used type. Crystals of HgCdTe today are mostly grown in thin epitaxial layers on infrared-transparent CdZnTe crystals. SWIR and MWIR material can also be grown on Si substrates with CdZnTe buffer layers. Growth of the epitaxial layers is by liquid phase melts, molecular beams, or by chemical vapor deposition. Substrate dimensions of CdZnTe crystals are in the 25 to 50 cm^2 range and Si wafers up to 5 to 6 in. (12.5 to 15 cm) in diameter have been used for this purpose. The device structure for a typical HgCdTe photodiode is shown in Figure 3.3.

FIGURE 3.7 Spectral response per watt of an InSb detector at 80 K.

FIGURE 3.8 Representative spectral response curves for a variety of HgCdTe alloy detectors. Spectral cutoff can be varied over the SWIR, MWIR, and LWIR regions.

FIGURE 3.9 Values of R_0A product as a function of wavelength for HgCdTe photodiodes. Note that the R_0A product varies slightly with illumination — 0° field-of-view compared with $f/2$ — especially for shorter-wavelength devices.

At 80 K the leakage current of HgCdTe is small enough to provide both MWIR and LWIR detectors that can be photon-noise dominated. Figure 3.9 shows the R_0A product of representative diodes for wavelengths ranging from 4 to 12 μm.

The versatility of HgCdTe detector material is directly related to being able to grow a broad range of alloy compositions in order to optimize the response at a particular wavelength. Alloys are usually adjusted to provide response in the 1 to 3 μm short wavelength infrared (SWIR), 3 to 5 μm MWIR, or the 8 to 12 μm LWIR spectral regions. Short wavelength detectors can operate uncooled, or with thermoelectric coolers that have no moving parts. Medium and long wavelength detectors are generally operated at 80 K using a cryogenic cooler engine. HgCdTe detectors in 256 × 256, 240 × 320, 480 × 640, and 512 × 640 formats are available from a number of vendors.

Quantum well infrared photodetectors (QWIPs) consist of alternating layers of semiconductor material with larger and narrower bandgaps [14–20]. This series of alternating semiconductor layers is deposited one layer upon another using an ultrahigh vacuum technique such as molecular beam epitaxy (MBE). Alternating large and narrow bandgap materials give rise to quantum wells that provide bound and quasi-bound states for electrons or holes [1–5].

Infrared Detectors and Detector Arrays

FIGURE 3.10 Quantum wells generate bound states for electrons in the conduction band. The conduction bands for a QWIP structure are shown consisting of $Al_xGa_{1-x}As$ barriers and GaAs wells. For a given pair of materials having a fixed conduction band offset, the binding energy of an electron in the well can be adjusted by varying the width of the well. With an applied bias, photoexcited electrons from the GaAs wells are transported and detected as photocurrent.

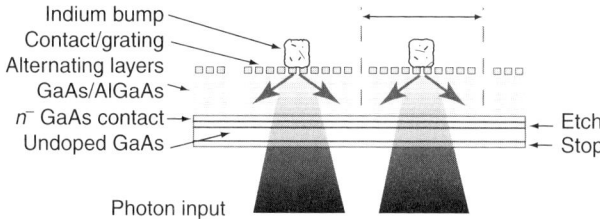

FIGURE 3.11 Backside illuminated QWIP structure with a top side diffraction grating/contact metal. Normally-incident light is coupled horizontally into the quantum wells by scattering off a diffraction grating located at the top of the focal plane array.

Many simple QWIP structures have used GaAs as the narrow bandgap quantum well material and $Al_xGa_{1-x}As$ as the wide bandgap barrier layers as shown in Figure 3.10. The properties of the QWIP are related to the structural design and can be specified by the well width, barrier height, and doping density. In turn, these parameters can be tuned by controlling the cell temperatures of the gallium, aluminum, and arsenic cells as well as the doping cell temperature. The quantum well width (thickness) is governed by the time interval for which the Ga and As cell shutters are left opened. The barrier height is regulated by the composition of the $Al_xGa_{1-x}As$ layers, which are determined by the relative temperature of the Al and Ga cells. QWIP detectors rely on the absorption of incident radiation within the quantum well and typically the well material is doped n-type at an approximate level of 5×10^{17}.

The QWIP detectors require that an electric field component of the incident radiation be perpendicular to the layer planes of the device. Imaging arrays use diffraction gratings as shown in Figure 3.11. In particular, the latter approach is of practical importance in order to realize two-dimensional detector arrays. The QWIP focal plane array is a reticulated structure formed by conventional photolithographic techniques. Part of the processing involves placing a two-dimensional metallic grating over the focal plane pixels. The grating metal is typically angled at 45° patterns to reflect incident light obliquely so as to couple the perpendicular component of the electric field into the quantum wells thus producing the photoexcitation. The substrate material (GaAs) is backside thinned and a chemical/mechanical polish is used to produce a mirrorlike finish on the backside. The front side of the pixels with indium bumps are flip-chip bonded to a readout IC. Light travels through the back side and is unabsorbed during its first pass through the epilayers; upon scattering with a horizontal propagation component from the grating some of it is then absorbed by the quantum wells, photoexciting carriers. An electric field is produced perpendicular to the layers by applying a bias voltage at doped contact layers. The structure then behaves as a photoconductor.

FIGURE 3.12 Representative spectral response of QWIP detectors.

The QWIP detectors require cooling to about 60 K for LWIR operation in order to adequately reduce the dark current. They also have comparatively low quantum efficiency, generally less than 10%. They thus require longer signal integration times than InSb or HgCdTe devices. However, the abundance of radiation in the LWIR band in particular allows QWIP detectors to still achieve excellent performance in infrared cameras.

The maturity of the GaAs-technology makes QWIPs particularly suited for large commercial focal plane arrays with high spatial resolution. Excellent lateral homogeneity is achieved, thus giving rise to a small fixed-pattern noise. QWIPs have an extremely small $1/f$ noise compared to interband detectors (like HgCdTe or InSb), which is particularly useful if long integration times or image accumulation are required. For these reasons, QWIP is the detector technology of choice for many applications where somewhat smaller quantum efficiencies and lower operation temperatures, compared to interband devices, are tolerable. QWIPs are finding useful applications in surveillance, night vision, quality control, inspection, environmental sciences, and medicine.

Quantum well infrared detectors are available in the 5- and 10-μm spectral region. The spectral response of QWIP detectors can be tuned to a wide range of values by adjusting the width and depth of quantum wells formed in alternating layers of GaAs and GaAlAs. An example of the spectral response from a variety of such structures is shown in Figure 3.12. QWIP spectral response is generally limited to fairly narrow spectral bandwidth — approximately 10 to 20% of the peak response wavelength. QWIP detectors have higher dark currents than InSb or HgCdTe devices and generally must be cooled to about 60 K for LWIR operation.

The quantum efficiencies of InSb, HgCdTe, and QWIP photon detectors are compared in Figure 3.13. With antireflection coating, InSb and HgCdTe are able to convert about 90% of the incoming photon flux to electrons. The QWIP quantum efficiencies are significantly lower, but work at improving them continues to occupy the attention of research teams.

We conclude this section with a description of Type-II superlattice detectors [21–26]. Although Type-II superlattice detectors are not yet used in arrays for in commercial camera system, the technology is briefly reviewed here because of its potential future importance. This material system mimics an intrinsic detector material such as HgCdTe, but is "bandgap engineered." Type-II superlattice structures are fabricated from multilayer stacks of alternating layers of two different semiconductor materials. Figure 3.14 illustrates the structure. The conduction band minimum is in one layer and the valence band minimum is in the adjacent layer (as opposed to both minima being in the same layer as in a Type-I superlattice).

The idea of using Type-II superlattices for LWIR detectors was originally proposed in 1977. Recent work on the MBE growth of Type-II systems by [7] has led to the exploitation of these materials for

FIGURE 3.13 Comparison of the quantum efficiencies of commercial infrared photon detectors. This figure represents devices that have been antireflection coated.

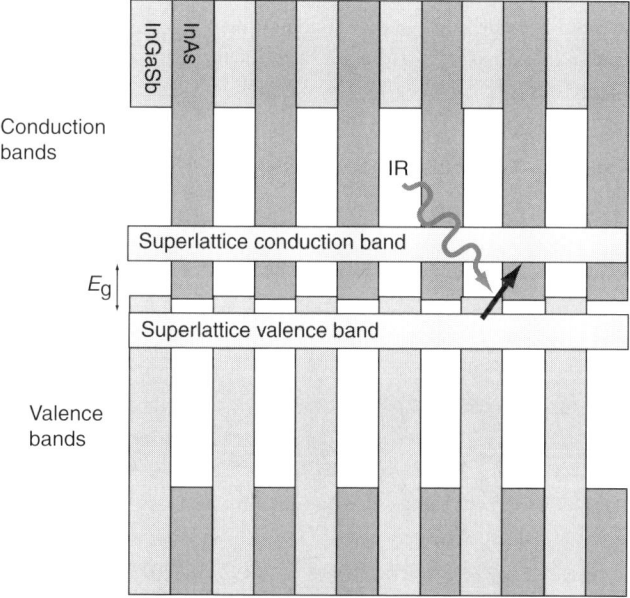

FIGURE 3.14 Band diagram of a short-period InAs/(In,Ga)Sb superlattice showing an infrared transition from the heavy hole (hh) miniband to the electron (e) miniband.

IR detectors. Short period superlattices of, for example, strain-balanced InAs/(Ga,In)Sb lead to the formation of conduction and valence minibands. In these band states heavy holes are largely confined to the (Ga,In)Sb layers and electrons are primarily confined to the InAs layers. However, because of the relatively low electron mass in InAs, the electron wave functions extend considerably beyond the interfaces and have significant overlap with heavy-hole wave functions. Hence, significant absorption is possible at the minigap energy (which is tunable by changing layer thickness and barrier height).

Cutoff wavelengths from 3 to 20 μm and beyond are potentially possible with this system. Unlike QWIP detectors, the absorption of normally incident flux is permitted by selection rules, obviating the need for grating structures or corrugations that are needed with QWIPs. Finally, Auger transition rates, which place intrinsic limits on the performance of these detectors and severely impact the lifetimes found in bulk, narrow-gap detectors, can be minimized by judicious choices of the structure's geometry and strain profile.

In the future, further advantages may be achievable by using the InAs/Ga(As,Sb) material system where both the InAs and Ga(As,Sb) layers may be lattice matched to InAs substrates. The intrinsic quality obtainable in these structures can be in principle superior to that obtained in InAs/(Ga,In)Sb structures. Since dislocations may be reduced to a minimum in the InAs/Ga(As,Sb) material system, it may be the most suitable Type-II material for making large arrays of photovoltaic detectors.

Development efforts for Type-II superlattice detectors are primarily focused on improving material quality and identifying sources of unwanted leakage currents. The most challenging problem currently is to passivate the exposed sidewalls of the superlattices layers where the pixels are etched in fabrication. Advances in these areas should result in a new class of IR detectors with the potential for high performance at high operating temperatures.

3.4 Detector Readouts

Detectors themselves are isolated arrays of photodiodes, photoconductors, or bolometers. Detectors need a readout to integrate or sample their output and convey the signal in an orderly sequence to a signal processor and display [27].

Almost all readouts are integrated circuits (ICs) made from silicon. They are commonly referred to as readout integrated circuits, or ROICs. Here we briefly describe the functions and features of these readouts, first for photon detectors and then for thermal detectors.

3.4.1 Readouts for Photon Detectors

Photon detectors are typically assembled as a hybrid structure, as illustrated in Figure 3.15. Each pixel of the detector array is connected to the unit cell of the readout through an indium bump. Indium bumps allow for a soft, low-temperature metal connection to convey the signal from the detector to the readout's input circuit.

FIGURE 3.15 Hybrid detector array structure consists of a detector array connected to a readout array with indium metal bumps. Detector elements are usually photodiodes or photoconductors, although photocapacitors are sometimes used. Each pixel in the readout contains at least one addressable switch, and more often a preampflifier or buffer together with a charge storage capacitor for integrating the photosignal.

Infrared Detectors and Detector Arrays

Commercial thermal imagers that operate in the MWIR and LWIR spectral regions generally employ a direct injection circuit to collect the detector signal. This is because this circuit is simple and works well with the relatively high photon currents in these spectral bands. The direct injection transistor feeds the signal onto an integrating capacitor where it stored for a time called the integration time. The integration time is typically around 200 μsec for the LWIR spectral band and 2 msec for the MWIR band, corresponding to the comparative difference in the photon flux available. The integration time is limited by the size of the integration capacitor. Typical capacitors can hold on the order of 3×10^7 electrons.

For cameras operating in the SWIR band, the lower flux levels typically require a more complicated input amplifier. The most common choice employs a capacitive feedback circuit, providing the ability to have significant gain at the pixel level before storage on an integrating capacitor.

Two readout modes are employed, depending upon the readout design:

- Snapshot
- Rolling frame

In the snapshot mode, all pixels integrate simultaneously, are stored, and then read out in sequence, followed by resetting the integration capacitors. In the rolling frame mode the capacitors of each row are reset after each pixel in that row is read. In this case each pixel integrates in different parts of the image frame. A variant of the rolling frame is an interlaced output. In this case the even rows are read out in the first frame and the odd rows in the next. This corresponds to how standard U.S. television displays function.

It is common for each column in the readout to have an amplifier to provide some gain to the signal coming from each row as it is read. The column amplifier outputs are then fed to the output amplifiers. Commercial readouts typically have one, two, or four outputs, depending upon the array size and frame rate. Most commercial cameras operate at 30 or 60 Hz.

Another common feature found on some readouts is the ability to operate at higher frame rates on a subset of the full array. This ability is called windowing. It allows data to be collected more quickly on a limited portion of the image.

3.4.2 Thermal Detector Readouts

Bolometer detectors have comparatively lower resistance than photon detectors and relatively slow inherent response times. This condition allows readouts that do not have to integrate the charge during the frame, but only need to sample it for a brief time. This mode is frequently referred to as pulse-biased.

The unit cell of the bolometer contains only a switch that is pulsed on once per frame to allow current to flow from each row in turn to the column amplifiers. Bias is supplied by the row multiplexer. Sample times for each detector are typically on the order of the frame time divided by the number of rows. Many designs employ differential input column amplifiers that are simultaneously fed an input from a dummy or blind bolometer element in order to subtract a large fraction of the current that flows when the element is biased.

The nature of bolometer operation means that the readout mode is rolling frame. Some designs also provide interlaced outputs for input to TV-like displays.

3.4.3 Readout Evolution

Early readouts required multiple bias supply inputs and multiple clock signals for operation. Today only two clocks and two bias supplies are typically required. The master clock sets the frame rate. The integration clock sets the time that the readout signal is integrated, or that the readout bias pulse is applied. On-chip clock and bias circuits generate the additional clocks and biases required to run the readout. Separate grounds for the analog and digital chip circuitry are usually employed to minimize noise.

Current development efforts are beginning to add on-chip analog-to-digital (A/D) converters to the readout. This feature provides a direct digital output, avoiding significant difficulties in controlling extraneous noise when the sensor is integrated with an imaging or camera system.

3.5 Technical Challenges for Infrared Detectors

Twenty-five years ago, infrared imagining was revolutionized by the introduction of the Probeye Infrared camera. At a modest 8 pounds, Probeye enabled handheld operation, a feature previously unheard of at that time when very large, very expensive IR imaging systems were the rule. Infrared components and technologies have advanced considerably since then. With the introduction of the Indigo Systems Omega camera, one can now acquire a complete infrared camera weighing less than 100 g and occupying 3.5 in.³

Many forces are at play enabling this dramatic reduction in camera size. Virtually all of these can be traced to improvements in the silicon IC processing industry. Largely enabled by advancements in photolithography, but additionally aided by improvements in vacuum deposition equipment, device feature sizes have been steadily reduced. It was not too long ago that the minimum device feature size was just pushing to break the 1-μm barrier. Today, foundries are focused on production implementation of 65 to 90 nm feature sizes.

The motivation behind such significant improvements has been the high-dollar/high-volume commercial electronics business. Silicon foundries have expended billions of dollars in capitalization and R&D aimed at increasing the density and speed of the transistors per unit chip area. Cellular telephones, personal data assistants (PDAs), and laptop computers are all applications demanding smaller size, lower power, and more features — performance — from electronic components. Infrared detector arrays and cameras have taken direct advantage of these advancements.

3.5.1 Uncooled Infrared Detector Challenges

The major challenge for all infrared markets is to reduce the pixel size while increasing the sensitivity. Reduction from a 50-μm pixel to a 25-μm pixel, while maintaining or even reducing noise equivalent temperature difference (NETD), is a major goal that is now being widely demonstrated (see Figure 3.16). The trends are illustrated by a simple examination of a highly idealized bolometer: the DC response of a detector in which we neglect all noise terms except temperature fluctuation noise, and the thermal conductance value is not detector area dependent (i.e., we are not at or near the radiation conductance limit). Using these assumptions, reducing the pixel area by a factor of four will reduce the SNR by a factor

FIGURE 3.16 Uncooled microbolometer pixel structures having noise-equivalent temperature difference (NEΔT) values <50 mK: single level for 2 mil (50 μm) pixels in a 240 × 320 format and double level for 1 mil (25 μm) pixels in a 480 × 640 format. (Courtesy of Raytheon Vision Systems.)

Infrared Detectors and Detector Arrays

of eight as shown below:

$$\Delta T_{signal|DCresponse} = \frac{P_{signalDC}}{G_{th}} = \frac{\gamma A_D I_{light}}{G_{th}} \qquad (3.22)$$

where $P_{signalDC}$ is the DC signal from IR radiation (absorbed power) [W], A_D is the detector area [m^2], I_{light} is the light intensity [W/m^2], G_{th} is the thermal conductance [W/K], and γ is a constant that accounts for reflectivity and other factors not relevant to this analysis.

For a detector in the thermal fluctuation limit, the root mean square temperature fluctuation noise is a function of the incident radiation and the thermal conductance of the bolometer bridge.

$$\Delta T_{noise} \sqrt{\langle \Delta T^2 \rangle} = \sqrt{\frac{kT^2}{C_{th}}} \qquad (3.23)$$

where T is the operating temperature in Kelvin, k is Boltzman's constant, and C_{th} is the total heat capacity of the detector in Joules per Kelvin [J/K].

The total heat capacity can be written as $C_{th} = c_p A_d Z_{bridge}$, where Z_{bridge} is the bolometer bridge thickness in meters and c_p is the specific heat of the detector in J/K-m^3.

The signal to noise (SNR) is then

$$\frac{\Delta T_{signal}}{\Delta T_{noise}} = \frac{\gamma A_D I_{light}}{G_{th}} \sqrt{\frac{c_p A_D Z_{bridge}}{kT^2}} = \frac{\gamma A_D I_{light}}{G_{th}} A_D^{3/2} \sqrt{\frac{c_p Z_{bridge}}{kT^2}} \qquad (3.24)$$

It can be seen that the SNR goes as the area to the three halves. Therefore, a 4× reduction in detector area reduces the SNR by a factor of eight for this ideal bolometer case. Thermal conductance is assumed constant, that is, the ratio of leg length to thickness remains constant as the detector area is reduced. In practical constructions, reducing the pixel linear dimensions by 2× also reduces the leg length by 2×, thus the thermal conductance increases and aggravates the problem. In order to improve the SNR caused by the 4× loss in area, one may be tempted to reduce the thermal conductance G_{th} by 8×. To accomplish this, the length of the legs must be increased and their thickness reduced. By folding the legs under the detector, as seen in Figure 3.10, one can achieve this result. However, an 8× reduction in thermal conductance would result in a detrimental increase in the thermal time constant.

The thermal time constant is given by $\tau_{thermal} = C_{th}/G_{th}$. The heat capacity is reduced by 4× because of the area loss. If G_{th} is reduced by a factor of 8×, then $\tau_{thermal} = 2C_{th}/G_{th}$ is increased by a factor of two. This image smear associated with this increased time constant would prove problematic for practical military applications.

In order to maintain the same time constant, the total heat capacity must be reduced accordingly. Making the detector thinner may achieve this result except that it also increases the temperature fluctuation noise. From this simple example one can readily see the inherent relationship between SNR and the thermal time constant.

We would like to maintain both an equivalent SNR and thermal time constant as the detector cell size is decreased. This can be achieved by maintaining the relationships between the thermal conductance, detector area, and bridge thickness as shown in the following.

The thermal time constant is given by:

$$\tau_{thermal} = \frac{C_{th}}{G_{th}} = \frac{c_p A_D Z_{bridge}}{G_{th}} \qquad (3.25)$$

Equating the thermal time constant of the large and small pixels equal and doing the same with the SNR leads to the following relationships, where the primed variables are the parameters required for the new

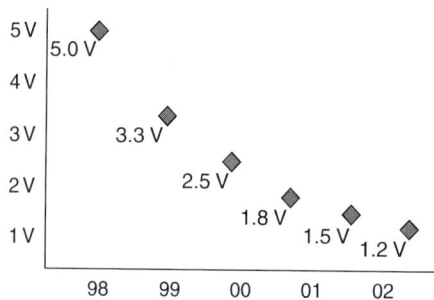

FIGURE 3.17 IC device core voltage vs. time

detector cell:

$$\tau_{\text{thermal}} = \frac{c_p A_D Z_{\text{bridge}}}{G_{\text{th}}} = \frac{c_p A'_D Z'_{\text{bridge}}}{G'_{\text{th}}} \quad (3.26)$$

$$\frac{\Delta T_{\text{signal}}}{\Delta T_{\text{noise}}} = \frac{\gamma A_D I_{\text{light}}}{G_{\text{th}}} \sqrt{\frac{c_p A_D Z_{\text{bridge}}}{kT^2}} = \frac{\gamma A'_D I_{\text{light}}}{G'_{\text{th}}} \sqrt{\frac{c_p A'_D Z'_{\text{bridge}}}{kT^2}} \quad (3.27)$$

Rearranging τ_{thermal} to find the ratio $G_{\text{th}}/G'_{\text{th}}$ and substituting into the SNR, we obtain:

$$\frac{Z'_{\text{bridge}}}{Z_{\text{bridge}}} = \frac{A'_D}{A_D}, \quad \text{and it follows that} \quad \frac{G'_{\text{th}}}{G_{\text{th}}} = \left(\frac{Z'_{\text{bridge}}}{Z_{\text{bridge}}}\right)^2 \quad (3.28)$$

So, it becomes evident that a 4× reduction in pixel cell area requires a 16×, and not an 8×, reduction in thermal conductance to maintain equivalent SNR and thermal time constant. This gives some insight into the problems of designing small pixel bolometers for high sensitivity. It should be noted that in current implementations, the state-of-the-art sensitivity is about 10× from the thermal limits.

3.5.2 Electronics Challenges

Specific technology improvements spawned by the commercial electronics business that have enabled size reductions in IR camera signal processing electronics include:

- Faster digital signal processors (DSPs) with internal memory ≥ 1 MB)
- Higher-density field-programmable gate arrays (FPGAs) (>200 K gates and with an embedded processor core
- Higher-density static (synchronous?) random access memory >4 MB
- Low-power, 14-bit differential A/D converters

Another enabler, also attributable to the silicon industry, is reduction in the required core voltage of these devices (see Figure 3.17). Five years ago, the input voltage for virtually all-electronic components was 5 V. Today, one can buy a DSP with a core voltage as low as 1.2 V. Power consumption of the device is proportional to the square of the voltage. So a reduction from 5- to 1.2-V core represents more than an order of magnitude power reduction.

The input voltage ranges for most components (e.g., FPGAs, memories, etc.) are following the same trends. These reductions are not only a boon for reduced power consumption, but also these lower power devices typically come in much smaller footprints. IC packaging advancements have kept up with the

FIGURE 3.18 Advancements in component packaging miniaturization together with increasing pin count that enables reduced camera volume.

higher-density, lower-power devices. One can now obtain a device with almost twice the number of I/Os in 25% of the required area (see Figure 3.18).

All of these lower power, smaller footprint components exist by virtue of the significant demand created by the commercial electronics industry. These trends will continue. Moore's law (logic density in bits/in.^{2} will double every 18 months) nicely describes the degree by which we can expect further advancements.

3.5.3 Detector Readout Challenges

The realization of tighter design rules positively affects reduction in camera size in yet another way. Multiplexers, or ROICs, directly benefit from the increased density. Now, without enlarging the size of the ROIC die, more functions can be contained in the device. On-ROIC A/D conversion eliminates the need for a dedicated, discrete A/D converter. On-ROIC clock and bias generation reduces the number of vacuum Dewar feedthroughs to yield a smaller package as well as reducing the complexity and size of the camera power supply. Putting the nonuniformity correction circuitry on the ROIC reduces the magnitude of the detector output signal swing and minimizes the required input dynamic range of the A/D converter. All of these increases in ROIC functionality come with the increased density of the silicon fabrication process.

3.5.4 Optics Challenges

Another continuing advancement that has helped reduced the size of IR cameras is the progress made at increasing the performance of the uncooled detectors themselves. The gains made at increasing the sensitivity of the detectors has directly translated to reduction in the size of the optics. With a sensitivity goal of 100 mK, an $F/1$ optic has traditionally been required to collect enough energy. Given the recent sensitivity improvements in detectors, achievement of 100 mK can be attained with an $F/2$ optic. This reduction in required aperture size greatly reduces the camera size and weight. These improvements in detector sensitivity can also be directly traceable to improvements in the silicon industry. The same photolithography and vacuum deposition equipments used to fabricate commercial ICs are used to make bolometers. The finer geometry line widths translate directly to increased thermal isolation and increased fill factor, both of which are factors in increased responsivity.

Reduction in optics' size was based on a sequence of NEDT performance improvements in uncooled VO_x microbolometer detectors so that faster optics $F/1.4$ to $F/2$ could be utilized in the camera and still maintain a moderate performance level. As indicated by Equations 3.29 to 3.33, the size of the optics is based on the required field-of-view (FOV), number of detectors (format of the detector array), area of the detector, and F# of the optics (see Figure 3.19). The volume of the optics is considered to be approximately a cylinder with a volume of $\pi r^2 L$. In Equations 3.29 to 3.33, FL is the optics focal length equivalent to L, D_o is the optics diameter and $D_o/2$ is equivalent to r, A_{det} is the area of the detector, F# is the f-number

FIGURE 3.19 Trade-off between optics size and volume and $f/\#$, array format, and pixel size.

of the optics and HFOV is the horizontal field-of-view.

$$\text{FL} = \frac{\text{\# horizontal detectors}}{\text{Tan(HFOV/2)}} = \frac{\sqrt{A_{\text{det}}}}{2} \tag{3.29}$$

$$D_o = \frac{\text{\# horizontal detectors}}{\text{Tan(HFOV/2)}} = \frac{\sqrt{A_{\text{det}}}}{2F\#} \tag{3.30}$$

$$F\# = \frac{\text{FL}}{D_o} \tag{3.31}$$

$$\text{Volume}_{\text{optics}} = \pi \left[\frac{D_o}{2}\right]^2 = \text{FL}$$
$$= \pi \left[\frac{(\text{\# horizontal detectors}/(\tan(\text{HFOV}/2))) = (\sqrt{A_{\text{det}}}/2F\#)}{2}\right]^2 = \text{FL} \tag{3.32}$$

$$\text{Volume}_{\text{optics}} = \pi \left[\frac{(\text{\# horizontal detectors}/(\tan(\text{HFOV}/2))) = \sqrt{A_{\text{det}}}}{32F\#^2}\right]^3 \tag{3.33}$$

Uncooled cameras have utilized the above enhancements and are now only a few ounces in weight and require only about 1 W of input power.

3.5.5 Challenges for Third-Generation Cooled Imagers

Third-generation cooled imagers are being developed to greatly extend the range at which targets can be detected and identified [28–30]. U.S. Army rules of engagement now require identification prior to attack. Since deployment of first- and second-generation sensors there has been a gradual proliferation of thermal imaging technology worldwide. Third-generation sensors are intended to ensure that U.S. Army forces maintain a technological advantage in night operations over any opposing force.

Infrared Detectors and Detector Arrays

FIGURE 3.20 Illustration of a simultaneous two-color pixel structure — cross section and SEM. Simultaneous two-color FPAs have two indium bumps per pixel. A 50-μm simultaneous two-color pixel is shown.

Thermal imaging equipment is used to first detect an object, and then to identify it. In the detection mode, the optical system provides a wide field-of-view (WFOV — $f/2.5$) to maintain robust situational awareness [31]. For detection, LWIR provides superior range under most Army fighting conditions. Medium wavelength infrared offers higher spatial resolution sensing, and a significant advantage for long-range identification when used with telephoto optics (NFOV — $f/6$).

3.5.5.1 Cost Challenges — Chip Size

Cost is a direct function of the chip size since the number of detector and readout die per wafer is inversely proportion to the chip area. Chip size in turn is set by the array format and pixel size. Third-generation imager formats are anticipated to be in a high-definition 16×9 layout, compatible with future display standards, and reflecting the soldier's preference for a wide field-of-view. An example of such a format is 1280×720 pixels. For a 30 μm pixel this format yields a die size greater than 1.5×0.85 in. (22×38 mm). This will yield only a few die per wafer, and will also require the development of a new generation of dewar-cooler assemblies to accommodate these large dimensions. A pixel size of 20 μm results in a cost saving of more than $2\times$, and allows the use of existing dewar designs.

3.5.5.1.1 Two-Color Pixel Designs

Pixel size is the most important factor for achieving affordable third-generation systems. Two types of two-color pixels have been demonstrated. Simultaneous two-color pixels have two indium–bump connections per pixel to allow readout of both color bands at the same time. Figure 3.20 shows an example of a simultaneous two-color pixel structure. The sequential two-color approach requires only one indium bump per pixel, but requires the readout circuit to alternate bias polarities multiple times during each frame. An example of this structure is illustrated in Figure 3.21. Both approaches leave very little area available for the indium bump(s) as the pixel size is made smaller. Advanced etching technology is being developed in order to meet the challenge of shrinking the pixel size to 20 μm.

3.5.5.2 Sensor Format and Packaging Issues

The sensor format was selected to provide a wide field-of-view and high spatial resolution. Target detection in many Army battlefield situations is most favorable in LWIR. Searching for targets is more efficient in a wider field-of-view, in this case $f/2.5$. Target identification relies on having 12 or more pixels across the target to adequately distinguish its shape and features. Higher magnification, $f/6$ optics combined with MWIR optical resolution enhances this task.

Consideration was also given to compatibility with future standards for display formats. Army soldiers are generally more concerned with the width of the display than the height, so the emerging 16:9 width to height format that is planned for high-definition TV was chosen.

A major consideration in selecting a format was the packaging requirements. Infrared sensors must be packaged in a vacuum enclosure and mated with a mechanical cooler for operation. Overall array size was therefore limited to approximately 1 in. so that it would fit in an existing standard advanced dewar

FIGURE 3.21 Illustration of a sequential two-color pixel structure — cross section and SEM. Sequential two-color FPAs have only one indium bump per pixel, helping to reduce pixel size. A 20 μm sequential two-color pixel is shown.

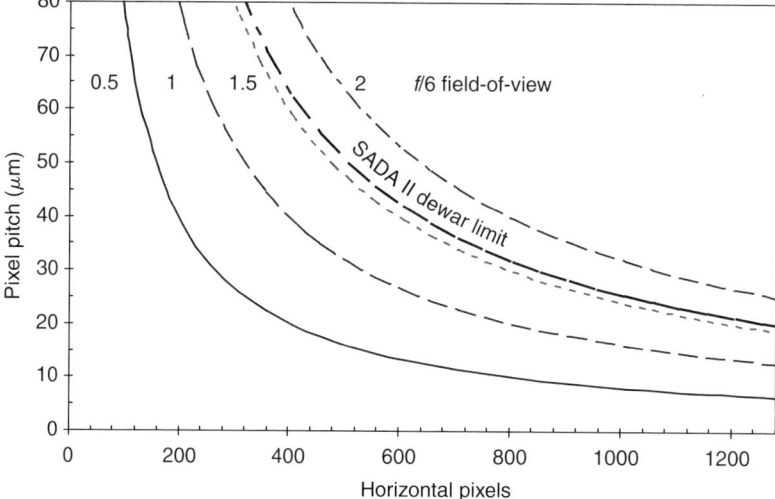

FIGURE 3.22 Maximum array horizontal format is determined by the pixel size and the chip size limit that will fit in an existing SADA dewar design for production commonality. For a 20-μm pixel and a 1.6° FOV, the horizontal pixel count limit is 1280. A costly development program would be necessary to develop a new, larger dewar.

assembly (SADA) dewar design. Figure 3.22 illustrates the pixel size/format/field-of-view trade within the design size constraints of the SADA dewar.

3.5.5.3 Temperature Cycling Fatigue

Modern cooled infrared focal plane arrays are hybrid structures comprising a detector array mated to a silicon readout array with indium bumps (see Figure 3.15).

Very large focal plane arrays may exceed the limits of hybrid reliability engineered into these structures. The problem stems from the differential rates of expansion between HgCdTe and Si, which results in large stress as a device is cooled from 300 K ambient to an operating temperature in the range of 77 to 200 K. Hybrids currently use mechanical constraints to force the contraction of the two components to closely match each other. This approach may have limits — when the stress reaches a point where the chip fractures.

Two new approaches exist that can extend the maximum array size considerably. One is the use of silicon as the substrate for growing the HgCdTe detector layer using MBE. This approach has shown excellent

Infrared Detectors and Detector Arrays

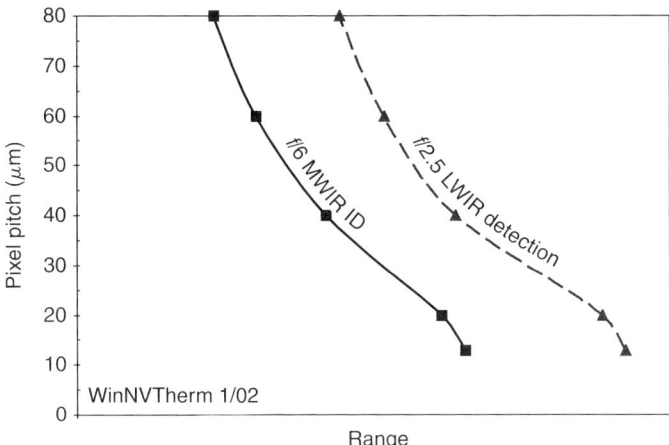

FIGURE 3.23 Range improves as the pixel size is reduced until a limit in optical blur is reached. In the examples above, the blur circle for the MWIR and LWIR cases are comparable since the f/number has been adjusted accordingly. D^* and integration time have been held constant in this example.

results for MWIR detectors, but not yet for LWIR devices. Further improvement in this approach would be needed to use it for Third-Generation MWIR/LWIR two-color arrays.

A second approach that has proven successful for InSb hybrids is thinning the detector structure. HgCdTe hybrids currently retain their thick, 500 μm, CdZnTe epitaxial substrate in the hybridized structure. InSb hybrids must remove the substrate because it is not transparent, leaving only a 10-μm thick detector layer. The thinness of this layer allows it to readily expand and contract with the readout. InSb hybrids with detector arrays over 2 in. (5 cm) on a side have been successfully demonstrated to be reliable.

Hybrid reliability issues will be monitored as a third-generation sensor manufacturing technology and is developed to determine whether new approaches are needed.

In addition to cost issues, significant performance issues must also be addressed for third-generation imagers. These are now discussed in the following section.

3.5.5.4 Performance Challenges

3.5.5.4.1 Dynamic Range and Sensitivity Constraints

A goal of third-generation imagers is to achieve a significant improvement in detection and ID range over Second-Generation systems. Range improvement comes from higher pixel count, and to a lesser extent from improved sensitivity. Figure 3.23 shows relative ID and detection range vs. pixel size in the MWIR and LWIR, respectively. Sensitivity (D^* and integration time) have been held constant, and the format was varied to keep the field-of-view constant.

Sensitivity has less effect than pixel size for clear atmospheric conditions, as illustrated by the clear atmosphere curve in Figure 3.24. Note that here the sensitivity is varied by an order of magnitude, corresponding to two orders of magnitude increase in integration time. Only a modest increase in range is seen for this dramatic change in SNR ratio. In degraded atmospheric conditions, however, improved sensitivity plays a larger role because the signal is weaker. This is illustrated in Figure 3.24 by the curve showing range under conditions of reduced atmospheric transmission.

Dynamic range of the imager output must be considered from the perspective of the quantum efficiency and the effective charge storage capacity in the pixel unit cell of the readout. Quantum efficiency and charge storage capacity determine the integration time for a particular flux rate. As increasing number of quanta are averaged, the SNR ratio improves as the square root of the count. Higher accuracy A/D converters are therefore required to cope with the increased dynamic range between the noise and signal levels. Figure 3.25 illustrates the interaction of these specifications.

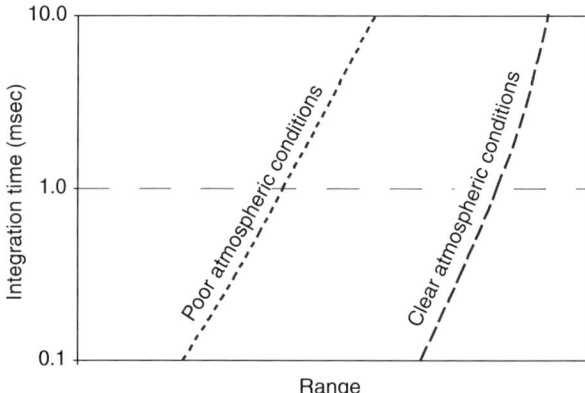

FIGURE 3.24 Range in a clear atmosphere improves only modestly with increased sensitivity. The case modeled here has a 20 μm pixel, a fixed D^*, and variable integration time. The 100× range of integration time corresponds to a 10× range in SNR. Improvement is more dramatic in the case of lower-atmospheric transmission that results in a reduced target signal.

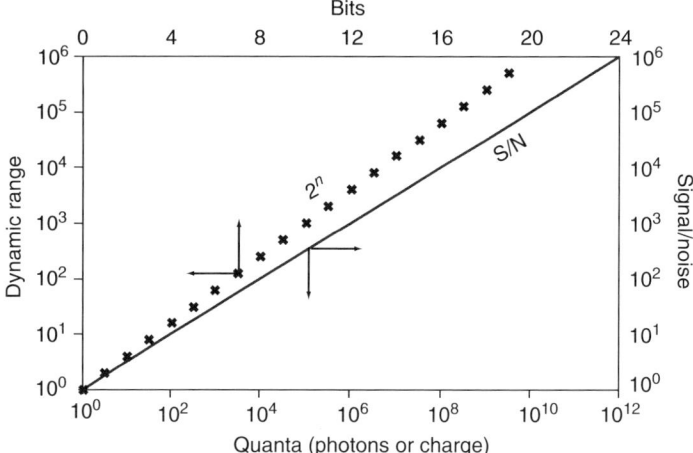

FIGURE 3.25 Dynamic range (2^n) corresponding to the number of digital bits (n) is plotted as a discrete point corresponding to each bit and referenced to the left and top scales. SNR ratio, corresponding to the number of quanta collected (either photons or charge) is illustrated by the solid line in reference to the bottom- and right-hand scales.

System interface considerations lead to some interesting challenges and dilemmas. Imaging systems typically specify a noise floor from the readout on the order of 300 μV. This is because system users do not want to encounter sensor signal levels below the system noise level. With readouts built at commercial silicon foundries now having submicrometer design rules, the maximum bias voltage applied to the readout is limited to a few volts — this trend has been downward from 5 V in the past decade as design rules have shrunk, as illustrated in Figure 3.26. Output swing voltages can only be a fraction of the maximum applied voltage, on the order of 3 V or less.

This means that the dynamic range limit of a readout is about 10,000 — 80 db in power — or less. Present readouts almost approach this constraining factor with 70 to 75 db achieved in good designs. In order to significantly improve sensitivity, the noise floor will have to be reduced.

If sufficiently low readout noise could be achieved, and the readout could digitize on chip to a level of 15 to 16 bits, the data could come off digitally and the system noise floor would not be an issue. Such developments may allow incremental improvement in third-generation imagers in the

Infrared Detectors and Detector Arrays

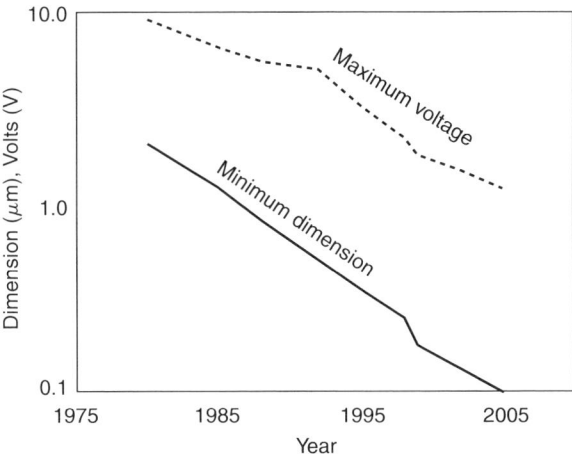

FIGURE 3.26 Trends for design rule minimum dimensions and maximum bias voltage of silicon foundry requirements.

FIGURE 3.27 Focal planes with on-chip A/D converters have been demonstrated. This example shows a 900 × 120 TDI scanning format array. (Photo supplied by Lester Kozlowski of Rockwell Scientific, Camarillo, CA.)

future. Figure 3.27 illustrates an example of an on-chip A/D converter that has demonstrated 12 bits on chip.

A final issue here concerns the ability to provide high charge storage density within the small pixel dimensions envisioned for third-generation imagers. This may be difficult with standard CMOS capacitors. Reduced oxide thickness of submicrometer design rules does give larger capacitance per unit area, but the reduced bias voltage largely cancels any improvement in charge storage density. Promising technology in the form of ferroelectric capacitors may provide much greater charge storage densities than the oxide-on-silicon capacitors now used. Such technology is not yet incorporated into standard CMOS foundries. Stacked hybrid structures* [32] may be needed as at least an interim solution to incorporate the desired charge storage density in detector-readout-capacitor structures.

3.5.5.4.2 High Frame Rate Operation

Frame rates of 30 to 60 fps are adequate for visual display. In third-generation systems we plan to deploy high frame rate capabilities to provide more data throughput for advanced signal processing functions

---

*It should be noted that the third-generation imager will operate as an on-the-move wide area step-scanner wit automated ATR versus second-generation systems that rely on manual target searching. This allows the overall narrower field of view for the third-generation imager.

FIGURE 3.28 Javelin cooler coefficient of performance vs. temperature.

such as automatic target recognition (ATR), and missile and projectile tracking. An additional benefit is the opportunity to collect a higher percentage of available signal. Higher frame rates pose two significant issues. First, output drive power is proportional to the frame rate and at rates of 480 Hz or higher, this could be the most significant source of power dissipation on the readout. Increased power consumption on chip will also require more power consumption by the cryogenic cooler. These considerations lead us to conclude that high frame rate capabilities need to be limited to a small but arbitrarily positioned window of 64 × 64 pixels, for which a high frame rate of 480 Hz can be supported. This allows for ATR functions to be exercised on possible target locations within the full field-of-view.

3.5.5.5.4.3 *Higher Operating Temperature*

Current tactical infrared imagers operate at 77 K with few exceptions — notably MWIR HgCdTe, which can use solid-state thermoelectric (TE) cooling. Power can be saved, and cooler efficiency and cooler lifetime improved if focal planes operate at temperatures above 77 K.

Increasing the operating temperature results in a major reduction of input cryogenic cooler power. As can be seen from Figure 3.28 the coefficient of performance (COP) increases by a factor of 2.4 from 2.5 to 6% as the operating temperature is raised from 80 to 120 K with a 320 K heat sink. If the operating temperature can be increased to 150 K, the COP increases fourfold. This can have a major impact on input power, weight, and size.

Research is underway on an artificial narrow bandgap intrinsic-like material — strained-layer superlattices of InGaAsSb — which have the potential to increase operating temperatures to even higher levels [33]. Results from this research may be more than a decade away, but the potential benefits are significant in terms of reduced cooler operating power and maintenance.

The above discussion illustrates some of the challenges facing the development of third-generation cooled imagers. In addition to these are the required advances in signal processing and display technologies to translate the focal plane enhancements into outputs for the user. These advances can be anticipated to not only help to increase the range at which targets can be identified, but also to increase the rate of detection and identification through the use of two-color cues. Image fusion of the two colors in some cases is anticipated to help find camouflaged targets in clutter. Improved sensitivity and two-color response is further anticipated to minimize the loss of target contrast now encountered because of diurnal crossover. Future two-color imagers together with novel signal processing methods may further enhance the ability to detect land mines and find obscured targets.

3.6 Summary

Infrared sensors have made major performance strides in the last few years, especially in the uncooled sensors area. Cost, weight, and size of the uncooled have dramatically been reduced allowing a greater proliferation into the commercial market. Uncooled sensors will find greater use in the medical community as a result. High-performance cooled sensors have also been dramatically improved including the development of multicolor arrays. The high-performance sensors will find new medical applications because of the color discrimination and sensitivity attributes now available.

References

[1] D.G. Crowe, P.R. Norton, T. Limperis, and J. Mudar, Detectors, in *Electro-Optical Components*, W.D. Rogatto, Ed., Vol. 3, ERIM, Ann Arbor, MI; *Infrared and Electro-Optical Systems Handbook*, J.S. Accetta and D.L. Schumaker, Executive Eds., SPIE, Bellingham, WA, 1993, revised 1996, Chapter 4, pp. 175–283.

[2] P.R. Norton, Detector focal plane array technology, in *Encyclopedia of Optical Engineering*, R.G. Driggers, Ed., Vol. 1, Marcel Dekker, New York, 2003, pp. 320–348.

[3] P.W. Kruse and D.D. Skatrud, Eds., Uncooled infrared imaging arrays and systems in *Semiconductors and Semimetals*, R.K. Willardson and E.R. Weber, Eds., Academic Press, New York, 1997.

[4] P. Norton, Infrared image sensors, *Opt. Eng.*, 30, 1649–1663, 1991.

[5] T. Ashley, I.M. Baker, T.M. Burke, D.T. Dutton, J.A. Haigh, L.G. Hipwood, R. Jefferies, A.D. Johnson, P. Knowles, and J.C. Little, *Proc. SPIE*, 4028, 2000, pp. 398–403.

[6] P.J. Love, K.J. Ando, R.E. Bornfreund, E. Corrales, R.E. Mills, J.R. Cripe, N.A. Lum, J.P. Rosbeck, and M.S. Smith, Large-format infrared arrays for future space and ground-based astronomy applications, *Proceedings of SPIE*; *Infrared Spaceborne Remote Sensing IX*, Vol. 4486–38; pp. 373–384, 29 July–3 August, 2001; San Diego, USA.

[7] The photoconductive and photovoltaic detector technology of HgCdTe is summarized in the following references: D. Long and J.L. Schmidt, Mercury-cadmium telluride and closely related alloys, in *Semiconductors and Semimetals* 5, R.K. Willardson and A.C. Beer, Eds., Academic Press, New York, pp. 175–255, 1970; R.A. Reynolds, C.G. Roberts, R.A. Chapman, and H.B. Bebb, Photoconductivity processes in 0.09 eV bandgap HgCdTe, in *Proceedings of the 3rd International Conference on Photoconductivity*, E.M. Pell, Ed., Pergamon Press, New York, p. 217, 1971; P.W. Kruse, D. Long, and O.N. Tufte, Photoeffects and material parameters in HgCdTe alloys, in *Proceedings of the 3rd International Conference on Photoconductivity*, E.M. Pell, Ed., Pergamon Press, New York, p. 233, 1971; R.M. Broudy and V.J. Mazurczyk (HgCd) Te photoconductive detectors, in *Semiconductors and Semimetals*, 18, R.K. Willardson and A.C. Beer, Eds., Chapter 5, Academic Press, New York, pp. 157–199, 1981; M.B. Reine, A.K. Sood, and T.J. Tredwell, Photovoltaic infrared detectors, in *Semiconductors and Semimetals*, 18, R.K. Willardson and A.C. Beer, Eds., Chapter 6, pp. 201–311; D. Long, Photovoltaic and photoconductive infrared detectors, in *Topics in Applied Physics* 19, *Optical and Infrared Detectors*, R.J. Keyes, Ed., Springer-Verlag, Heidelberg, pp.101–147, 1970; C.T. Elliot, infrared detectors, in *Handbook on Semiconductors* 4, C. Hilsum, Ed., Chapter 6B, North Holland, New York, pp. 727–798, 1981.

[8] P. Norton, Status of infrared detectors, *Proc. SPIE*, 2274, 82–92, 1994.

[9] I.M., Baker, Photovoltaic IR detectors in *Narrow-gap II–VI Compounds for Optoelectronic and Electromagnetic Applications*, P. Capper, Ed., Chapman and Hall, London, pp. 450–73, 1997.

[10] P. Norton, Status of infrared detectors, *Proc. SPIE*, 3379, 102–114, 1998.

[11] M. Kinch., HDVIP® FPA technology at DRS, *Proc. SPIE*, 4369, pp. 566–578, 1999.

[12] M.B. Reine., Semiconductor fundamentals — materials: fundamental properties of mercury cadmium telluride, in *Encyclopedia of Modern Optics*, Academic Press, London, 2004.

[13] A. Rogalski., HgCdTe infrared detector material: history, status and outlook, *Rep. Prog. Phys.* 68, 2267–2336, 2005.

[14] S.D. Guanapala, B.F. Levine, and N. Chand, *J. Appl. Phys.*, 70, 305, 1991.

[15] B.F. Levine, *J. Appl. Phys.*, 47, R1–R81, 1993.

[16] K.K. Choi., *The Physics of Quantum Well Infrared Photodetectors*, World Scientific, River Edge, New Jersey, 1997.

[17] S.D. Gunapala, J.K. Liu, J.S. Park, M. Sundaram, C.A. Shott, T. Hoelter, T.-L. Lin, S.T. Massie, P.D. Maker, R.E. Muller, and G. Sarusi, 9 μm Cutoff 256×256 GaAs/AlGaAs quantum well infrared photodetector hand-held camera, *IEEE Trans. Elect. Dev.*, 45, 1890, 1998.

[18] S.D. Gunapala, S.V. Bandara, J.K. Liu, W. Hong, M. Sundaram, P.D. Maker, R.E. Muller, C.A. Shott, and R. Carralejo, Long-wavelength 640×480 GaAs/AlGaAs quantum well infrared photodetector snap-shot camera, *IEEE Trans. Elect. Dev.*, 44, 51–57, 1997.

[19] M.Z. Tidrow et al., Device physics and focal plane applications of QWIP and MCT, *Opto-Elect. Rev.*, 7, 283–296, 1999.

[20] S.D. Gunapala and S.V. Bandara, Quantum well infrared photodetector (QWIP) focal plane arrays, in *Semiconductors and Semimetals*, R.K. Willardson and E.R. Weber, Eds., 62, Academic Press, New York, 1999.

[21] G.A. Sai-Halasz, R. Tsu, and L. Esaki, *Appl. Phys. Lett.*, 30, 651, 1977.

[22] D.L. Smith and C. Mailhiot, Proposal for strained type II superlattice infrared detectors, *J. Appl. Phys.*, 62, 2545–2548, 1987.

[23] S.R. Kurtz, L.R. Dawson, T.E. Zipperian, and S.R. Lee, Demonstration of an InAsSb strained-layer superlattice photodiode, *Appl. Phys. Lett.*, 52, 1581–1583, 1988.

[24] R.H. Miles, D.H. Chow, J.N. Schulman, and T.C. McGill, Infrared optical characterization of InAs/GaInSb superlattices, *Appl. Phys. Lett.* 57, 801–803, 1990.

[25] F. Fuchs, U.Weimar, W. Pletschen, J. Schmitz, E. Ahlswede, M. Walther, J. Wagner, and P. Koidl, *J. Appl. Phys. Lett.*, 71, 3251, 1997.

[26] Gail J. Brown, Type-II InAs/GaInSb superlattices for infrared detection: an overview, *Proceedings of SPIE*, 5783, pp. 65–77, 2005.

[27] J.L. Vampola, Readout electronics for infrared sensors, in *electro-optical components*, Chapter 5, Vol. 3, W.D. Rogatto, Ed., *Infrared and Electro-Optical Systems Handbook*, J.S. Accetta and D.L. Schumaker, Executive Eds., ERIM, Ann Arbor, MI and SPIE, Bellingham, WA, pp. 285–342, 1993, revised 1996.

[28] D. Reago, S. Horn, J. Campbell, and R. Vollmerhausen, Third generation imaging sensor system concepts, *SPIE*, 3701, 108–117, 1999.

[29] P. Norton*, J. Campbell III, S. Horn, and D. Reago, Third-generation infrared imagers, *Proc. SPIE*, 4130, 226–236, 2000.

[30] S. Horn, P. Norton, T. Cincotta, A. Stoltz, D. Benson, P. Perconti, and J. Campbell, Challenges for third-generation cooled imagers, *Proc. SPIE*, 5074, 44–51, 2003.

[31] S. Horn, D. Lohrman, P. Norton, K. McCormack, and A. Hutchinson, Reaching for the sensitivity limits of uncooled and minimally cooled thermal and photon infrared detectors, *Proc. SPIE*, 5783, 401–411, 2005.

[32] W. Cabanskia, K. Eberhardta, W. Rodea, J. Wendlera, J. Zieglera, J.Fleißnerb, F. Fuchsb, R. Rehmb, J. Schmitzb, H. Schneiderb, and M. Walther, 3rd gen focal plane array IR detection modules and applications, *Proc. SPIE*, 5406, 184–192, 2004.

[33] S. Horn, P. Norton, K. Carson#, R. Eden, and R. Clement, Vertically-integrated sensor arrays — VISA, *Proc. SPIE*, 5406, 332–340, 2004.

[34] R. Balcerak and S. Horn, Progress in the development of vertically-integrated sensor arrays, *Proc. SPIE*, 5783, 384–391, 2005.

4
Infrared Camera Characterization

Joseph G. Pellegrino
Jason Zeibel
Ronald G. Driggers
Philip Perconti
U.S. Army CERDEC Night Vision and Electronic Sensors Directorate

4.1	Dimensional Noise	4-3
4.2	Noise Equivalent Temperature Difference	4-5
4.3	Dynamic Range	4-6
4.4	Modulation Transfer Function	4-8
4.5	Minimum Resolvable Temperature	4-8
4.6	Spatial Resolution	4-9
	Pixel Size	
References		4-10

Many different types of infrared (IR) detector technology are now commercially available and the physics of their operation has been described in an earlier chapter. IR imagers are classified by different characteristics such as scan type, detector material, cooling requirements, and detector physics. Thermal imaging cameras prior to the 1990s typically contained a relatively small number of IR photosensitive detectors. These imagers were known as *cooled scanning systems* because they required cooling to cryogenic temperatures and a mechanical scan mirror to construct a two-dimensional (2D) image of the scene. Large 2D arrays of IR detectors, or staring arrays, have enabled the development of *cooled staring systems* that maintain sensitivity over a wide range of scene flux conditions, spectral bandwidths, and frame rates. Staring arrays consisting of small bolometric detector elements, or microbolometers, have enabled the development of *uncooled staring systems* that are compact, lightweight, and low power (see Figure 4.1).

FIGURE 4.1 Scanning and staring system designs.

The sensitivity, or thermal resolution, of uncooled microbolometer focal plane arrays has improved dramatically over the past decade, resulting in IR video cameras that can resolve temperature differences under nominal imaging conditions as small as twenty millidegrees Kelvin using $f/1.0$ optics. Advancements in the manufacturing processes used by the commercial silicon industry have been instrumental in this progress. Uncooled microbolometer structures are typically fabricated on top of silicon integrated circuitry (IC) designed to readout the changes in resistance for each pixel in the array. The silicon-based IC serves as an electrical and mechanical interface for the IR microbolometer.

The primary measures of IR sensor performance are sensitivity and resolution. When measurements of end-to-end or human-in-the-loop (HITL) performance are required, the visual acuity of an observer through a sensor is included. The sensitivity and resolution are both related to the hardware and software that comprises the system, while the HITL includes both the sensor and the observer. Sensitivity is determined through radiometric analysis of the scene environment and the quantum electronic properties of the detectors. Resolution is determined by analysis of the physical optical properties, the detector array geometry, and other degrading components of the system in much the same manner as complex electronic circuit/signals analysis. The sensitivity of cooled and uncooled staring IR video cameras has improved by more than a factor of ten compared to scanning systems commercially available in the 1980s and early 1990s [1,2].

Sensitivity describes how the sensor performs with respect to input signal level. It relates noise characteristics, responsivity of the detector, light gathering of the optics, and the dynamic range of the sensor. Radiometry describes how much light leaves the object and background and is collected by the detector. Optical design and detector characteristics are of considerable importance in sensor sensitivity analysis. In IR systems, noise equivalent temperature difference (NETD) is often a first order description of the system sensitivity. The three-dimensional (3D) noise model [1] describes more detailed representations of sensitivity parameters. The sensitivity of scanned long-wave infrared (LWIR) cameras operating at video frame rates is typically limited by very short detector integration times on the order of tens or hundreds of microseconds. The sensitivity of staring IR systems with high quantum efficiency detectors is often limited by the charge integration capacity, or well capacity, of the readout integrated circuit (ROIC). The detector integration time of staring IR cameras can be tailored to optimize sensitivity for a given application and may range from microseconds to tens of milliseconds.

The second type of measure is resolution. Resolution is the ability of the sensor to image small targets and to resolve fine detail in large targets. Modulation transfer function (MTF) is the most widely used resolution descriptor in IR systems. Alternatively, it may be specified by a number of descriptive metrics such as the optical Rayleigh Criterion or the instantaneous field-of-view of the detector. Where these metrics are component-level descriptions, the system MTF is an all-encompassing function that describes the system resolution. Sensitivity and resolution can be competing system characteristics and they are the most important issues in initial studies for a design. For example, given a fixed sensor aperture diameter, an increase in focal length can provide an increase in resolution, but may decrease sensitivity [2]. A more detailed consideration of the optical design parameters is included in the next chapter.

Quite often metrics, such as NETD and MTF, are considered separable. However, in an actual sensor, sensitivity and resolution performance are interrelated. As a result, minimum resolvable temperature difference (MRT or MRTD) has become a primary performance metric for IR systems.

This chapter addresses the parameters that characterize a camera's performance. A website advertising IR camera would in general contain a specification sheet that contains some variation of the terms that follow. A goal of this section is to give the reader working knowledge of these terms so as to better enable them to obtain the correct camera for their application:

- Three-dimensional noise
- NETD (Noise equivalent temperature difference)
- Dynamic range
- MTF

Infrared Camera Characterization

- MRT (minimum resolvable temperature) and MDT (minimum detectable temperature)
- Spatial resolution
- Pixel size

4.1 Dimensional Noise

The 3D noise model is essential for describing the sensitivity of an optical sensor system. Modern imaging sensors incorporate complex focal plane architectures and sophisticated postdetector processing and electronics. These advanced technical characteristics create the potential for the generation of complex noise patterns in the output imagery of the system. These noise patterns are deleterious and therefore need to be analyzed to better understand their effects upon performance. Unlike classical systems where "well behaved" detector noise predominates, current sensor systems have the ability to generate a wide variety of noise types, each with distinctive characteristics temporally, as well as along the vertical and horizontal image directions. Earlier methods for noise measurements at the detector preamplifier port that ignored other system noise sources are no longer satisfactory. System components following the stage that include processing may generate additional noise and even dominate total system noise.

Efforts at the Night Vision and Electronic Sensor Directorate to measure 2nd generation IR sensors uncovered the need for a more comprehensive method to characterize noise parameters. It was observed that the noise patterns produced by these systems exhibited a high degree of directionality. The data set is 3D with the temporal dimension representing the frame sequencing and the two spatial dimensions representing the vertical and horizontal directions within the image (see Figure 4.2).

To acquire this data cube, the field of view of a camera to be measured is flooded with a uniform temperature reference. A set number n (typically around 100) of successive frames of video data are then collected. Each frame of data consists of the measured response (in volts) to the uniform temperature source from each individual detector in the 2D focal plane array (FPA). When many successive frames of data are "stacked" together, a uniform source data cube is constructed. The measured response may be either analog (RS-170) or digital (RS-422, Camera Link, Hot Link, etc.) in nature depending on the camera interface being studied.

To recover the overall temporal noise, first the temporal noise is calculated for each detector in the array. A standard deviation of the n measured voltage responses for each detector is calculated. For an h by v array, there are hv separate values where each value is the standard deviation of n voltage measurements. The median temporal noise among these hv values is stated as the overall temporal noise in volts.

Following the calculation of temporal noise, the uniform source data cube is reduced along each axis according to the 3D noise procedure. There are seven noise terms as part of the 3D noise definition. Three components measure the average noise present along on each axis (horizontal, vertical, and temporal) of the data cube (σ_h, σ_v, and σ_t). Three terms measure the noise common to any given pair of axes in the data cube (σ_{tv}, σ_{th}, and σ_{vh}). The final term measures the uncorrelated random noise (σ_{tvh}). To calculate

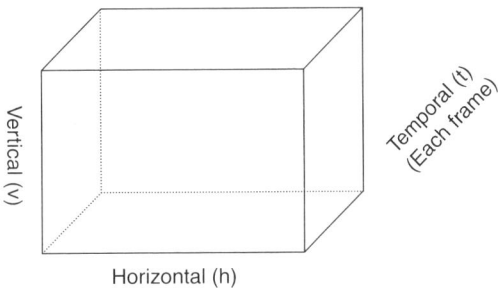

FIGURE 4.2 An example of a uniform source data cube for 3D noise measurements. The first step in the calculation of 3D noise parameters is the acquisition of a uniform source data cube.

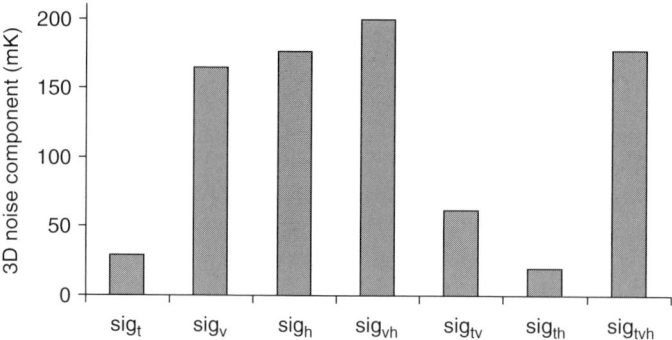

FIGURE 4.3 The 3D noise values for a typical data cube. The spatial nonuniformity can be seen in the elevated values of the spatial only 3D noise components σ_h, σ_v, and σ_{vh}. The white noise present in the system (σ_{tvh}) is roughly the same magnitude as the spatial 3D noise components.

FIGURE 4.4 An example of a camera system with high spatial noise components and very low temporal noise components.

the spatial noise for the camera, each of the 3D noise components that are independent of time (σ_v, σ_h, and σ_{vh}) are added in quadrature. The result is quoted as the spatial noise of the camera in volts.

In order to represent a data cube in a 2D format, the cube is averaged along one of the axes. For example, if a data cube is averaged along the temporal axis, then a time averaged array is created. This format is useful for visualizing purely spatial noise effects as three of the components are calculated after temporal averaging (σ_h, σ_v, and σ_{vh}). These are the time independent components of 3D Noise. The data cube can also be averaged along both spatial dimensions. The full 3D Noise calculation for a typical data cube is shown in Figure 4.3.

Figure 4.4 shows an example of a data cube that has been temporally averaged. In this case, many spatial noise features are present. Column noise is clearly visible in Figure 4.4, however the dominant spatial noise component appears to be the "salt and pepper" fixed pattern noise. The seven 3D Noise components are shown in Figure 4.5. σ_{vh} is clearly the dominant noise term, as was expected due to the high fixed pattern noise. The column noise σ_h and the row noise σ_v are the next dominant. In this example, the overall bulls-eye variation in the average frame dominates the σ_v and σ_h terms. Vertical stripes present in the figure add to σ_v, but this effect is small in comparison, leading to similar values for σ_v and σ_h.

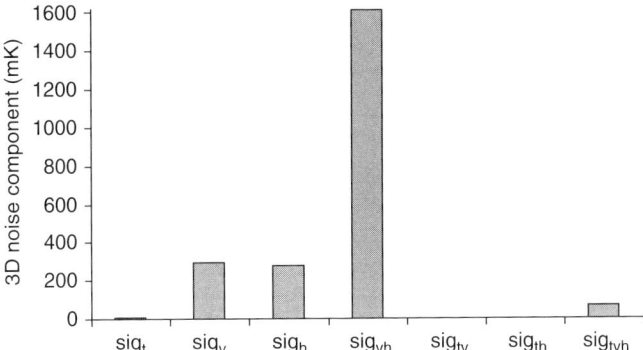

FIGURE 4.5 The 3D noise components for the data cube used to generate. Note that the amount of row and column noise is significantly smaller than the fixed pattern noise. All the 3D noise values with a temporal component are significantly smaller than the purely spatial values.

In this example, the temporal components of the 3D noise are two orders of magnitude lower than σ_{vh}. If this data cube were to be plotted as individual frames, we would see that successive frames would hardly change and the dominant spatial noise would be present (and constant) in each frame.

4.2 Noise Equivalent Temperature Difference

In general, imager sensitivity is a measure of the smallest signal that is detectable by a sensor. For IR imaging systems, noise equivalent temperature difference (NETD) is a measure of sensitivity. Sensitivity is determined using the principles of radiometry and the characteristics of the detector. The system intensity transfer function (SITF) can be used to estimate the noise equivalent temperature difference. NEDT is the system noise rms voltage over the noise differential output. It is the smallest measurable signal produced by a large target (extended source), in other words the minimum measurable signal.

Equation below describes NETD as a function of noise voltage and the system intensity transfer function. The measured NETD values are determined from a line of video stripped from the image of a test target, as depicted in Figure 4.10. A square test target is placed before a blackbody source. The delta T is the difference between the blackbody temperature and the mask. This target is then placed at the focal point of an off axis parabolic mirror. The mirror serves the purpose of a long optical path length to the target, yet relieves the tester from concerns over atmospheric losses to the temperature difference. The image of the target is shown in Figure 4.6. The SITF slope for the scan line in Figure 4.6 is the $\Delta\Sigma/\Delta T$, where $\Delta\Sigma$ is the signal measured for a given ΔT. The N_{rms} is the background signal on the same line.

$$\text{NETD} = \frac{N_{rms}\,[\text{volts}]}{\text{SITF\_Slope}\,[\text{volts/K}]}$$

After calculating both the temporal and spatial noise, a signal transfer function (SiTF) is measured. The field of view of the camera is again flooded with a uniform temperature source. The temperature of the source is varied over the dynamic range of the camera's output while the mean array voltage response is recorded. The slope of the resulting curve yields the SiTF responsivity in volts per degree Kelvin change in the scene temperature. Once both the SiTF curve and the temporal and spatial noise in volts are known, the NETD can be calculated. This is accomplished by dividing the temporal and spatial noise in volts by the responsivity in volts per degree Kelvin. The resulting NETD values represent the minimum discernable change in scene temperature for both spatial and temporal observation.

The SiTF of an electro-optical (EO) or IR system is determined by the signal response once the dark offset signal has been subtracted off. After subtracting off the offset due to non flux effects, the SiTF

FIGURE 4.6 Dynamic range and system transfer function.

plots the counts output relative to the input photon flux. The SiTF is typically represented in response units of voltage, signal electrons, digital counts, etc. vs. units of the source: blackbody temperature, flux, photons, and so on. If the system behaves linearly within the dynamic range then the slope of the SiTF is constant. The dynamic range of the system, which may be defined by various criteria, is determined by the minimum (i.e., signal to noise ratio = 1) and maximum levels of operation.

4.3 Dynamic Range

The responsivity function also provides dynamic range and linearity information. The camera dynamic range is the maximum measurable input signal divided by the minimum measurable signal. The NEDT is assumed to be the minimum measurable signal. For AC systems, the maximum output depends on the target size and therefore the target size must be specified if dynamic range is a specification. Depending upon the application, the maximum input value may be defined by one of several methods. One method for specifying the dynamic range of a system involves having the ΔV_{sys} signal reach some specified level, say 90% of the saturation level as shown in Figure 4.7. Another method to assess the maximum input value is based on the signal's deviation from linearity. The range of data points that fall within a specified band is designated as the dynamic range. A third approach involves specifying the minimum SiTF of the system.

For most systems, the detector output signal is adjusted both in gain and offset so that the dynamic range of the A/D converter is maximized. Figure 4.8 shows a generic detector system that contains an 8-bit A/D converter. The converter can handle an input signal between 0 and 1 volt and an output between 0 and 255 counts. By selecting the gain and offset, any detector voltage range can be mapped into the digital output. Figure 4.9 shows 3 different system gains and offsets. When the source flux level is less than Φ_{min},

Infrared Camera Characterization

FIGURE 4.7 Dynamic range defined by linearity.

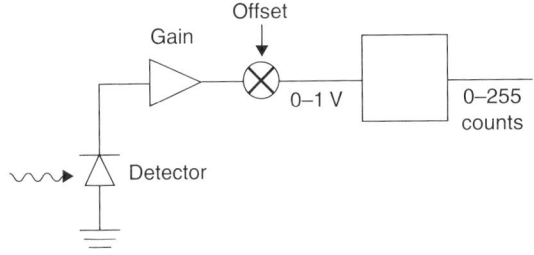

FIGURE 4.8 System with 8-bit A/D converter.

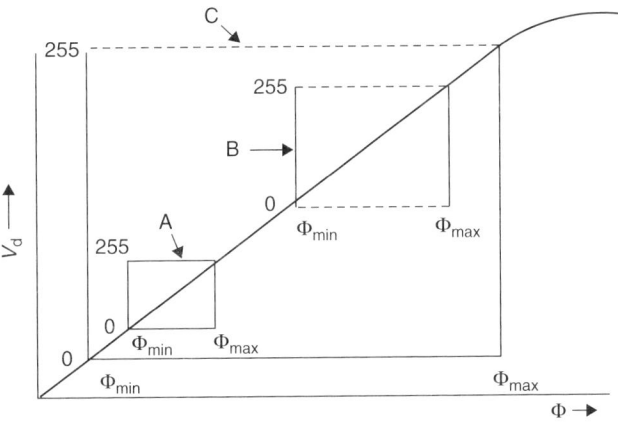

FIGURE 4.9 Different gains and voltage offsets affect the input-to-output transition.

the source will not be seen (i.e., it will appear as 0 counts). When the flux level is greater than Φ_{max}, the source will appear as 255 counts, and the system is said to be saturated. The gain parameters, Φ_{min} and Φ_{max} are redefined for each gain and offset level setting.

Output A below occurs with maximum gain. Point B occurs with moderate gain and C with minimum gain. For the various gains, the detector output gets mapped into the full dynamic range of the A/D converter.

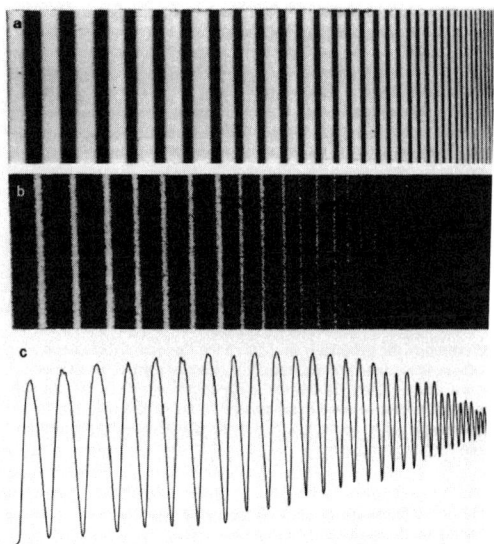

FIGURE 4.10 This figure shows the falloff in MTF as spatial frequency increases. Panel a is a sinusoidal test pattern, panel b is the optical system's (negative) response, and panel c shows the contrast as a function of spatial frequency.

4.4 Modulation Transfer Function

The modulation transfer function (MTF) of an optical system measures a system's ability to faithfully image a given object. Consider for example the bar pattern shown in Figure 4.10, with the cross section of each bar being a sine wave. Since the image of a sine wave light distribution is always a sine wave, no matter how bad the aberrations may be, the image is always a sine wave. The image will therefore have a sine wave distribution with intensity shown in Figure 4.10.

When the bars are coarsely spaced, the optical system has no difficulty faithfully reproducing them. However, when the bars are more tightly spaced, the contrast,

$$\text{Contrast} = \frac{\text{bright} - \text{dark}}{\text{bright} + \text{dark}}$$

begins to fall off as shown in panel c. If the dark lines have intensity $= 0$, the contrast $= 1$, and if the bright and dark lines are equally intense, contrast $= 0$. The contrast is equal to the MTF at a specified spatial frequency. Furthermore, it is evident that the MTF is a function of spatial frequency and position within the field.

4.5 Minimum Resolvable Temperature

Each time a camera is turned on, the observer subconsciously makes a judgement about image quality. The IR community uses the MRT and the MDT as standard measures of image quality. The MRT and MDT depend upon the IR imaging system's resolution and sensitivity. MRT is a measure of the ability to resolve detail and is inversely related to the MTF, whereas the MDT is a measure to detect something. The MRT and MDT deal with an observer's ability to perceive low contrast targets which are embeddedd in noise.

MRT and MDT are not absolute values rather they are temperature differentials relative to a given background. They are sometimes referred to as the minimum resolvable temperature difference (MRTD) and the minimum detectable temperature difference (MDTD).

Infrared Camera Characterization

The theoretical MRT is

$$\mathrm{MRT}(f_x) = \frac{k \cdot (\mathrm{NEDT})}{\mathrm{MTF}_{\mathrm{perceived}}(f_x)} \cdot \sqrt{\{\beta_1 + \cdots + \beta_n\}}$$

where $\mathrm{MTF}_{\mathrm{perceived}} = \mathrm{MTF}_{\mathrm{SYS}}\, \mathrm{MTF}_{\mathrm{MONITOR}}\, \mathrm{MTF}_{\mathrm{EYE}}$. The $\mathrm{MTF}_{\mathrm{system}}$ is defined by the product $\mathrm{MTF}_{\mathrm{sensor}}$ $\mathrm{MTF}_{\mathrm{optics}}\, \mathrm{MTF}_{\mathrm{electronics}}$. Each β_i in the equation is an eye filter that is used to interpret the various components of noise. As certain noise sources increase, the MRT also increases. MRT has the same ambient temperature dependence as the NEDT; as the ambient temperature increases, MRT decreases. Because the MTF decreases as spatial frequency increases, the MRT increases with increasing spatial frequency. Overall system response depends on both sensitivity and resolution. The MRT parameter is bounded by sensitivity and resolution. Figure shows that different systems may have different MRTs. System A has a better sensitivity because it has a lower MRT at low spatial frequencies. At mid-range spatial frequencies, the systems are approximately equivalent and it can be said that they provide equivalent performance. At higher frequencies, System B has better resolution and can display finer detail than system A. In general, neither sensitivity, resolution, nor any other single parameter can be used to compare systems; many quantities must be specified for complete system-to-system comparison.

4.6 Spatial Resolution

The term resolution applies to two different concepts with regard to vision systems. Spatial resolution refers to the image size in pixels—for a given scene, more pixels means higher resolution. The spatial resolution is a fixed characteristic of the camera and cannot be increased by the frame grabber of post-processing techniques. Zooming techniques, for example, merely interpolate between pixels to expand an image without adding any new information to what the camera provided. It is easy to decrease the resolution, however, by simply ignoring part of the data. National Instruments frame grabbers provide for this with a "scaling" feature that instructs the frame grabber to sample the image to return a 1/2, 1/4, 1/8, and so on, scaled image. This is convenient when system bandwidth is limited and you don't require any precision measurements of the image.

The other use of the term "resolution" is commonly found in data acquisition applications and refers to the number of quantization levels used in A/D conversions. Higher resolution in this sense means that you would have improved capability of analyzing low-contrast images. This resolution is specified by the A/D converter; the frame grabber determines the resolution for analog signals, whereas the camera determines it for digital signals (the frame grabber must have the capability of supporting whatever resolution the camera provides, though).

4.6.1 Pixel Size

Camera pixel size consists of the tiny dots that make up a digital image. So let us say that a camera is capable of taking images at 640×480 pixels. A little math shows us that such an image would contain 307,200 pixels or 0.3 megapixels. Now let's say the camera takes 1024×768 images. That gives us 0.8 megapixels. So the larger the number of megapixels, the more image detail you get. Each pixel can be one of 16.7 million colors.

The detector pixel size refers to the size of the individual sensor elements that make up the detector part of the camera. If we had two charge-coupled devices (CCDs) detectors with equal Quantum Efficiency (QEs) but one has 9 μm pixels and the other has 18 μm pixels (i.e., the pixels on CCD#2 are twice the linear size of those on CCD #1) and we put both of these CCDs into cameras that operate identically, then the image taken with CCD#1 will require 4X the exposure of the image taken with CCD#2. This seeming discrepancy is due in its entirety to the area of the pixels in the two CCDs and could be compared to the effectiveness of rain gathering gauges with different rain collection areas: A rain gauge with a 2-in. diameter throat will collect 4X as much rain water as a rain gauge with a 1-in. diameter throat.

References

[1] J. D'Agostino and C. Webb, 3-D analysis framework and measurement methodology for imaging system noise. *Proc. SPIE*, 1488, 110–121 (1991).

[2] R.G. Driggers, P. Cox, and T. Edwards, *Introduction to Infrared and Electro-Optical Systems*, Artech House, Boston, MA, 1998, p. 8.

5
Infrared Camera and Optics for Medical Applications

Michael W. Grenn
Jay Vizgaitis
Joseph G. Pellegrino
Philip Perconti
U.S. Army CERDEC Night Vision and Electronic Sensors Directorate

5.1	Infrared Sensor Calibration	5-4
5.2	Gain Detector	5-6
	Nonuniformity Calibration	
5.3	Operational Considerations	5-7
5.4	Infrared Optical Considerations	5-8
	Resolution	
5.5	Spectral Requirement	5-10
	Depth of Field	
5.6	Selecting Optical Materials	5-11
	Special Considerations • Coatings • Reflective Optics	
Acknowledgments		5-14
References		5-14
Further Information		5-14

The infrared radiation emitted by an object above 0 K is passively detected by infrared imaging cameras without any contact with the object and is nonionizing. The characteristics of the infrared radiation emitted by an object are described by Planck's blackbody law in terms of spectral radiant emittance.

$$M_\lambda = \varepsilon(\lambda) \frac{c_1}{\lambda^5 (e^{c_2/\lambda T} - 1)} \text{ W/cm}^2 \, \mu\text{m}$$

where c_1 and c_2 are constants of 3.7418×10^4 W $\mu\text{m}^4/\text{cm}^2$ and 1.4388×10^4 μm K. The wavelength, λ, is provided in micrometers and $\varepsilon(\lambda)$ is the emissivity of the surface. A blackbody source is defined as an object with an emissivity of 1.0, so that it is a perfect emitter. Source emissions of blackbodies at nominal terrestrial temperatures are shown in Figure 5.1. The radiant exitance of a blackbody at a 310 K, corresponding to a nominal core body temperature of 98.6°F, peaks at approximately 9.5 μm in the LWIR. The selection of an infrared camera for a specific application requires consideration of many factors including sensitivity, resolution, uniformity, stability, calibratability, user controllability, reliability, object of interest phenomenology, video interface, packaging, and power consumption.

Planck's equation describes the spectral shape of the source as a function of wavelength. It is readily apparent that the peak shifts to shorter wavelengths as the temperature of the object of interest increases.

FIGURE 5.1 Planck's blackbody radiation curves.

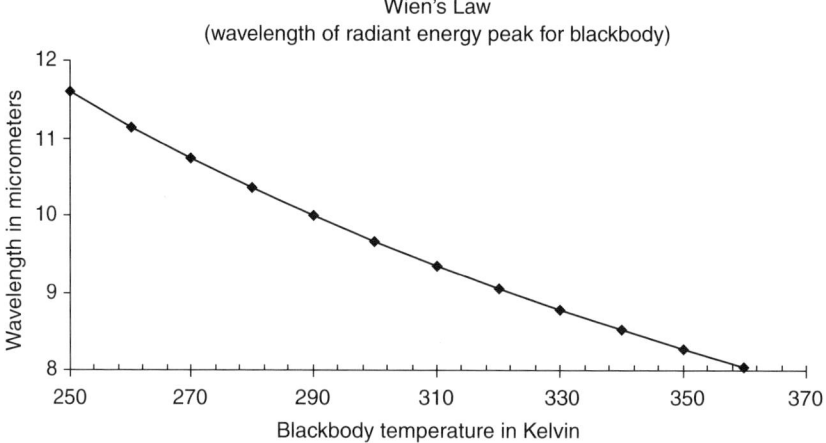

FIGURE 5.2 Location of peak of blackbody radiation, Wien's Law.

If the temperature of a blackbody approaches that of the sun, or 5900 K, the peak of the spectral shape would shift to 0.55 μm or green light. This peak wavelength is described by Wien's displacement law

$$\lambda_{\max} = 2898/T \ \mu m$$

Figure 5.2 shows the radiant energy peak as a function of temperature in the LWIR. It is important to note that the difference between the blackbody curves is the "signal" in the infrared bands. For an infrared sensor, if the background temperature is 300 K and the object of interest temperature is 302 K, the signal is the 2 K difference in flux between these curves. Signals in the infrared ride on very large amounts of background flux. This is not the case in the visible. For example, consider the case of a white object on a black background. The black background is generating no signal, while the white object is generating a maximum signal assuming the sensor gain is properly adjusted. The dynamic range may be fully utilized in a visible sensor. For the case of an IR sensor, a portion of the dynamic range is used by the large background flux radiated by everything in the scene. This flux is never a small value, hence sensitivity and dynamic range requirements are much more difficult to satisfy in IR sensors than in visible sensors.

A typical infrared imaging scenario consists of two major components, the object of interest and the background. In an IR scene, the majority of the energy is emitted from the constituents of the scene. This emitted energy is transmitted through the atmosphere to the sensor. As it propagates through the atmosphere it is degraded by absorption and scattering. Obscuration by intervening objects and additional energy emitted by the path also affect the target energy. This effect may be very small in short range imaging applications under controlled conditions. All these contributors, which are not the object of interest, essentially reduce one's ability to discriminate the object. The signal is further degraded by the optics of the sensor. The energy is then sampled by the detector array and converted to electrical signals. Various electronics amplify and condition this signal before it is presented to either a display for human interpretation or an algorithm like an automatic target recognizer for machine interpretation. A linear systems approach to modeling allows the components' transfer functions to be treated separately as contributors to the overall system performance. This approach allows for straightforward modifications to a performance model for changes in the sensor or environment when performing tradeoff analyses.

The photon flux levels (photons per square centimeter per second) on Earth is 1.5×10^{17} in the daytime and around 1×10^{10} at night in the visible. In the MWIR, the daytime and nighttime flux levels are 4×10^{15} and 2×10^{15}, respectively, where the flux is a combination of emitted and solar reflected flux. In the LWIR, the flux is primarily emitted where both day and night yield a 2×10^{17} level. At first look, it appears that the LWIR flux characteristics are as good as a daytime visible system, however, there are two other factors limiting performance. First, the energy bandgaps of infrared sensitive devices are much smaller than in the visible, resulting in significantly higher detector dark current. The detectors are typically cooled to reduce this effect. Second, the reflected light in the visible is modulated with target and background reflectivities that typically range from 7 to 20%.

In the infrared, where all terrestrial objects emit, a two-degree equivalent blackbody difference in photon flux between object and background is considered high contrast. The flux difference between two blackbodies of 302 K compared to 300 K can be calculated in a manner similar to that shown in Figure 5.1. The flux difference is the signal that provides an image, hence the difference in signal compared to the ambient background flux should be noted. In the LWIR, the signal is 3% of the mean flux and in the MWIR it is 6% of the mean flux. This means that there is a large flux pedestal associated with imaging in the infrared.

There are two major challenges accompanying the large background pedestal in the infrared. First, the performance of a typical infrared detector is limited by the background photon noise and this noise term is determined by the mean of the pedestal. This value may be relatively large compared to the small signal differences. Second, the charge storage capacity of the silicon input circuit mated to each infrared detector in a staring array limits the amount of integrated charge per frame, typically around 10^7 charge carriers. An LWIR system in a hot desert background would generate 10^{10} charge carriers in a 33 msec integration time. The optical f-number, spectral bandwidth, and integration time of the detector are typically tailored to reach half well for a given imaging scenario for dynamic range purposes. This well capacity limited condition results in a sensitivity, or noise equivalent temperature difference (NETD) of 10 to 30 times below the photon limited condition. Figure 5.3 shows calculations of NETD as a function of background temperature for MWIR and LWIR staring detectors dominated by the photon noise of the incident IR radiation. At 310 K, the NETD of high quantum efficiency MWIR and LWIR focal plane arrays (FPAs) is nearly the same, or about 3 millidegrees K, when the detectors are permitted to integrate charge up to the frame time, or in this case about 33 msec. The calculations show the sensitivity limits from the background photon shot noise only and does not include the contribution of detector and system temporal and spatial noise terms. The effects of residual spatial noise on NETD are described later in the chapter. The well capacity assumed here is 10^9 charge carriers to demonstrate sensitivity that could be achieved under large well conditions. The MWIR device is photon limited over the temperature range and begins to reach the well capacity limit near 340 K. The 24 μm pitch 9.5 μm cutoff LWIR device is well capacity limited over the entire temperature range. The 18 μm pitch 9.5 μm cutoff LWIR device becomes photon limited around 250 K. Various on-chip signal processing techniques, such as charge skimming and

FIGURE 5.3 Background limited NETD for high quantum efficiency MWIR and LWIR detectors.

charge partitioning, have been investigated to increase the charge capacity of these devices. In addition, as the minimum feature sizes of the input circuitry decreases, more real estate in the unit cell can be allocated to charge storage.

Another major difference between infrared and visible systems is the size of the detector and diffraction blur. Typical sizes for MWIR and LWIR detectors, or pixels, range from 20 to 50 μm. Visible detectors less than 6 μm are commercially available today. The diffraction blur for the LWIR is more than ten times larger than the visible blur and MWIR blur is eight times larger than visible blur. Therefore, the image blur due to diffraction and detector size is much larger in an infrared system than a visible system. It is very common for infrared staring arrays to be sampling limited where the sample spacing is larger than the diffraction blur and the detector size. Dither and microscanning are frequently used to enhance performance. A more detailed discussion of the optical considerations of infrared sensors is provided later in the chapter.

Finally, infrared staring arrays consisting of cooled photon detectors or uncooled thermal detectors may have responsivities that vary dramatically from pixel to pixel. It is common practice to correct for the resulting nonuniformity using a combination of factory preset tables and user inputs. The nonuniformity can cause fixed pattern noise in the image that can limit the performance of the system even more than temporal noise and these effects are demonstrated in the next section.

5.1 Infrared Sensor Calibration

Significant advancement in the manufacturing of high-quality FPAs operating in the SWIR, MWIR, and LWIR has enabled industry to offer a wide range of affordable camera products to the consumer. Commercial applications of infrared camera technology are often driven by the value of the information it provides and price points set by the marketplace. The emergence of uncooled microbolometer FPA cameras with sensitivity less than 0.030°C at standard video rates has opened many new applications of the technology. In addition to the dramatic improvement in sensitivity over the past several years, uncooled microbolometer FPA cameras are characteristically compact, lightweight, and low power. Uncooled cameras are commercially available from a variety of domestic and foreign vendors including Agema, BAE Systems, CANTRONIC Systems, Inc., DRS and DRS Nytech, FLIR Systems, Inc., Indigo Systems, Inc.,

FIGURE 5.4 Windows-based GUI developed at NVESD for an uncooled medical imaging system.

Electrophysics Corp., Inc., Infrared Components Corp., IR Solutions, Inc., Raytheon, Thermoteknix Systems Ltd., ompact, low power The linearity, stability, and repeatability of the SiTF may be measured to determine the suitability of an infrared camera for accurate determination of the apparent temperature of an object of interest. LWIR cameras are typically preferred for imaging applications that require absolute or relative measurements of object irradiance or radiance because emitted energy dominates the total signal in the LWIR. In the MWIR, extreme care is required to ensure the radiometric accuracy of data. Thermal references may be used in the scene to provide a known temperature reference point or points to compensate for detector-to-detector variations in response and improve measurement accuracy. Thermal references may take many forms and often include temperature controlled extended area sources or uniformly coated metal plates with contact temperature sensors. Depending on the stability of the sensor, reference frames may be required in intervals from minutes to hours depending on the environmental conditions and the factory presets. Many sensors require an initial turn-on period to stabilize before accurate radiometric data can be collected. An example of a windows-based graphical user interface (GUI) developed at NVESD for an uncooled imaging system for medical studies is shown in Figure 5.4. The system allows the user to operate in a calibrated mode and display apparent temperature in regions of interest or at any specified pixel location including the pixel defined by the cursor. Single frames and multiple frames at specified time intervals may be selected for storage. Stability of commercially available uncooled cameras is provided earlier.

The LTC 500 thermal imager had been selected as a sensor to be used in a medical imaging application. Our primary goal was to obtain from the imagery calibrated temperature values within an accuracy of approximately a tenth of a degree Celsius. The main impediments to this goal consisted of several sources of spatial nonuniformity in the imagery produced by this sensor, primarily the spatial variation of radiance across the detector FPA due to self heating and radiation of the internal camera components, and to a lesser extent the variation of detector characteristics within the FPA. Fortunately, the sensor provides a calibration capability to mitigate the effects of the spatial nonuniformities.

We modeled the sensor FPA as a 2D array of detectors, each having a gain G and offset K, both of which are assumed to vary from detector to detector. In addition we assumed an internally generated radiance Y for each detector due to the self-heating of the internal sensor components (also varying from detector to detector, as well as slowly with time). Lastly, there is an internally programmable offset C for each detector which the sensor controls as part of its calibration function. Therefore, given a radiance X incident on some detector of the FPA from the external scene, the output Z for that detector is given by:

$$Z = GX + GY + K + C$$

5.2 Gain Detector

Individual detector gains were calculated by making two measurements. First, the sensor was allowed to run for several hours in order for the internal temperatures to stabilize. A uniform blackbody source at temperature T_1 (20°C) was used to fill the field of view (FOV) of the sensor and an output image Z_1 was collected. Next the blackbody temperature was set to T_2 (40°C) and a second output image Z_2 was collected. Since the measurement interval was small (<1 to 2 min) we assume the Y values remain constant, we have (for each detector):

$$Z_1 = GX_1 + GY + K + C$$

$$Z_2 = GX_2 + GY + K + C$$

where X_1 and X_2 refer to the external scene radiance corresponding to temperatures T_1 and T_2 incident on the detector and were calculated by integrating Planck's blackbody function over the 8 to 12 μm spectral band of the sensor. Taking the difference, we have (for each detector):

$$G = \frac{Z_2 - Z_1}{X_2 - X_1}$$

where the numbers here refer to measurements at different temperatures and, again, the value G (as well as Z and X) are assumed to vary from detector to detector (detector subscripts were omitted for clarity).

5.2.1 Nonuniformity Calibration

The LTC 500 provides the capability for nonuniformity calibration that allows the user to remove nonuniformities across the FPA assuming they do not change too rapidly with time. The procedure involves placing a uniform blackbody source across the FOV of the sensor and pressing the calibrate button. At this point, the sensor internally adjusts the value of a programmable offset for each detector so that the output Z of each detector is equal to a constant that we will denote Z_{CAL} (which the sensor sets to the midpoint of the digital pixel range, i.e., 16384).

Let D_1 and D_2 be two detectors selected from the 2D FPA, the outputs Z_1, Z_2 are then given by:

$$Z_1 = G_1 X_1 + G_1 Y_1 + K_1 + C_1$$

$$Z_2 = G_2 X_2 + G_2 Y_2 + K_2 + C_2$$

where now the numbers refer to different detectors, and as before G is gain, X is the incident radiance from the external scene, Y is the internal self heating radiance on the detectors, K is a possible offset variation from detector to detector, and C represents the programmable calibration offset for each detector. If we fill the FOV with a uniform blackbody at some temperature (T_{CAL}) producing a uniform radiance X_{CAL} on the FPA and activate the calibration function, we have:

$$Z_1 = Z_{CAL} = G_1 X_{CAL} + G_1 Y_1 + K_1 + C_1$$

$$Z_2 = Z_{CAL} = G_2 X_{CAL} + G_2 Y_2 + K_2 + C_2$$

so

$$C_1 = Z_{CAL} - G_1 X_{CAL} - G_1 Y_1 - K_1$$

$$C_2 = Z_{CAL} - G_2 X_{CAL} - G_2 Y_2 - K_2$$

where X_{CAL} is calculated by spectrally integrating Planck's function from 8 to 12 μm at $T = T_{CAL}$. C_1 and C_2 will now retain these values until the sensor is either recalibrated or powered down. Now, for some arbitrary externally supplied radiance X_1, X_2 on the FPA we have:

$$Z_1 = G_1 X_1 + G_1 Y_1 + K_1 + C_1$$

$$Z_1 = G_1 X_1 + G_1 Y_1 + K_1 + Z_{CAL} - G_1 X_{CAL} - G_1 Y_1 - K_1$$

$$Z_1 = G_1 X_1 + Z_{CAL} - G_1 X_{CAL}$$

$$Z_1 = G_1 (X_1 - X_{CAL}) + Z_{CAL}$$

and, similarly

$$Z_2 = G_2 (X_2 - X_{CAL}) + Z_{CAL}$$

therefore, the output of each detector depends only on the individual detector gain (which we know) and the external radiance incident on the detector. The spatially varying components (Y and K) have been removed.

Rearranging to solve for radiance input X as a function of the output intensity Z we have:

$$X = \frac{(Z - Z_{CAL})}{G} + X_{CAL}$$

Given a precomputed look up table RAD2TEMP of T, X pairs we can take the radiance value X and look up the corresponding temperature T for any pixel in the image. Hence we have computed temperature T_C as a function of radiance X on any detector:

$$T_C = \text{RAD2TEMP}[X]$$

5.3 Operational Considerations

Upon testing the system in a scenario that more accurately reflected the operational usage anticipated (i.e., with up to 10 ft between the sensor and the measured object), we encountered an unexpected discrepancy between the computed temperature values and the actual values as reported by the blackbody temperature display. We decided to assume that actual temperature values would vary linearly with the values computed by the above method. Therefore, we added a second step to the calibration procedure that requires the user to collect an image at a higher temperature than the calibration temperature T_{CAL}. Also, this second measurement would be made at a sensor to blackbody distance of approximately 10 ft. So now, we have two computed temperatures and two actual corresponding temperatures. Then we compute a slope and y-intercept describing the (assumed) linear relationship between the computed and actual temperatures.

$$T_A = M T_C + B$$

where

$$M = \frac{T_{A_2} - T_{A_1}}{T_{C_2} - T_{C_1}}$$

and

$$B = T_{A_1} - M T_{C_1}$$

FIGURE 5.5 Gain calculation, (a) *low temperature*: uniform 30°C black body source, calibrated at 30°, $\mu = 16381$, $\sigma = 1.9$ (raw counts). (b) *High temperature*: uniform 40°C black body source, calibrated at 30°, $\mu = 16842$, $\sigma = 11.3$ (raw counts). (c) *Processed using uniform gain*: uniform 35°C black body source, calibrated at 30°, $\mu = 34.74$, $\sigma = 0.12$ (°C). (d) *Processed using computed gain*: uniform 35°C black body source, calibrated at 30°, $\mu = 34.74$, $\sigma = 0.04$ (°C).

where T_A is the adjusted temperature, T_C is the computed temperature from the previously described methodology. M and B are recomputed during each nonuniformity calibration.

From a camera perspective, the system intensity transfer function (SiTF) in digital counts for a $DC = A + B \varepsilon T^4$.

$$T = \left(\frac{DN - A}{B\varepsilon} \right)^{1/4}$$

By adding this second step to the calibration process, we were able to improve the accuracy of the computed temperature to within a tenth of a degree for the test data set (Figure 5.5).

5.4 Infrared Optical Considerations

This section focuses mainly on the MWIR and LWIR since optics in the NIR and SWIR and very similar to that of the visible. This area assumes a basic knowledge of optics, and applies that knowledge to the application of infrared systems.

5.4.1 Resolution

Designing an IR optical system is first initiated by developing a set of requirements that are needed. These requirements will be used to determine the focal plane parameters and desired spectral band. These parameters in turn drive the first order design, evolving into the focal length, entrance pupil diameter, FOV, and f/number.

If we start with the user inputs of target distance, size, cycle criteria (or pixel criteria), and spectral band, we can begin designing our sensor. First we calculate the minimum resolution angle (α, in radians). This parameter is also known as the instantaneous field of view (IFOV), and can be calculated by

$$\alpha = \frac{\text{Size}_{\text{tar}}}{(\text{Range})(2 \times \text{Cycles})}$$

or

$$\alpha = \frac{\text{Size}_{\text{tar}}}{(\text{Range})(\text{Pixels})}$$

Based on the wavelength, we can determine the minimum entrance pupil diameter that is necessary to distinguish between the two blur spots.

$$\text{EPD} = \frac{1.22\lambda}{\alpha}$$

Knowing the detector size and pixel pitch we can then determine the minimum focal length based on our IFOV that is required to meet our resolution requirements. Longer focal lengths will provide better spatial resolution.

$$\text{EFL} = \frac{\text{Pitch}}{\alpha}$$

Once we know our focal length, we can determine our FOV based on the height of the detector and the focal length. The vertical and horizontal fields of view are calculated separately based on their respective dimensions.

$$\theta = 2\tan\left[\frac{0.5h}{\text{EFL}}\right]$$

where h is the full detector height (or width). Depending on the system requirements, the size of the FPA may want to be scaled to match the desired FOV. Arrays with more pixels provide for greater resolution for a given FOV. However, smaller arrays cost less. Scaling an optical system to match the FOV for a different array format results in the scaling of the focal length, and thus the resolution.

The f/number is then calculated as the ratio of the focal length to the entrance pupil diameter.

$$f/\text{number} = \frac{\text{EFL}}{\text{EPD}}$$

The f/number of the system can be further optimized based on two parameters: the sensitivity and the blur circle. The minimum f/number is already set based on the calculated minimum entrance pupil diameter and focal length. The f/number can be adjusted to improve sensitivity by trying to optimize the blur circle to match the diagonal dimension of the detector pixel. This method provides a way to maximize the amount of energy on the pixel while minimizing aliasing.

$$f/\text{number} = \frac{\text{Pixel}_{\text{diagonal}}}{2.44\lambda}$$

A faster f/number is good in many ways as it can improve the resolution by reducing the blur spot and increasing the optics cutoff frequency. It also allows more signal to the detector and gives a boost in the signal to noise ratio. A fast f/number is absolutely necessary for uncooled systems because they have to overcome the noise introduced from operation at warmer temperatures. Faster f/numbers also help in environments with poor thermal contrast. However, a faster f/number also means that the optics will be larger, and the optical designs will be more difficult. Faster f/numbers introduce more aberrations into each lens making all aberrations more difficult to correct, and a diffraction limited system harder to achieve. A cost increase may also occur due to larger optics and tighter tolerances. A tradeoff has to occur to find the optimal f/number for the system. The table below shows the tradeoffs between optics diameter, focal length, resolution and FOV.

5.5 Spectral Requirement

The spatial resolution is heavily dependent on the wavelength of light and the f/number. Diffraction limits the minimum blur size based on these two parameters.

$$d_{\text{spot}} = 2.44\lambda(f/\text{number})$$

The table given below compares blur sizes for various wavelengths and f/numbers:

f/number	Spot size (μm)			
	$\lambda = 0.6$	$\lambda = 2$	$\lambda = 4$	$\lambda = 10$
1	1.5	4.9	9.8	24.4
2.5	3.7	12.2	24.4	61.0
4	5.9	19.5	39.0	97.6
5.5	8.1	26.8	53.7	134.2
7	10.2	34.2	68.3	170.8

First Order Parameters Resolution

	f/number	Focal length	Field of view	Entrance pupil diameter
Impact resolution	A faster f/number results in a smaller optics blur due to diffraction. The result is an improved diffraction limit, and thus better spatial resolution. However, two things can adversely impact this improvement. Aberrations increase with faster f/number, potentially moving a system out of being diffraction limited, in which case the faster f/number can potentially hurt you. Also, a fixed front aperture system will have to reduce its focal length to accommodate the faster f/number, thus reducing spatial resolution through a change in focal length	Increasing the focal length will increase spatial resolution. However, the amount of improvement may be limited by the size of the allowed aperture, as having to go to a slower f/number can reduce some of the gains. Longer focal lengths also result in narrower FOVs, which can be limited by stabilization issues	Narrower FOVs are the direct result of longer focal lengths. Longer focal lengths result in improved spatial resolution. The Field of view can also vary by changing the size of the FPA. If all other parameters are maintained, and the FPA size is increased merely through the addition of more pixels, then the FOV increases without impacting resolution. If the number of pixels stay the same, but the pixel size is increased. then resolution is decreased. If pixel size is constant, number of pixels is increased, and focal length is scaled to maintain a constant FOV, then the resolution scales with the focal length	The entrance pupil diameter (EPD) can impact the resolution in three ways. Increasing the EPD while maintaining focal length improves resolution by utilizing a faster f/number. Increasing the EPD while maintaining a constant f/number results in a longer focal length, and thus increase spatial resolution. Maintaining a constant EPD while increasing focal length results in an improved spatial resolution due to the focal length, but a reduced resolution due to diffraction. The point where there is no longer significant improvement is dependent on the pixel size

5.5.1 Depth of Field

It is often desired to image targets that are located at different distances in object space. Two targets that are separated by a distance will both appear to be equally in focus if they fall within the depth of field

Infrared Camera and Optics for Medical Applications

(DOF) of the optics. A target that is closer to the optics than the DOF will appear defocused. In order to bring the out-of-focus target back in focus, it is required to refocus the optics so that the image plane shifts back to the location of the detector. Far targets focus shorter than near targets. If it is assumed that the optics are focused for an infinite target distance, the near DOF, known as the hyperfocal distance (HFD), can be found by

$$\text{HFD} = \frac{D^2}{2\lambda}$$

where D is the entrance pupil diameter, and λ is the wavelength in the same units as the diameter. This approximation can be made in the infrared because we can assume that we are utilizing a diffraction limited system.

This formula is dependent only on the aperture diameter and wavelength. It is easily seen that shorter wavelengths and larger apertures have larger HFDs. This relationship is based on the Rayleigh limit which states that as long as the wavefront error is within a $\frac{1}{4}$ wavelength of a true spherical surface, it is essentially diffraction limited. The depth of field can then be improved by focusing the optics to be optimally focused at the HFD. The optics are then in focus from that point to infinity based on the $\frac{1}{4}$ wave criteria, but also for a $\frac{1}{4}$ wave near that target distance. The full DOF of the system then becomes half the HFD to infinity. This is approximated by

$$\text{DOF} = \frac{D^2}{4\lambda}$$

If the region of interest is not within these bounds, it is possible to approximate the near and far focus points for a given object distance with

$$Z_{\text{near}} = \frac{\text{HFD} \times Z_o}{\text{HFD} + (Z_o - f)}$$

$$Z_{\text{far}} = \frac{\text{HFD} \times Z_o}{\text{HFD} - (Z_o - f)}$$

where X is the object distance that the objects are focused for and f is the focal length of the optics.

Work has been done with digital image processing techniques to improve the DOF by applying a method known as Wavefront Coding, developed by Cathey and Dowksi at the University of Colorado. This effectiveness of this technique has been well documented and demonstrated for the visible spectral band. Efforts are underway to demonstrate the effectiveness with LWIR uncooled cameras.

5.6 Selecting Optical Materials

The list of optical materials that transmit in the MWIR and LWIR spectrum is very short compared to that found in the visible spectrum. There are 21 crystalline materials and a handful chalcogenide glasses that transmit radiation at these wavelengths. Of the 21 crystalline materials, only six are practical to use in the LWIR, and nine are usable in the MWIR. The remaining possess poor characteristics such as being hygroscopic, toxic to the touch, etc., making them impractical for use in a real system. The list grows shorter for multi-spectral applications as only four transmit in the visible, MWIR, and LWIR. The chalcogenide glasses are an amorphous conglomerate of two or three infrared transmitting materials. A table of the practical infrared materials is listed along with a chart of their spectral bands. Transmission losses due to absorption can be calculated from the absorption coefficient of the material at the specified wavelength.

$$T_{\text{abs}} = e^{-at}$$

Transmission range for common IR materials

Table of Infrared Optical Materials

Material	Refractive Index		dn/dT (K^{-1})	Spectral range (μm)
	4 μm	=10 μ		
Germanium	4.0243	4.0032	0.000396	2.0–17.0
Gallium arsenide	3.3069	3.2778	0.000148	0.9–16.0
ZnSe	2.4331	2.4065	0.000060	0.55–20.0
ZnS (cleartran)	2.2523	2.2008	0.000054	0.37–14.0
AMTIR-1	2.2514	2.4976	0.000072	0.7–14.0
AMTIR-3	2.6200	2.6002	0.000091	1.0–14.0
AMTIR-4	2.6487	2.6353	−0.000030	1.0–14.0
GASIR 1	2.5100	2.4944	0.000055	1.0–14.0
GASIR 2	2.6038	2.5841	0.000058	1.0–14.0
Silicon	3.4255	N/A	0.000160	1.2–9.0
Sapphire	1.6753	N/A	0.000013	0.17–5.5
BaF$_2$	1.4580	1.4014	−0.000015	0.15–12.5
CaF$_2$	1.4097	1.3002	−0.000011	0.13–10.0
As$_2$S$_3$	2.4112	2.3816	−0.0000086	0.65–8.0
MgO	1.6679	N/A	0.000011	0.4–8.0

5.6.1 Special Considerations

In the LWIR, germanium is by far the best material to use for color correction and simplicity of design due to its high index of refraction and low dispersion. It is possible to design entire systems with germanium, but there are some caveats to this choice. Temperature plays havoc on germanium in two ways. It has a very high dn/dT (0.000396 K^{-1}), defocusing a lens that changes temperature of only a few degrees. It also has an absorption property in the LWIR for temperatures greater than 57°C. As the optic temperature rises above this point, the absorption coefficient increases, reducing the transmission. The high cost of germanium can also be a factor. It is not always good choice for a low-cost sensor, as the lens may end

Infrared Camera and Optics for Medical Applications

up costing more than the FPA. A good thermal match to compensate for the dn/dT of germanium is AMTIR-4. Its negative dn/dT provides for an excellent compensator for the germanium. It is possible to design a two lens germanium/AMTIR-4 lens system that does not require refocusing for over a 60°C temperature range.

The low-cost optics are silicon, ZnS, and the chalcogenide glasses. Silicon is only usable in the MWIR, and although the material is very inexpensive, its hardness can make it very difficult to diamond turn, and thus expensive. Although it does not diamond turn well, it does grind and polish easily, providing a very inexpensive solution when complex surfaces such as aspheres and diffractives are not used. ZnS is relatively inexpensive to germanium and ZnSe, but is relatively expensive to silicon and the chalcogenide glasses. The chalcogenide glasses are by far the least expensive to make and manufacture making them an excellent solution for low-cost system design. There are three types of the chalcogenide glasses that are moldable. AMTIR-4, a product of Amorphous Materials, Inc., has a lower melting point that the other chalcogenides making it the easiest to mold. Another material GASIR1 and GASIR2, products of Umicore, have also been demonstrated as being moldable. They have similar optical properties to that of AMTIR-1 and AMTIR-3.

5.6.2 Coatings

The high indices of refraction of most infrared materials lead to large fresnel losses, and thus require AR coatings. The transmission for a plane uncoated surface is shown below. In air, $n_1 = 1$.

$$T = 1 - \left(\frac{n_1 - n_2}{n_1 + n_2}\right)^2$$

The total reflectance off both sides of an uncoated plate is the multiplication of the two surfaces. This is in turn multiplied by the transmission of the material due to absorption. An example is given below:

Example
Uncoated Zinc Selenide flat, $n = 2.4$ in air, $t = 1.5$ cm thickness, absorption $= 0.0005$.

$$\text{Total transmission through both sides} = (0.83)(0.999)(0.83) = 0.688$$

Standard AR coatings are readily available for all of the materials previously listed. Generally, better than 99% can be expected for an AR-coated lens for either the MWIR or LWIR. If dual band operation is required, expect this performance to drop to 96%, and for the price to go up. The multispectral coatings are more difficult to design, and result in having many more layers. Infrared beamsplitter coatings can be difficult and expensive to manufacture. Care should be taken in specifying both the transmission and reflection properties of the beamsplitter. Specifications that are too stringent often lead to huge costs and schedule delays. Also, it is very important to note that the choice of which wavelength passes through and which wavelength is reflected can make a significant impact on the performance of a beamsplitter. In general, transmitting the longer wavelength and reflecting the shorter wavelength will boost performance and reduce cost.

5.6.3 Reflective Optics

Reflective optics can be a very useful and effective design too in the infrared. Reflective optics have no chromatic aberrations, and allow for diffraction limited solutions for very wide spectral bands. However, the use of reflective optics is somewhat limited to narrow FOVs and have difficulty with fast f/numbers. In addition, the type of reflective system can impact the performance fairly significantly for longer wavelengths. The most common type of design, the Cassegrain, two mirrors that are aligned on the same optical axis. The secondary mirror acts as an obscuration to the primary, which results in a degraded MTF due to diffraction around the obscuration. This effect is not apparent in most wavebands because the MTF loss occurs after the Nyquist frequency of the detector. However, this is not the case for the LWIR where the MTF drop occurs before Nyquist. To overcome this effect, most reflective systems used in the LWIR are off-axis reflective optics. These optics will provide diffraction limited MTF as long as the f/numbers do not get too fast, and the FOVs do not get too large. The off-axis nature makes these reflective systems hard to align, and expensive to manufacture.

Acknowledgments

Thanks to John O'Neill, Jason Zeibel, Tim Mikulski, Kent McCormack for data. EO-IR Measurements, Inc. for developing the graphical user interface for the medical infrared imaging camera. Leonard Bonnell, Vipera Systems, Inc., for development of the infrared endoscope.

References

[1] J. D'Agostino and C. Webb, 3-D analysis framework and measurement methodology for imaging system noise. *Proc. SPIE*, 1488, 110–121 (1991).
[2] R.G. Driggers, P. Cox, and T. Edwards, *Introduction to Infrared and Electro-Optical Systems*. Artech House, Boston, MA, p. 8 (1998).
[3] G.C. Holst, *Electro-Optical Imaging System Performance*. JCD Publishing, Winter Park, FL, p. 347 (1995).
[4] M.W. Grenn, Recent advances in portable infrared imaging cameras. *Proc. IEEE–EMBS*, Amsterdam (1996).
[5] M.W. Grenn, Performance of portable staring infrared cameras. *Proc. IEEE/EMBS* Oct. 30–Nov. 2, Chicago, IL, USA (1997).

Further Information

D'Agostino, J. and Webb, C. 3-D analysis framework and measurement methodology for imaging system noise. *Proc. SPIE*, 1488, 110–121 (1991).
Holst, G.C. *Electro-Optical Imaging System Performance*. JCD Publishing, Winter Park, FL, p. 432 (1995).
Johnson, J. Analysis of image forming systems. *Proc. IIS*, 249–273 (1958).
Ratches, J.A. NVL Static Performance Model for Thermal Viewing Systems, USA Electronics Command Report ECOM 7043, AD-A011212 (1973).
Schade, O.H. Electro-optical characteristics of television systems. *RCA Review*, IX(1–4) (1948).
Sendall, R. and Lloyd, J.M. Improved specifications for infrared imaging systems. *Proc. IRIS*, 14, 109–129 (1970).
Vollmerhausen, R.H. and Driggers, R.G. NVTHERM: next generation night vision thermal model. *Proc. IRIS Passive Sensors*, 1 (1999).

6
Physiology of Thermal Signals

6.1	Overview	**6**-1
6.2	Skin Thermal Properties in Response to Stress	**6**-2
6.3	Regulation of Skin Blood Flow for Heat Transfers	**6**-3
6.4	Heat Transfer Modeling Equations for Microcirculation	**6**-4
6.5	Cutaneous Circulation Measurement Techniques.....	**6**-5
	Procedures and Techniques • Dyes and Stains • Plethysmography • Doppler Measurement • Clearance Measurement • Thermal Skin Measurement • Measurement Techniques and Procedures Summary	
6.6	Objective Thermography..............................	**6**-7
	Efficiency of Heat Transport in the Skin of the Hand (Example 6.1) • Effect of a Reduced Blood Flow (Example 6.2) • Median Nerve Block in the Hand (Example 6.3) • Infrared-Thermography and Laser Doppler Mapping of Skin Blood Flow (Example 6.4) • Use of Dynamic IR-Thermography to Highlight Perforating Vessels (Example 6.5) • Reperfusion of Transplanted Tissue (Example 6.6) • Sports Medicine Injury (Example 6.7) • Conclusions	
	Acknowledgments...	**6**-17
	References	**6**-18

David D. Pascoe
Auburn University

James B. Mercer
University of Tromsø

Lois de Weerd
University Hospital of North Norway

6.1 Overview

William Herschel first recognized heat emitted in the infrared (IR) wave spectrum in the 1800s. Medical infrared, popularly known as IR-thermography has utilized this heat signature since the 1960s to measure and map skin temperatures. Our understanding of the regulation of skin blood flow, heat transfers through the tissue layers, and skin temperatures has radically changed during these past 40 years, allowing us to better interpret and evaluate these thermographic measurements. During this same period of time, improved camera sensitivity coupled with advances in focal plan array technology and new developments in computerized systems with assisted image analysis have improved the quality of the noncontact, noninvasive thermal map or thermogram [1–3]. In a recent electronic literature search in Medline using the keywords "thermography" and "thermogram" more than 5000 hits were found [4]. In 2003 alone, there were 494 medical references, 188 basic science, 148 applied science (14 combined with Laser Doppler and

28 combined with ultrasound research), and 47 in biology including veterinary medicine [5]. Further databases and references for medical thermography since 1987 are available [6].

This review will highlight some of the literature and applications of thermography in medical and physiological settings. More specifically, infrared thermography and the structure and functions of skin thermal microcirculation can provide a better understanding of (1) thermoregulation and skin thermal patterns (e.g., comfort zone, influences of heat, cold, and exercise stressors, etc.), (2) assess skin blood perfusion (e.g., skin grafts), (3) observe and diagnose vascular pathologies that manifest thermal disturbances in the cutaneous circulation, (4) evaluate thermal therapies, and (5) monitor patient/subject/athlete's recovery as evidenced by the resumption of normal thermal patterns during the rehabilitation process for some musculoskeletal injuries.

At the outset, it needs to be stressed that an IR image is a visual map of the skin surface temperature that can provide accurate thermal measurement but cannot quantify measurements of blood flow to the skin tissue. It is also important to stress that recorded skin temperatures may represent heat transferred from within the core through various tissue layers to the skin that may be the result of conductive or radiant heat provided from an external thermal stressor. In order to interpret thermographic images and thermal measurement, a basic understanding of physiological mechanisms of skin blood flow and factors that influence heat transfers to the skin must be considered to evaluate this dynamic process. With this understanding, objective data from IR-thermography can add valuable information and complement other methodologies in the scientific inquiry and medical practices.

6.2 Skin Thermal Properties in Response to Stress

The thermal properties of the skin surface can change dramatically to maintain our core temperature within a narrowly defined survival range (cardiac arrest at 25°C to cell denaturation at 45°C) [7]. This remarkable task is accomplished despite a large variability in temperatures both from the hostile environment and internal production of heat from metabolism. Further perturbations to core and skin temperature may result from thermal stressors associated with injury, fever, hormonal milieu, and disease. The skin responds to these thermal challenges by regulating skin perfusion.

During heat exposure or intense exercise, skin blood flow can be increased to provide greater heat dissipating capacity. The thermal properties of the skin combined with increased cutaneous circulation operate as a very efficient radiator of heat (emitted radiant heat of 0.98 compared to a blackbody source of 1.0) [8]. Evaporative cooling of sweat on the skin surface further enhances this heat dissipating process. Under hyperthermic conditions, the skin masterfully combines anatomical structure and physiological function to protect and defend the organism from potentially lethal thermal stressors by regulating heat transfers between core, skin, and environment. When exposed to a cold environment, the skin surface nearly eliminates blood flow and becomes an excellent insulator. Under these hypothermic conditions, our skin functions to conserve our body's core temperature. It accomplishes this by reducing convective heat transfers, minimizing heat losses from the core and lessening the possibility of excessive cooling from the environment.

The ability of the skin to substantially increase blood flow, far in excess of the tissue's metabolic needs, alludes to the tissue's role and potential in heat transfer mechanisms. The nutritive needs of skin tissue has been estimated at 0.2 ml/min per cubic centimeter of skin [9], which is considerably lower than the maximal rate of 24 ml/min per cubic centimeter of skin (estimated from total forearm circulatory measurement during heat stress) [10]. If one were to approximate skin tissue as 8% of the forearm, then skin blood would equate to 250 to 300 ml/100 ml of skin per minute [11]. Applying this flow rate to an estimated skin surface of 1.8 m^2 (average individual), suggests that approximately 8 liters of blood flow could be diverted to the skin to dissipate heat at rate of 1750 W to the environment [12,13]. This increased blood flow required for heat transfers from active muscle tissue and skin blood flow for thermoregulation is made available through the redistribution of blood flow (splanchnic circulatory beds, renal tissues) and increases in cardiac output [14]. The increased cardiac output has been suggested to account for two-thirds of the increased blood flow needs, while redistribution provides the remaining one-third [15]. Several good reviews are available regarding cutaneous blood flow, cardiovascular function, and thermal stress [14–19].

6.3 Regulation of Skin Blood Flow for Heat Transfers

In the 1870s, Goltz, Ostromov, and others injected atropine and pilocaprine into the skin to help elucidate the sympathetic neural innervation of the skin tissue for temperature, pressure, pain, and the activation of the sweat glands [20]. The reflex neural regulation of skin blood flow relies on both sympathetic vasoconstrictor and vasodilator controls to modulate internal heat temperature transfers to the skin. The vasoconstrictor system is responsible for eliminating nearly all of the blood flow to the skin during exposure to cold. When exposed to thermal neutral conditions, the vasoconstrictor system maintains the vasomotor tone of the skin vasculature from which small changes in skin blood flow can elicit large changes in heat dissipation. Under these conditions, the core temperature is maintained; mean skin temperature is stable, but dependent upon the extraneous influences of radiant heat, humidity, forced convective airflow, and clothing. A naked individual in a closed room with ambient air temperature between 27 and 28°C can retain thermal equilibrium without shivering or sweating [21]. Slightly dressed individuals are comfortable in a neutral environment with temperatures between 20 and 25°C. This thermoneutral zone provides the basis for the clinical testing standards for room temperatures being set at 18–25°C during infrared thermographic studies. Controlling room test conditions is important when measuring skin temperature responses as changes in ambient temperatures can alter the fraction of flow shared between the musculature and skin [19]. Under the influence of whole body hyperthermic conditions, removal of the vasomotor vasoconstrictor tone can account for 10–20% of cutaneous vasodilation, while the vasodilator system provides the remaining skin blood flow regulation [10]. Alterations in the threshold (onset of vascular response and sweating) and sensitivity (level of response) in vasodilation blood flow control can be related to an individual's level of heat acclimation [22], exercise training [22], circadian rhythm [23,24], and women's reproductive hormonal status [10]. Recent literature suggests that some observed shifts in the reflex control are the result of female reproductive hormones. Both estrogen and progesterone have been linked to menopausal hot flashes [10].

Skin blood flow research has identified differences in reflex sympathetic nerve activation for various skin surface regions. In 1956, Gaskell demonstrated that sympathetic neural activation in the acral regions (digits, lips, ears, cheeks, and palmer surfaces of hands and feet) is controlled by adrenergic vasoconstrictor nerve activity [20]. In contrast, I.C. Roddie in 1957 demonstrated that in nonacral regions, the adrenergic vasoconstrictor activity accounts for less than 25% of the control mechanism [25]. In the nonacral region, the sympathetic nervous system has both adrenergic (vasoconstriction) and nonadrenergic (vasodilator) components. While the vasodilator activity in the nonacral region is well accepted, the vasoconstrictor regulation is not fully understood and awaits the identification of neural cotransmitters that mediate the reductions in blood flow. For a more in-depth discussion of regional sympathetic reflex regulation, see Charkoudian [10] and Johnson and Proppe [13].

A further distinction in blood flow regulation can be found in the existence of arteriovenous anastamoses (AVA) that are principally found in acral tissues but not commonly found in nonacral tissues of the legs, arms, and chest regions [10,26,27]. The AVAs are thick walled, low resistance vessels that provide a direct blood flow route from arterioles to the venules. The arterioles and AVA, under sympathetic adrenergic vasoconstrictor control, modulate and substantially control flow rates to the skin vascular plexuses in these areas. When constricted, blood flow into subcutaneous venous plexus is reduced to a very low level (minimal heat loss); while, when dilated, extremely rapid flow of warm blood into the venous plexus is allowed (maximal heat loss). The skin sites where these vessels are found are among those where skin blood flow changes are discernible to the IR-thermographer. While the AVA are most active during heat stress, their thick walls and high velocity flow rates do not support their significant role in heat transfers to adjoining skin tissue [12].

Localized cooling of the skin surface can cause skin blood flow vasoconstriction induced by the stimulation of the nonadrenergic sympathetic nerves. This localized cooling or challenge can be used as a diagnostic tool by infrared thermographers to identify clinically significant alterations in skin blood flow response. Using a cold challenge test, Francis Ring developed a vasoplasticity test for Raynaud's syndrome based on the temperature gradient in the hand following a cold water immersion (20°C for 60 sec) [28]. Challenge testing and IR imaging has also been used to evaluate blood flow thermal patterns in patients with carpal tunnel syndrome pre- and post-surgery [29]. Skin blood flow vasodilation in response to local heating is stimulated by the release of sensory nerve neuropeptides or the nonneural stimulation of the cutaneous arteriole by nitric oxide. Thermographic imagers have exploited this localized warming response to provide a skin blood flow challenge [10].

As stated earlier, conditions of thermal stress from heat exposure and increased metabolic heat from exercise necessitate increases in skin blood flow to transfer the heat to the environment. This could have serious blood pressure consequences if it were not for baroreflex modulation of skin blood flow in regulating both sympathetic vasoconstriction and vasodilation [30,31]. With mild heat stress for 1 h (38 and 46°C, 42% relative humidity), cardiac output was not significantly impacted [32–34]. When exposing the individual to longer duration bouts and higher temperatures, significant changes in cardiac output have been observed. During these hyperthermic bouts, skin blood flow will withdraw vasodilation in nonacral regions in response to situations that displace blood volumes to the legs (lower body negative pressure or upright tilting) [35]. In contrast, under normothermic conditions, skin blood flow will demonstrate a sympathetic vasoconstriction to these same blood volume situations. Thus, it appears that the baroreceptor response can activate either sympathetic pathway. Withdrawing vasodilation under normothermic conditions was not an option in this inactive system [36].

In summary, skin blood flow during whole body thermal stress is regulated by neural reflex control via sympathetic vasoconstriction and vasodilation. There are structural (AVA) and neural mechanisms (vasoconstriction vs. vasodilation) differences between the acral and nonacral regions. During local thermal stress, stimulation of the sensory afferent nerve, nitric oxide stimulation of cutaneous arteriole, and inhibition of sympathetic vasoconstrictor system regulate changes in local blood flow. During thermal stress and increased heat from exercise metabolism, the skin blood flow can be dramatically increased. This increase in skin blood flow is matched to increased cardiac output and peripheral resistance to maintain blood pressure.

6.4 Heat Transfer Modeling Equations for Microcirculation

The capacity and ability of blood to transfer heat through various tissue layers to the skin can be predicted from models. These models are based on calculations from tissue conductivity, tissue density, tissue specific heat, local tissue temperature, metabolic or externally derived heat sources, and blood velocity. Many current models were derived from the 1948 Pennes model of blood perfusion, often referred to as the "bioheat equation" [9]. The bioheat equation calculates volumetric heat that is equated to the proportional volumetric rate of blood perfusion. The Pennes model assumed that thermal equilibrium occurs in the capillaries and venous temperatures were equal to local tissue temperatures. Both of these assumptions have been challenged in more recent modeling research. The assumption of thermal equilibrium within capillaries was challenged by the work of Chato [37] and Chen and Holmes in 1980 [38]. Based on this vascular modeling for heat transfer, thermal equilibrium occurred in "thermally significant blood vessels" that are approximately 50 to 75 μm in diameter and located prior to the capillary plexus. These thermally significant blood vessels derive from a tree-like structure of branching vessels that are closely spaced in countercurrent pairs. For a historical perspective of heat transfer bioengineering, see Chato in Reference 37 and for a review of heat transfers and microvascular modeling, see Baish in Reference 39.

This modeling literature provides a conceptual understanding of the thermal response of skin when altered by disease, injury, or external thermal stressors to skin temperatures (environment or application of cold or hot thermal sources, convective airflow, or exercise). From tissue modeling, we know that tissue is only slightly influenced by the deep tissue blood supply but is strongly influenced by the cutaneous circulation. With the use of IR-thermography, the skin temperatures can be accurately quantified and the thermal pattern mapped. However, these temperatures cannot be assumed to represent thermal conditions at the source of the thermal stress. Furthermore, the thermal pattern only provides a visual map of the skin surface in which heat is dissipated throughout the skin's multiple microvascular plexuses.

6.5 Cutaneous Circulation Measurement Techniques

A brief review of some of the techniques and procedures that have been employed to reveal skin tissue structure, rates and variability of perfusion, and factors that provide regulatory control of blood flow are provided. This serves to inform the reader as to how these measurement techniques have molded our understanding of skin structure and function. It is also important to recognize the advantages and disadvantages each technique brings to our experimental investigations. It is the opinion of the authors that IR-thermography can provide complimentary data to information obtained from these other methodologies.

6.5.1 Procedures and Techniques

Visual and microscopic views of skin have provided scientists with a structural layout of skin layers and blood flow. Despite our understanding of the structural organization, we still struggle to understand the regulation and functioning of the skin as influenced by the multitude of external and internal stressors. Since ancient times, documents have recorded visible observations made regarding changes to skin color and temperature that underscore some of the skin's functions. These observations include increased skin color and temperature when someone is hyperthermic, skin flushing when embarrassed, and the appearance of skin reddening when the skin is scratched. In contrast, decreases of skin color and temperature are observed during hypothermia, when blood flow is occluded, or during times of circulatory shock. In addition to observations, testing procedures and techniques have been employed in search of an understanding of skin function. Skin blood flow has provided one of the greatest challenges and has been notoriously difficult to record quantitatively in terms of ml/min per gram of skin tissue.

6.5.2 Dyes and Stains

Stains and dyes have been a useful tool to investigate the structure of various histological tissue preparations. In 1889 Overton used Florescin, a yellow dye that glows in visible light, to visualize the lipid bilayer membrane structure [40]. Florescin is still used today to illuminate the blood vessel in various tissues. In the early 1900s, August Krogh was able to identify perfused capillaries by staining them with writer's ink before the tissue was excised and observed under the microscope. Using a different approach to observe the structure of skin blood flow, Michael Salmon in the 1930s developed a radio-opaque preservative mixture that was injected into fresh cadavers and produced detailed pictures of the arterial blood flow to skin tissue regions which were mapped for the entire skin surface [41]. Scientists have also used Evans Blue Dye to investigate changes in blood volume by calculating the dilution factor of pre- and post-samples. Evans Blue and Pontamine Sky Blue dyes have also been used to investigate skin microvascular permeability and leakage as induced by various stimuli [42]. A more recent staining technique involves the use of an IR absorbing dye, indocyanine green (ICG). The dye ICG fluoresces with invisible IR light when captured by special cameras sensitive to these light wavelengths. Recent publications have suggested that ICG video angiographies provide qualitative and quantitative data from which clinicians may assess tissue blood flow in burn wounds [43,44].

6.5.3 Plethysmography

The rationale for venous occlusion plethysmography (VOP) is that a partially inflated cuff around a limb exceeds the pressure of venous blood flow but does not interfere with arterial blood flow to the limb.

This can be effectively accomplished when the cuff is inflated to a pressure just below diastolic arterial pressure. Consequently, portions of the limb distal to the cuff will swell as blood accumulates. The original VOP technology relied on measuring the rate of swelling as indicated by the displacement volume of the water-filled chamber around the limb. Later, gauges were used to record changes in limb circumference as the limb expanded. Either way, the geometric forces allows one to express the changes in terms of a starting volume, thus scales are labeled as ml/min per 100 ml in the illustrations of VOP data. Unfortunately, the 100 ml reference quantity refers to the whole limb (not the quantity of the skin) and the VOP technique provides discontinuous measurement, usually four measurements per minute. Currently, VOP represents the most reliable quantitative measure of skin blood flow. More recently, a modified plethysmography technique has been developed that equates changes in blood flow to the changes in electrical impedance, when a mild current is introduced into the blood flow and recorded by serially placed electrodes along the limb.

6.5.4 Doppler Measurement

The Doppler Effect describes the shift in wave length frequency or pitch that result when sound or light from any portion of the electromagnetic spectrum are influenced by the distance and directional movement of the object. Both ultrasound and laser Doppler techniques rely on this physical principle to make the skin blood flow measurement. A continuous wave Doppler ultrasound emits a high frequency sound wave from which reflected or echo sounds can be used to calculate the direction of flow and velocity of moving objects (circulating blood cells). When ultrasound equipment is pulsated, the depth of the circulatory flow vessel can be identified. The blood flow is assessed in Doppler units or volts and can be continuously monitored over a small surface area. Similar measurements can be made with the laser Doppler technique, but neither technique is able to yield quantitative blood flow values except through reference data obtained by VOP.

6.5.5 Clearance Measurement

In the 1930s, scientists relied on the thermal conductance method for determining blood flow in tissues. This methodology was based on measurement of heat dissipation in blood flow downstream from a known heat source (thermocouple). The accuracy of the methodology was assumed through strong correlations made with direct drop counting from isolated sheep spleens. However, these blood flow measurements had problems related to trauma associated with the obstruction and insertion of the thermocouple. During the 1950s and 1960s, injection of small amounts of radioactive isotopes was used in an attempt to better quantify skin blood flow [45]. In order to accurately measure skin blood flow, the isotopes had to be freely diffusible and able to cross the capillary endothelium to enter the blood stream. The blood flow measurement (ml blood flow per 100 g of tissue) obtained through this methodology was not reproducible and subjects were exposed to injected radioactive isotope substances.

6.5.6 Thermal Skin Measurement

Physicians and parents have often relied upon touching a child's forehead to identify a fever or elevated temperature. While this is a crude measure of skin temperature, it has demonstrated practical importance. The development of the thermistor has provided quantifiable measurements of the skin surface. This has been extensively used in research related to thermoregulation and in research in which the skin temperature for a particular physiological perturbation must be quantified. Mean skin temperature formulas have been developed in which various regional temperatures (3 to 15 sites) are combined or a weighted mean based on the DuBois formula for surface area is calculated from the regions measured. When measuring skin temperatures under the influence of colder environments, skin temperature distribution is heterogeneous, especially in the acral regions [46]. Under these conditions, the various placements of the thermistor will provide different temperature measurement that may not be indicative of the mean skin temperature for that region. In contrast, the skin surface temperature is more homogeneous under warm environmental conditions. To provide an accurate measurement, physiologists investigating mean skin temperatures have modified the number of thermistors required during testing as dictated by environmental temperatures [46]. Thermistor attachment to the skin surface is problematic as it creates a microenvironment between the probe, skin, and adhering tape and exerts a pressure on the site. Furthermore, one site placement of the thermistor cannot represent variable responses under conditions and within regions that demonstrate heterogeneous temperature distributions.

Infrared thermography provides a thermal map of the skin surface area by measuring the radiant heat that is emitted. Current IR-thermography machines provide accurate skin surface temperatures (<0.05°C) that are noninvasive, noncontact measurements through the use of stable detectors. These systems produce high speed–high resolution images from which thermal data can be pictorially and quantitatively stored and analyzed. While IR-radiation begins at wavelengths of 0.7 μm, current IR-thermographic imagers are operating at either the mid-range (3–5 μm) or long range (8–14 μm) wavelengths [1–3]. At these wavelengths the skin's ability to emit the radiant heat is 0.98 on a scale of 1.0 for a perfect radiator, blackbody surface [8]. IR-thermographers sometimes rely on "challenge tests" in which the skin thermal response is evaluated after cold or hot water immersion, convective airflow, or an exercise bout that alters skin blood flow. Under these thermally challenging conditions, the clinical importance of abnormalities of skin blood flow may be more apparent. However, one must also recognize that as the heat is being transferred through the various layers of skin, some of the heat is dissipated into the adjoining tissues. The heat decay as the blood traverses the layers of tissue and its dispersion pattern within the circulatory plexus of the skin may disguise the origin of the tissue producing the abnormal thermal response.

6.5.7 Measurement Techniques and Procedures Summary

Since ancient times, significant progress has been made in the quest to understand the anatomy and physiology of skin blood flow and the thermal heat transfers that are dissipated to the skin surface. Current measurement technologies are unable to quantify skin blood flow per skin tissue area (ml/min per 100 ml skin). At this time, our best estimations of skin blood flow come from venous occlusion plethysmography. VOP provides discontinuous blood flow measurements based on tissue perfusion of a whole limb extremity. In recent years, laser Doppler blood flow measures have been popular when investigating more localized tissue areas, but this technique must be calibrated through the data obtained by plethysmography. In the quest to understand skin surface heat transfers, noncontact IR-thermography provides researchers with accurate measures of skin temperature for specific locations and thermal maps of regions of interest. Thermographic images provide spatial and temporal changes in skin temperature that are representative of spatial and temporal changes in perfusion. However, the scientist and clinician should be aware of blood–skin heat transfer properties prior to interpreting and evaluating the thermal responses of skin perfusion or investigating pathologies that are thermally transferred to the skin.

6.6 Objective Thermography

The main focus of this section is to present some specific examples to show that IR thermal imaging is a useful, objective tool for medical and physiological-based investigations. Although IR thermal imaging cannot determine quantitative measurements of blood flow, this imaging can quantify skin thermal measurement that can be correlated to qualitative evaluations of skin blood flow. As with any technique, it is imperative for the IR-thermographer to understand the anatomical and dynamic physiological features (e.g., vasomotor activity) of the blood vessels involved in skin circulation in order to interpret skin temperature responses. This is particularly important in situations where skin blood flow and temperature are responding to some external or internal thermal stress (e.g., clinician's cold challenge testing, exercise, environment, etc.) or nonthermal stimuli (e.g., disease, injury, medications, etc.). When properly assessed, skin temperature can provide researchers, scientists, and physicians with valuable information about the blood flow and thermal regulation of organs and tissues (see Examples 6.6.1 to 6.6.7).

6.6.1 Efficiency of Heat Transport in the Skin of the Hand (Example 6.1)

The AVA are specialized vascular structures within acral regions. At normal body temperature, sympathetic vasoconstrictor nerves keep these anastomoses closed. However, when the body becomes overheated, sympathetic discharge is greatly reduced so that the anastomoses dilate allowing large quantities of warm blood to flow into the subcutaneous venous plexus, thereby promoting heat loss from the body (Figure 6.1a). In thermal physiology, hands and feet are well recognized as effective thermal windows. By controlling the amount of blood perfusing through these extremities, the temperature of the skin surface can change over a wide range of temperatures. It is at such peripheral sites that the effect of changes in blood flow, and therefore skin temperature are most clearly discernable.

The following example demonstrates how efficient skin blood flow in the hand is dissipating a large incoming radiant heat load. The radiant heat load was provided by a Hydrosun® type 501 water-filtered infrared-A (wIRA) irradiator. The Hydrosun® allows a local regional heating of skin tissue with a higher penetration depth than that of conventional IR therapy. The unique principle of operation involves the use of a hermetically sealed water filter in the radiation path to absorb those IR wavelengths emitted by conventional IR lamps which would otherwise harm the skin (OH-group at 0.94, 1.18, 1.38, and 1.87 μm). The total effective radiation from the Hydrosun® lamp was 400 mW/cm^2, which is about three times the intensity of the IR-A radiation from the sun. Throughout the time course of the experiment (Figure 6.1a), sequential digital IR-thermal images were taken every 2 sec. With the image analysis software, five points within the radiation field of each image were selected for temperature measurement and used to construct temperature curves shown in Figure 6.1b.

In the experiment (Figure 6.1b) a rubber mat with an emissivity close to 1.0 was irradiated with the Hydrosun® wIRA lamp for a period of 25 min at a standard distance of 25 cm. At this distance the circular irradiation field had a diameter of about 16 cm. Since the rubber material has a high emissivity it rapidly absorbs heat from the lamp. As can be seen from the time course of the five temperature curves in Figure 6.2 (five fixed measuring points within the radiation field), the center of the irradiated rubber mat rapidly reached temperatures over 90°C during the first 10 min of irradiation. After the first 10 min of irradiation, the hand of a healthy 54-year-old male subject was abruptly placed on the irradiated rubber mat and kept there for a further 10 min, before being removed. When the hand was placed onto the irradiation field, three of the five fixed temperature-measuring sites now measured skin temperature on the dorsal skin surface. Based on the temperature curves in Figure 6.1b, skin temperature on the surface of the hand directed toward the irradiator never rose higher than 40°C, while the two remaining temperature-measuring points on the rubber mat remained at their original high values. The patient suffered no thermal discomfort from placing his hand on the "hot" rubber mat, even though the temperature of the center of the rubber mat was more than 90°C before the hand was placed on it. This was presumably due to a combination of the low heat capacity of the rubber material combined with a high rate of skin blood flow that is capable of rapidly dissipating heat. The visual data created from the IR-thermal images coupled with the temperature curves which were calculated from sequential IR-thermal images clearly demonstrates the large heat transporting capacity of the skin.

6.6.2 Effect of a Reduced Blood Flow (Example 6.2)

During exposure to cold, heat loss from the extremities is minimized by reducing blood flow (vasoconstriction). In cool environments, this vasomotor tone results in a heterogeneous distribution of skin surface temperatures; while in a warm environment the skin surface becomes more homogeneous (see Figure 6.2a). The importance of the integrity of blood flow in a limb as a whole can also be demonstrated at room temperature by totally cutting off the blood supply to the limb with the aid of a pressure cuff. This is demonstrated in the experiment shown in Figure 6.2b. In this experiment, skin surface on the back of the left hand of a 60-year-old healthy male subject was irradiated for a 10-min period with a wIRA lamp (see description in Section 6.6.1). The fingers were not heated. The heating was repeated twice. In the upper panel (Figure 6.2b) intact blood supply is demonstrated. In the lower panel (Figure 6.2b),

Physiology of Thermal Signals

FIGURE 6.1 (See color insert at the back of the book.) (a) A Thermogram of a healthy 52-year-old male subject in a cold environment (ca. 15°C; left panel) and in a warm environment (ca. 25°C; right panel). In the cold environment arteriovenous anastomoses in the nose and the auricle region of the ears are closed, resulting in low skin temperatures at these sites. Also note reduced blood flow in the cheeks but not on the forehead, where the blood vessels in the skin are unable to vasoconstrict. (b) Efficiency of skin blood flow as a heat transporter. The photograph in the upper left panel shows a rubber mat being heated with a water-filtered infrared-A irradiator at high intensity (400 mW/cm^2) for a period of 20 min. In the lower panel the time course of surface temperature of the mat at five selected spots as measured by an IR-camera is given. During the last 10 min of the 20-min heating period, the left hand of a healthy 54-year-old male subject was placed on the mat. Note that skin surface temperature of the hand remains below 39°C.

(a) 30 min equilibration in cool environment (20°C, 30% rh)

30 min equilibration in warm environment (41°C, 30% rh)

Range of temperature (°C) within regions at two climatic conditions.

	Anterior torso	Posterior torso	Anterior arms	Posterior arms	Palmer hands	Dorsal hands
Cool 20°C	5.0	5.1	6.3	4.5	5.2	4.0
Warm 41°C	3.0	3.2	3.2	3.6	4.0	3.5

FIGURE 6.2 (**See color insert.**) (a) A thermoregulatory response of the torso when exposed to a cool or warm environment. Note the heterogeneous temperature distribution in the cool environment as opposed to the more homogeneous temperature distribution in the warm environment. Different colors represent different temperatures. One might recognize the difficulty related to choosing one point (thermocouple data) as the reference value in a region.

thermal response to heating of the limb while blood flow was totally restricted using a blood pressure cuff is presented. The time course of the temperature curves shown in the upper panel of Figure 6.2b demonstrates a gradual increase in skin temperature, eventually stabilizing just below 39°C. The finger skin temperature on the heated hand only showed a minor increase during the heating period. When the lamp was switched off the accumulated heat was rapidly dissipated and skin temperature of the heated area returned to the preheating level. In the lower panel the experiment was repeated, but as the heater was turned on, a pressure cuff placed around the upper arm was inflated to above systolic pressure to totally cut off blood supply to the arm. As can be seen, the rate of rise of skin temperature over the heated skin area was quite rapid, soon reaching a level deemed to be uncomfortably hot, after which the heater was turned off (at this stage the pressure cuff was still inflated). During the heating period finger skin temperature on the same hand steadily decreased (i.e., the fingers were passively cooling due to lack of circulation). After the heater was turned off the temperature of the back of the left hand also began to decrease indicating a passive cooling. When the pressure cuff was reopened and blood flow to the arm reestablished, the rate of cooling on the back of the hand increased (active cooling) and the skin temperature of the cooled fingers also rapidly returned to normal.

While the same result could have been gained by using other methods to measure skin temperature, such as thermocouples, the visual effect gained by using IR-thermography provides much more information

FIGURE 6.2 (Continued) (**See color insert.**) (b) Skin heating with and without intact circulation in a 65-year-old healthy male subject. The two panels on the right show the time course of 6 selected measuring sites (4 spot measurements and 2 area measurements) of skin temperatures as determined by IR-thermography before, during, and after a period in which the skin surface on the back of the left hand was heated with a water-filtered infrared-A irradiator at high intensity (400 mW/cm^2) in two separate experiments. The results shown in the upper right panel were performed under a situation with a normal intact blood circulation, while the results shown in the lower left panel were made during total occlusion of circulation in the right arm by means of an inflated pressure cuff placed around the upper arm. The time of occlusion is indicated. The IR-thermogram on the left was taken just prior to the end of the heating period in the experiment described in the upper panel. The location of the temperature measurement sites on the hand (4 spot measurements [Spot 1 to Spot 4] and the average temperature within a circle [Areas 5 and 6]) are indicated on the thermogram.

than a single point measurement. Various points or areas of interest can be investigated during and after the experimental procedures. Modern digital image processing software provides endless possibilities, especially with systems allowing the recording of sequential IR-images. Today modern fire-wire technology permits one to record IR-images at very high frequencies (100 Hz and greater).

6.6.3 Median Nerve Block in the Hand (Example 6.3)

The nervous supply to the hand is via three main nerves: radial, ulnar, and median nerve. The approximate distribution of the sensory innervation by these nerves is shown in Figure 6.3a. With a sudden removal (or disruption) of the sympathetic discharge to one of the main nerves, a maximal vasodilatation of blood vessels in the area supplied by the nerve is observed. Such a vasodilatation will result in a significant increase in skin blood flow to that area and therefore in a rise in skin temperature. The IR-thermogram in Figure 6.3b shows such a response. The subject is a 40-year-old female suffering from excessive sweating in the palms of her hands, a condition known as hyperhidrosis palmaris. Excessive sweating causes cooling of the skin surface. The blue color in Figure 6.3b represents areas of excessive sweating as well as areas of lowest skin temperature. Hyperhidrosis palmaris is treated by subcutaneous injections of Botulinum Toxin. The skin in the palm of the hand is very sensitive and anesthesia is therefore required. A very effective way to provide adequate anesthesia is the median nerve block. At the level of the wrist, a local anesthetic is injected around the median nerve and blocks the nervous activity in the median nerve.

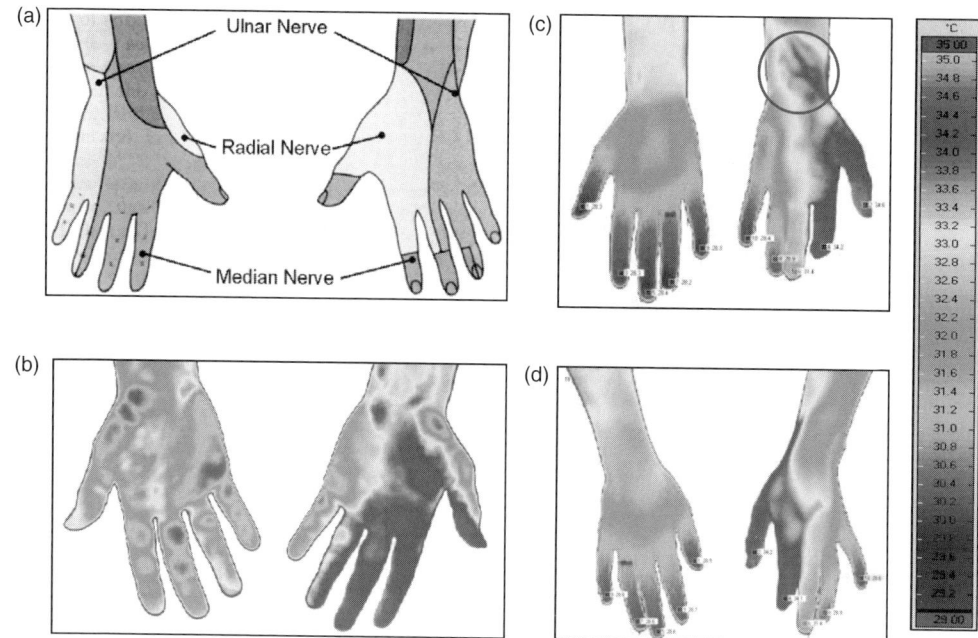

FIGURE 6.3 (See color insert.) (a) The distribution of cutaneous nerves to the hand. (b) IR-thermogram of a 40-year-old female patient following a successful nerve block of the left median nerve. (c) and (d) IR-thermograms of the hands of a 36-year-old female patient whose left wrist (middle of the red circle) was punctured with a sharp object resulting in partial nerve damage (motor and sensory loss). The strong vasodilatory response resulting from partially severed nerves can be easily seen.

The resulting increase in skin temperature on the palmar side of the left hand after such an injection is clearly seen in Figure 6.3b. One sees that part of the thumb and half of the fourth finger show no increase in temperature, closely matching the predicted area of distribution for this nerve in Figure 6.3a. Although a median nerve block was applied to the right hand, neither vasodilatation nor a change in skin temperature was seen. The Botulinum Toxin injections on this side were painful. The placement of the anesthetic was therefore incorrect, and as a result, normal nervous activity in the right hand was observed. In Figure 6.3c,d, the thermograms show the hands of a 36-year-old female patient. Her left wrist (middle of the red circle) was punctured with a sharp object, resulting in partial nerve damage. The strong vasodilatory response, due to the nerve damage, results in an increased skin temperature as shown in Figure 6.3d.

The diagnosis of acute nerve damage can be a challenge for a surgeon. In the acute situation, pain makes a proper physical examination often impossible. To evaluate the extent of the nerve injury, cooperation of the patient is necessary and the use of local anesthesia can mask the extent of the injury. IR-thermography proves to be a helpful, noninvasive diagnostic tool by visualizing changes in skin temperature and, indirectly blood flow to the skin, due to the nerve injury.

6.6.4 Infrared-Thermography and Laser Doppler Mapping of Skin Blood Flow (Example 6.4)

As mentioned in the introduction above, one of the drawbacks of using IR-thermography to indirectly indicate changes in skin blood flow is being able to decide, for example, if an increase in skin temperature is due to a parallel increase in skin blood flow. One way to verify whether observed skin temperature changes are related to changes in skin blood flow is to combine IR-thermography with a more direct measurement technique of skin blood flow. Laser Doppler can ascertain the direction of skin blood flow

Physiology of Thermal Signals

FIGURE 6.4 (See color insert.) IR-thermograms, temperature profiles, scanning laser doppler (SLD) scans, and blood flow profiles (perfusion units PU) of the abdominal area of a 44-year-old healthy female subject before (a), immediately after (b), and 5 min (c), 10 min (d) and 20 min (e) after a 20 min heating of the right side of the abdomen with a water-filtered infrared-A irradiation lamp. The blue horizontal lines in the IR-thermograms indicate the position of the temperature profiles. The red horizontal lines in the SLD scans indicate the position of the blood flow profiles. In IR-thermogram (b) the white color indicates skin temperatures greater than 36°C.

but these measurements are restricted to small surfaces and blood flow is not quantified but reported as changes in Doppler units or volts [45]. With IR-thermography rapid changes in skin temperature over a large area can be easily measured. Laser-Doppler mapping involves a scanning technique using a lower power laser beam in a raster pattern and requires time to complete a scan (up to minutes depending on the size of the scanned area). During the time it takes to complete a scan it is possible that the skin blood flow has changed in the skin area examined at the start compared to the skin area being examined at the end of each scan. This is most likely to happen in dynamic situations where skin blood flow is rapidly changing. Despite this draw back, the use of IR-thermography and laser Doppler mapping can provide a complimentary investigative view of this dynamic process.

In Figure 6.4, both IR-thermography and scanning laser Doppler mapping have been simultaneously used to examine a healthy 44-year-old female subject. In this experiment the subject was submitted to a 20 min heating of the right side of the abdomen using a water filtered IR-A irradiation lamp (see Section 6.6.1). During the period of heating, the left side of the abdomen was covered with a drape to prevent this side of the body from being heated. At predetermined intervals prior to, during, and

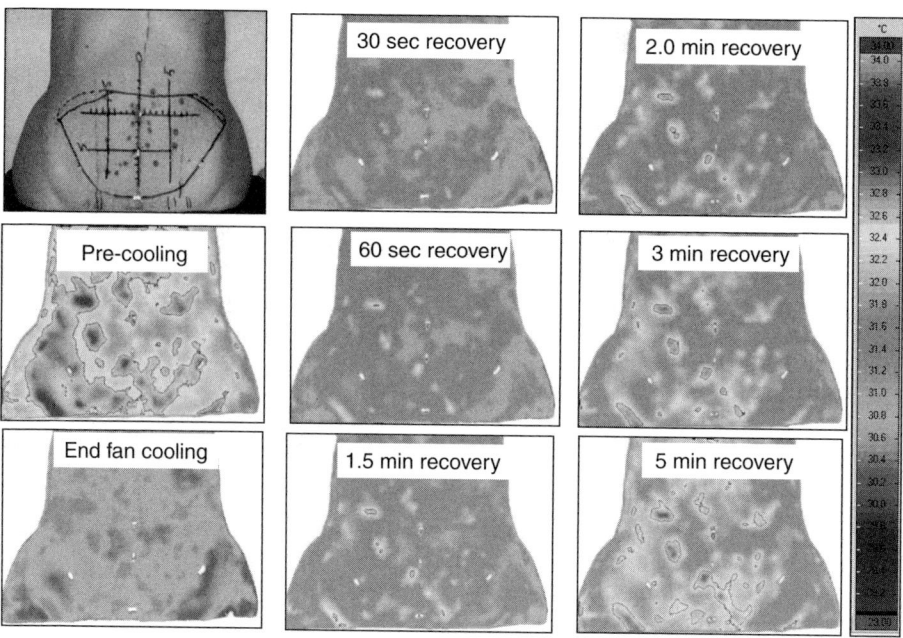

FIGURE 6.5 (See color insert.) Abdominal cooling in a 32-year-old female patient prior to breast reconstruction surgery. In this procedure skin and fat tissue from the abdominal area was used to reconstruct a new breast. The localization of suitable perforating vessels for reconnection to the mammary artery is an important part of the surgical procedure. In this sequence of thermograms the patient was first subjected to a mild cooling of the abdominal skin (2 min fan cooling). IR-thermograms of the skin over the entire abdominal area were taken prior to, immediately after, and at various time intervals during the recovery period following the cooling period. To help highlight the perforating vessels, an outline function has been employed in which all skin areas having a temperature greater than 32.5°C are enclosed in solid lines.

after the heating period both IR-thermal images and laser Doppler mapping images were recorded, the latter with a MoorLDI^{TM} laser Doppler imager (LDI-1), Moor Instruments, England. As can be seen in Figure 6.5, the wIRA heating lamp causes a large increase in skin temperature on the irradiated side of the abdomen. After the end of the heating period, the temperature of the heated area gradually decreases. These changes nicely correspond with the laser Doppler mapping images. A semi quantitative value of blood flow (perfusion units) for each LDI image was also calculated (right panels in Figure 6.5). Each blood flow profile corresponds well with their respective temperature profiles.

6.6.5 Use of Dynamic IR-Thermography to Highlight Perforating Vessels (Example 6.5)

The procedure of dynamic thermography involves promoting changes in skin blood flow by local heating or cooling. In the example shown in Figure 6.5, a mild cooling (2 min period of fan cooling) of the skin overlying the abdominal area of a 36-year-old female patient prior to undergoing breast reconstruction surgery was performed in order to highlight perforating blood vessels [41]. These blood vessels originate in deeper lying tissue and course their way toward the skin surface, although they may not necessarily reach the skin surface. By invoking a local cooling, a temporary vasoconstrictor response is initiated in skin blood vessels. Blood flow in the perforating blood vessels is little affected and following the end of the cooling period they rapidly contribute to the skin rewarming. During the rewarming process the localization of the "hot-spots" caused by these perforating vessels becomes more diffuse as heat from them spreads into neighboring tissue. This technique allows one to more easily identify so-called perforator vessels of the medial and lateral branches of the deep inferior epigastric artery, one or more of which will be selected for reconnection to the internal mammary artery (the usual recipient vessel) during reconstruction of a new breast from this abdominal tissue.

6.6.6 Reperfusion of Transplanted Tissue (Example 6.6)

With the development of microvascular surgery, it has become possible to connect (anastomose) blood vessels with a diameter as small as 0.5 mm to each other. Transplantation of tissue from one place to another place in the same patient (autologous transplantation) or from one individual to another (allologous transplantation) has become daily practice in medicine. The technique requires high surgical skills. During the operation, blood supply to the transplant is completely severed and the blood vessels to the transplant are later connected to recipient vessels. These recipient blood vessels will supply blood to the transplant at the new site. Kidney transplantation is a well-known example of allologous transplantation. Here, a patient with a nonfunctional kidney receives a donor kidney to provide normal renal function. Nowadays, autologous tissue transplantation is an integrated part in trauma surgery and cancer surgery. The successful reperfusion of the transplant is obviously essential for its survival. A nonsuccessful operation causes psychological stress for the patient and is indeed an inefficient use of resources stress. IR-thermography provides an ideal noninvasive and rapid method for monitoring the reperfusion status of transplanted tissue.

Autologous breast reconstruction is a critical part of the overall care plan for patients faced with a diagnosis of breast cancer and a plan that includes removal of the breast. The deep inferior epigastric perforator (DIEP) flap is the state of the art in autologous breast reconstruction today. The technique uses skin and fatty tissue from the lower abdomen for reconstruction of a new breast (Figure 6.6). The fatty tissue and skin on the lower abdomen are supplied by many blood vessels. By using this tissue as a DIEP flap in autologous breast reconstruction, the blood supply to this tissue is reduced to one single artery and veins, each with a diameter of 1.0 to 1.5 mm. A critical period during the operative procedure is the connection (anastomosing) of the flap to the recipient vessels. The blood vessels of the DIEP flap are anastomosed to the internal mammary vessels to provide blood supply to the flap. Blood circulation to the newly reconstructed breast is dependent on the viability of the microvascular anastomosis. The series of IR-thermograms shown in Figure 6.6 were taken at various time intervals after reestablishing the blood supply to the flap in a patient undergoing autologous breast reconstruction with a DIEP flap.

During the operation, there is a period (ca. 50 min) with no blood supply to the dissected flap, and as a result, it cools down. The rate and pattern of rewarming of the flap after anastomoses to the recipient vessels provides the surgeon with important information on the blood circulation in the transplanted flap. With a successful and adequate outcome of the anastomosis, the rewarming response was found to be rapid and well distributed (Figure 6.6). A poor rewarming response often made an extra venous anastomosis necessary to improve venous drainage (the most common problem). In such cases, IR-thermography provides an excellent method to quickly verify improvement in the blood flow status in the flap. In addition, in the days following surgery, examination of the skin temperatures using IR-thermography of the newly reconstructed breast was found to be a quick and easy way to monitor its blood flow status. The peripheral areas of the new breast can suffer from diminished blood circulation. Improvement in blood circulation could be seen during post surgery.

6.6.7 Sports Medicine Injury (Example 6.7)

Thermal images of an injury sustained by an 18-year-old American football player after a helmet impacted the superior portion of his right shoulder. X-ray and MRI immediately post game showed no structural damage. IR images were taken 12 h post-injury in a controlled environment (22°C, 30% rh, after 20 min equilibration). Upon examination, the athlete was unable to lift his right arm above shoulder level. Note the disruption in the thermal pattern in the right side torso view (T4 spinal region on left side of image)

FIGURE 6.6 (See color insert.) Infrared thermal images of an abdominal skin flap during breast reconstruction surgery. The sequence of IR-thermal images demonstrates the return of heat to the excised skin flap following reestablishing its blood supply (anastomizing of a mammary artery and vein to a single branch of the deep inferior epigastric artery and a concomitant vein). Prior to this procedure the excised skin flap had been without a blood supply for about 50 min and consequently cooled down. The photograph in the upper left panel shows the skin flap in position on the chest wall prior to being shaped into a new breast.

and the very cold temperatures and pattern extending down the left arm. After 3 weeks of rehabilitation, the weakness experienced in the shoulder and arm was resolved. IR imaging confirmed a return to normal symmetrical thermal pattern in the back torso and warmer arm temperatures.

6.6.8 Conclusions

As pointed out in the introduction to this section the main objective of this article is to try and persuade those who are not familiar with IR-thermography that this technology can provide objective data, which makes clinical sense. The reader has to be aware that the examples presented above only represent a tiny fraction of the possibilities that this technology provides. It is important to realize that an IR-thermal image of a skin area under examination will more often not provide the examiner with a satisfactory result. It is important to keep in mind that blood flow is a very dynamic event and in many situations useful clinical information can only be obtained by manipulating skin blood flow, for example by local cooling. Thus, the need to have a basic understanding of the physiological mechanisms behind the control of skin blood flow cannot be overemphasized. One also has to realize that this technology should be thought of as an aid to making a clinical diagnosis and in many cases should, if possible, be combined with other complementary techniques. For example, IR-thermography does not have the ability to pinpoint the location of a tumor in the breast. Consequently, IR-thermography's role is in addition to mammography, ultrasound and physical examination, not in lieu of. IR-thermography does not replace mammography and mammography does not replace IR-thermography, the tests complement each other.

FIGURE 6.7 (See color insert.) An American football player who suffered a helmet impact to the right shoulder (left side of image). The athlete was unable to flex his arm above shoulder level. Note the asymmetrical torso pattern in the posterior torso.

Acknowledgments

Examples of IR images from patients and volunteers (Figures 6.1, 6.2b, 6.3 to 6.7) from the Department of Medical Physiology, Faculty of Medicine, University of Tromsø, Norway and the Department of Clinical Physiology, Hillerød Hospital, Hillerød, Denmark. The IR images in these examples were taken using two different IR-cameras: A Nikon Laird S270 cooled camera and a FLIR ThermaCAM® PM695 uncooled bolometer. The respective image analysis software used was ThermaCAM researcher ver. 2.1 and PicWin-IRIS, (EBS Systemtechnik GmbH, Munich, Germany). The studies described in Examples 6.1 and 6.2 were carried out at the Department of Clinical Physiology, Hillerød Hospital, Hillerød, Denmark in collaboration with consultant Dr Stig Pors Nielsen. The assistance of Master student Lise Bøe Setså in the studies described in Examples 6.5 and 6.6 is also acknowledged. Examples of IR images (Figures 6.2a and 6.8) come from the Thermal Lab, Auburn University, Alabama, United States, utilizing a Computerized Thermal

Imager 2000. We would like to acknowledge the assistance of JohnEric Smith and Estevam Strecker in these projects.

References

[1] Jones B.F. and Plassmann P. Digital infrared thermal imaging of human skin. *IEEE Eng. Med. Biol.* 21, 41–48, 2002.

[2] Otsuka K., Okada S., Hassan M., and Togawa T. Imaging of skin thermal properties with estimation of ambient radiation temperature. *IEEE Eng. Med. Biol.* 21, 65–71, 2002.

[3] Head J.F. and Elliott R.L. Infrared imaging: making progress in fulfilling its medical promise. *IEEE Eng. Med. Biol.* 21, 80–85, 2002.

[4] Park J.Y., Kim S.D., Kim S.H., Lim D.J., and Cho T.H. The role of thermography in clinical practice: review of the literature. *Thermol. Int.* 13, 77–78, 2003.

[5] Ammer K. Thermology 2003—a computer-assisted literature survey with a focus on nonmedical applications of thermal imaging. *Thermol. Int.* 14, 5–36, 2004.

[6] Abernathy M. and Abernathy T.B. *International Bibliography of Medical Thermology.* Vol. 2, Washington DC, American College of Thermology, Georgetown University Medical Center, 1987.

[7] Pascoe D.D., Bellinger T.A., and McCluskey B.S. Clothing and exercise II: influence of clothing during exercise/work in environmental extremes. *Sports Med.* 18, 94–108, 1994.

[8] Flesch, U. Physics of skin-surface temperature. In *Thermology Methods*. Engel J.M., Flesch U., and Stüttgen G. (eds), translated by Biederman–Thorson M.A. Federal Republic of Germany Weinheim, pp. 21–37, 1985.

[9] Pennes H.H. Analysis of tissue and arterial blood temperatures in resting human forearm. *J. Appl. Physiol.* 1, 93–102, 1948.

[10] Charkoudian N. Skin blood flow in adult thermoregulation: how it works, when it does not, and why. *Mayo Clin. Proc.* 78, 603–612, 2003.

[11] Greenfield A.D.M. The circulation through the skin. In *Handbook of Physiology—Circulation*. Hamilton W.P. (ed.), Washington DC, American Physiological Society, Sec. 3, Vol. 2 (Chapter 39), pp. 1325–1351, 1963.

[12] Johnson J.M., Brenglemann G.L., Hales J.R.S., Vanhoutte M., and Wenger C.B. Regulation of the cutaneous circulation. *Fed. Proc.* 45, 2841–2850, 1986.

[13] Johnson J.M. and Proppe D.W. Cardiovascular adjustments to heat stress. In *Handbook of Physiology—Environmental Physiology*. Fregly M.J. and Blatteis C.M. (eds), Oxford, Oxford University Press/American Physiological Society, pp. 215–243, 1996.

[14] Rowell L.B. Human cardiovascular adjustments to exercise and thermal stress. *Physiol. Rev.* 54, 75–159, 1974.

[15] Rowell L.B. Cardiovascular adjustments in thermal stress. In *Handbook of Physiology. Section 2 Cardiovascular System, Vol. 3 Peripheral Circulation and Organ Flow*, J.T. Shepard and F.M. Abboud (Eds), Bethesda MD, American Physiological Society, pp. 967–1024, 1983.

[16] Rowell L.B. *Human Circulation: Regulation During Physiological Stress*. New York, Oxford University Press, 1986.

[17] Sawka M.N. and Wenger C.B. Physiological responses to acute exercise–heat stress. In *Human Performance Physiology and Environmental Medicine at Terrestrial Extremes*. Pandolf K.B., Sawka M.N., and Gonzales R.R. (eds), Indianapolis, IN, Benchmark Press, pp. 97–151, 1988.

[18] Johnson J.M. Circulation to the skin. In *Textbook of Physiology*. Patton H.D., Fuchs A.F., Hille B., Scher A.M., and Steiner R. (eds), Philadelphia, W.B. Saunders Co. Vol. 2 (Chapter 45), 1989.

[19] Johnson J.M. Exercise and the cutaneous circulation. *Exercise Sports Sci. Rev.* 20, 59–97, 1992.

[20] Garrison F.H. *Contributions to the History of Medicine*. New York, Hafner Publishing Co., Inc., p. 311, 1966.

[21] Kirsh K.A. Physiology of skin-surface temperature. In *Thermology Methods.* Engel J.M., Flesch U., and Stüttgen G. (eds), translated by Biederman–Thorson M.A., Federal Republic of Germany/Weinheim, pp. 1–9, 1985.

[22] Roberts M.P., Wenger C.B., Stölwik, and Nadel E.R. Skin blood flow and sweating changes following exercise training and heat acclimation. *J. Appl. Physiol.* 43, 133–137, 1977.

[23] Stephenson L.A. and Kolka M.A. Menstrual cycle phase and time of day alter reference signal controlling arm blood flow and sweating. *Am. J. Physiol.* 249, R186–R192, 1985.

[24] Aoki K., Stephens D.P., and Johnson J.M. Diurnal variations in cutaneous vasodilator and vasoconstrictor systems during heat stress. *Am. J. Physiol. Regul. Integr. Comp. Physiol.* 281, R591–R595, 2001.

[25] Rodie I.C., Shepard J.T., and Whelan R.F. Evidence from venous oxygen saturation that the increase in arm blood flow during body heating is confined to the skin *J. Physiol.* 134, 444–450, 1956.

[26] Gaskell P. Are there sympathetic vasodilator nerves in the vessels of the hands? *J. Physiol.* 131, 647–656, 1956.

[27] Fox R.H. and Edholm O.G. Nervous control of the cutaneous circulation. *J. Appl. Physiol.* 57, 1688–1695, 1984.

[28] Ring E.E.J. Cold stress testing in the hand. In *The Thermal Image in Medicine and Biology.* Ammer K. and Ring E.E.J. (eds), Wein, Uhlen-Verlag, pp. 237–240, 1995.

[29] Pascoe D., Purohit R., Shanley L.A., and Herrick R.T. Pre and post operative thermographic evaluations of CTS. In *The Thermal Image in Medicine and Biology.* Ammer K. and Ring E.E.J. (eds), Wein, Uhlen-Verlag, pp. 188–190, 1995.

[30] Faithfull N.S., Reinhold P.R., van den Berg A.P., van Roon G.C., Van der Zee J., and Wike-Hooley J.L. Cardiovascular challenges during whole body hyperthermia treatment of advanced malignancy. *Eur. J. Appl. Physiol.* 53, 274–281, 1984.

[31] Finberg J.P.M., Katz M., Gazit H., and Berlyne G.M. Plasma rennin activity after acute heat exposure in non-acclimatized and naturally acclimatized man. *J. Appl. Physiol.* 36, 519–523, 1974.

[32] Carlsen A., Gustafson A., and Werko L. Hemodynamic influence of warm and dry environment in man with and without rheumatic heart disease. *Acta Med. Scand.* 169, 411–417, 1961.

[33] Damato A.N., Lau S.H., Stein E., Haft J.I., Kosowsky B., and Cohen S.J. Cardiovascular response to acute thermal stress (hot dry environment) in unacclimatized normal subjects. *Am. Heart J.* 76, 769–774, 1968.

[34] Sancetta S.M., Kramer J., and Husni E. The effects of "dry" heat on the circulation of man. I. General hemodynamics. *Am. Heart J.* 56, 212–221, 1958.

[35] Crandall C.G., Johnson J.M., Kosiba W.A., and Kellogg D.L. Jr. Baroreceptor control of the cutaneous active vasodilator system. *J. Appl. Physiol.* 81, 2192–2198, 1996.

[36] Kellogg D.L. Jr, Johnson J.M., and Kosiba, W.A. Baroreflex control of the cutaneous active vasodilator system in humans. *Cir. Res.* 66, 1420–1426, 1990.

[37] Chato J.C. A view of the history of heat transfer in bioengineering. In *Advances in Heat Transfer.* Cho Y.J. (ed.), Academic Press, Inc./Harcourt Brace Jovanovich Publishers, Boston, Vol. 22, pp. 1–19, May 1981.

[38] Chen M.M. and Holmes K.R. Microvascular contributions in tissue heat transfer. In *Thermal Characteristics of Tumors: Applications in Detection and Treatment.* Jain R.K. and Guillino P.M. (eds), *Ann. N.Y. Acad. Sci.* 335, 137, 1980.

[39] Baish J.W. Microvascular heat transfer. In *The Biomedical Engineering Handbook.* Bronzino J.D. (ed.), Boca Raton, FL, CRC Press/IEEE Press, Vol. 2, 98, pp. 1–14, 2000.

[40] Hille B. Membranes and ions: introduction to physiology of excitable cells. In *Textbook of Physiology.* Patton H.D., Fuchs A.F., Hille B., Scher A.M. and Steiner R. (eds), Philadelphia, W.B. Saunders Co., pp. 2–4, 1989.

[41] Taylor G.I. and Tempest M.N. (eds), *Michael Salmon: Arteries of the Skin.* London, Churchill Livingstone, 1988.

[42] He S. and Walls A.F. Human mast cell trypase: a stimulus of micorvascular leakage and mast cell activation. *Eur. J. Pharmacol.* 328, 89–97, 1997.

[43] Kalmolz L.P., Haslik A.H., Donner A., Winter W., Meissl G., and Frey M. Indocyanine green video angiographics help identify burns requiring operating. *Burns* 29, 785–791, 2003.

[44] Flock S.T. and Jacques S.L. Thermal damage of blood vessels in a rat skin-flap window chamber using indocyanine green and pulsated alexandrite laser: a feasibility study. *Lasers Med. Sci.* 8, 185–196, 1993.

[45] Ryan T.J., Jolles B., and Holti G. *Methods in Microcirculation Studies.* London, HK Lewis and Co., Ltd, 1972.

[46] Olsen B.W. How many sites are necessary to estimate a mean skin temperature? In *Thermal Physiology.* Hales J.R.S. (ed.), New York, Raven Press, pp. 33–38, 1984.

7
Quantitative Active Dynamic Thermal IR-Imaging and Thermal Tomography in Medical Diagnostics

7.1	Introduction...	7-1
	Thermal Tomography	
7.2	Thermal Properties of Biological Tissues	7-3
7.3	Thermal Models and Equivalent/Synthetic Parameters	7-7
7.4	Measurement Procedures	7-8
7.5	Measurement Equipment	7-11
7.6	Procedures of Data and Image Processing	7-12
	Pulsed Thermography • Active Dynamic Thermal IR-Imaging • Pulse Phase Thermography • Thermal Tomography	
7.7	Experiments and Applications	7-17
	Organization of Experiments • Results and Discussion • Skin Burns • Clinics • Cardiac Surgery • Clinics	
7.8	Conclusions	7-25
	Acknowledgments...	7-27
	References	7-27

Antoni Nowakowski
Gdansk University of Technology

7.1 Introduction

Static infrared (IR) thermal imaging has a number of attractive properties for its practical applications in industry and medicine. The technique is noninvasive and harmless as there is no direct contact of the diagnostic tool to an object under test, the data acquisition is simple and the equipment is transportable and well adapted to mass screening applications. There are also some fundamental limitations concerning this technique. Only processes characterized by changes in temperature distribution on external surfaces directly accessible by an IR-camera can be observed. The absolute value of temperature measurement is usually not very accurate due to generally limited knowledge of the emission coefficient. Many harmful processes are not inducting any changes in surface temperature, for example, in industrial applications material corrosion or cracks are usually not visible in IR thermographs, in medicine in mammography inspection a cyst may mask cancer, etc. For such cases active dynamic thermal imaging methods with sources of external excitations are helpful. Therefore the nondestructive evaluation (NDE) of materials using active dynamic thermal IR-imaging is extensively studied; see, for example, proceedings of QIRT [1]. The method is already well developed in some of industrial applications but in medicine this technique is almost unknown.

Active dynamic thermal (ADT) IR-imaging, known in industry either as *infrared-nondestructive testing* (IR-NDT), or as thermographic nondestructive testing (TNDT or just NDT), is under intensive development during at least the last 20 years [1,2]. The concept of material testing by active thermography is based on delivery of external energy to a specimen and observation of the thermal response. In ADT imaging only thermal transients are studied. Such approach allows visualization of material subsurface abnormalities or failures and has already gained high recognition in technical applications [1,2]. In medicine it was applied probably for the first time also around 20 years ago [3,4]. Microwave excitation was applied to evidence breast cancer. Unfortunately, after early experiments the research was suspended, probably due to poor control of microwave energy dissipation. Again some proposals to use ADT in medicine have been published at the end of the last years of the twentieth century [5–7].

The visualization of affected regions needs some extra efforts therefore the role and practical importance of the use of synthetic pictures in ADT for medical applications should be underlined [8–10]. In this case equivalent thermal model parameters are defined and calculated for objective quantitative data visualization and evaluation.

Potential role of medical applications of ADT is clearly visible from experiments on phantoms, and *in vivo* on animals as well as in clinical applications [11,12].

7.1.1 Thermal Tomography

Another concept based on ADT is *thermal tomography* (TT). Vavilow et al. [13–15] dealing with IR-NDTs, proposed this term almost 20 years ago. Even today, the concept is not new this modality may be regarded as being still at the early development stage in technical applications, especially taking into account the limited number of practical applications published up to now. The first proposals to apply the concept of thermal tomography in medicine are just under intensive development in the Department of Biomedical Engineering TUG [16–18]. The main differences comparing TT to simple ADT arise due to necessity of advanced reconstruction procedures applied for determination of internal structure of tested objects.

Tomography is known in medical diagnostics as the most advanced technology for visualization of tested object internal structures. X-rays—CT (computed tomography), NMR—MRI (nuclear magnetic resonance imaging), US—ultrasound imaging, SPECT (single-photon emission computed tomography), PET (positron-emission tomography) are the modalities of already established position in medical diagnostics. There are three additional tomography modalities, still in the phase of intensive research and development—optical tomography (OT), electroimpedance tomography (EIT), and TT. Here we concentrate our notice on ADT and TT. The aim of this chapter is discussion of potential applications of the both modalities in medical diagnostics and analysis of existing limitations.

General concept of tomography requires collection of data received in so-called projections—measurements performed for a specific direction of applied excitation; data from all projections form a scan. Having a model of a tested object the inverse problem is solved showing internal structure of the object. In the oldest tomographic modality—CT—the measurement procedure requires irradiation of a tested object from different directions (projections), all possible projections giving one scan. Then, basing on realistic model of a tested object, a reconstruction procedure based on solving the inverse problem allows visualization of external structure of the object. In early systems, a 2D picture of internal organs was shown; nowadays more complex acquisition systems allow visualization of 3D cases. More or less similar procedures are applied in all other tomography modalities, including TT, OT, and EIT. The main advantages of TT, OT, and EIT technologies are fully safe interaction with tested objects (organisms) and relatively low cost of instrumentation.

The concept and problems of validity in medical diagnostics of ADT imaging as well as of TT are here discussed. In both cases practically the same instrumentation is applied and only the data treatment and object reconstruction differs. Also, the sources of errors influencing quality of measurements and limiting accuracy of reconstruction data are the same. Main limitations are due to the necessity of using proper thermal models of living tissues, which are influenced by physiological processes from one side and are not very accurate due to hardly controlled experiment conditions from the other side.

The main element allowing quantitative evaluation of tested objects is the use of realistic thermal equivalent models. The measurement procedure requires use of heat sources, which should be applied to the object under test (OUT). Thermal response at the surface of OUT to external excitation is recorded using IR-camera. Usually the natural recovery to initial conditions gives reliable data for further analysis. The dynamic response recorded as a series of IR pictures allows reconstruction of properties of the OUT equivalent thermal model. Either thermal properties of the model elements (for defined structure of OUT) or the internal structure (for known material thermal properties) may be determined and recognized. The main problem is correlation of thermal and physiological properties of living tissues, which may strongly differ for *ex vivo* and *in vivo* data. Practical measurement results from phantoms and *in vivo* animal experiments as well as from clinical applications of ADT performed in the Department of Biomedical Engineering Gdansk University of Technology (TUG), Poland and in co-operating clinics of the Medical University of Gdansk are taken into account for illustration of this chapter. The studies in this field are concentrated on applications of burns, skin transplants, cancer visualization, and open-heart surgery, evaluation and diagnostics [19–26].

In following subchapters all elements of the ADT and TT procedures are described. First, thermal tissue properties are defined. Then basic elements of thermal model construction are described. Following is description of the experiment of active dynamic thermography based on OUT excitation (pulse) and infrared recording. Finally the procedures of model identification are described basing on phantom and *in vivo* experiments. Some clinical applications illustrate practical value of the described modalities.

7.2 Thermal Properties of Biological Tissues

What is the basic difference between IR-thermography (IRT) and ADT and TT?

In IRT, main information is the absolute value of temperature, T, and distribution of thermal fields, $T(x, y)$. Therefore regions of high temperature (hot spots) or low temperature (cold spots) are determined giving usually data of important diagnostic value. Unfortunately the accuracy of temperature measurements is limited. It is mainly due to limited accuracy of IR-cameras; due to limited knowledge of the emission coefficient, as individual features of living tissues may be strongly diversified; finally due to hardly controlled conditions of the environment, what may strongly influence temperature distribution at the surface and its absolute values. Additionally surface temperature does not always properly reflects complicated processes, which may exist underneath or in the tissue bulk or which may be masked by fat or other biological structures.

In ADT and TT basic thermal properties of tissues are quantitatively determined; the absolute value of temperature practically is not interesting. Only thermal flows are important. We ask the question—how fast are thermal processes? In ADT, specific equivalent parameters are defined and visualized. In TT directly either spatial distribution of thermal conductivity is of major importance or for known tissue properties the geometry of the structure is determined.

Basic thermal properties (Figures of Merit) of materials and tissues important in ADT and in TT are following:

- k—Thermal conductivity—(W m^{-1} K^{-1}), it describes ability of a material (tissue) to conduct heat in the steady state conditions
- c_p—Specific heat—(J kg^{-1} K^{-1}), describes ability of a material to store the heat energy. It is defined by the amount of heat energy necessary to raise the temperature of a unit mass by 1 K
- ρ—Density of material—(kg m^{-3})
- ρc_p—Volumetric specific heat—(J m^{-3} K^{-1})
- α—Thermal diffusivity—(m^2 sec^{-1}); is defined as

$$\alpha = \frac{k}{\rho \cdot c_p} \tag{7.1}$$

Volumetric specific heat and thermal conductivity are responsible for thermal transients described by the equation

$$\frac{\partial T}{\partial t} = \alpha \nabla^2 T \tag{7.2}$$

For one directional heat flow (what describes the case of infinite plate structures composed of uniform layers and uniformly excited at the surface) this may be rewritten in the form:

$$\frac{\partial T}{\partial t} = \frac{k}{\rho \cdot c_p} \cdot \frac{\partial^2 T}{\partial x^2} \tag{7.3}$$

Thermal diffusivity describes heat flow and is equivalent to the reciprocal of the time constant τ describing the electrical RC circuit:

$$\alpha = \frac{k}{\rho \cdot c_p} \leftrightarrow \frac{1}{\tau} = \frac{1}{RC} \tag{7.4}$$

Basing on this analogy, materials are frequently described by equivalent thermal model composed of thermal resistivity R_{th} and thermal capacity C_{th}, which are responsible for the value of the thermal time constant, τ_{th},

$$\tau_{th} = R_{th} C_{th} \tag{7.5}$$

Those are the most frequently used equivalent parameters. Determination of such parameters is easy basing on measurements of thermal transients and using fitting procedures for determination of the applied model parameters.

Additionally one may define thermal inertia as $k \cdot \rho \cdot c_p$.

Useful may be also introducing the definition of thermal effusivity β, defined as the root-square of the thermal inertia—(J m^{-2} K^{-1} sec$^{-1/2}$) or (W sec$^{1/2}$ m^{-2} K^{-1}).

$$\beta^2 = k \cdot \rho \cdot c_p \tag{7.6}$$

Importance of IRT and ADT/TT in medical diagnostics is complementary. Regions of abnormal vascularization are detected in IRT as *hot spots* in the cases of intensive metabolic processes or as *cold spots* for regions of affected vascularization or necrosis. The same places may represent higher or lower thermal conductivity, but this is not a rule. Thermal properties of tissues may differ significantly depending on the vascularization, physical structure, water content, and so on. Knowledge of thermal properties and geometry of tested objects may be used in medical diagnostics if correlation of thermal properties and specific physiological features are known. Important is character of the data allowing objective quantitative description of tissues or organs.

The main advantage of thermal tissue parameter characterization comparing to absolute temperature measurements is relatively low dependence on external conditions, for example, ambient temperature, what usually is of a great importance in IRT. The main disadvantage is still limited knowledge of thermal tissue properties and very complicated structure of biological organs. Although the first results of thermal tissue properties have been published at the end of nineteenth century, the main data, still broadly cited, were collected around 30 years ago [27–30]. Unfortunately, literature data of thermal tissue properties should be treated as not very reliable, because measurement conditions are not always known [31], *in vivo* and *ex vivo* data are mixed, etc. Table 7.1 illustrates this problem. Detailed description of measurement methods of biological tissue thermal parameters is given in References 18, 31, and 32.

In Table 7.2 basic thermal tissue properties—mean values of data given by different studies and for different tissues taken *in vitro* at 37°C—are collected [18].

It has to be underlined that thermal tissue properties are temperature dependent (typically around 0.2–1 %/°C). In most of ADT and TT measurements this effect may be neglected as being not significant for data interpretation, as possible temperature differences are usually limited. The differences of temperature in *in vivo* experiments may be usually neglected as not important at all. Also there is a strong influence of water content and blood perfusion, see, for example, results of Valvano et al., 1985 in Reference 33. Usually effective thermal conductivity and diffusivity are applied to overcome this problem in modeling of thermal processes. Additionally, in subtle analysis one should remember that some tissues might be anisotropic [18,31].

For mixture of N substances, each characterized by thermal conductivity $k_1, \ldots, k_N$, the effective thermal conductivity is the mean value of the volumetric content of components:

$$k_{tk} = \frac{\sum_{i=1}^{N} k_i \cdot V_i}{\sum_{i=1}^{N} V_i} = \rho_{tk} \sum_{i=1}^{N} k_i \frac{m_i}{m_{tk}} \cdot \frac{1}{\rho_i} \qquad (7.7)$$

where the index tk concerns all tissue, and the index i—ith component. Analogically, one may calculate effective specific heat either as the mean value of mass components

$$c_{wtk} = \frac{\sum_{i=1}^{N} c_{wi} \cdot m_i}{\sum_{i=1}^{N} m_i} \qquad (7.8)$$

TABLE 7.1 Thermal Properties of Muscle Tissue

Muscle	Conditions	Author	Thermal conductivity (W m^{-1} K^{-1})	Diffusivity (m^2 sec^{-1})
Heart	37°C	Bowman (1981)	0.492–0.562	No data
Heart	37°C	Valvano et al. (1985)	0.537	1.47×10^{-7}
Heart	5–20°C	Cooper, Trezek (1972)	No data	1.41–1.57×10^{-7}
Heart (dog)	*In vivo*	Chen et al. (1981)	0.49	No data
Heart (dog)	37°C	Valvano et al. (1985)	0.536	1.51×10^{-7}
Heart (dog)	21°C	Bowman et al. (1974)	No data	1.47–1.55×10^{-7}
Heart (swine)	38°C	Valvano et al. (1986)	0.533	No data
Skeletal	37°C	Bowman (1981)	0.449-0,546	No data
Skeletal (dog)	No data	Bowman et al. (1974)	No data	1.83×10^{-7}
Skeletal (cow)	30°C	Cherneeva (1956)	No data	1.25×10^{-7}
Skeletal (cow)	24–38°C	Poppendiek (1966)	0.528	No data
Skeletal (swine)	30°C	Cherneeva (1956)	No data	1.25×10^{-7}
Skeletal (ship)	21°C	Balasubramaniam, Bowman (1977)	No data	1.51–1.67×10^{-7}

TABLE 7.2 Mean Values of Thermal Tissue Properties Taken *In Vitro*

Parameter unit of measure symbol	Density (kg m^{-3}) ρ	Thermal conductivity [W/(m K)] k	Specific heat [J/(kg K)] c	Volumetric specific heat [J/(m^3 K)] $\rho \cdot c \, (\times 10^6)$	Diffusivity (m^2 sec^{-1}) $\alpha \, (\times 10^{-7})$	Effusivity [J/(m^2 K sec$^{1/2}$)] β
Soft tissues						
Heart muscle	1060	0.49–0.56	3720	3.94	1.24–1.42	1390–1490
Skeletal muscle	1045	0.45–0.55	3750	3.92	1.15–1.4	1330–1470
Brain	1035	0.50–0.58	3650	3.78	1.32–1.54	1375–1480
Kidney	1050	0.51	3700	3.89	1.31	1410
Liver	1060	0.53	3500	3.71	1.27–1.43	1320–1400
Lung	1050	0.30–0.55	3100	3.26	0.92–1.69	990–1340
Eye	1020	0.59	4200	4.28	1.38	1590
Skin superficial layer	1150	0.27	3600	4.14	0.65	1060
Fat under skin	920	0.22	2600	2.39	0.92	725
Hard tissues						
Tooth-enamel	3000	0.9	720	2.16	4.17	1400
Tooth-dentine	2200	0.45	1300	2.86	1.57	1130
Cancellous bone	1990	0.4	1330	2.65	1.4–1.89	990–1150
Trabecular bone	1920	0.3	2100	4.03	0.92–1.26	1220–1430
Marrow	1000	0.22	2700	2.70	0.82	770
Fluids						
Blood; 44% HCT	1060	0.49	3600	3.82	1.28	1370
Plasma	1027	0.58	3900	4.01	1.45	1520

Source: From Hryciuk M., Ph.D. Dissertation—Investigation of layered biological object structure using thermal excitation (in Polish), *Politechnika Gdanska*, 2003. Shitzer A. and Eberhart R.C., *Heat Transfer in Medicine and Biology*, Plenum Press, 1985.

TABLE 7.3 Thermal Properties for the Equivalent Three-Component Model

Quantity unit	Density [kg/m^3]	Thermal conductivity [W/(m K)] K		Specific heat [J/(kg K)]	Specific heat (volumetric) [J/(m^{3}K)]
Symbol	ρ	see Reference 28		c_w	$\rho \cdot c_w \, (\times 10^6)$
Water	1000	0.628	0.6	4200	4.2
Fat	815	0.231	0.22	2300	1.87
Proteins	1540	0.117	0.195	1090	1.68

Source: From Marks R.M. and Bartan S.P., *The Physical Nature of the Skin*, MTP Press, Boston, 1998.

or as the mean value of volumetric components

$$\rho_{tk} c_{wtk} = \frac{\sum_{i=1}^{N} \rho_i c_{wi} \cdot V_i}{\sum_{i=1}^{N} V_i} \tag{7.9}$$

Marks and Burton [34] propose a thermal model, composed of three components—water, fat, and proteins—using the values collected in the Table 7.3. Though, it was suggested that more realistic values of thermal conductivity are given by Bowman [18,28].

7.3 Thermal Models and Equivalent/Synthetic Parameters

Basic analysis of existing thermal processes in correlation with physiological processes is necessary to understand significance of thermal flows in medical diagnostics. Thermal models are very useful to study such problems. It should be underlined that ADT and TT are based on analysis of thermal models of tested objects. Solution of the so-called direct problem while external excitation (determination of temperature distribution in time and space for assumed boundary conditions and known model parameters) involves simulation of temperature distribution in defined object under test. It allows study on thermal tomography concept, simulation of heat exchange and flows using optimal excitation methods, analysis of theoretical, and practical limitations of proposed methods, etc.

Direct problems may be properly solved only for realistic thermal models. Having such a model, one can compare the results of experiments and can try to solve the reverse problem. This responds to the question—what is the distribution of thermal properties in the internal structure of a human body? Such knowledge may be directly used in clinical diagnostics if the correlation of thermal and physiological properties is high.

In biologic applications solution of the direct problem is basic to see relationship between excitation and temperature distribution at the surface of a tested object, what is a measurable quantity. This requires solution of the heat flow in 3D space. Equation 7.10, representing the general parabolic heat flow [35] describes this problem mathematically:

$$\text{div}(k \cdot \text{grad} T) - c_p \rho \frac{\partial T}{\partial t} = -q(P, t) \tag{7.10}$$

where T is the temperature in K; k the thermal conductivity in W m^{-1} K^{-1}, c_p the specific heat in J g^{-1} K^{-1}; ρ the material (tissue) density in g m^{-3}, t the time in sec, and $q(P, t)$ is the volumetric density of generating or dissipated power in W m^{-3}. For biologic tissues Pennes [36] defined "the biologic heat flow equation":

$$c_p \rho \frac{\partial T(x, y, z, t)}{\partial t} = k \nabla^2 T(x, y, z, t) + q_b + q_m + q_{ex} \tag{7.11}$$

where $T(x, y, z, t)$ is the temperature distribution at the moment t, q_b (W/m^3) the heat power density delivered or dissipated by blood, q_m the heat power density delivered by metabolism, and q_{ex} is the heat power density delivered by external sources. Solving of this equation, including all processes influencing tissue temperature, is very complicated and analytically even impossible. Generally there are three approaches in analysis and solving of heat transfers and distribution of temperature.

The first one is analytic, usually very simplified description of an object, typically using the Fourier series method. Analytical solutions of heat flows are known only for very simple structures of well-defined shapes, what usually is not the case acceptable for analysis of biological objects. The simplest solution assumes one directional flow of energy, as it is for multilayer, infinite structures, thermally uniformly excited. Distribution of temperature, if several sources exist, may be solved assuming the superposition method.

The second option is the use numerical methods, usually based on finite element method (FEM); to model more complicated structures. There are several commercial software packages broadly known and used for solving problems of heat flows, usually combining a mechanical part, including generator of a model mesh as well as modules solving specific thermal problems, for example References 37 and 38. Also general mathematical programs, as Matlab [39] or Mathematica [40], contain proper tools allowing thermal analysis. FEM methods allow solution of 3D heat flow problems in time. Functional variability of thermal properties and nonlinear parametric description of tested objects may be easy taken into consideration. Again, there are basic limitations concerning the dimension of a problem to be solved (complexity and number of model elements), which should be taken into account from the point of view of the computational costs.

The solution of the Equations 7.10 and 7.11 may be given in the explicit form:

$$T_n^{i+1} = \frac{\Delta t}{\rho c_p V_n}\left[\sum_m k_{nm} T_m^i + \left(\frac{\rho c_w V_n}{\Delta t} - \sum_m k_{nm} T_m^i\right) + q_n V_n\right] \quad (7.12)$$

or in the implicit form:

$$T_n^{i+1} - T_n^i = \frac{\Delta t}{\rho c_p V_n}\left[\sum_m k_{nm}\left(T_m^{i+1} - T_n^i\right) + q_n V_n\right] \quad (7.13)$$

where i indicates moment of time, Δt is the time step, n the position in space (node number), V_n the volume of the n node, m indicates neighboring nodes, k_{nm} is thermal conductivity between the nodes n and m, T_n^i the temperature of a node at the beginning of a time step, T_n^{i+1} the temperature of a node at the end of the time step, and q_n is the power density representing generation of heat per unit volume at the nth node. Each node represents a specific part of the modeled structure defined by mass, dimensions, and physical properties. The node is assumed to be thermally uniform and isotropic. Boundary conditions may be assumed discretional, depending on real conditions of experiments to be performed (under analysis). Usually adiabatic or isothermic conditions and a value of excitation power are assumed. The boundary conditions, the value of excitation power as well as individual properties of any node may be modified with time!

In the explicit method the temperature of each node is determined at the end of the time step, taking into account the heat balance based on temperature, heat generation, and thermal properties at the beginning of the time step. Assuming neither proper time step nor model geometry may effect in lack of stable solution or poor accuracy of analysis.

In the implicit method, the increase of temperature in each node is calculated from the heat balance resulting from temperatures, heat generation, and thermal properties during the time step. The solution is stable. The duration of a time step may be modified in the adaptation procedure assuming several conditions, for example, maximum rise of temperature in any of nodes. Increase of iteration steps followed by the need of many possible modifications of parameters during iterations may lead to unacceptable rise of the computation time. Still, the mesh geometry may influence accuracy of analysis.

The numerical modeling is preferable in cases where solution of the direct problem may be sufficient, for example, in analysis of methods of investigation, because it allows easy and accurate modifications of important factors influencing measurements. The forward problem may be solved for any configuration of mesh and tissue as well as excitation parameters. Unfortunately, limited knowledge of living tissue properties is reducing possibility of using simulation methods for reliable *in vivo* case analysis.

The third approach is to build simple equivalent models of tested tissues or organs based on such synthetic parameters as thermal resistivity (conductivity) and thermal capacity. This solution, as the simplest one, seems to be the most useful practically. A medical doctor may accept relatively simple, still reliable description, based on synthetic parameters easily determined for such simple models. As an example, thermal structure of the skin may be represented by three equivalent layers described by the $R_{th}(1-3)C_{th}(1-3)$ model. Values of such simple model parameters may be relatively easily determined from experimental data using fitting procedures and well correlated to physical phenomena, for example, depth of burns. This is also probably the easiest method to be applied for solving the inverse problem and therefore the best offer for modern computer technology based diagnostic tools. Also, correlation of model parameters coefficients is not as complicated as in the case of the FEM approach.

7.4 Measurement Procedures

Study of heat transfer enables quantification of thermo-physical material properties such as thermal diffusivity or conductivity and finally detection of subsurface defects. The main drawback of thermal measurement methods is limitation in number of contact sensors distributed within a tested object or

IR-Imaging and Thermal Tomography in Medical Diagnostics

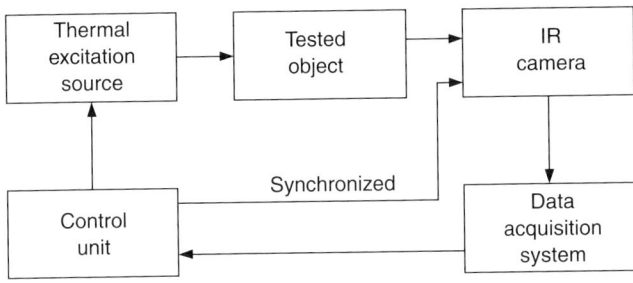

FIGURE 7.1 Schematic diagram of ADT and TT instrumentation.

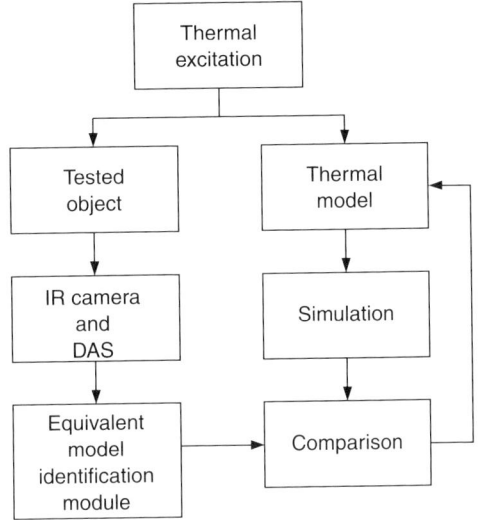

FIGURE 7.2 Model-based identification of a tested structure (object).

application of IR-methods of temperature measurements, allowing observation of the surface temperature distribution only, what in both cases results in limited accuracy of analysis.

The ADT and TT are based on IR technology. The general concept of measurements performed in such applications is shown in Figure 7.1. External thermal excitation source (heating or cooling) is applied to a tested object (TO). First, steady state temperature distribution on TO surface is registered using the IR-camera. The next step requires thermal excitation application, and registration of temperature transients on the TO surface. The control unit synchronizes the processes of excitation and registration. All data are stored in the data acquisition system (DAS) for further computer analysis.

To allow quantitative evaluation of TO properties, the procedures of both, ADT and TT, are based on determination of thermal models of TO. Typical procedure of model parameter estimation is shown in Figure 7.2. For the measurement structure shown in Figure 7.1 an equivalent model of TO must be assumed (developed and applied in the procedure). In this case usually a simple model, for example, the three layers $R_{th}(1-3)C_{th}(1-3)$, is applied. Thermal excitation (from a physical source as well as simulated for the assumed model), applied simultaneously to TO and to its model, results in thermal transients, registered at the surface of TO by the IR-camera (applied and simulated for the model). For each pixel, the registered temperature course is identified (typically the least square approximation—LSA and exponential model for thermal transients are applied). The result (measured thermal course) is compared with the simulated transient and if necessary the thermal model is modified to fit to experimental results.

The registration process is illustrated in Figure 7.3. An example for a pulse excitation and registration of temperature only during the recovery phase (in this case—cooling, after heating excitation) is shown.

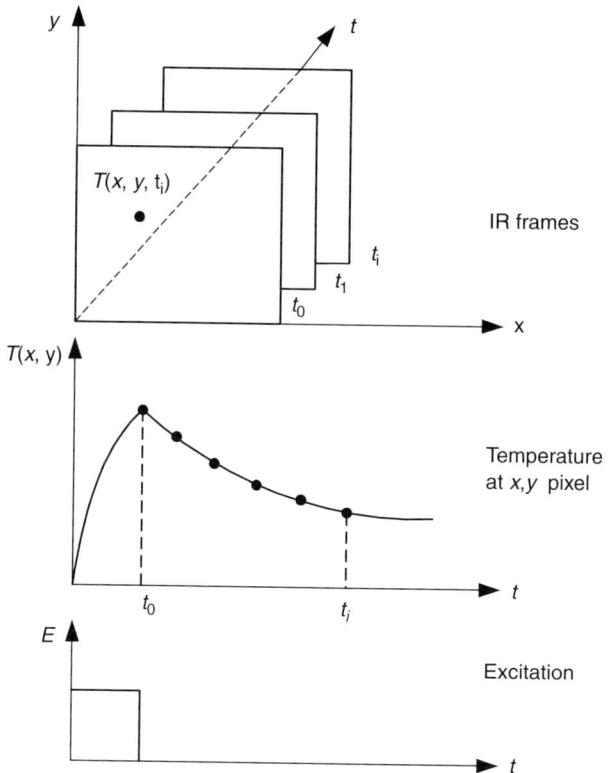

FIGURE 7.3 Registration procedure—after thermal excitation (here heating), a series of IR frames are recorded in controlled moments, starting just at the moment of switching the excitation off; temperature of each pixel is recorded to calculate time constants specific in each pixel.

This is a typical case of practical measurements using optical excitation. Each pixel showing the temperature distribution at the TO surface is represented by an equivalent model, therefore single excitation and registration of transient temperatures at the position x, y allows identification of the structure *in depth*, resulting in 3D picture of TO.

There are several procedures of nondestructive evaluation of defects by observation of temperature changes of an inspected sample surface using IR-imaging [2]:

1. Continuous heating of a tested object and observation of surface temperature changes during thermal stimulation (step heating, long pulse); the main drawback of the method is limited possibility of quantitative measurements. The information may be similar to classical static thermography with enhancement of specific defects.
2. Sinusoidal heating and synchronized observation of temperature distribution during stimulation (lock-in technique); this is the most accurate NDT–ADT method but not practical in medical applications as the experiment is rather difficult and time consuming.
3. Pulse excitation (e.g., heating using optical excitation, air fan for cooling, etc.) and observation during the heating and/or the cooling phases. Several procedures are possible, as pulsed ADT, multi-frequency binary sequences (MFBS) technique, pulse phase thermography (PPT), and other. The description in the following text is concentrating on a single pulse excitation, because this experiment is relatively simple, fast and of accuracy acceptable in medical applications. The time of excitation may be set short enough to eliminate biofeedback interactions, which are otherwise difficult in interpretation.

7.5 Measurement Equipment

Typical measurement set is shown in Figure 7.4. The main elements of the set are shown: an IR-camera; a fast data acquisition system; a set of excitation sources with a synchronized driving unit.

The better are the camera properties the higher accuracy measurements are possible, what is a condition for proper reconstruction of thermal properties of TO. Minimal technical requirements for an IR-camera are: repetition rate 30 frames/sec; MRTD better than $0.1°C$; LW—long wavelengths range preferable; FOV dependent on application—typically in clinical conditions measurements taken from around 1 m distance to a patient are advisable. Still application of a cooled FPA camera with higher registration speed and better MRTD would be advisable. SW cameras may be used for other than optical excitations or for analysis of the recovery phase only (time when the excitation is switched off).

Very important is the use of proper excitation sources. Application of optical halogen lamps, laser sources, microwave applicators, even ultrasound generators for heating and air fans or cold sprays for cooling, and some other has been noted [41–44]. As a heating source, an optical or IR lamp, a laser beam, a microwave generator, or an ultrasonic generator can be used. Electromagnetic or mechanical irradiation generated by a source (usually distant) is illuminating a tested object and generating a heating wave proportional to the irradiation energy and to the absorption rate, specific for a tested object material and varying with wavelength of excitation. Microwave irradiation, ultrasonic excitation or electric current flow might generate heat inside a specimen proportional to its dielectric or mechanical properties. For the microwave excitation the main role in the heating process plays the electrical conductivity of a tested object. For the ultrasonic excitation the thermo-elastic effect and mechanical hysteresis are responsible for temperature changes proportional to the applied stress tensor. For the optical irradiation the absorption coefficient is describing the rate of energy converted into heat.

In ADT, the basic information is connected with time dependent reaction of tested structures therefore it is very important to know the switching properties of the heating or cooling sources, especially the raising and the falling time of generated pulses. Dynamic properties of heating or cooling sources must be taken into account during modeling the different shapes of excitation. Some extra measures should be practically adopted, for example, to avoid the interaction between a lamp, which is self-heated during experiments, and a tested object; sometimes a special shutter is needed to assure proper shape of a heating signal. For microwave excitation the applicator must be directly connected to a tested object therefore a time for mechanical removing of an applicator from the heated object to allow thermographic observation is additionally needed what practically eliminates application of such sources in medical applications.

FIGURE 7.4 Measurement set—tested object is exposed to external thermal excitation; the IR-camera, synchronically with excitation records, surface temperature distribution in time.

TABLE 7.4 Wavelengths and Penetration Depths of the Microwave Source 2.45 GHz for Typical Tissue with Low and High Water Content

Water content	λ—In air (cm)	λ—In tissue (cm)	σ—Tissue conductivity (S/m)	Penetration depth (cm)
High (muscle, skin)	12.2	1.76	2.21	1.70
Low (fat, bones)	12.2	5.21	0.96–2.13	11.2

Source: From Duek A.F., *Physical Properties of Tissue*, Academic Press, London, 1990.

There are several conclusions regarding application of different sources of thermal excitation:

1. We are dealing with biological objects; therefore heating should be limited to a safe level, not exceeding 42°C; while cooling temperature of a living tissue should not be lower than 4°C.
2. Thermal excitation should be as uniform as possible; nonuniform excitation results in decrease of accuracy and misinterpretation of measurement data. It is relatively easy to fulfil this condition for optical excitation but very difficult for ultrasonic or microwave methods, even using specially developed applicators.
3. The other important factor is the depth of heat penetration. For different sources of excitation the energy penetration can vary from superficial only absorption to millimeters for some laser beams or even up to a few centimeters for microwave excitation. Ultrasounds are not applicable for biological tissues but of rigid structures only. As an example the data concerning microwave penetration are shown in the Table 7.4. High heat penetration may be very interesting for discrimination of deep regions; unfortunately control of microwave energy absorption practically is impossible being dependent on tissue electrical properties. This feature makes the use of microwave sources in medical applications very problematic.
4. Temperature interactions should be limited to periods not affected by biological feedback; additionally to assure proper data treatment special care should be devoted to fast switching the excitation power on and off. For optical sources mechanical shutters are advisable, as electrical switching is effective in the visible range but also other elements as, for example, housing may be heated to a level influencing sensitive IR-camera.
5. Noncontact methods, as optical, seem to be especially appreciated, as septic conditions are easy to be secured.
6. Concluding—optical excitation for heating and air fan for cooling seem to be the best options for daily practice in medical diagnostics.

Even ADT is not so sensitive to external conditions as the classical IRT still there are several conditions to be assured. Generally, patients should be prepared for experiments and all "golden standards" valid for classical thermography here should be also applied [46].

7.6 Procedures of Data and Image Processing

Depending on the method of excitation several procedures may be adopted to process the measurement data and then to extract diagnostic information. Here we concentrate only on pulse excitation as is at it is shown in Figure 7.3. Measurements of transients during the heating and the cooling phases allow further use of procedures developed for pulsed thermography (PT), ADT IR-imaging, pulse phase thermography (PPT), and TT. In all four cases, excitation and registration of thermal transients is performed in the same way using IR-camera. Visualization data differ as it is expressed respectively by thermal contrast images in PT; thermal time constants in ADT and phase shift images in PPT, finally thermal conductivity distribution in TT.

7.6.1 Pulsed Thermography

Pulsed thermography applies calculation of *the maximal thermal contrast index*—$C(t)$ [2].

$$C(t) = \frac{T_d(t) - T_d(0)}{T_s(t) - T_s(0)} \qquad (7.14)$$

where T is the temperature, t the time; for $t = 0$ the sample temperature is maximal, d, s are the subscripts indicating the defect and the sample. With given number of temperature images acquired during PT, the thermal contrast image may be expressed also as

$$C(x, y, t) = \frac{T(x, y, t) - T(x_0, y_0, t)}{T(x_0, y_0, t)} \qquad (7.15)$$

where x, y is the pixel coordinates and x_0, y_0 the pixel coordinates of the reference point in the chosen defect area.

To calculate contrast images, a defect template or a reference point should be defined. In medical applications, it is almost impossible to indicate such templates therefore to overcome this limitation estimation of the behavior of living tissues in PT conditions is possible. As an example, heat transfer caused by blood flow is different in normal and affected (e.g., cancerous) tissues. During the heating process the affected tissues usually are heated more than the normal tissues, what is caused by reduced thermoregulation. Further image processing (segmentation) allows discrimination of so-called *hot spots* and *cold spots* images. Another possibility is to define *the normalized differential PT index* (NDPTI) [47]:

$$\text{NDPTI}(x, y, t) = \frac{T(x, y, 0) - T(x, y, t)}{T(x, y, 0) + T(x, y, t)} \qquad (7.16)$$

Automatic processing requires definition of thresholds, which can extract only "hot spots" or "cold spots" in the image (i.e., pixels with a value lower than the threshold will compose an image background, while pixels with a value equal or greater than the threshold will compose—"hot spots"). Because popular indexes are constructed to indicate higher probability of detected elements by a higher index value (low values—"cold spots"; high values—"hot spots") it is possible to calculate a negative NDPTI image, too.

$$\text{NPTI}(x, y, t) = 1 - \text{NDPTI}(x, y, t) = \frac{2 * T(x, y, t)}{T(x, y, 0) + T(x, y, t)} \qquad (7.17)$$

The signal to noise ratio (SNR) of this technique is rather small. It can be improved by averaging images, repeating the pulse excitation with time interval long enough for proper cooling.

As an example Figure 7.5a is a photograph of the burns caused by fire. Figure 7.5b,c show fields of IIa/b degree burn evidenced at the first and the second day after the accident. The effect of treatment is also very well visible comparing the results of measurements done day by day. In the related example the burn area was small enough to avoid grafting.

FIGURE 7.5 Patient with burn wound, first day after the accident—photograph of the burn (a), NDPTI image of the same field (b), and the NDPTI image at the second day (c).

7.6.2 Active Dynamic Thermal IR-Imaging

The ADT is based on comparison of measurements with a simple multilayer thermal model described by Equations 7.4 and 7.5 giving a simplified description of parametric images of thermal time constants, which values are correlated with internal structure of tested objects [11,48]. Recorded in time thermal transients at a given pixel are described by exponential models. Here, the two exponential models are describing the process of natural cooling after switching the heating pulse off.

$$T(t) = T_{\min} + \Delta T_1 e^{-t/\tau_{1c}} + \Delta T_2 e^{-t/\tau_{2c}} \tag{7.18}$$

Model based identification of a tested structure (object) is performed as it is shown in Figure 7.2. The recorded thermal response is fitted to a model. In many cases the two exponential description is fully sufficient for practical applications. As an example, typical transient in time for a single pixel (e.g., from Figure 7.5) is shown in Figure 7.6, with fitting procedure applied to one and two exponential models.

The two exponential models, as Equation 7.18, are fully sufficient for the data of accuracy available in the performed experiment. Some more pictures and examples of the ADT procedure are shown in following paragraphs, especially in skin burn evaluation [49,50]. It should be underlined that time constants for the heating phase τ_h and for the cooling phase τ_c usually are different due to different heat flow paths.

7.6.3 Pulse Phase Thermography

The procedure of PPT [2,51] is based on Fourier transform. The sequence of infrared images is obtained as in conventional PT experiments, Figure 7.7. Next, for each pixel (x, y) in every of N images the temporal evolution $g_i(t)$ is extracted and then the discrete Fourier transform is performed using the formula:

$$F_i(f) = \frac{1}{N} \sum_{n=0}^{N-1} g_i(t) \exp\left(\frac{-j2\pi f t}{N}\right) = \text{Re}_i(f) + j\text{Im}_i(f) \tag{7.19}$$

$$\varphi_i(f) = \text{atan}\left(\frac{\text{Im}_i(f)}{\text{Re}_i(f)}\right); \qquad A_i(f) = \sqrt{\text{Re}_i(f)^2 + \text{Im}_i(f)^2}$$

More valuable diagnostic information is given in the phase shift; therefore this parameter is of major interest.

Interesting characteristics of PPT are evident since it combines the speed of PT with the features of lock-in approach (the phase and the magnitude image). The condition to get reliable results is application of fast and very high quality IR-cameras.

As this method was not applied in medicine, yet, we do not show any examples, but extensive discussion of the validity of the procedure may be found in Reference 51.

7.6.4 Thermal Tomography

Thermal tomography should allow tomographic visualization of 3D structures, solving the real inverse problem—find distribution of thermal conductivity inside a tested object. This attempt is fully successful in the case of skin burn evaluation [16–18], giving a powerful tool in hands of medical doctors allowing reliable quantitative evaluation of the burn depth [52–54]. Other applications are under intensive research [55–57].

In TT the first step is determination of thermal properties of a tested object, necessary for development of its thermal equivalent model, to be applied for further data treatment. A typical procedure allowing the model parameters determination is shown in Figure 7.8. The forward problem is solved and assumed model parameters are modified to satisfy a chosen criterion for model and measurement data comparison.

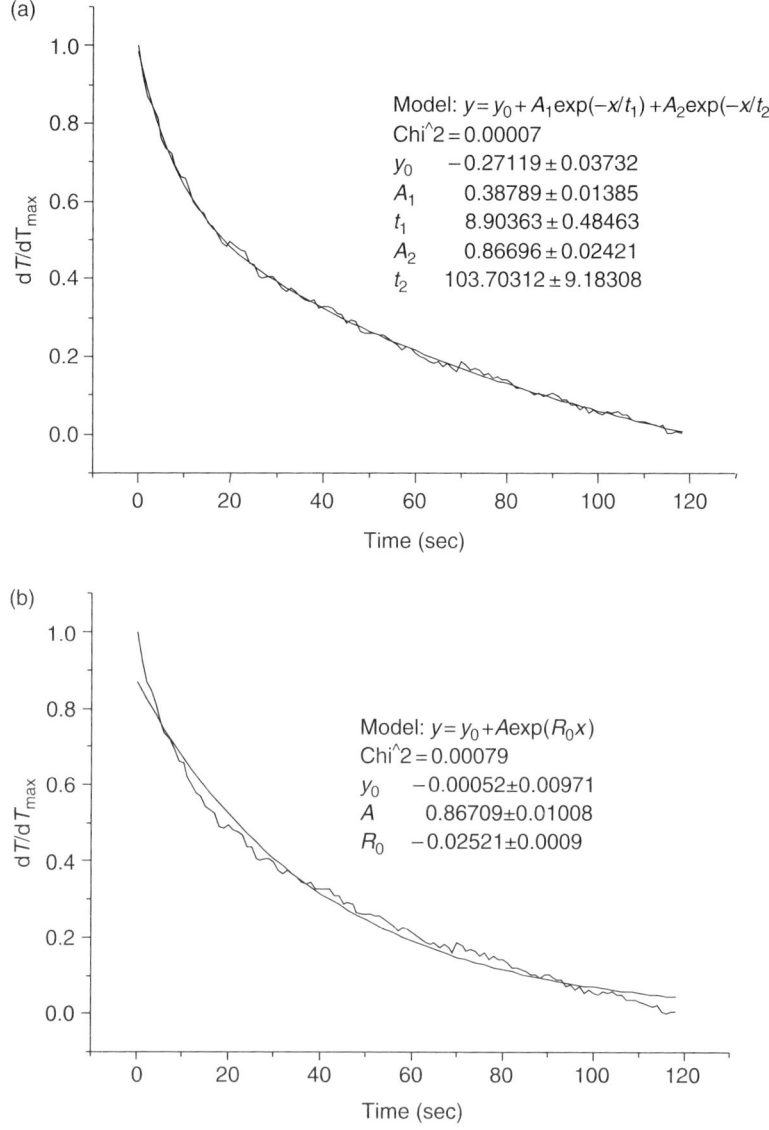

FIGURE 7.6 Fitting of the models to the measurement data—5-parameter model (a) and 3-parameter model (b).

The second step is organization of an active dynamic thermography experiment and registration of thermal transients forced by external excitation.

The next step requires advanced calculations to solve the inverse problem. The information of the correlation of the calculated figure of merit with a specific diagnostic feature is necessary to take a proper diagnostic decision based on the performed measurements. The decision function is directed to determine the internal thermal structure of the tested object basing on thermal transients at its surface. In this case, a real inverse problem has to be solved. We perform this procedure using Matlab scripts [17,18]. As the result a multilayer structure of different thermal properties may be reconstructed. To solve this problem additional assumptions, as number of layers, values of thermal properties or dimensions, are necessary because in general the problem is mathematically ill posed and nonlinear.

The method allows, under some conditions, not only to calculate the thermal effusivity, but also to reconstruct thermal diffusivity distribution in a layered structure. It is done using the nonlinear least

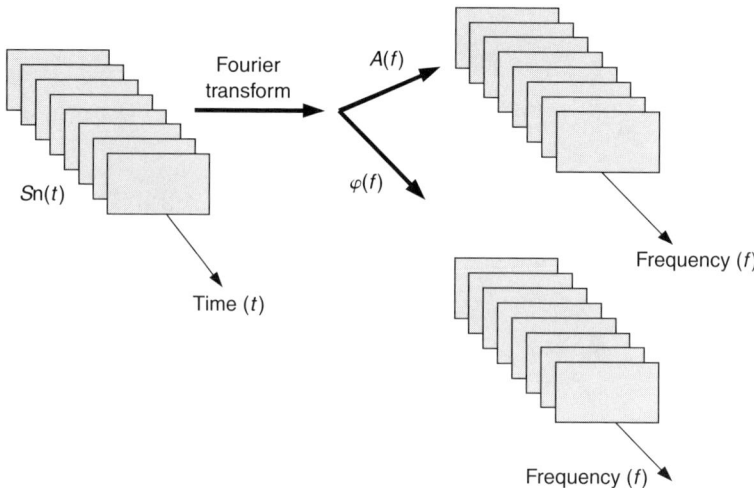

FIGURE 7.7 Procedure of calculation of synthetic pictures in PPT.

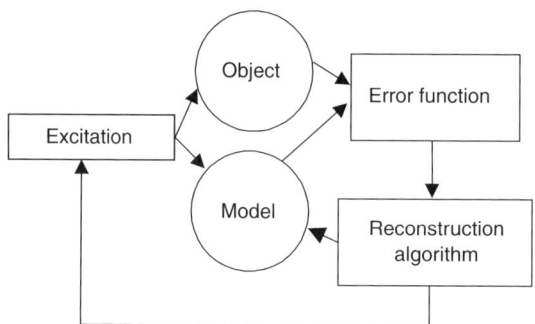

FIGURE 7.8 Determination of model parameters, based on comparison of measurement and simulation data, valid for all kind of tomography.

square optimization algorithm in inversion of direct problem:

$$\left.\begin{array}{l} T_0(x) \\ T_{\text{exc}} \\ \Phi(0,t) \\ k(0) \end{array}\right\} \Longrightarrow \alpha(x) \qquad (7.20)$$

where $T_0(x)$ is the initial temperature distribution in the object, T_{exc} the temperature of the heater, $\Phi(0,t)$ the heat flux at the surface, and $k(0)$ is the thermal conductivity of the outermost layer. In medical diagnostics of burn depth determination the problem is defined in a discrete form allowing determination of the parameter D, describing the depth of specific thermal properties, for example, depth of the burned tissue (the unknown parameter is local thickness of the tested object $d = D \cdot \Delta x$):

$$\left.\begin{array}{l} T_m^1, \quad m = 1, \ldots, M \\ \Phi_{\text{exc}} \\ T_1^p, \quad p = 1, \ldots, P \\ {[k_m, \rho c_m]}|_{m \leq D} = [k_{\text{rub}}, \rho c_{\text{rub}}] \\ {[k_m, \rho c_m]}|_{D < m < M} = [k_{\text{air}}, \rho c_{\text{air}}] \end{array}\right\} \Longrightarrow D \qquad (7.21)$$

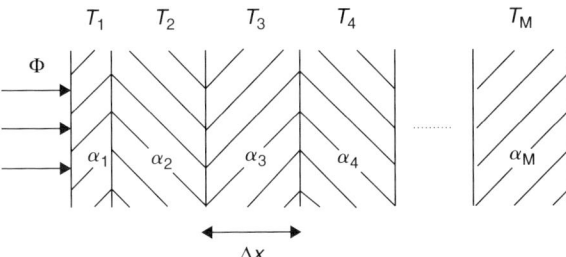

FIGURE 7.9 Spatial discretization of the properties of a multilayer object under test.

where the upper indexes describe the time domain and lower—the space domain. The inverse problem allows solution for which the direct simulation of temperature distribution is closest to the experiment results. This is by solving the problem, which is set by the goal function $F(D)$:

$$F(D) = \sum_{p=1}^{P}(T_{\text{dir}}^p(D) - T_{\text{meas}}^p)^2 \xrightarrow{D} \min \qquad (7.22)$$

where T_{dir}^p is the surface temperature for simulation performed for assumed value of the parameter D and T_{meas}^p the values measured. In the following examples the Matlab *lsqnonlin* function was adopted to solve this problem basing on modified interior-reflective Newton method [18]. Description of multilayer structures is also possible and may be defined in the form illustrated in Figure 7.9 [18,54]. One directional flow of heat energy is assumed.

What should be underlined is that the TT procedure requires advanced calculations and very reliable data, both from measurements as well as for modeling. Comparing to ADT this is much more demanding method, therefore it seems that typical for ADT description using thermal time constants at present stage of development seems to be easier accepted by medical staff.

7.7 Experiments and Applications

There are three groups of study performed:

1. On phantoms, for evaluation of technical aspects of instrumentation to be applied for *in vivo* experiments
2. On animals, *in vivo* experiments, for reference data
3. Clinical, for evaluation of the practical meaning of applied procedures

As the ADT as well as TT methods are new in medical diagnostics here we show some results of animal *in vivo* experiments and a few clinical cases. Described applications concern burns diagnostics and evaluation of cardiosurgery interventions. Results of phantom experiments and some other clinical applications were described in other cited publications, for example, References 22, 26, and 43.

7.7.1 Organization of Experiments

The clinical trials are done in *the Department of Plastic Surgery and Burns Treatment*, and in *the Department of Cardiac Surgery and Cardiology* of the Medical University of Gdansk. The leading medical personnel had all necessary legal rights for carrying the experiments, approved by the local ethical commission. All clinical experiments were done during normal diagnostic or treatment procedures, as the applied PT, ADT, and TT are noninvasive, aseptic, and safe. The excess of evoked surface temperature rise is around 2 to 4°C and the observation by the IR-camera is taken from a distance of 1 m. For skin temperature

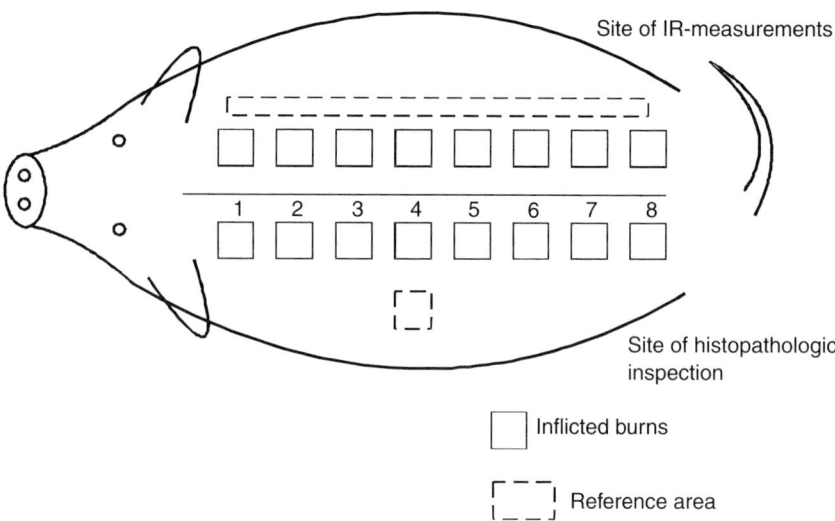

FIGURE 7.10 Location of experimental burns.

measurements illuminated area usually is kept wet using a thin layer of ointment to satisfy condition of constant evaporation from a tested surface and a constant value of emissivity coefficient. In cardiac surgery experiments with open chest, the surface of the heart is observed where the conditions of emissivity are regarded as constant. The IR-camera is located in a way not disturbing any activity of a surgeon.

The *in vivo* experiments on domestic pigs were performed in *the Department of Animal Physiology, Gdansk University*. The research program received a positive opinion of the institutional board of medical ethics. Housing and care of animals were in accordance with the national regulations concerning experiments on living animals. The choice of animals was intentional. No other animals have skin, blood, or heart properties so close to the human organs than pigs do [45]. Therefore, the experimental data carrying important medical information are of direct relationship to human organ properties.

Our burn experiments were based on the research of Singer et al. [58] and his methodology on standardized burn model. Following his experiment more than 120 paired sets of burns were inflicted on the back skin of 14 young domestic anesthetized pigs using aluminum and copper bars preheated in water in the range from 60 to 100°C. Typical distribution of burns is shown in Figure 7.10. Each pair was representing different conditions of injury giving a set of controlled burn depths. Additionally, each of measuring points was controlled by full-thickness skin biopsies and followed by histopathologic analysis of burn depth. The results of skin burn degree are in good accordance to the data given by Singer. The pigs were maintained under a surgical plane of anesthesia in conditioned environment of 24°C. The back skin was clipped before creation of burns. The total body surface area of the burns in each pig was approximately 4%. The animals were observed and treated against pain or discomfort.

After the "burns" experiment completed the same pigs were anesthetized, intubated and used for experimental myocardial infarction by closing the left descending artery. This experiment was lasting 5 h to evidence the nonreciprocal changes of the heart muscle. Full histopathology investigation was performed for objective evaluation of necrosis process.

Basic measurement set-up used in our experiments is composed of instruments shown in Figure 7.4. It is consisting the Agema 900 thermographic camera system; IR incandescent lamps of different power or a set of halogen lamps (up to 1000 W) with mechanical shutter or an air-cooling fan as thermal excitation sources; a control unit for driving the system. Additionally a specially designed meter of tissue thermal properties is used to determine the contact reference data necessary for reliable model of the skin or other tissue.

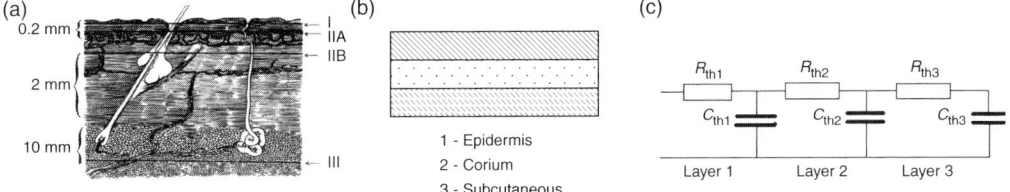

FIGURE 7.11 (a) Anatomy of the skin [59], (b) three-layer structural model, and (c) equivalent thermo-electric model.

The initial assumptions applied for reconstruction of a tested structure using ADT and TT procedures:

- Tested tissue is a 2- or 3-D medium with two- or three-layer composite structure (e.g., for skin—epidermis, dermis, subcutaneous tissue); (but for simplicity and having limited performance instrumentation even one layer model may be useful for diagnostic use in tissue evaluation).
- Tissue properties are independent on its initial temperature.

For skin and under-skin tissues an equivalent three-layer thermal model was developed [11]. For the assumed model its effective parameters have been reconstructed basing on the results of transient thermal processes. For known thermal diffusivity and conductivity of specific tissues the local thickness of a two- or three-layer structure may be calculated. In the structural model, each layer should correspond to the anatomy structure of the skin (see Figure 7.11). But in the case of a well developed burn a two-layer model is sufficient as the skin is totally changed and the new structure is determined by the died burned layer and modified by injury internal structure of thermal properties drastically different comparing the pre-injury state.

7.7.2 Results and Discussion

The related results are divided into groups covering clinical measurements of skin burns and heart surgery and equivalent measurements on pigs. The animal experiments are especially valuable to show importance of the discussed methods. Such experiments assure conditions which may be regarded as reference because fully controlled interventions and objective histopathologic investigations have been performed in this case.

7.7.3 Skin Burns

7.7.3.1 *In Vivo* Experiments on Pigs

The measurements were performed approximately 0.5 h after the burn creation and were repeated after 2 and 5 h and every 24 h during 5 consecutive days after the injury. As the ADT and TT experiments are new in medicine there are several notices concerning methodology of experiments. Especially some biological factors are of high importance. The pigs are growing in extremely fast; therefore the conditions of measurements are constantly changed. Also the hairs grow anew changing the measurement conditions and cannot be clipped again as the area is affected by injury. This was especially important for direct contact measurements but was not influencing IR measurements. The position of animals in consecutive days was not always the same causing some problems with data interpretation. The results of biopsy and histopathologic observations are used as the reference data of the skin burn thickness. We indicated the same set of parameters as given by Singer, what is shown in Figure 7.12 for exemplary burns of one of the pigs. The affected thickness of skin is dependent on the temperature and time of the aluminum and copper bars application. The plots are showing relative thickness of a burn with respect to the thickness of the skin. Such normalization may be important as the skin is of different thickness along the body. All affected points have full histopathologic description. Here only one example

FIGURE 7.12 Relative thickness of the burned skin for several aluminum bar temperatures for time of application equal 30 sec—different indicators describing burns are listed (biopsy results).

FIGURE 7.13 (**See color insert at the back of the book.**) Classical thermogram (a) and PT normalized differential thermography index pictures of burns (b) and (c).

is shown for points of the aluminum bar applications of different temperature but constant 30 sec time of application.

Some thermographic data of one of pigs taken 5 h after the burn injury are shown in Figure 7.13a [11]. A thermogram while heating is switched off with indicated six measurement areas is shown. Two bottom fields are uninjured reference points, four other are burns made using the aluminum bar—from the left: 100°C/30 sec; 100°C/10 sec and 90°C/30 sec; 80°C/30 sec. The set of halogen lamps was applied for PT and ADT experiment. The result of NDPTI pictures show temperature distribution 100 and 200 msec after the excitation Figure 7.13b,c. The burns are clearly visible and the relative temperature rise is very strongly correlated to the condition of the injury. For the indicated areas the mean value of temperature changes are calculated. This is shown for the first phase of cooling in Figure 7.14. The data might be fitted to thermal models giving ADT specific synthetic pictures of thermal time constants. The quality of the fitting procedure of measurement data to the equivalent model parameters is shown as an example in Figure 7.6a,b for one and two layer models.

There is a possibility to transform each of pixels into the equivalent model descriptor. In Figure 7.15a to f thermograms taken in consecutive days are transformed according to the formula $A \exp(-R_0 t)$. Distribution of the parameter—the thermal time constant—is shown.

Diagnostic importance of thermal transients is especially clearly visible in Figure 7.16 [18], where different injuries are responding differently to thermal excitation. The line mode of the IR-camera is here applied for fast data registration (>3000 scans/sec), allowing reduction of noise.

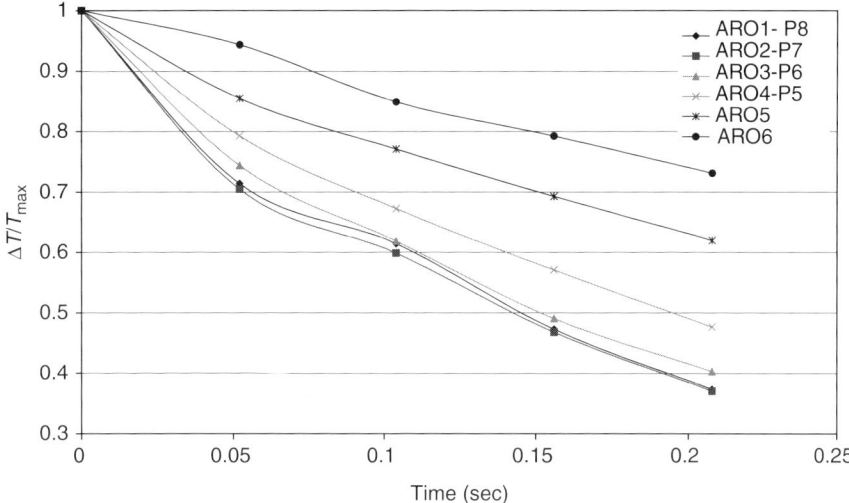

FIGURE 7.14 The normalized averaged temperature changes at the first phase after the excitation is switched off for indicated in Figure 7.13a points.

Basing on the same material TT procedure and reconstruction of thermal conductivity is also possible [18,54]. Assuming that we know the initial state of the object, the value of excitation flux, thermal response on the surface and spatial distribution of volumetric specific heat within the object it is possible to find the distribution of thermal conductivity:

$$\left.\begin{array}{l} T_m^1, \quad m=1,\ldots,M \\ \Phi_{exc} \\ T_1^p, \quad p=1,\ldots,P \\ \rho c_m, \quad m=1,\ldots,M \end{array}\right\} \Longrightarrow k_m, \quad m=1,\ldots,M \qquad (7.23)$$

The inverse problem defined by Equation 7.23 is highly justified due to practical reasons: the volumetric specific heat of biological tissues is much less dependent on water and fat content and other physiological factors than thermal conductivity is (especially effective thermal conductivity, which includes blood perfusion) [45]. Hence, the distribution of $\rho c(x)$ may be regarded with good approximation as known, and irregularities in thermal conductivity distribution should be searched for.

Figure 7.17 presents the results of minimization based on measurements taken during experiments with controlled degree burn fields as it was shown in Figure 7.16. The distribution of specific heat has been assumed identical with the healthy tissue, because of its low dependency on burn [18]. On the reconstructed thermal tomogram, a distinct layered structure of the skin can be seen, as well as the changes in its thermal structure caused by burns. The outermost two slices (0–0.2 mm) represent the epidermis and have thermal conductivity close to 0.3 W m^{-1} K^{-1}, which is almost not affected by burns. Fundamental changes in thermal properties induced by burns may be noticed in the next four slices (0.2–0.5 mm). From the anatomical point of view, this region represents the superficial plexus and adjacent layer of the dermis. As one can expect, for superficial burns we observe increase of k in this region, and decrease of k for severe burns. Based on this observation, quantitative classification criteria can be proposed [18].

For examination of skin burns is seems optimal to implement the expression 7.23. It allows obtaining thermal tomography images, which reflect pathologic changes in thermal conductivity distribution up to 2 to 3 mm.

FIGURE 7.15 Thermal time constant representation for the same case as showed in Figures 7.13 and 7.14 in consecutive days, starting from the moment of injury (upper left) and ending on the 5th day (bottom right). The placement of injures seems to be shifted due to different positions of the animal from day-to-day. Specific burn areas are easy recognizable. Additional studies are necessary for making full diagnostic medical recognition of injury, as there are two factors influencing each other—healing process and fast growth of the animal.

7.7.4 Clinics

We have examined around 100 patients with different skin injuries. Burn injuries were formed in different accidents as a result of flame action directly on skin, hands and faces, and on burning clothes, thorax. The investigations were performed during the first 5 days following an accident. To illustrate the clinical importance of the discussed methods an example of burns caused by an accident is shown in Figure 7.5. The well-determined area of the second-degree burn is evident. The next step—after rising more clinical data—will be quantitative classification based on data of the burn thickness. Long lasting effects of treatment and scars formation are still studied and not related here, yet. Already we claim that the value of the thermal time constant taken at the second day after the accident allows quantitative, objective discrimination between IIa and IIb burn [Renkielska, to be published].

7.7.5 Cardiac Surgery

7.7.5.1 *In Vivo* Experiments on Pigs

Understanding of thermal processes existing during the open chest heart operations is essential for proper surgical interventions, performed for saving the life. Experiments on pigs may be giving answers to several

FIGURE 7.16 (**See color insert.**) Thermal transients of burn fields of degree: I, IIa, IIb, IIb.

FIGURE 7.17 Results of the reconstruction of thermal conductivity distribution in burn fields.

important questions impossible to be responded in clinical situations. This especially may concern sudden heart temperature changes and proper interpretation of the causes.

Clamping the left descending artery and evoking a heart infarct performs the study. Temperature changes have been correlated with the histopathologic observations. The macroscopic thickness of the necrosis was evaluated. This was confirmed by the microscopic data. In Figure 7.18a anatomy of the

FIGURE 7.18 (**See color insert.**) Pig's heart after heart infarct evoked by the indicated clamp (a), the cross section of the heart with visible area of the stroke (the necrosis of the left ventricle wall—under the finger—is evidenced by darker shadow) (b) and the micro-histopathologic picture showing the cell necrosis (c).

FIGURE 7.19 (**See color insert.**) Thermograms of the heart: before (a) and after the evoked infarct (b). The change of the PT/ADT pictures in time (indicated in the subscript of the thermogram) 0.5 h after the LAD clamping (the tissue is still alive) (c), and 3 h later (the necrosis is evidenced by the change of thermal properties of the tissue) (d).

heart with the clamp is shown. The cross-section line is visible. In the Figure 7.18b the macroscopic cross-section is shown and the evidence of tissue necrosis is by the microscopic histopathology is shown in Figure 7.18c. The widths of the left and right ventricle as well as septum were also measured. The mass of the necrosis tissue was calculated. The evident correlation between the thickness of the left and right ventricle walls and the thermographic data are found. Thermographic views of this heart are shown in Figure 7.19a,b respectively before and after application of the clamp. The left ventricle wall is cooling faster than the right one as the left ventricle wall thickness is bigger and the heating effect caused by the flowing blood (of the same temperature in both ventricles) is here weaker. The cooling process of the heart caused by stopping the blood flow in LAD is shown in Figure 7.20—the mean temperature changes of the indicated in Figure 7.18a regions AR01 and AR02 are plotted.

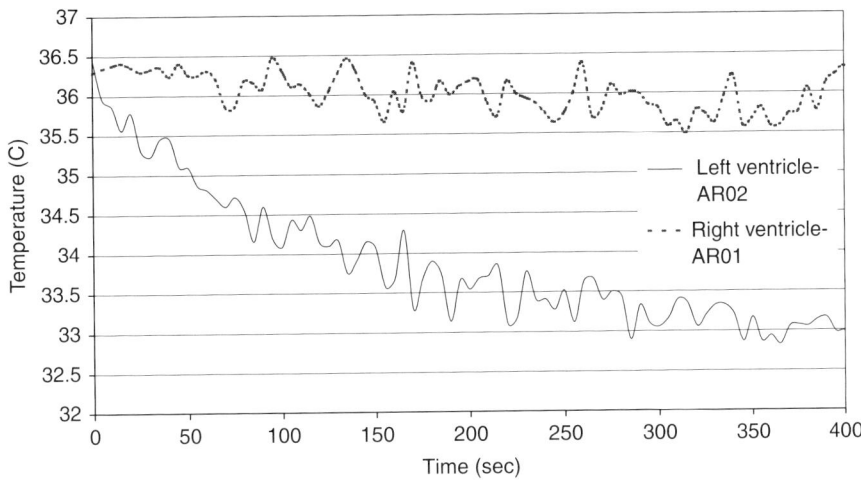

FIGURE 7.20 Temperature changes of the left and right ventricle after the LAD clamping related to Figure 7.19a,b.

The PT/ADT picture 0.5 h after the clamp was applied (Figure 7.19c) is still showing that thermal properties of the walls are unchanged even the temperature of the left ventricle wall is evidently decreased (Figure 7.19b). Progressing in time the necrosis process is changing thermal tissue properties what is clearly visible after 3 h in Figure 7.19d.

7.7.6 Clinics

Operation under extracorporeal circulation is normally a typical clinical situation. Two cases before and after CABG—coronary artery by-pass grafting—are shown for ADT in Figure 7.21a,b respectively. Areas of necrosis and of ischemia as well as volume of the healthy heart muscle were evaluated in respect to coronaroangiographic and radioisotope data showing high correlation. The observations performed before and after CABG show evident recovery of heart functioning. It is evidenced by smaller temperature rise after optical excitation of the heart in the same conditions. ADT shows the level and efficiency of revascularisation. The region of heart muscle dysfunction due to heart stroke was possible to be differentiated using both—normal thermography as well as ADT method—what leads to the conclusion that both modalities should be taken into account for diagnostics. The application of thermography for instant evaluation of the quality of the CABG intervention is prompt—the patency of the LIMA—LAD graft is unbeatable by any other method [60], but thermal tissue properties reflecting real state of the tissue is given only by ADT.

Application of all discussed modalities PT, ADT, PPT, and TT during the cardiosurgical interventions gives important indications how to improve surgical procedures.

7.8 Conclusions

The study shows that ADT as well as TT have been successfully used in medical applications giving not only qualitative improvement of diagnostics but in several applications allowing also quantitative evaluation of affected structures.

The importance of active dynamic thermal imaging and thermal tomography applied to burn evaluation and in the inspection of the open chest cardiology interventions was verified. Most probably there are also other attractive fields of medical applications of ADT and TT as, for example, cancer diagnostics [60]. ADT can by applied in medical procedures for monitoring the state of the skin and subdermal tissue structure during burns treatment giving objective, measurable ratings of the treatment procedure.

FIGURE 7.21 (**See color insert.**) ADT picture of clinical intervention—before the CABG (a) and after the operation (b). Important is more uniform temperature distribution after the operation proving that intervention was fully successful.

The moment of thermal investigation after an accident is of the highest significance. The most valuable results are obtained during the first and the second days following an accident. The clinical valuable features of the method in skin burns evaluation are the early objective determination of the burn depth—up to two days after an accident and possibility of quantitative evaluation of burn surface and depth as well as objective classification of burn degree. Also, the monitoring role of the method in interoperation of cardiac protection seems to be unbeatable. Changes of tissue vascularisation are important for prediction of treatment progress. In all applications, the method is noncontact, noninvasive, clean and nonstressed, allows wide area of investigation and clear and objective documentation of diagnoses and treatment process.

The use of different excitation sources should be limited to those of the best measurement properties. Basing on the described experiments most handy are optical sources of irradiation but probably cooling may give even better results in terms of higher signal to noise ratio. The operation of such sources is safe, harmful, and easy. The distribution of light may be relatively uniform; the control of irradiated power is also easy.

The work in the field of ADT and TT is still under fast development. Important is extensive IR instrumentation progress giving radical imaging improvement. The problem to be solved is development of a method of noncontact automatic determination of basic properties of thermal parameters of affected tissue what is one of main tasks for the future. Special software is under development for objective and automatic generation of affected tissue depth maps. Important will be to find not only qualitative information but also application of quantitative measures; to describe ratings of the burn wounds or calculate the thickness of affected heart tissues. Still more experiments giving statistically significant knowledge are necessary.

One of important goals is combination of different modalities and application of automatic classification procedures for improved diagnostics. This requires some progress in standardization of IR imaging, which still is not offered in the DICOM standard. For sure, distant consultation of images and automatic data retrieval will be pushing proper work in this field.

Acknowledgments

The author thanks his co-workers and Ph.D. students, who participated in development of ADT & TT in medicine and who produced the presented data. Most of the reported *in vivo* experiments have been performed with the help of Dr M. Kaczmarek, Dr M. Hryciuk, A. Galikowski and others from the Department of Biomedical Engineering, Gdansk University of Technology. Participation of medical staff: Dr A. Renkielska and Dr J. Grudziński (from the Department of Plastic Surgery and Burns Treatment), Prof. J. Siebert (from the Department of Cardiac Surgery and Cardiology, Medical University of Gdansk) and others are highly appreciated. *In vivo* animal experiments have been performed at the Department of Animal Physiology, Gdansk University with the main assistance of Dr W. Stojek. Others are listed in the attached bibliography as coauthors of common publications. The work was supported by several grants from KBN (Polish Ministry of Science and Information).

References

[1] *Proc. Quantitative InfraRed Thermography:* Chatenay-Malabary-1992, Naples-94, Stuttgart-1996, Lodz-1998, Venice-2000, Reims-2002, and Brussels-2004. See also QIRT Journal, 2004.

[2] Maldague X.P.V. *Theory and Practice of Infrared Technology for Nondestructive Testing*, John Wiley & Sons, Inc., New York, 2001.

[3] Van Denhaute E., Ranson W., Cornelis J., Barel A., and Steenhaut O., Contrast enhancement of IR thermographic images by microwave heating in biomedical applications, *Application mikro- und-optolelktronischer Systemelemente*, pp. 71–75, 1985.

[4] Steenhaut O., Van Denhaute E., and Cornelis J., Contrast enhancement in IR-thermography by application of microwave irradiation applied to tumor detection, *MECOMBE '86*, pp. 485–488, 1986.

[5] Nowakowski A. and Kaczmarek M., Dynamic thermography as a quantitative medical diagnostic tool, *Med. Biol. Eng. Comput. Incorporate Cell. Eng.* 37, Suppl. 1, Part 1, pp. 244–245, 1999.

[6] Kaczmarek M., Rumiński J., and Nowakowski A., Measurement of thermal properties of biological tissues—comparison of different thermal NDT techniques, *Proceedings of the Advanced Infrared Technology and Application*, Venice, 1999, pp. 322–329, 2001.

[7] Rumiński J., Kaczmarek M., and Nowakowski A., Data Visualization in dynamic thermography, *J. Med. Inform. Technol.*, 5, pp. IT29–IT36, 2000.

[8] Rumiński J., Nowakowski A., Kaczmarek M., and Hryciuk M., Model-based parametric images in dynamic thermography, *Polish J. Med. Phys. Eng.*, 6, pp. 159–164, 2000.

[9] Rumiński J., Kaczmarek M., and Nowakowski A., Medical active thermography—a new image reconstruction method, *Lecture Notes in Computer Science*, LNCS 2124, Springer, Berlin-Heidelberg, pp. 274–281, 2001.

[10] Nowakowski A., Kaczmarek M., and Rumiński J., Synthetic pictures in thermographic diagnostics, *Proceedings of the EMBS-BMES Conference*, CD, Houston, pp. 1131–1132, 2002.

[11] Nowakowski A., Kaczmarek M., Rumiński J., Hryciuk M., Renkielska A., Grudziński J., Siebert J., Jagielak D., Rogowski J., Roszak K., and Stojek W., Medical applications of model based dynamic thermography, Thermosense XIII, Orlando, *Proc. SPIE*, 4360, pp. 492–503, 2001.

[12] Sakagami T., Kubo S., Naganuma T., Inoue T., Matsuyama K., and Kaneko K., Development of a new diagnosis method for caries in human teeth based on thermal images under pulse heating, Thermosense XIII, Orlando, *Proc. SPIE*, 4360, pp. 511–515, 2001.

[13] Vavilov V., and Shirayev V., Thermal Tomograph—USSR Patent no. 1.266.308, 1985.

[14] Vavilov V.P., Kourtenkov D., Grinzato E., Bison P., Marinetti S., and Bressan C., Inversion of experimental data and thermal tomography using "Thermo Heat" and "Termidge" Software, *Proc. QIRT'94*, pp. 273–278, 1994.

[15] Vavilov V.P., 1D–2D–3D transition conditions in transient IR thermographic NDE, Seminar 64—Quantitative Infra-Red Thermography—QIRT'2000, Reims, 74, 2000.

[16] Hryciuk M., Nowakowski A., and Renkielska A., Multi-layer thermal model of healthy and burned skin, *Proc. 2nd European Medical and Biological Engineering Conference*, EMBEC'02, Vol. 3, Pt. 2., pp. 1614–1617, Vienna, 2002.

[17] Nowakowski A., Kaczmarek M., and Hryciuk M., Tomografia Termiczna, pp. 615–696, in Chmielewski L., Kulikowski J.L., and Nowakowski A., *Obrazowanie Biomedyczne*, (Biomedical Imaging—*in Polish*) Biocybernetyka i Inżynieria Biomedyczna 2000, 8, Akademicka Oficyna Wydawnicza EXIT, Warszawa, 2003.

[18] Hryciuk M., Badanie struktury biologicznych obiektów warstwowych z wykorzystaniem pobudzenia cieplnego (Ph.D. Dissertation—Investigation of layered biological object structure using thermal excitation, *in Polish*), *Politechnika Gdanska*, 2003.

[19] Kaczmarek M., Nowakowski A., and Renkielska A., Rating burn wounds by dynamic thermography, in D. Balageas, J. Beaudoin, G. Busse, and G. Carlomagno, eds., *Quantitative InfraRed Thermography* 5, pp. 376–381, Reims, 2000.

[20] Kaczmarek M., Nowakowski A., Renkielska A., Grudziński J., and Stojek W., Investigation of skin burns based on active thermography, *Proc. 23rd Annual International Conference IEEE EMBS*, CD-ROM, Istanbul, 2001.

[21] Nowakowski A, Kaczmarek M., Wtorek J., Siebert J., Jagielak D., Roszak K., and Topolewicz J., Thermographic and electrical measurements for cardiac surgery inspection, *Proc. of 23rd Annual International Conference IEEE EMBS*, CD-ROM, Istanbul, 2001.

[22] Nowakowski A., Kaczmarek M., Hryciuk M., and Rumiński J., *Postępy termografii–aplikacje medyczne*, Wyd. Gdańskie (Advances of thermography–medical applications, *in Polish*), Gdańsk, 2001.

[23] Hryciuk M. and Nowakowski A., Multi-layer thermal model of healthy and burned skin, *Proc. 2nd European Medical and Biological Engineering Conference*, EMBEC'02, Vol. 3, Pt. 2., pp. 1614–1617, Vienna, 2002.

[24] Hryciuk M. and Nowakowski A., Evaluation of thermal diffusivity variations in multi-layered structures, *Proc. 6 QIRT*, Zagreb, pp. 267–274, 2003.

[25] Kaczmarek M. and Nowakowski A., Analysis of transient thermal processes for improved visualization of breast cancer using IR imaging, *Proc. IEEE EMBC*, Cancun, pp. 1113–1116, 2003.

[26] Kaczmarek M., Modelowanie właściwości tkanek żywych dla potrzeb termografii dynamicznej, (Ph.D. dissertation—Modeling of living tissue properties for dynamic thermography, *in Polish*) Politechnika Gdañska, 2003.

[27] Chato J.C., A method for the measurement of the thermal properties of biological materials, thermal problems in biotechnology, *ASME Symp.*, pp. 16–25, 1968.

[28] Bowman H.F., Cravalho E.G., and Woods M., Theory, measurement and application of thermal properties of biomaterials, *Ann. Rev. Biophys. Bioeng.*, No. 4, pp. 43–80, 1975.

[29] Chen M.M., Holmes K.R., and Rupinskas V., Pulse-decay method for measuring the thermal conductivity of living tissues, *J. Biomech. Eng.*, 103, pp. 253–260, 1981.

[30] Balasubramaniam T.A. and Bowman H.F., Thermal conductivity and thermal diffusivity of biomaterials: a simultaneous measurement technique, *J. Biomech. Eng.*, 99, pp. 148–154, 1977.

[31] Shitzer A. and Eberhart R.C., *Heat Transfer in Medicine and Biology*, Vols. 1, 2, Plenum Press, 1985.

[32] Balageas D.L., Characterization of living tissues from the measurement of thermal effusivity, *Innov. Tech. Biol. Med.*, Vol. 12, 1991.

[33] Valvano J.W., Cochran J.R., and Diller K.R., Thermal conductivity and diffusivity of biomaterials measured with self-heating thermistors, *Int. J. Thermophys.*, No. 6, pp. 301–311, 1985.

[34] Marks R.M. and Barton S.P., *The Physical Nature of the Skin*, Boston, MTP Press, 1998.

[35] Janna W.S., *Engineering Heat Transfer*, CRC Press, Washington DC, 2000.

[36] Pennes H.H., Analysis of tissue and arterial blood temperatures in the resting human forearm, *J. Appl. Physiol.*, No. 1, pp. 93–122, 1948.

[37] IDEAS operating manual.

[38] NASTRAN operating manual.

[39] Matlab operating manual.

[40] Mathematica operating manual.
[41] Salerno A., Dillenz A., Wu D., Rantala J., and Busse G., Progress in ultrasound lock-in thermography, *Proc. QIRT'98*, pp. 154–160, Lodz, 1998.
[42] Maldague X. and Marinetti S., Pulse phase thermography, *J. Appl. Phys.*, 79, (5), pp. 2694–2698, 1996.
[43] Nowakowski A., Kaczmarek M., and Dêbicki P., Active thermography with microwave excitation, D. Balageas, J., Beaudoin, G., Busse, G., and Carlomagno, eds., *Quantitative InfraRed Thermography*, 5, pp. 387–392, 2000.
[44] Nowakowski A., Kaczmarek M., Renkielska A., Grudziński J., and Stojek J., Heating or cooling to increase contrast in thermographic diagnostics, *Proc. EMBS-BMES Conference*, CD, Houston, pp. 1137–1138, 2002.
[45] Duck A.F., *Physical Properties of Tissue*, Academic Press, London, 1990.
[46] Ring E.F.J., Standardization of Thermal Imaging Technique, *Thermology Oesterrich*, 3, pp. 11–13, 1993.
[47] Rumiński J., Kaczmarek M., Nowakowski A., Hryciuk M., and Werra W., Differential analysis of medical images in dynamic thermography, *Proc. V National Conference on Application of Mathematics in Biology and Medicine*, Zawoja, pp. 126–131, 1999.
[48] Nowakowski A., Kaczmarek M., and Rumiński J., Synthetic pictures in thermographic diagnostics, *Proc. EMBS-BMES Conf.* 2002, CD, pp. 1131–1132, Houston, 2002.
[49] Kaczmarek M., Nowakowski A., and Renkielska A., Rating burn wounds by dynamic thermography, D. Balageas, J. Beaudoin, G. Busse, and G. Carlomagno, eds., *Quantitative InfraRed Thermography*, Vol. 5, pp. 376–381, 2000.
[50] Kaczmarek M., Rumiński J., Nowakowski A., Renkielska A., Grudziński J., and Stojek W., In-vivo experiments for evaluation of new diagnostic procedures in medical thermography, *Proceedings of 6th International Conference on Quantitative Infrared thermography*, Proc. Quantitative Infrared Thermography 6-QIRT'02, pp. 260–266, Zagreb, 2003.
[51] Ibarra-Castanedo C. and Maldague X., Pulsed phase thermography reviewed, *QIRT J.*, 1(1), pp. 47–70, 2004.
[52] Hryciuk M. and Nowakowski A., Multilayer thermal model of healthy and burned skin, *Proc. 2nd European Medical and Biological Engineering Conference*, EMBEC'02, Vol. 3, Pt. 2., pp. 1614–1617, Vienna, 2002.
[53] Hryciuk M. and Nowakowski A., Evaluation of thermal diffusivity variations in multi-layered structures, *Proceedings of 6th International Conference on Quantitative Infrared thermography*, Proc. Quantitative Infrared Thermography 6-QIRT'02, pp. 267–274, Zagreb, 2003.
[54] Hryciuk M. and Nowakowski A., Formulation of inverse problem in thermal tomography for burns diagnostics, *Proc. SPIE*, 5505, pp. 11–18, 2004.
[55] Kaczmarek M., Rumiński J., and Nowakowski A., Data processing methods for dynamic medical thermography, *Proceedings of International Federation for Medical and Biological Engineering*, EMBEC'02, pp. 1098–1099, Vienna, 2002.
[56] Nowakowski A., Kaczmarek M., Siebert J., Rogowski J., Jagielak D., Roszak K., Topolewicz J., and Stojek W., Role of thermographic inspection in cardiosurgery, *Proc. Int. Federation for Medical and Biological Engineering*, EMBEC'02, pp. 1626–1627, Vienna, 2002.
[57] Kaczmarek M. and Nowakowski A., Analysis of transient thermal processes for improved visualization of breast cancer using IR imaging, *25th Annual International Conference of the IEEE Engineering in Medicine and Biology Society* "A New Beginning for Human Health," Cancun, Mexico, CD, 2003.
[58] Singer A.J., Berruti L., Thode HC J.R., and McClain S.A., Standardized burn model using a multiparametric histologic analysis of burn depth. *Academic Emergency Medicine*, 7(1), pp. 1–6, 2000.
[59] Eberhart C. *Heat Transfer in Medicine and Biology, Analysis and Applications*, Vol. 1. Plenum Press, London, 1985
[60] Kaczmarek M., Nowakowski A., Siebert J., and Rogowski J., Infrared thermography—applications in heart surgery, *Proc. SPIE*, 3730, pp. 184–188, 1999.

8
Dynamic Thermal Assessment

8.1	Introduction...	**8-1**
8.2	Biomedical Dynamic Thermal Assessment	**8-2**
	Early History • "Quantitative Dynamic Area Telethermometry in Medical Diagnosis and Management": An Imaginative Speculative Treatise • Considering the Realities	
8.3	DTA Experimentation (1997–2001).....................	**8-7**
	Early DTA Experimentation • Research at the Millard Fillmore Hospital at Buffalo • Preliminary DTA Findings on Melanoma and Diabetes	
8.4	Recent DTA Studies (2000–2005).......................	**8-11**
	Detection of and Treatment of Malignancy • Use of DTI in the Study of Brain Function and Brain Malignancies • Use of DTI Intraoperatively in Other Surgical Procedures • Clinical Applications of DTI in Other Fields	
8.5	Conclusion	**8-16**
References		**8-17**

Michael Anbar
University at Buffalo (SUNY)

8.1 Introduction

The purpose of this chapter is not just to summarize studies on dynamic thermal assessment (DTA) [aka *dynamic infrared imaging* (DIRI) or *dynamic thermal imaging* (DTI)] published since 1987, but to present this topic from a general, critical perspective, focusing on studies published since 2000, which have significantly extended the scope of this promising biomedical technique. The latter most interesting achievements have not been reviewed up-to-date in the context of DTI. This chapter is not a tutorial on DTI or DTA, replicating previously published reviews. Interested readers are, therefore, encouraged to consult appropriate review papers pointed out below. Further, since this chapter is likely to be the last first-hand account of the history of DTI, written by the person who conceptualized and initiated this field of endeavor, it will include historical details that were not published before. The nature of this chapter also allows the author to include personal views on some of the topics discussed.

To bring readers up to speed, they must understand the concept of DTA as compared with classical *static thermal imaging*. Whereas the former methodology monitors or quantitatively measures temporal *changes* in temperature over areas of interest, the latter technique involves observation of temperature distribution over such areas. Thermal changes can be *monotonic*—warming or cooling of areas of interest or parts thereof—or they can be *periodic*, manifested as temperature *modulation*. Monitoring of either kind of temperature change over an area can be done just by one kind of technology—using infrared cameras, preferably in the 8 to 12 μm range, to monitor the blackbody radiation of the areas of interest. Consequently, one can describe this technique as dynamic *infrared* monitoring or *DIRI*. In brief, whenever we use in this review the terms DTI or DTA, it is implied that the measurement of temperature was done remotely using infrared detection.

Certain clinical applications of DTI have been monitoring monotonic temperature changes—warming of organs following a cold challenge, following surgical reperfusion, or cooling of organs following perfusion with a cold fluid (used occasionally in cardiac surgery). Such slow monotonic warming or cooling processes can be visually monitored in real-time. This is one kind of DTI—display of sequential thermal images over a period of time to be observed visually. These sequential observations can also be represented by single images of the *rates* of gradual temperature change, which may be different for different subareas of the region of interest (ROI). The spatial distribution of rates over the ROI can be displayed on color-coded bitmaps.

Physiological processes that affect the temperature of live surfaces (e.g., skin, cornea, or the surface of the brain) are generally *periodic*, resulting in *temperature modulation*. Observing gradual warming of biological surfaces ignores the minute underlying modulations and averages them out. However, those minute modulations, which generally require higher precision of temperature measurement, convey important physiological information. Moreover, those modulations can be monitored when no gross changes in average surface temperature take place. In fact, the use of DTI in this mode, with no prior thermal challenge, is generally far more informative, as it monitors physiology noninvasively under *undisturbed* conditions.

Quantitative assessment of temperature modulation requires accumulation of hundreds or even thousands of sequential thermal images acquired at a significantly higher rate than the frequencies of the physiological or pathophysiological temperature modulation monitored. Presented generally to the end user is the spatial distribution of amplitudes of temperature modulation at discrete frequencies or range of frequencies. This modulation amplitude vs. frequency presentation is derived from fast Fourier transformation (FFT) of the observed periodic temperature changes. This spatial distribution can be displayed as color bitmaps of *amplitudes* distribution or of the *microhomogeneity of amplitude* distribution [1], at a given frequency or range of frequencies. These can then be visually spatially correlated with anatomical features over the ROI.

With the exception of real-time continuous DTI, generally used in surgical intraoperative applications, DTI "images" do not represent spatial distribution of infrared radiation flux or of temperature, but are a computerized presentation of periodic temperature *changes*. Furthermore, certain applications of "DIRI" that monitor well-defined anatomical features, requiring no anatomic spatial correlation, do not require display of any images altogether. Thus the term "imaging" in these cases is an utter misnomer.

Notwithstanding semantic finesse, while discussing DTA, we will often use the term "DTI" interchangeably with DTA, because "*thermal*" imaging," that is, imaging of thermal phenomena, which are generally *dynamic*, is distinct from classical *static* thermographic "*temperature* imaging."

8.2 Biomedical Dynamic Thermal Assessment

8.2.1 Early History

DTA was conceptualized in the late 1980s by Michael Anbar [2–5]. Anbar discovered that rapid *changes* in human skin temperature convey valuable physiological and pathophysiological information, information that cannot be derived from static temperature mapping (i.e., measurement of temperature distribution over areas of skin). These ideas crystallized further on the basis of rudimentary experimental studies in the early 1990s [1,6–18].

Since under physiological conditions the temperature of skin depends on blood supply to cutaneous and subcutaneous tissues, blood being the heat exchange fluid, skin temperature manifests a variety of hemodynamic processes. These processes are modulated by pulsatile cardiogenic changes in blood flow as well as by neuronal control of blood flow in the vasculature and microvasculature. Since blood perfusion affects skin temperature differently at different areas of skin, depending on the underlying vascular anatomy, assessment of these processes requires repeated temperature imaging of ROI at frequencies higher than the highest frequency of measurable blood supply modulation. In brief, DTI of ROI can provide new information on the anatomy of the vasculature, on systemic changes in blood flow due to both heart function and neuronal systemic and local control of vascular blood flow and perfusion of the capillary bed.

In addition to useful anatomic and physiologic information, DTI can also be clinically useful. Pathologies that affect any anatomic or physiologic parameters of blood supply can be diagnosed by this technique. For these discoveries Anbar was awarded the President's Award of the American Academy of Thermology for 1990.

The only thermometric technique that can attain the spatial resolution, thermal sensitivity, and speed of data acquisition of skin temperature is infrared imaging with a large ($\geq 256 \times 256$) solid-state detector array in the 8 to 12 μm range (temperature can be measured also by infrared sensors in the 3 to 5 μm range—however, at a significantly lower sensitivity and subject to substantial reflectivity artifacts). In the early 1990s, infrared detection technology was still in its infancy (multidetector two-dimensional arrays were still on the drawing board) and thus it could not meet the requirement of a practical dynamic diagnostic technique. Anbar's early experiments were, therefore, rudimentary, far from offering a practical solution to any clinical problem. Medical technology had to wait, therefore, for additional developments in infrared detection and image-processing technologies.

8.2.2 "Quantitative Dynamic Area Telethermometry in Medical Diagnosis and Management": An Imaginative Speculative Treatise

In 1994, Anbar summarized his ideas and preliminary experimental research in this new field in a monograph titled "Quantitative Dynamic Area Telethermometry in Medical Diagnosis and Management" [19]. The term "area telethermometry" was used to distinguish remote, noncontact, infrared thermal imaging from the, now obsolete, contact thermometric imaging methods (e.g., liquid crystals, thermistor arrays). Today the term "thermal imaging" implies *infrared* imaging. That monograph described the scientific background of this imaging technique, which is uniquely suited for dynamic applications.

The book projected a large variety of clinical applications that would be feasible using DTI.

It describes potential clinical uses of DTA in a variety on neurological disorders that affect circulatory behavior and/or cutaneous perfusion. These include carpal tunnel syndrome and Raynaud's syndrome, complex regional pain syndrome (earlier named "reflex sympathetic dystrophy"), backpain and leg pain due to spinal stenosis or herniation, as well as migraines and other headaches involving vasospasms.

Among other neurological effects that can be monitored by DTI the book describes sympathetic nervous response to mental stress. The latter entails numerous potential clinical applications in psychiatry both as a diagnostic as well as therapeutic tool (using biofeedback). DTI could as well effectively monitor mental stress induced by deception ("lie detection"). Since sympathetic vasoconstriction or vasodilatation are much more sensitive manifestations of mental stress than perspiration, Anbar suggested that remote monitoring of subjects by DTI (which also readily measures heart rate) is likely to be a far more effective "lie detector" than the best of polygraphs.

Vascular disorders are the next group of clinical applications of DTI discussed in the book. These include occlusions (including peripheral vascular occlusive disease) and aneurysms, as well as vascular effects of diabetes. Anbar suggested that DTI could distinguish between diabetic neuropathies and diabetic vascular occlusive disease, helping optimize treatment of diabetes mellitus.

Then Anbar's book discusses how DTI can be useful in the differential diagnosis and monitoring of treatment of inflammatory processes, including rheumatic disease, local infections, and burns.

Potential surgical applications of DTI are the next topic discussed in the 1994 book. These include monitoring of reperfusion of transplanted organs (e.g., kidneys) and of the heart following cardioplegia in open heart surgery, reperfusion of skin grafts and skin flaps in plastic surgery, and monitoring reperfusion following reconnection of blood vessels and of intestines or in colostomy. It also suggests the use of DTI in monitoring anesthesia.

"Quantitative Dynamic Area Telethermometry" suggests the use of DTI to monitor metabolic processes also at the cellular level. Metabolic processes are either endothermic or exothermic. At the cellular level they are periodical, that is, oscillatory, owing to thermal and nonthermal autocatalysis, as well as because of the complex interactive kinetics of diffusion of nutrients, oxygen, and metabolites through cellular membranes and cytoplasm. Anbar suggested to monitor the metabolism of mammalian cells in tissue cultures and thus rapidly detect, using DTI, changes in cellular metabolism (a physiological approach) due to the effect of antimetabolites or toxins, instead of waiting for the effects manifested in replication (essentially an anatomic approach).

Clinical applications of the cellular DTI methodology include rapid evaluation of the effect of chemotherapeutic agents on cells extracted by biopsy from malignant tumors, rapid evaluation of the effect of antigens on such cells, and rapid evaluation of their radiation sensitivity. Another potential clinical application of DTI discussed in the book was rapid determination of the sensitivity of bacteria or fungi to antibiotics, without the needed follow-up *in vitro* of proliferation of such pathogens.

A preliminary study done at the University at Buffalo by the author in collaboration with Dr. Malcolm Slaughter indicates the feasibility of cellular DTI. In a study on the thermal behavior of live retinal neurons *in vitro*, retinas of newts were isolated and their thermal behavior was dynamically observed with the aid of a 1:1 germanium macro lens (AIM, Infrarot Module, Heilbrunn, Germany). The study tried to find out if temperature modulation of the neurons (4 neurons per pixel), due to cellular metabolism, observed in the 2 to 8 Hz range, was altered by pulsed light stimulation. The findings were positive though not sufficiently reproducible because of experimental limitations (mainly spatial resolution at 256×256 pixels). However, this has been the first attempt to monitor *in vitro* cellular metabolism by DTI. Commercially available equipment with 16 times higher spatial resolution could be used today to verify DTI's potential in this field.

Cellular DTI could be extended to detection of viral infection of cells in tissue cultures because the metabolism of affected cells changes dramatically owing to the effect of the virus on their transcriptive apparatus. Cellular DTI could be much faster than radiotracer uptake studies. This might allow rapid detection of viruses and testing the effectiveness of antiviral drugs. Although Anbar discussed in his book the use of DTI for detecting viral infections *in vivo*, due to their effect on macrophages, which locally generate nitric oxide (NO) very much like cancerous cells (see below), he overlooked, at the time, this potentially highly important *in vitro* application of cellular DTI in clinical virology. This is, therefore, a new idea whose time will hopefully come soon.

Among the most exciting of the potential clinical applications of DTI discussed by Anbar were those related to oncology. Neoplastic lesions are generally associated with angiogenesis and subsequent local hypervascularization. This by itself must produce aberration in the local anatomy of perfusion. Moreover, newly formed neoplastic blood vessels are likely to be sparsely innervated, if at all, and therefore their response to neuronal vascular control is likely to be abnormal and therefore detectable by DTI, which monitors neuronal modulation of vascular flow. However, even a more specific feature of neoplastic lesions from the standpoint of potential detection and management of cancer by DTI is their generation of NO.

Back in 1978, Anbar has discovered that humans and other mammals produce and carry measurable amounts of endogenic NO in their blood [20]. The physiologic function of this highly reactive substance was unknown at the time and remained unknown until the late 1980s and early 1990s, when it was shown to be a neurotransmitter that induces vasodilatation [21–23]. Since it had been well documented that neoplastic disease is associated with local hyperthermia of the overlying skin, Anbar showed in 1994 by quantitative analysis that this phenomenon must be associated with local vasodilatation [24]. He then advanced a hypothesis that this manifestation of neoplasms is due to generation of NO by cancerous tissues.

He showed that this abnormality of neoplastic cells gives them a substantial advantage over normal cells by enhancing blood supply to the neoplastic tissue (before it induces angiogenesis) and by enhancing potential metastasis [25]. This hypothesis has been experimentally corroborated independently already in 1994 in different types of cancerous cell lines [26–28].

Since it was known by 1994 that NO is a chemical messenger in regulation of vascular tone, Anbar speculated that NO produced by cancerous lesions will interfere with vasomotor regulation of perfusion. Thus Anbar's hypothesis predicted not only that cancerous lesions will enhance regional vascular perfusion but also that perfusion in the surrounding tissues will not be normally modulated. The corollary of this hypothesis is that DTI might detect the effect of cancer-produced NO on the neuronal modulation of perfusion, and thereby detect cancerous lesions more effectively than by just monitoring local hyperthermia. A recent thermographic study confirmed Anbar's conclusion that breast-cancer-induced hyperthermia is not due to local hypervascularity [29], and it must, therefore, be associated with local vasodilatation.

An important parameter conceptualized by Anbar and described in his monograph is the microhomogeneity of temperature modulation or spatial thermal homogeneity (STH = 1/SD (standard deviation) of temperature values of spots in a given subarea) [1]. Quantitative DTI can also measure the modulation of local homogeneity of subareas at any given frequency or range of frequencies. The latter parameter measures the level of perfusion of a given subcutaneous region: that is, when the region's perfusion reaches a maximum so does the microhomogeneity.

Finally, another novel concept highlighted by Anbar already in 1994 was the direct *objective* use of digital data in clinical diagnosis. DTI is essentially not an anatomic imaging technique but a physiological one. It produces its findings on the oscillatory behavior of the temperature of biological surfaces in terms of frequencies and their relative amplitudes (following FFT, as demonstrated by Anbar in 1991). DTI expresses pathology or biological abnormalities as frequency–amplitude aberrations, analogously to electrocardiogram (ECG) or electroencephalogram (EEG). When these aberrations are monitored over large areas of skin their spatial distribution can be bitmapped, color coded, and visually evaluated by the human eye. However, these are not images of temperature but images of the distribution of temperature *changes*. This is the only meeting point between DTI and anatomy. Now, in many clinical applications the anatomical information is absolutely unnecessary, because the physiological data contain all the diagnostics information. As these data are digital to begin with, they can be processed further to provide *objective* diagnostic measures of pathology, or of the probability of pathology. DTI can therefore become a forerunner of computerized medicine in the twenty-first century.

In brief, at the risk of repetition, it must be concluded that in spite of its common name, DTI is essentially not an imaging technique. Clinical imaging techniques require always evaluation of images by experts to achieve a diagnosis. DTA is, therefore, more than an imaging technique.

Back in 1994, all these scores of novel-computerized clinical applications were essentially just a glimpse in the eye of the author. At that time, this well-documented, scientific book with hundreds of references was still not far from being good science fiction, because none of the applications envisioned there had been reduced to practice. Like Jules Verne in his time or Arthur Clarke, Anbar recognized the potential of a new technology in an entirely different field. In this case it was infrared imaging, which was likely to rapidly develop so to meet emerging needs of military surveillance and targeting. Anbar foresaw that this technology will meet the sensitivity and speed requirements of clinically useful DTI. Also computational speed and computer memory available in 1994 were insufficient to process DTI data in any practical manner. This did not deter Anbar from projecting that these will be available when infrared technology will meet DTI requirements. Many of these "dreams" were realized within less than a decade.

After publicizing his new ideas on DTA [30,31], and extending the ideas on the mechanism of breast cancer hyperthermia [25,32], Anbar advanced a hypothesis on the role of NO in pathophysiological pain, explaining the mechanism of hyperthermia associated with pain [33,34]. Yet all these plausible speculations awaited experimental verification.

8.2.2.1 Hypothesis on the Effect of Cancer on Perfusion Confirmed

Anbar's hypothesis that NO generated in neoplastic cells affects vascular behavior in the vicinity of solid tumor has been confirmed already in the following 3 years [35–39]. The role of NO in cancer biology has been demonstrated in breast cancer [40–42], cancer of the colon [43–45], squamous cell carcinomas of the head and neck [46–48], brain malignancies [49–52], melanoma [53–55], lung cancer [56–58], cancer of the prostate [59], ovarian cancer [60], cancer of the pancreas [61], chondrosarcoma [62], cancer of the bladder [63,64; see, however, 65], and gastric cancer [66,67]. In brief, the production of NO in malignant tissues has been well established, corroborating Anbar's prediction [24,25], as has been its vasodilatatory effect. (For a more detailed discussion see the introduction in Reference 68.)

What remained to be demonstrated was to what extent can the specific effect of solid tumors on the modulation of tissue perfusion be detected at skin level by DTI, refining the information on the tumor-associated local skin hyperthermia (an effect that has been well known for decades—although its mechanism remained obscure before the NO mechanism has been elucidated) [24].

8.2.3 Considering the Realities

The 1994 publication of Anbar's monograph was a landmark in the history of DTI, but this technique would have been forgotten if not for his research efforts to make his dream come through. In making DTI a practical technique one must consider its scope and limitations.

After discussing the wide scope of DTI's potential applications, we must consider also the limitations of this technique when applied to the live human body. It must be realized that because of the very high absorption coefficient of skin tissue to photons in the 8 to 10 μm range, blackbody radiation emitted from the skin and detectable by infrared cameras represents the temperature of a layer less than 0.1 mm thick of skin. Since no temperature changes can occur intrinsically within that thin skin layer, any modulation in local skin temperature of the upper layer of skin represents temperature modulation of subcutaneous tissues, including blood vessels, conducted to the skin's surface. The modulation of skin temperature is due to modulation of perfusion of the subcutaneous capillary bed as well as modulation of blood flow through vessels in proximity of the skin. These modulations are driven by two processes—cardiogenic pulses and neurological modulation of the vascular tone (i.e., vasodilatation and vasoconstriction). Locally elevated or lower temperature due to hypermetabolism or hypometabolism of tissues, respectively, or to environmental factors, are not expected to manifest any modulation below 0.001 Hz and will not be detectable by appropriately programmed computerized DTI.

Further, modulation of perfusion of tissues or vasculature situated deep (>10 mm) below the skin is unlikely to be detectable at skin level because of heat dissipation, which results in impedance of the modulated thermal signal. The latter effect will result in blurred modulated images of deep vessels detectable at skin level; the deeper the vessel the more blurred will be its modulated thermal image until it fades into the background. Since the impedance of temperature modulation increases with frequency, only low frequency modulation of heat sources situated deep under the skin will be detectable at skin level. It can be expected that temperature modulation of heat sources below, say, 10 mm, will not be detectable at all at skin level even if unmodulated skin temperature might be higher in a given area due to a low-lying heat source. The level of detectable modulation depends obviously on the precision of temperature measurement. The higher the precision the more sensitive will be the detection of modulation due to perfusion of deeper structures.

In brief, the higher the frequency of the modulation the more pronounced will be the attenuation of the heat dissipated signals. Consequently, we expect to detect high frequency modulation (>1 Hz) only of modulated cutaneous microvasculature or over superficially situated large vessels. However, temperature modulation of large vessels will be predominantly driven by cardiogenic pulses with only minor effects of vasodilatation or vasoconstriction that occur at other frequencies. In any case, temperature modulation at the skin surface is necessarily a biased representation of the modulation of subcutaneous tissue perfusion. While modulation frequencies >2 Hz can occasionally be detectable at skin surface (excluding FFT artifactual harmonics of cardiac pulsation) most useful DTI information is expected in the below the 2 Hz frequency region. These may include low frequency waves due to reflection and interference of cardiogenic waves and to beats of interference between higher frequency neurogenic vasoconstriction or vasodilatation modulations.

It must be concluded, therefore, that assessment of perfusion dynamics by DTI is rather limited in spite of the relative simplicity of measurement, and more precise information on perfusion dynamics of deeper tissues might be obtained by other technologies, such as Laser Doppler flowmetry, Doppler ultrasound, or MRI. Yet all the basic predictions developed by Anbar regarding the diagnostic usefulness of monitoring *modulation* of blood perfusion (described above) are valid irrespective of the monitoring technique. It must also be realized that the limitations on DTI of skin do not apply to DTI of cells in tissue cultures or of microorganisms.

8.3 DTA Experimentation (1997–2001)

8.3.1 Early DTA Experimentation

Modulation of skin temperature due to hemodynamic effects is of the order of 10 mK [69], which requires a precision of temperature measurement better than 2 mK. If the hemodynamic modulation frequencies of interest are 2 to 10 Hz, a data acquisition rate of at least 100 Hz is required as is a stability of 1 mK over >30 min—the duration of a complete multi-image DTI study [70]. Anbar's attempts from 1992 till mid-1997 to experimentally use different commercial infrared camera systems available at that time to verify basic concepts of quantitative DTA on human subjects have ended with ambiguous results because of the inadequate sensitivity, reproducibility, and speed of those systems. None of those failed experiments were published.

Finally, by the end of 1996 Anbar became aware of the new type of fast and sensitive Ga/As 256 × 256 array quantum-well infrared photodetectors (QWIP) developed by Gunapala *et al.* [71,72] at the Jet Propulsion Laboratory (JPL) in Pasadena. The availability of a sensitive 256 × 256 focal plane detector array has been a minimal prerequisite for meaningful DTA biomedical applications. At the time, that camera could be transferred to and used in a DOD laboratory only. Consequently, Anbar joined Dr. Kaveh Zamani at the Walter Reed Army Institute of Research (WRAIR) in Washington DC and explored a variety of potential biomedical uses of DTA with this unique camera.

These studies included demonstration of monitoring cardiac pulsatile hemodynamics and measurement of blood flow rate in peripheral vasculature [69,73], and demonstration of DTA use in assessment of cutaneous lesions and neuropathies caused by chemicals and of observation of significant changes in facial perfusion under mental stress [74]. Shortly later, DTI was also applied, though with less advanced equipment, to study joint inflammation and pain, presumably mediated by NO [75–77].

Following the promising preliminary findings at WRAIR Dr. Gunapala loaned his camera to facilitate preliminary DTI clinical studies at Buffalo. At the Erie County Hospital, in collaboration with Dr. William Flynn of the Deptartment of Surgery, Anbar demonstrated the effective use of DTI in assessment of microsurgical attachment of a severed penis. Then, in collaboration with Dr. Kenneth Eckert, he demonstrated, at the Windsong Clinic of Buffalo, the use of DTA in assessment of hemodynamic behavior of cancerous breasts [78]. These brief preliminary demonstration studies with borrowed equipment confirmed the potential usefulness of DTA in the clinic. The conclusions of these preliminary findings were then summarized in review papers that pointed out the instrumental and software requirements of this technique [70,79–81].

8.3.2 Research at the Millard Fillmore Hospital at Buffalo

By 1999 Anbar received from a company (OmniCorder Technologies Inc., now Advanced Biophotonics Inc., East Setauket, New York) a state-of-the-art commercial fast digital infrared camera with a QWIP 8 to 9 μm 256 × 256 detector array, operating at a rate of 100 frames/s (AIM, Infrarot Module, Heilbrunn, Germany). That camera incorporated a highly reliable and stable Stirling helium cooler, which is essential for meaningful DTA studies (because the of the high temperature dependence of the sensitivity of QWIP detectors). Anbar received this camera, placed at the Millard Fillmore University Hospital in Buffalo, for experimental DTA studies on breast cancer.

The goal of the research project at Buffalo was twofold:

1. Develop algorithms that will *objectively* differentiate between cancerous and cancer-free breasts without the need for human expertise of "reading" bitmaps of DTI modulation amplitudes. In other words, alleviate *imaging* from DTI and make it a genuine DTA computerized technique. DTI, which is essentially a wholly computerized technique, which produces FFT-generated modulation amplitude spectra for each pixel of the image, lends itself uniquely to the latter end when the whole organ in question, or well-defined regions of it, are treated as an anatomically undifferentiated region of interest [68,70,82].
2. Establish the feasibility of using the algorithms developed meeting the fist goal to *objectively* detect breast cancer in patients who have had suspicious x-ray mammograms before undergoing exploratory biopsy, that is, to distinguish between true- and false-positive x-ray mammograms; the DTA findings were to be compared with the pathology of calcified biopsied tissue as the "gold standard."

Using algorithms developed by Dr. Lorin Milescu [83,84], Anbar's group studied DTI data of a total of 100 breasts, 64 free of cancer and 36 with biopsy-confirmed breast cancers (three DTI views were taken for each breast), of patients examined at the Millard Fillmore Hospital at Buffalo and at the Department of Radiology, University Hospital and Medical Center at Stony Brook, New York [68,85]. That was the first study to demonstrate the potential use of DTA as an *objective* quantitative diagnostic technique. Because of this and since this may be the last time this study will be reviewed in the general context of DTA, we shall include here certain clarifying details and somewhat newer and more effective computational analysis procedures used in the last phase of this 3-year research effort.

To summarize, the objective of that study was to demonstrate that DTA can effectively differentiate between cancerous breasts (irrespective of the type of the cancer) and breasts free of cancer. Once this objective has been achieved, a follow-on study would have had to use the criteria developed in the first study to test the effectiveness of the new methodology under clinical field conditions. Although the objective of the first study has been fully achieved [68,85], unfortunately, no follow up clinical study under similar experimental and computational conditions was implemented up-to-date.

8.3.2.1 Methodology of Assessment

The working hypothesis of the Buffalo study was that the skin of cancerous breasts will manifest significantly lower temperature modulation because of higher perfusion, primarily owing to the vasodilatatory effect of NO.

The following DTA methodology was developed to quantify the temperature modulation of the surface of breasts and identify breasts with low modulation.

Following the acquisition of 1200 sequential thermal images at a rate of 100 frames/s, the projected area of the thermal image of the breast was subdivided into square subareas (spots) of 4×4 pixels each, corresponding to approximately 16 mm^2 of skin. The total area of interest delineated manually on the primary thermal image, comprised of about 1700$\pm$ spots, depending on the size of the breast. The average temperature of each of those spots was then calculated, and a time series of 1024 temperature values was obtained for each spot. After linear regression eliminated slow (<0.1 mHz) temperature changes, and after correction for spurious modulation of the camera or of the environment (common interference removal), each time series underwent FFT analysis [69,83]. Using the FFT data of 160 intervals, 50 mHz each, in the frequency range 2 to 10 Hz, the modulation amplitude of each spot at each of these 160 discrete frequencies was obtained. The cardiogenic modulation frequencies (0.5 to 2 Hz) were excluded, primarily because their assessment would require longer observation times, exacerbating motion artifacts (primarily patient breathing).

For each discrete frequency a subarea (or subareas) of spots with lowest modulation amplitudes (≥ 24 spots in the published study) was (were) identified. Such a subarea was named a *cluster* of low amplitude spots. These clusters were identified and demarcated as follows: all the spots that represented the area of interest (the whole demarcated breast) were rank ordered by their amplitudes (the spot with the lowest amplitude first, the spot with the second lowest second, up to the spot with the highest amplitude).

Spots with low amplitude, owing to one or more "dead" pixels, caused by corresponding inactive detector elements, were excluded from the ranking. The position of the spots with the lowest amplitudes was then registered. If these spots were adjacent to other such spots, a cluster of two or more low amplitude spots was identified. Then spots with the next to lowest amplitude were identified and those in the proximity of a spot with the lowest amplitude were counted as members of a recognized cluster.

This computerized process was continued until a cluster of low amplitude spots with a specified size was identified (24 spots in this study, corresponding approximately to 4 cm^2 (that number could be larger than 24 because the last step could have added more than one sequential spot to the low amplitude cluster, or more than a single cluster with more than 24 spots was formed in the last step of clustering). The amplitude of the spot with the highest amplitude in the identified cluster was then registered. Then the ratio between the number of spots in the identified low amplitude cluster (or clusters with $\geq$24 spots) and all the other spots (nonclustered or less clustered) that, at that frequency, had amplitudes smaller or equal to the spot with the highest amplitude value in the identified low amplitude cluster was determined. That ratio was defined as "first cluster ratio" (FCR).

Another differentiating parameter used was the "first cluster amplitude ratio" (FCA) = the ratio between the average amplitude of the first cluster and the average of the amplitudes of all the spots over the whole demarcated area of interest (the whole breast). The working hypothesis was that both FCR and FCA in a cancerous breast will be significantly lower than in a cancer-free breast.

As discussed earlier, computerized DTA produced information on modulation of both temperature and STH [1,68]; thus we computed in parallel also FCR and FCA values for STH of the spots.

For each case studied and for each of its three views, the computerized output was a spectrum of FCR and FCA values of both temperature and homogeneity for each of the 160 frequencies analyzed.

This large data matrix was statistically analyzed to find out if these parameters can differentiate between cancerous and cancer-free breasts.

The working hypothesis predicted cancerous breasts to have higher FCR and FCA values, at least at certain frequencies, because local attenuation of modulation by extravascular, cancer-produced NO is expected to result in larger clusters with attenuated temperature amplitudes and greater homogeneity compared with breasts free of cancerous lesions. This hypothesis could by tested by a statistical analysis of the FCR and FCA values obtained for the 100 breasts studied.

8.3.2.2 Statistical Analysis and Findings

Using a macroprocedure, a computer sequentially processed each of the image series (cases) in our database, that is, each of the views of each case. For each view, the researchers obtained as the output four ASCII files that listed the FCR(temp), FCR(STH), FCA(temp), and FCA(STH) values for each of the 160 discrete frequencies analyzed. This output could be displayed as a spreadsheet with 160 columns (frequencies), with each row corresponding to a single case (a single view of a specified breast). The same spreadsheet also contained demographic and clinical data. These spreadsheets were then fed to a statistical program, developed at Buffalo by Dr. Aleksey Naumov, for further analysis. The statistical analysis, described before for other DTA-derived parameters [85], reaches the same conclusion—DTA can highly effectively differentiate between cancerous and cancer-free breasts; sensitivities and diagnostic powers >0.95 were obtained, with STH data providing a somewhat higher significance. It was also found that frontal views of cancerous breasts yield significantly higher sensitivity and specificity values than lateral views of the same breast. A description of the statistical procedures and findings are, however, outside the purview of this review chapter.

8.3.2.3 Limitations

The Buffalo study was limited to assessing only high-frequency modulation >2 Hz because the motion artifacts limited the acquisition time to 12 s. While the discrete structures of the average spectra and the highly significant difference between the averages of the two groups of subjects indicates manifestation of hemodynamic process in the 2 to 8 Hz region [68,85], it is regrettable that no reliable information could be produced at lower frequencies. (This limitation has been recently removed by sophisticated motion correction algorithms to be published soon, and those algorithms have already been used to process data in a very recent breast cancer study [86]; see below.)

Removal of motion artifacts will evidently revolutionize many of DTI's clinical applications, especially its use in breast cancer detection. It is now possible to study the hemodynamic behavior of the breast or other tissues down to 0.01 Hz. This could open up a new era in the application of DTA to breast cancer detection and evaluation.

8.3.2.4 Physiological Considerations and Their Implications

From the physiological mechanistic standpoint, the positive findings of the Buffalo study pose interesting questions. While it is expected that a hyperperfused breast will appear warmer, as found in classical thermal imaging, how could changes in perfusion modulation kinetics of a tumor situated, say 20 mm below the skin, affect temperature modulation and the homogeneity of temperature distribution at the skin level. It must be concluded, therefore, that the presence of a cancerous lesion inside the breast affects the behavior of the cutaneous capillary bed. Were it only due to the higher heat dissipation of cancerous breasts, DTI would not have had a higher sensitivity, and especially specificity, of breast cancer detection than classical thermography. Moreover, ductal carcinoma *in situ* (DCIS) that is unlikely to affect the heat dissipation of the whole breast would not have been detectable as it was by DTA [68,85]. We must advance the hypothesis that the NO produced in a tumor inside the breast affects *cutaneous* perfusion dynamics measurable by DTI.

Then one must ask whether it is NO that diffuses from the cancerous lesion to the cutaneous capillary bed and, if so, how does it diffuse? Is it carried in the arterial blood supply? This is rather unlikely in view of its short lifetime in the presence of hemoglobin. Does it diffuse through the lymphatic system or in the interstitial space? This again is not very plausible in view of the rate of oxidation of NO in aqueous media.

We venture here the hypothesis that cancerous breasts build up a significant level of NO in their fat wherein the half-life of NO is likely to be quite long. Then the NO diffuses slowly from the fat into the cutaneous capillary bed, affecting its hemodynamic behavior. This hypothesis awaits, evidently, experimental verification. The fact that cancerous breasts were identified irrespective of the size of the tumors by examining temperature modulation over the whole breast, irrespective of the site of the tumor, supports this new hypothesis, presented here for the first time.

The NO–fat hypothesis implies that subcutaneous fat of cancerous breasts retrieved by needle liposuction will have a significant NO content, while fat of cancer-free breasts would be virtually free of NO. This suggests a quasi-invasive preliminary test of breasts that were found suspicious by x-ray mammography. Such a test could be an attractive alternative to exploratory biopsy, which has a significant level of false negatives, in addition to its invasiveness and costs. It is noteworthy that the presence of NO in subcutaneous fat is less dependent on the locale and nature of the cancerous lesion and might be, therefore, a highly sensitive and specific test, actually alleviating the need for DTI for this clinical problem. Furthermore, if this test proved reliable, it could be streamlined to become the first-line diagnostic test to be followed by surgery. If this hypothesis was verified and such a diagnostic test was found effective, it can be considered a conceptual offshoot of the Buffalo DTI study, justifying inclusion of this suggestion in this review paper.

8.3.3 Preliminary DTA Findings on Melanoma and Diabetes

Although the main trust of DTA studies at Buffalo were on breast cancer patients, two other exploratory studies done there warrant being mentioned. Preliminary studies of patients with osteosarcoma and melanoma undergoing chemotherapy gave encouraging results. In the first study, carried out in collaboration with Dr. C. Karakousis of the Department of Surgery, it was found that cancer induced characteristic DTI "signatures" of melanoma disappeared following chemotherapy, suggesting that inoperative metastatic tumors lost their capacity of NO production as a result of chemotherapy, as a result of their metabolic arrest. In other patients DTI was also able to pick up indication of the presence of residual malignant tissue following excision of the primary lesion.

The other preliminary study was done by Dr. C. Carthy in collaboration with Dr. P. Dandona on diabetic patients. These investigators explored the use of DTI in staging of diabetes mellitus by examining the perfusion of the extremities. The preliminary findings, though promising, however, were not conclusive.

8.4 Recent DTA Studies (2000–2005)

8.4.1 Detection of and Treatment of Malignancy

Following the preliminary findings in Buffalo there have been a number of attempts in different clinical research centers to use DTI in oncology. This included detection of malignant lesions as well as follow-up of treatment of cancer.

Janicek et al. [87] studied the response of soft tissue sarcomas to chemotherapy with DTI, in parallel with CT and PET. DTA detected the malignancy in superficially located sarcomas, and the findings were reported to correlate well with assessments by the two other imaging modalities. Janicek et al. [88–90] showed enhanced temperature modulation, probably due to hypervascularization since they monitored in the 0.8 to 2 Hz range, also in the case of metastatic gastrointestinal stromal tumors; the finding correlated well with those of Doppler ultrasound. Similar results were observed also in the case of malignant lymphomas. The malignant lesions studied by Janicek et al. [91] might have been too deep to exhibit frequencies higher than 2 Hz; thus only the cardiogenic pulsatile modulation were observable. The conclusion of these preliminary clinical studies and suggestions to use DTI in other than breast cancer studies were summarized in 2003.

Lately, a research project was undertaken by Dr. Johan Nilsson at the Karolinska Institute in Stockholm to explore the use of DTI in the detection of metastatic melanoma. In a preliminary series of tests on two patients, melanoma metastases were detectable as spots of enhanced modulation on DTI temperature amplitude bitmaps, both in the cardiogenic frequency range of 0.9 to 1.7 Hz and in the low vasomotor frequency range of 0.05 to 0.2 Hz. The DTI detected melanoma metastases, some of which were visible on the skin and palpable, and confirmed *prior* to the DTI study by thin needle aspiration biopsy. Unfortunately, this preliminary study was not extended to include detection of lesions that were not known beforehand, like in the case of the prebiopsy breast cancer study in Buffalo. These preliminary measurements in the <2 Hz modulation frequency range complement Anbar's earlier observations (see above) on the effect of melanoma metastases on localized temperature modulation in the 2 to 8 Hz range. This far an optimal frequency range for detection of melanoma by DTI has yet to be established.

Following the Buffalo study, there have been just two more DTI studies aimed at breast cancer detection. A major multicenter study by Parisky et al. [92] involved close to a thousand prebiopsy patients. These investigators tried to identify emerging characteristic thermal patterns on thermal images of breasts, in response to external cooling by a stream of cold air. In this study Parisky used hundreds of sequential thermal images. This subset of what has been done in Buffalo 4 years earlier is based on Anbar's hypothesis that vasculature surrounding cancerous lesions is less likely to respond to sympathetic vasoconstriction induced by cold stimuli. The findings corroborated this hypothesis. Unfortunately this extensive study was limited by inferior IR equipment that lacked the sensitivity and speed necessary to monitor temperature modulation. The other limitation of this study was the use of human "experts" in evaluating the computerized images. As was pointed out by Moskowitz [93], the usefulness of this subjective DTI protocol is rather limited.

Another study on breast cancer detection was done by Button et al. [94] at Stony Brook University Hospital. Button used up-to-date equipment and computational procedures in his study of temperature modulation in the cardiogenic frequency range. His findings on a limited number of prebiopsy patients were indicative but nonconclusive, partially because he, like Parisky, used trained human "experts" to evaluate the DTI images.

The latest use of DTI in breast oncology has been in a study by Fanning et al. [86] at the Cleveland Clinic. In their preliminary experiments they assessed the effect of chemotherapeutic agents on established cancerous lesions, on the basis of the assumption that as the viability of the lesion diminishes so will the effect of the NO on temperature modulation. Their preliminary findings were encouraging. However, this use of DTI has limited sensitivity because NO is also produced by phagocytes during the necrosis of the shrinking tumors [33].

In summary, in spite of several encouraging attempts by several groups, the use of DTA in breast oncology still awaits extensive, well-designed clinical trials. A major obstacle to acquisition of reliable DTA data over a wide range of frequencies has been recently removed by motion corrections algorithms. However, this new promising approach to detection of breast cancer has yet to be tested in large-scale clinical studies. Such studies are warranted in view of independent experimental findings that confirmed the vascular effect of cancer-produced NO.

Button et al. [94] have shown in an animal study that the generation of NO by a neoplastic lesion can be detected by DTI. Mice were implanted subcutaneously with human epithelial caner cells. Once these cells established a viable neoplastic lesion 7 days after implantation, the lesion was unambiguously manifested on a DTI bitmap. This manifestation was totally abolished by administration of a conventional NO synthesis inhibitor (LNAME) but reappeared 3 days later, when the effect of the inhibitor abated. This study also demonstrated detection by DTI of the vasodilatatory effect of NO on the vasculature of mice following topical treatment with nitroglycerin.

8.4.2 Use of DTI in the Study of Brain Function and Brain Malignancies

Up to this point we discussed only DTI studies of skin, the huge exposed organ of the body. However, the exposed parenchyma of any other organ could be studied by DTI if its blackbody radiation can be exposed to an IR camera. During open brain surgery for intracranial vascular repair or removal of malignant or benign space occupying lesions, the outer surface of the brain is exposed, allowing infrared imaging, including DTI.

Alexander Gorbach conceptualized the idea of using infrared imaging to monitor the brain already in 1993 when he was still in Russia [95]. Gorbach persisted with his studies in this field at NIH and has published since 2002 a series of highly impressive studies, starting with animal experimentation [96] and ending with numerous clinical open brain intraoperative investigations. Gorbach's studies covered two major aspects:

1. Monitoring the physiology of neurological functions in different regions of the brain by manifestations of changes in local perfusion and metabolic activity [97,98].
2. Clinical uses of DTI, including real-time follow up of reperfusion in the course of vascular neurosurgery, and localization of benign or malignant space occupying lesions by their abnormal vascular structure and perfusion dynamics, allowing then following up of their surgical removal [96,99,100].

Gorbach has shown that local metabolism even in hypermetabolic brain tissues is just a minor contributor of temperature change follwing mental stimulation compared with enhanced perfusion of the region of interest [97,98]; this confirmed Anbar's conclusion regarding the metabolism vs. perfusion in cancerous breasts [24]. Gorbach's findings on regional perfusional changes in response to somatosensory stimulation have been most recently independently confirmed [101].

Unlike Anbar, Gorbach used a 3 to 5 μm camera with a lower thermal sensitivity and stability, and lower acquisition rate, as well as lower accuracy because of the need for a much greater correction for the reflectivity of the monitored surface. These studies were limited, therefore, to monitoring of changes in brain surface temperature following stimulation or surgical manipulations rather than changes in modulation amplitudes of perfusion. In view of these limitations Gorbach's beautifully designed experiments and their unambiguous conclusions are even more praiseworthy. Moreover, Gorbach did not limit his studies to visual observations of temperature change or of the rate of temperature change (which are generally sufficient for neurosurgeons), but he used computerized data processing, similar to that used by Anbar 4 years earlier [83], to receive off-line *objective* information [97]. Since we believe that this is going to be a major advantage of DTA, the independent use of similar algorithms in processing DTI data is quite gratifying.

In parallel with Gorbach's studies of the brain at NIH, Ecker et al. [102] at the Mayo Clinic in Rochester, MN, carried out a DTI study using up-to-date IR imaging equipment and superior data processing software. The superior equipment used at the Mayo clinic allowed demonstration of the same clinical uses of DTI demonstrated at NIH, that is, visualization of brain reperfusion following vascular operations and localization of brain tumors by their abnormal perfusion patterns and vascular dynamics. The equipment used by Ecker et al. [102] (200 frames/s) and its FFT algorithms allowed detection of pathology with a much higher sensitivity and resolution. This demonstrated again the pronounced advantages of computerized analysis of temporal temperature modulation at high spatial resolution.

Ecker's study, independently corroborated by Gorbach's later findings, unambiguously indicates the use DTI in neurosurgery. What is preventing today the routine use of this modality are not the cost of the equipment (<$300,000 for a surgical procedure costing >$20,000 each) or its sophistication (it can be fully automated). What is needed is a multicenter clinical study that will demonstrate the added value, in terms of outcomes of open brain surgical procedures, of using DTI as a tool. From the commercial standpoint, such a multimillion dollar study is not attractive because of the relatively limited commercial market for such equipment (brain surgery is not a common medical procedure). Also from the standpoint of public health, problems that call for brain surgery are not very common compared to other public health care problems. Therefore, expenditure of millions on this problem might be of low priority. Neurosurgeons will have to wait, therefore, for manufacturers of DTI equipment to build up a sufficiently large market for their products in other clinical fields to be in position to sponsor an outcome-driven clinical study in cranial neurosurgery, so as to open up another, though limited, market for their equipment.

Amazingly, Ecker's paper does not refer at all to Gorbach's closely related work, whereas Gorbach refers only once to Ecker's study. In the closely knit community of neurosurgeons of the top institutions in the United States, including NIH and the Mayo Clinic, people must have been aware of the parallel efforts. It seems that science calls for more collegial information exchange and collaboration. It is perhaps equally surprising that Ecker, who unlike Gorbach was not a pioneer in this field, did not refer also to Anbar's monograph, which summarized in detail the history of uses of IR imaging in neurosurgery up to 1993 and strongly recommends the use of DTI in this clinical field. Chances are that Ecker got the idea of using DTI in his clinic from that book, as he used Anbar's algorithms in his study (which he does refer to). Moreover, Ecker's paper's title starts with the pretentious phrase: "Vision of the Future": Whose vision has this been to begin with? It is quite conceivable that Ecker would never have undertaken his study without having been made aware of Anbar's monograph by the distributor of the IR equipment he used.

This teaches us something about the sociology of science, studied by Anbar many years earlier [103]. Academicians are often more ready to give due credit to developers of new hardware or software, or to producers of new data, rather than to people who conceptualized new ideas. However, new ideas are those that have driven science through the ages. Scientists ought to be recognized and rewarded for their ideas first of all.

To summarize, the clinical use of DTI in neurosurgery is one of the first to have verified Anbar's vision on the potential clinical value of this science-based approach.

8.4.3 Use of DTI Intraoperatively in Other Surgical Procedures

There are numerous potential uses of DTI used in surgery. We discussed in Section 8.3.2 neurosurgical applications separately, because open cranial surgery has yielded substantial new physiological neurological information, in addition to is potential clinical uses. Other surgical applications to be discussed next are primarily of clinical value only.

Different surgical applications were suggested in Anbar's monograph, based predominantly on previous static infrared imaging studies. All surgical applications of DTI are based on intraoperative monitoring of perfusion. Two groups of surgical applications of DTI have been recently reduced to practice in well-documented clinical studies—uses in reconstructive and vascular surgery (which have been first demonstrated by Anbar in 1998; see above) and uses in cardiac and transplant surgery. These uses will be described below.

8.4.3.1 Reconstructive and Vascular Surgery

Intraoperative DTI is potentially an ideal tool for reconstructive and vascular surgery, as it allows to assess perfusion and reperfusion in real-time and thus provide the surgeon immediate feedback. Surgeons can thus take corrective action when it is most effective. Zeroing in on and displaying bitmaps of the spatial distribution of cardiogenic frequency modulation in real-time enhances significantly the sensitivity of the technique. DTI can also be a highly useful preoperative and postoperative evaluation tool.

In addition, DTI at cardiogenic frequency allows the precise localization of perforator vessels, which perfuse subcutaneous tissue from below, preoperatively, and thus significantly improving the outcome of grafting. The currently used laser Doppler flowmetry has inferior capacity to provide information on the vasculature over large areas of skin. The application of DTI to this important surgical problem, which has been first demonstrated by Binzoni et al. [104] at the University of Geneva, is likely to be adopted by plastic surgeons as a routine preoperative procedure once a broad scale multicenter clinical study demonstrates its usefulness in a controlled outcome study.

While the use of DTI in reconstructive and vascular surgery is self-evident, it is surprising that only two other clinical studies have been published in this field in recent years. In addition to the pioneering study in Geneva, a study on the intraoperative use of DTI in vascular surgery was carried out in Dundee University in Scotland [105]. A study at Tohoku University demonstrated the advantage of long-wave IR cameras in DTI-assisted vascular surgery [106]. Those three demonstration studies are expected to be just a beginning to a highly beneficial array of routine uses of DTI in these surgical specialties.

8.4.3.2 Cardiac and Transplant Surgery

The use of DTI in open heart surgery is an obvious clinical application, as it involves perfusion and reperfusion of a highly vascular organ. It also involves grafting of vessels (discussed in Section 8.4.3.1). Mohr et al. [109] demonstrated this application on a large number of patients and documeted improved outcomes when this technique was used [107,108]. Mohr actually extended the use of DTI in cardiac surgery he pioneered in 1989, using later much better equipment. The former study was cited in Anbar's 1994 monograph as a model for surgical uses of DTI. Surprisingly, in spite of these well-documented positive clinical results, no other studies on the use of DRI in cardiac surgery in other clinical centers were published to date.

Another surgical application that depends on assessment of reperfusion is transplant surgery. Gorbach et al. [110] have demonstrated the effectiveness of using DTI in kidney transplant surgery. They showed the rate of reperfusion to be an important predictive parameter of the success of transplantation, especially in the case of allografts from cadavers that have been subjected to extended periods of ischemic cooling. The history of this application of thermal imaging, which dates back to the early 1970s, was reviewed in Anbar's 1994 monograph. Yet only modern DTI equipment enabled a reproducible quantitative noninvasive assessment of perfusion rates, making this an attractive procedure for routine kidney transplant surgery, as well as for other transplant situations. Like in the case of cardiac surgery, there has been so far no other follow-up studies of these pioneering efforts.

It seems that introduction of a new technology into surgical suits requires more than just good clinical demonstration studies. Surgery is a relatively conservative discipline, and changes in protocol take a considerable effort, especially when they involve the installation of substantial instrumentation in the operating room. It is often easier to find an enthusiastic research clinician to test a new technological modality and get academic credit for it, than to convince a hospital administrator to acquire a new instrument for a clinic with the sole benefit of better clinical outcomes. As long as there is no competition that forces a hospital to modernize, modernization is less likely. Moreover, the use of any new technique in the clinic requires appropriate compensation by medical insurance, Medicare in particular. Insurance companies are, obviously, reluctant to approve new technology unless it cuts the cost of hospitalization. In the case of cardiac surgery it can be readily claimed that early detection of failure in vascular grafting or of rejection in the case of transplant surgery will cut hospitalization costs. Yet we see how slow has been the acceptance of routine use of DTI even in these surgical procedures.

8.4.4 Clinical Applications of DTI in Other Fields

The use of infrared imaging to monitor reperfusion of tissues, of the extremities in particular, is as old as classic infrared imaging [19]. DTI in its most rudimentary mode—quantitative assessment of warming rates at different subareas of the region of interest—makes this methodology of clinical value. After our review of its uses in surgery (see above), we shall discuss a few recent studies that have used this approach in nonsurgical clinical situation.

Gold et al. [111] have recently used DTI to diagnose upper extremity musculoskeletal disorders, including carpal tunnel syndrome, by following the perfusion dynamics of hands during and after a standardized typing task. The findings were consistent with earlier ones [19], but the more precise DTI assessment allowed meaningful statistical evaluation. It remains to be seen if this technique, which has been known for decades among neurologists, will become more accepted with more precise computerized equipment available today. As was pointed out by Anbar already in 1994, it is conceivable that more precise differential diagnosis could be achieved if temperature modulation was monitored in addition to gross cooling or warm-up rates.

Rewarming of extremities following brief immersion (10 s) in cold water has been used as a diagnostic test also for neurovascular damage resulting from type 2 diabetes mellitus [112]. Since the test performed used classic thermal imaging at 5-min intervals, it can hardly be classified as a DTI procedure. A similar study, though more sophisticated and precise, was carried out more recently on type 1 diabetes patients by Zotter et al. [113] at the University of Graz. In this study differential diagnosis was based on the relative rewarming rates of different toes, adding an anatomic dimension to the test.

Regretfully, up-to-date, no studies have confirmed the value of DTI in differential diagnosis between diabetes-induced vascular occlusions and vascular neuropathies, which should be possible by comparing thermal modulation of the skin of extremities in the cardiogenic and vasomotor frequency ranges, respectively [19]. This could be done without thermal stress, although response to a transient thermal stress could add diagnostic information. Also no attempts have been made so far to use DTI as a management tool to stage diabetes and monitor the effectiveness of treatment.

The same limitations on the acceptance of DTI routinely in surgery, discussed above, apply also to its use in diabetic clinics. Feasibility studies are first needed, and then large-scale clinical tests must prove the added value of the diagnostic technique, before a new technology reaches routine clinical use.

Finally, in the field of peripheral neuronal diseases we will cite a recent quantitative DTI study on complex regional pain syndrome [115]. Huygen et al. [115] at Rotterdam, studied the dynamics of temperature change in the hands of patients following systemic major thermal challenge by a themosuit. While the DTI temperature imaging was done at 10 min intervals, their computerized diagnostic test allowed *objective* evaluation of patients, as in Anbar's diagnostic test on breast cancer [83]. Moreover, this application of DTA has been among those suggested by Anbar 10 years earlier [19].

Other early DTI studies have had recent follow-ups. Fifteen years after Anbar had first demonstrated the use of DTI in monitoring the temperature of the cornea [11,114], a 2005 review recommends the use of dynamic ocular thermography in ophthalmology [116]. The early use of DTI in pain assessment [33,76] have been recently followed in patients with postoperative neuralgia [117]. The results in this group of patient have shown, however, no correlation between cutaneous blood flow and tactile induced pain, unlike pain in rheumatic inflammation [76], suggesting that the former pain is not due to a local vasoactive process. The latter suggestion has been corroborated by another independent thermographic study [118].

Completing the review of thermal imaging warm-up studies since 1999, one has to mention a study on the warm up of teeth and gingival tissue following a brief cooling period with a stream of cold air, to assess the perfusion and thereby the vitality of teeth [119,120]. This study essentially establishes that all normal teeth in a patient's mouth have a similar warm-up pattern, implying that an affected tooth will show a lower rate of thermal recovery. The competing technology is, however, laser Doppler flowmetry (LDF), which can provide the same information at a lower cost. This study is an example of an unjustified use of DTI. Since the area of interest is quite small and DTI equipment is bulkier and more expensive than LDF, there is no justification for the use of DTI for this specific dental problem. It is not surprising, therefore, that there has been no follow-up to this study. However, DTI has a potential use in dental surgery (example, in the management of TMJ pain [75,76]).

8.5 Conclusion

It has been both a gratifying experience and a disappointment for me writing this chapter. I found that the ideas I advanced in the early 1990s, summarized in my 1994 monograph, on the potential advantages of physiology-based DTI as a clinical tool have merit. Many investigators, most of them new users of thermal imaging, have accepted and adopted these notions. At the same time, static, anatomic thermal imaging, which has been around since the early 1970s, has failed to gain acceptance by the medical community. By now it has been universally recognized that thermal imaging manifests physiology and it must, therefore, measure the *dynamics* of physiological processes. A fair number of clinical applications of DTI suggested in my 1994 monograph have been successfully demonstrated since 2000, when appropriate computerized infrared monitoring equipment became commercially available. By now DTI is a recognized domain in medical technology. This has been truly gratifying.

On the other hand, this far none of those applications has reached the stage of routine use in a clinical setting. This may not be as disappointing as it looks, compared with the long time it took to get ultrasonic imaging or even MRI into routine clinical use. In either of these two cases it took time until major medical equipment manufacturers realized the potential of those technologies and marketed them on a large scale. It all boils down to marketing. DTI has not yet reached this stage.

However, it has become more difficult with time to market new medical technologies because of economic constraints. One must prove that the benefits of using a new technology (in terms of better clinical outcomes—patients' survival and quality of life, days of hospitalization, patients' pain and suffering, etc.) outweigh its costs (including the equipment, space, training of personnel, risks, etc.). Moreover, the benefit/cost of the given technology must exceed those of competing technologies. For reasons I pointed out already in 1994 [19], classic clinical thermal imaging has not met these criteria over 30+ years of its existence, in spite of a few successful preliminary attempts. It was left behind, while ultrasound imaging, CT and MRI have flourished.

Will DTI be more successful? For one, it is based on firmer biomedical grounds (users can understand what they are measuring in physiological terms), it is quantitative and is potentially the most *objective* among all medical imaging techniques (as described above, computerized DTA can be used without *any* imaging output), and its hardware costs a fraction of that of CT, PET, or MRI. It also exceeds competing technologies—Laser Doppler flowmetry and Ultrasound Doppler imaging—in its ability to acquire information extremely rapidly on large anatomical areas. Moreover, while DTI can become an invaluable tool in surgery by providing real-time information on facets unavailable to the clinician in any other way, DTA allows completely automated objective diagnosis, as I have demonstrated. DTA heralds therefore a new paradigm in clinical medicine alleviating the need for imaging experts, thus substantially reducing heath care costs. It must be realized that DTA poses a threat to radiologists, the experts who interpret clinical images, and it might be fought by them for obvious reasons. In spite of this, DTI and especially DTA are, with all likelihood, going to become someday a mainstream biomedical technology. This may take more time, possibly not during the lifetime of this reviewer.

The author is comforted by another personal experience. In the late 1950s Anbar pioneered the use of F^{18} in nuclear medicine [121,122], and demonstrated its use in brain tumor localization by coincidence detection of positrons [123–125]. This was long before computers allowed CT to develop. It took more than 30+ years revolutionary developments in computer technology before PET scanners became clinically useful. Hopefully, DTA will have a similar fate.

The author wishes to conclude this review with a personal note.

Note: In his desire to make this review of DTI as inclusive as possible, the author covered all relevant papers that have appeared up to January 2006 in the National Library of Medicine database, in the European *EMbase* (Excerpta

Medica). Also covered were *Thermology* (discontinued), *Thermology International* (and its discontinued predecessors *Thermologie Osterreich* and *European Journal of Thermology*), and *Biomedical Thermology* (Japan), which are not covered in full in the international medical databases. The author also consulted Prof. K. Ammer and Prof. K. Mabuchi, the editors of the two latter current journals. Consequently, publications on DTI outside these resources could have been left out.

Note: Review papers are demarcated by an asterisk (*).

References

[1] Anbar M. and Haverly R.F. Local "micro" variance in temperature distribution evaluated by digital thermography. *Biomedical Thermology*, 13, 173–187, 1994. Also in *Advanced Techniques and Clinical Applications in Biomedical Thermology*. Mabuchi K., Mizushina S. and Harrison B. (eds.) Chur, Harwood Academic Publishers, 173–187, 1994.

[2] Anbar M. Computerized thermography. The emergence of a new diagnostic imaging modality. *International Journal of Technology Assessment in Health Care*, 3, 613–621, 1987.

[3] Montoro J. and Anbar M. New modes of data handling in computerized thermography. *Proceedings of the 10th Annual International Conference of the IEEE Engineering in Medicine and Biology Society*, Harris G. and Walker C. (eds.), Vol. 10, 845–847, 1988.

[4] Montoro J., Hershey L.A. and Anbar M. Enhancement of interpretation of thermograms through on-line software. *Thermology*, 3, 121–124, 1989.

[5] Montoro J., Lee K.-H. and Anbar M. Study of regulation of skin temperature using dynamic digital thermal imaging. *Proceedings of the 11th Annual International Conference of the IEEE Engineering in Medicine and Biology Society*. Seattle, WA, 1158–1159, 1989.

[6] Montoro J., Lee K.-H., Spangler R.A. and Anbar M. Assessment of skin temperature regulation by dynamic digital thermal imaging. *Proceedings of the 34th Annual Meeting of the Biophysical Society. Biophysical Journal*, 57, 280a, 1990.

[7] Montoro J., Lee K.-H. and Anbar M. Skin temperature regulation parameters derived from temporal studies of infrared images. *The FASEB Journal*, Abstracts Part I, 4, A698, 1990.

[8] Montoro J. and Anbar M. Visualization and analysis of dynamic thermographic changes. *Proceedings of the First Conference on Visualization in Biomedical Computing*, Atlanta, GA, 486–489, 1990.

[9] Montoro J., D'Arcy S. and Anbar M. Temporal analysis of thermal images. *Proceedings of the 12th Annual International Conference of the IEEE Engineering in Medicine and Biology Society*, 12, 1578–1579, 1990.

[10] Anbar M. Objective assessment of clinical computerized thermal images. *SPIE Proceedings* 1445, 479–484, 1991.

[11] Montoro J.C., Haverly R.F., D'Arcy S. J., Gyimesi I.M., Coles W.H., Spangler R.A. and Anbar M. Use of digital infrared imaging to objectively assess thermal abnormalities in the human eye. *Thermology* 3, 242–248, 1991.

[12] Anbar M., Montoro J.C., Lee K.-H. and D'Arcy S.J. Manifestation of neurological abnormalities through frequency analysis of skin temperature regulation. *Thermology*, 3, 234–241, 1991.

[13] Anbar M., D'Arcy S. and Montoro J. Characteristic frequencies of human skin temperature regulation derived from temporal analysis of infrared images. *The FASEB Journal*, 5, 4303, 1991.

[14] Anbar M. and D'Arcy S. Localized regulatory frequencies of human skin temperature derived from the analysis of series of infrared images. *Proceedings of the 4th Annual IEEE Symposium on Computer Based Medical Systems (CBMS '91)*, 184–191, 1991.

[15] Anbar M. Recent technological developments in thermology and their impact on clinical applications. *Biomedical Thermology*, 10, 270–276, 1992.

[16] Anbar M. Thermoregulatory processes affecting skin temperature derived from time series of infrared images. *Thermologie Osterreich*, 2S, 18, 1992.

[17]* Anbar M. Dynamic area telethermometry—a new field in clinical thermology Part I. *Medical Electronics*, 146, 62–73, 1994.

[18]* Anbar M. Dynamic area telethermometry—a new field in clinical thermology Part II. *Medical Electronics*, 147, 73–85, 1994.
[19]* Anbar M. *Quantitative Dynamic Telethermometry in Medical Diagnosis and Management.* Boca Raton, FL, CRC Press Inc., 1994.
[20] Freeman G., Dyer R.L., Juhos L., St. John G.A. and Anbar M. Identification of nitric oxide (NO) in human blood. *Archives of Environmental Health*, 33, 19–23, 1978.
[21] Moncada S. The first Robert Furchgott lecture: from endothelium-dependent relaxation to the L-arginine: NO pathway. *Blood Vessels*, 27, 208–217, 1990.
[22] Luscher T.F. Endothelium-derived nitric oxide: the endogenous nitrovasodilator in the human cardiovascular system. *European Heart Journal*, 12, Suppl E, 2–11, 1991.
[23] Moncada S. and Higgs A. The L-arginine-nitric oxide pathway. *New England Journal of Medicine*, 329, 2002–2012, 1993.
[24] Anbar M. Hyperthermia of the cancerous breast—analysis of mechanism. *Cancer Letters*, 84, 23–29, 1994.
[25] Anbar M. Mechanism of hyperthermia of the cancerous breast. *Biomedical Thermology*, 15, 135–139, 1995.
[26] Thomsen L.L., Lawton F.G., Knowles R.G., Beesley J.E., Riveros-Moreno V. and Moncada S. Nitric oxide synthase activity in human gynecological cancer. *Cancer Research*, 54, 1352–1354, 1994.
[27] Fujisawa H., Ogura T., Kurashima Y., Yokoyama T., Yamashita J. and Esumi H. Expression of two types of nitric oxide synthase mRNA in human neuroblastoma cell lines. *Journal of Neurochemistry*, 63, 140–145, 1994.
[28] Jenkins D.C., Charles I.G., Baylis S.A., Lelchuk R., Radomski M.W. and Moncada S. Human colon cancer cell lines show a diverse pattern of nitric oxide synthase gene expression and nitric oxide generation. *British Journal of Cancer*, 70, 847–849, 1994.
[29] Xie W., McCahon P., Jakobsen K. and Parish C. Evaluation of the ability of digital infrared imaging to detect vascular changes in experimental animal tumours. *International Journal of Cancer*, 108, 790–794, 2004.
[30]* Anbar M. Quantitative and dynamic telethermometry—a fresh look at clinical thermology. *IEEE Engineering in Medicine and Biology Magazine*, 14, 15–16, 1995.
[31]* Anbar M. Dynamic area telethermometry and its clinical applications. *SPIE Proceedings*, 2473, 312–322, 1995.
[32] Anbar M. The role of nitric oxide as a synchronizing chemical messenger in the hyperperfusion of the cancerous breast. In *The Biology of Nitric Oxide Part 5*, Moncada S. et al. (eds.), London, Portland Press, pp. 288a–288d, 1996.
[33] Anbar M. and Gratt B.M. Role of nitric oxide in the physiopathology of pain. *Journal of Pain and Symptom Management*, 14, 225–254, 1997.
[34] Anbar M. Mechanism of the association between local hyperthermia and local pain in joint disorders. *European Journal of Thermology*, 7, 173–188, 1997.
[35] Jenkins D.C., Charles I.G., Thomsen L.L., Moss D.W., Holmes L.S., Baylis S.A., Rhodes P., Westmore K., Emson P.C. and Moncada S. Roles of nitric oxide in tumor growth. *Proceedings of the Natural Academy of Science USA*, 92, 4392–4396, 1995.
[36] Maeda H., Noguchi Y., Sato K. and Akaike T. Enhanced vascular permeability in solid tumor is mediated by nitric oxide and inhibited by both new nitric oxide scavenger and nitric oxide synthase inhibitor. *Japan Journal of Cancer Research*, 85, 331–334, 1994.
[37] Tozer G.M., Prise V.E. and Bell K.M. The influence of nitric oxide on tumour vascular tone. *Acta Oncology*, 34, 373–377, 1995.
[38] Tozer G.M., Prise V.E. and Chaplin D.J. Inhibition of nitric oxide synthase induces a selective reduction in tumor blood flow that is reversible with L-arginine. *Cancer Research*, 57, 948–955, 1997.
[39] Fukumura D. and Jain R.K. Role of nitric oxide in angiogenesis and microcirculation in tumors. *Cancer Metastasis Review*, 17, 77–89, 1998.

[40] Thomsen L.L., Miles D.W., Happerfield L., Bobrow L.G., Knowles R.G. and Moncada S. Nitric oxide synthase activity in human breast cancer. *British Journal Cancer*, 72, 41–44, 1995.

[41] Zeillinger R., Tantscher E., Schneeberger C., Tschugguel W., Eder S., Sliutz G. and Huber J.C. Simultaneous expression of nitric oxide synthase and estrogen receptor in human breast cancer cell lines. *Breast Cancer Research Treatment*, 40, 205–207, 1996.

[42] Duenas-Gonzalez A., Isales C.M., del Mar Abad-Hernandez M., Gonzalez-Sarmiento R., Sangueza O. and Rodriguez-Commes J. Expression of inducible nitric oxide synthase in breast cancer correlates with metastatic disease. *Modern Pathology* 10, 645–649, 1997.

[43] Blachier F., Selamnia M., Robert V., M'Rabet-Touil H. and Duee P.H. Metabolism of L-arginine through polyamine and nitric oxide synthase pathways in proliferative or differentiated human colon carcinoma cells. *Biochimica et Biophysica Acta*, 1268, 255–262, 1995.

[44] Ambs S., Merriam W.G., Bennett W.P., Felley-Bosco E., Ogunfusika M.O, Oser S.M., Klein S., Shields P.G., Billiar T.R. and Harris C.C. Frequent nitric oxide synthase-2 expression in human colon adenomas: implication for tumor angiogenesis and colon cancer progression. *Cancer Research*, 58, 334–341, 1998.

[45] Kojima M., Morisaki T., Tsukahara Y., Uchiyama A., Matsunari Y., Mibu R. and Tanaka M. Nitric oxide synthase expression and nitric oxide production in human colon carcinoma tissue. *Journal of Surgical Oncology*, 70, 222–229, 1999.

[46] Rosbe K.W., Prazma J., Petrusz P., Mims W., Ball S.S. and Weissler M.C. Immunohistochemical characterization of nitric oxide synthase activity in squamous cell carcinoma of the head and neck. *Otolaryngology Head and Neck Surgery*, 113, 541–549, 1995.

[47] Gallo O., Masini E., Morbidelli L., Franchi A., Fini-Storchi I., Vergari W.A. and Ziche M. Role of nitric oxide in angiogenesis and tumor progression in head and neck cancer. *Journal of Natural Cancer Institute*, 90, 587–596, 1998.

[48] Gavilanes J., Moro M.A., Lizasoain I., Lorenzo P., Perez A., Leza J.C. and Alvarez-Vicent J.J. Nitric oxide synthase activity in human squamous cell carcinoma of the head and neck. *Laryngoscope*, 109, 148–152, 1999.

[49] Cobbs C.S., Brenman J.E., Aldape K.D., Bredt D.S. and Israel M.A. Expression of nitric oxide synthase in human central nervous system tumors. *Cancer Research*, 55, 727–730, 1995 and *British Journal of Cancer*, 73, 189–196, 1996.

[50] Ellie E., Loiseau H., Lafond F., Arsaut J. and Demotes-Mainard J. Differential expression of inducible nitric oxide synthase mRNA in human brain tumours. *Neuro Report*, 7, 294–296, 1995.

[51] Whittle I.R., Collins F., Kelly P.A., Ritchie I. and Ironside J.W. Nitric oxide synthase is expressed in experimental malignant glioma and influences tumour blood flow. *Acta Neurochir (Wien)*, 138, 870–875, 1996.

[52] Bakshi A., Nag T.C., Wadhwa S., Mahapatra A.K. and Sarkar C. The expression of nitric oxide synthases in human brain tumours and peritumoral areas. *Journal of Neurology Science*, 155, 196–203, 1998.

[53] Joshi M., Strandhoy J. and White W.L. Nitric oxide synthase activity is up-regulated in melanoma cell lines: a potential mechanism for metastases formation. *Melanoma Research*, 6, 121–126, 1996.

[54] Joshi M. The importance of L-arginine metabolism in melanoma: an hypothesis for the role of nitric oxide and polyamines in tumor angiogenesis. *Free Radical Biology and Medicine*, 22, 573–578, 1997.

[55] Ahmad N., Srivastava R.C., Agarwal R. and Mukhtar H. Nitric oxide synthase and skin tumor promotion. *Biochemical and Biophysical Research Communication*, 232, 328–331, 1997.

[56] Edwards P., Cendan J.C., Topping D.B., Moldawer L.L., MacKay S., Copeland E.M. and Lind D.S. Tumor cell nitric oxide inhibits cell growth *in vitro*, but stimulates tumorigenesis and experimental lung metastasis *in vivo*. *Journal of Surgical Research*, 63, 49–52, 1996.

[57] Liu C.Y., Wang C.H., Chen T.C., Lin H.C., Yu C.T. and Kuo H.P. Increased level of exhaled nitric oxide and up-regulation of inducible nitric oxide synthase in patients with primary lung cancer. *British Journal of Cancer*, 78, 534–541, 1998.

[58] Fujimoto H., Ando Y., Yamashita T., Terazaki H., Tanaka Y., Sasaki J., Matsumoto M., Suga M. and Ando M. Nitric oxide synthase activity in human lung cancer. *Japan Journal of Cancer Research*, 88, 1190–1198, 1997.

[59] Klotz T., Bloch W., Volberg C., Engelmann U. and Addicks K. Selective expression of inducible nitric oxide synthase in human prostate carcinoma. *Cancer*, 82, 1897–1903, 1998.

[60] Thomsen L.L., Sargent J.M., Williamson C.J. and Elgie A.W. Nitric oxide synthase activity in fresh cells from ovarian tumour tissue: relationship of enzyme activity with clinical parameters of patients with ovarian cancer. *Biochemical Pharmacology*, 56, 1365–1370, 1998.

[61] Hajri A., Metzger E., Vallat F., Coffy S., Flatter E., Evrard S., Marescaux J. and Aprahamian M. Role of nitric oxide in pancreatic tumour growth: *in vivo* and *in vitro* studies. *British Journal of Cancer*, 78, 841–849, 1998.

[62] Di Cesare P.E., Carlson C.S., Attur M., Kale A.A., Abramson S.B., Della Valle C., Steiner G. and Amin A.R. Up-regulation of inducible nitric oxide synthase and production of nitric oxide by the Swarm rat and human chondrosarcoma. *Journal of Orthopaedic Research*, 16, 667–674, 1998.

[63] Swana H.S., Smith S.D., Perrotta P.L., Saito N., Wheeler M.A. and Weiss R.M. Inducible nitric oxide synthase with transitional cell carcinoma of the bladder. *Journal of Urology*, 161, 630–634, 1999.

[64] Morcos E., Jansson O.T., Adolfsson J., Kratz G. and Wiklund N.P. Endogenously formed nitric oxide modulates cell growth in bladder cancer cell lines. *Urology*, 53, 1252–1257, 1999.

[65] Jansson O.T., Morcos E., Brundin L., Bergerheim U.S., Adolfsson J. and Wiklund N.P. Nitric oxide synthase activity in human renal cell carcinoma. *Journal of Urology*, 160, 556–560, 1998.

[66] Eroglu A., Demirci S., Ayyildiz A., Kocaoglu H., Akbulut H., Akgul H. and Elhan H.A. Serum concentrations of vascular endothelial growth factor and nitrite as an estimate of *in vivo* nitric oxide in patients with gastric cancer. *British Journal of Cancer*, 80, 1630–1634, 1999.

[67] Goto T., Haruma K., Kitadai Y., Ito M., Yoshihara M., Sumii K., Hayakawa N. and Kajiyama G. Enhanced expression of inducible nitric oxide synthase and nitrotyrosine in gastric mucosa of gastric cancer patients. *Clinical Cancer Research*, 5, 1411–1415, 1999.

[68] Anbar M., Naumov A., Milescu L. and Brown C. Objective detection of breast cancer by DAT—an update. *Thermology International*, 11, 11–18, 2001.

[69] Anbar M., Grenn M.W., Marino M.T., Milescu L. and Zamani K. Fast dynamic area telethermometry (DAT) of the human forearm with a Ga/As quantum well infrared focal plane array camera. *European Journal of Thermology*, 7, 105–118,1997.

[70]* Anbar M. and Milescu L. Hardware and software requirements of clinical DAT. *SPIE Proceedings*, 3698, 63–74, 1999.

[71] Gunapala S.D., Liu J.K., Sundaram M., Bandara S.V, Shott C.A., Hoelter T.R., Maker P.D. and Muller R.E. Long-wavelength 256 × 256 QWIP hand-held camera. *SPIE Proceedings*, 2746, 124–133, 1996.

[72] Gunapala S.D., Liu J.K., Park J.S., Sundaram M., Shott C.A., Hoelter T., Lin T.-L., Massie S.T., Maker P.D., Muller R.E. and Sarusi G. 9 μm cutoff 256 × 256 GaAs/AlxGal-xAs quantum well infrared photodetector hand-held camera. *IEEE Transactions of Electron Devices*, 44, 51–57, 1997.

[73] Anbar M., Milescu L., Grenn M.W., Zamani K. and Marino M.T. Study of skin hemodynamics with fast dynamic area telethermometry (DAT). *Proceedings of the 19th IEEE EMBS International Conference*, 644–648, 1997.

[74] Zamani K., Marino M.T., Bonner M. and Anbar M. Assessment of mental stress as well as neurological effects of chemical warfare agents by dynamic area telethermometry. *Proceedings of the 21th Army Science Conference*, 125–130, 1998.

[75] Gratt B.M. and Anbar M. Thermology and facial thermography: Part II. Current and future clinical applications in dentistry. *Journal of Dentomaxillofacial Radiology*, 27, 68–74, 1998.

[76] Anbar M. and Gratt B.M. The possible role of nitric oxide in the physiopathology of pain associated with temporomandibular disorders. *Journal of Oral and Maxillofacial Surgery*, 56, 872–882, 1998.

[77] Anbar M. and Zamani K. A DAT study of a painful knee—comparison with MRI findings. *Proceedings of the 4th Congress of the International College of Thermology* and *27th Annual Meeting of the American Academy of Thermology*, Fort Lauderdale, FL, 25, 1998.

[78] Anbar M., Eckhert K.H. Jr. and Milescu L. Preliminary study of women's breasts with dynamic area telethermometry (DAT). *Proceedings of the 4th Congress of the International College of Thermology* and *27th Annual Meeting of the American Academy of Thermology*, Fort Lauderdale, FL, 27–28, 1998.

[79]* Anbar M. Clinical thermal imaging today—shifting from phenomenological thermography to pathophysiologically based thermal imaging. *IEEE EMBS Magazine*, 17, 25–33, 1998.

[80] Anbar M. and Milescu L. Scope and limitations of dynamic area telethermometry (DAT). *Proceedings of the 20th IEEE EMBS International Conference*, Hong Kong, HK, 928–931, 1998.

[81] Anbar M., Brown C.A., Milescu L. and Babalola J.A. Clinical applications of DAT using a QWIP FPA camera. *SPIE Proceedings*, Orlando, FL, 3698, 93–104, 1999.

[82] Anbar M., Brown C.A., Milescu L., Babalola J.A. and Gentner L. Potential applications of dynamic area telethermometry (DAT) in assessment of cancer in the breasts. *IEEE EMBS Magazine*, 19, 58–62, 2000.

[83] Anbar M., Brown C.A. and Milescu L. Objective identification of cancerous breasts by dynamic area telethermometry (DAT). *Thermology International*, 9, 137–143, 1999.

[84] Anbar M., Brown C.A. and Milescu L. Objective detection of beast cancer by dynamic area telethermometry. *Proceedings of the 21st Annual International Conference of EMBS*, 1115–1116, 1999.

[85] Anbar M., Milescu L., Naumov A., Brown C.A., Button T., Carty C. and AlDulaimi K. Detection of cancerous breasts by dynamic area telethermometry (DAT). *IEEE EMBS Magazine*, 20, 80–91, 2001.

[86] Fanning S.R., Short S., Coleman K., Andresen S., Budd G.T., Moore H., Rim A., Crowe J. and Weng D.E. Correlation of dynamic infrared imaging with radiologic and pathologic response for patients treated with primary systemic therapy for locally advanced breast cancer. *American Society of Clinical Oncology (ASCO) Annual Meeting*, Atlanta, GA, 2006.

[87] Janicek M.J., Waxman A., Janicek M.R. and Demetri G.D. Assessment of early response to therapy in sarcomas: dynamic infrared imaging (DIRI), computerized tomography (CT) and F-18 FDG positron emission tomography (PET). *American Society of Clinical Oncology (ASCO) Annual Meeting*, 2001, Abstract #1390.

[88] Janicek M.J., van Sonnenberg E. and Demetri G.D. Monitoring of early response to treatment in metastatic gastrointestinal stromal tumor (gist): model of multimodality approach including f-18 fdg pet, infrared imaging and Doppler ultrasound. *SGR (Society of Gastrointestinal radiologists) Abdominal radiology Conference*, 2001.

[89] Janicek M.J., Janicek M.R., Merriam P., Potter A., Silberman S., Dimitrijevic S., Fauci M. and Demetri G.D. Imaging responses to Imatinib mesylate (Gleevec, STI571) in gastrointestinal stromal tumors (GIST): Vascular perfusion patterns with Doppler ultrasound (DUS) and dynamic infrared imaging (DIRI). *American Society of Clinical Oncology (ASCO) Annual Meeting*, 2002, Abstract #333.

[90] Janicek M.J., Demetri G.D., Janicek M.R., Shaffer K. and Fauci M.A. Dynamic infrared imaging of newly diagnosed malignant lymphoma compared with Gallium-67 and Fluorine-18 fluorodeoxyglucose (FDG) positron emission tomography. *Cancer Research and Treatment*, 2, 571–578, 2003.

[91] Janicek M.J., Demetri G., Janicek M.R., Shaffer K. and Fauci M.A. Dynamic infrared imaging of newly diagnosed malignant lymphoma compared with gallium-67 and fluorine-18 fluorodeoxyglucose (FDG) positron emission tomography. *Technology in Cancer Research and Treatment*, 2, 71–77, 2003.

[92] Parisky Y.R., Sardi A., Hamm R., Hughes K., Esserman L., Rust S. and Callahan K. Efficacy of computerized infrared imaging analysis to evaluate mammographically suspicious lesions. *American Journal of Roentgenology*, 180, 263–269, 2003.

[93] Moskowitz M. Efficacy of computerized infrared imaging. *American Journal of Roentgenology*, 180, 596, 2003.

[94] Button T.M., Li H., Fisher P., Rosenblatt R., Dulaimy K., Li S., O'Hea B., Salvitti M., Geronimo V., Geronimo C., Jambawalikar S., Carvelli P. and Weiss R. Dynamic infrared imaging for the detection of malignancy. *Physics in Medicine and Biology*, 49, 3105–3116, 2004.

[95] Gorbach A.M. Infrared imaging of brain function. *Advances in Experimental Medicine and Biology*, 333, 95–123, 1993.

[96] Watson J.C., Gorbach A.M., Pluta R.M., Rak R., Heiss J.D. and Oldfield E.H. Real-time detection of vascular occlusion and reperfusion of the brain during surgery by using infrared imaging. *Journal of Neurosurgery*, 96, 918–923, 2002.

[97] Gorbach A.M., Heiss J., Kufta C., Sato S., Fedio P., Kammerer W.A., Solomon J. and Oldfield E.H. Intraoperative infrared functional imaging of human brain. *Annals of Neurology*, 54, 297–309, 2003.

[98] Gorbach A.M. Local alternated temperature gradients as footprints of cortical functional activation. *Journal of Thermal Biology*, 29, 589–598, 2004.

[99] Gorbach A.M., Heiss J.D., Kopylev L. and Oldfield E.H. Intraoperative infrared imaging of brain tumors. *Journal of Neurosurgery*, 101, 960–969, 2004.

[100] Gorbach A.M., Ntziachristos V. and Perelman L. Advances in optical imaging of cancer. In *New Techniques in Oncologic Imaging*, Padhani A.M. and Choyke P.L. (eds), New York, Taylor and Francis, Chapter 18, pp. 351–370, 2005.

[101] Trubel H.K., Sacolik L.I. and Hyder F. Regional temperature changes in the brain during somatosomatic stimulation. *Journal Cerebral Blood Flow and Metabolism*, 26, 68–78, 2006.

[102] Ecker R.D., Goerss S.J., Meyer F.B., Cohen-Gadol A.A., Britton J.W. and Levine J.A. Vision of the future: initial experience with intraoperative real-time high-resolution dynamic infrared imaging. *Journal of Neurosurgery*, 97, 1460–1471, 2002.

[103] Cohen B.P., Kruse R.J. and Anbar M. The social structure of scientific research teams. *Pacific Sociological Review*, 25, 205–245, 1982.

[104] Binzoni T., Leung T., Delpy D.T., Fauci M.A. and Rufenacht D. Mapping human skeletal muscle perforator vessels using a quantum well infrared photodetector (QWIP) might explain the variability of NIRS and LDF measurements. *Physics in Medicine and Biology*, 49, N165–N173, 2004.

[105] Campbell P.A., Cresswell A.B., Frank T.G. and Cuschieri A. Real-time thermography during energized vessel sealing and dissection. *Surgical Endoscopy*, 17, 1640–1645, 2003.

[106] Nakagawa A., Hirano T., Uenohara H., Utsunomiya H., Suzuki S., Takayama K., Shirane R. and Tominaga T. Use of intraoperative dynamic infrared imaging with detection wavelength of 7–14 μm in the surgical obliteration of spinal arteriovenous fistula: case report and technical considerations. *Minimally Invasive Neurosurgery*, 47, 136–139, 2004.

[107] Falk V., Walther T., Philippi A., Autschbach R., Krieger H., Dalichau H. and Mohr F.W. Thermal coronary angiography for intraoperative patency control of arterial and saphenous vein coronary artery bypass grafts: results in 370 patients. *Journal of Cardiac Surgery*, 10, 147–160, 1995.

[108] van Son J.A., Falk V., Walther T., Diegeler A. and Mohr F.W. Thermal coronary angiography for intraoperative testing of coronary patency in congenital heart defects. *Annals of Thoracic Surgery*, 64, 1499–1500, 1997.

[109] Mohr F.W. and Falk V. Thermal coronary angiography: a method for assessing graft patency and coronary anatomy in coronary bypass surgery. *Annals of Thoracic Surgery*, 47, 441–449, 1989. Updated in 1997 *Annals of Thoracic Surgery*, 63, 1506–1507.

[110] Gorbach A., Simonton D., Hale D.A., Swanson S.J. and Kirk A.D. Objective, real-time, intraoperative assessment of renal perfusion using infrared imaging. *American Journal of Transplantation*, 3, 988–993, 2003.

[111] Gold J.E., Cherniack M. and Buchholz B. Infrared thermography for examination of skin temperature in the dorsal hand of office workers. *European Journal of Applied Physiology*, 93, 245–251, 2004.

[112] Fujiwara Y., Inukai T., Aso Y. and Takemura Y. Thermographic measurement of skin temperature recovery time of extremities in patients with type 2 diabetes mellitus. *Experimental and Clinical Endocrinology and Diabetes*, 108, 463–469, 2000.

[113] Zotter H., Kerbl R., Gallistl S., Nitsche H. and Borkenstein M. Rewarming index of the lower leg assessed by infrared thermography in adolescents with type 1 diabetes mellitus. *Journal of Pediatric Endocrinology Metabolism*, 16, 1257–1262, 2003.

[114] Haverly R.F. and Anbar M. A telethermometric study of the age dependence of corneal temperature. *Biomedical Thermology*, 14, 10–26, 1994.

[115] Huygen F.J., Niehof S., Klein J. and Zijlstra F.J. Computer-assisted skin videothermography is a highly sensitive quality tool in the diagnosis and monitoring of complex regional pain syndrome type I. *European Journal of Applied Physiology*, 91, 516–524, 2004.

[116] Purslow C. and Wolffsohn J.S. Ocular surface temperature: a review. *Eye Contact Lens*, 31, 117–123, 2005.

[117] Besson M., Brook P., Chizh B.A. and Pickering A.E. Tactile allodynia in patients with postherpetic neuralgia: lack of change in skin blood flow upon dynamic stimulation. *Pain*, 117, 154–191, 2005.

[118] Kemppainen P., Forster C. and Handwerker H.O. The importance of stimulus site and intensity in differences of pain-induced vascular reflexes in human orofacial regions. *Pain*, 91, 331–338, 2001.

[119] Kells B.E., Kennedy J.G., Biagioni P.A. and Lamey P.J. Computerized infrared thermographic imaging and pulpal blood flow: Part 1. A protocol for thermal imaging of human teeth. *International Endodontic Journal*, 33, 442–447, 2000.

[120] Kells B.E., Kennedy J.G., Biagioni P.A. and Lamey P.J. Computerized infrared thermographic imaging and pulpal blood flow: Part 2. Rewarming of healthy human teeth following a controlled cold stimulus. *International Endodontic Journal*, 33, 448–462, 2000.

[121] Anbar M., Guttmann S. and Lewitus Z. The accumulation of fluoroborate ions in thyroid glands of rats. *Endocrinology*, 66, 888–890, 1960.

[122] Anbar M. Application of fluorine 18 in biological studies with special reference to bone physiology. In *Production and Use of Short Lived Radioisotopes*, Vienna, IAEA, Vol. II, pp. 227–245, 1963.

[123] Anbar M., Kosary I., Laor Y., Guttmann S., Lewitus Z. and Askenasy H. The localization of intracranial tumors by positron emitting F18 labelled fluoborate. *Proceedings of the Beilinson Hospital*, 10, 50–52, 1961.

[124] Askenasy H., Kosary I., Toledo E., Lewitus Z. and Anbar M. The use of radioisotopes in the detection of brain tumors. *Proceedings of the Beilinson Hospital*, 10, 53–58, 1961.

[125] Ashkenazy H.M., Anbar M., Laor Y., Kosary I.Z. and Guttmann S. The localization of intracranial space-occupying lesions by fluoroborate ions labelled with fluorine 18. *American Journal of Roentgenology and Nuclear Medicine*, 88, 350–354, 1962.

Infrared Imaging of the Breast: A Review

Prologue		9-1
9.1	Introduction	9-2
9.2	Fundamentals and Standards in Infrared Breast Imaging	9-2
	Physics • Equipment Considerations • Laboratory and Patient Preparation Protocols • Imaging • Special Tests • Image Interpretation • Correlation between Pathology and Infrared Imaging	
9.3	The Role of Infrared Imaging in the Detection of Cancer	9-9
9.4	Infrared Imaging as a Risk Indicator	9-11
9.5	Infrared Imaging as a Prognostic Indicator	9-12
9.6	Breast Cancer Detection and Demonstration Project	9-13
	Poor Study Design • Untrained Personnel and Protocol Violations	
9.7	Mammography and Infrared Imaging	9-15
9.8	Current Status of Breast Cancer Detection	9-16
9.9	Future Advancements in Infrared Imaging	9-17
9.10	Conclusion	9-17
References		9-18

William C. Amalu
Pacific Chiropractic and Research Center

William B. Hobbins
Women's Breast Health Center

Jonathan F. Head
Robert L. Elliot
Elliot-Elliot-Head Breast Cancer Research and Treatment Center

Prologue

The use of infrared imaging in health care is not a recent phenomenon. However, its utilization in breast cancer screening is seeing renewed interest. This attention is fueled by research that clearly demonstrates the value of this procedure and the tremendous impact it has on the mortality of breast cancer.

Since the late 1950s, extensive research has been performed on the use of infrared imaging in breast cancer screening. Over 800 papers can be found in the indexed medical literature. In this database, well over 300,000 women have participated as study subjects. The numbers of participants in many studies are very large and range from 10,000 to 85,000 women. Some of these studies have followed patients for up to 12 years in order to investigate and establish the technology's unique ability as a risk marker.

With strict standardized interpretation protocols having been established for over 15 years, infrared imaging of the breast has obtained an average sensitivity and specificity of 90%. As a future risk indicator for breast cancer, a persistent abnormal thermogram carries a 22 times higher risk and is 10 times more significant than a first order family history of the disease. Studies clearly show that an abnormal infrared image is the single most important risk marker for the existence of or future development of breast cancer.

9.1 Introduction

The first recorded use of thermobiological diagnostics can be found in the writings of Hippocrates around 480 BC [1]. A mud slurry spread over the patient was observed for areas that would dry first and was thought to indicate underlying organ pathology. Since this time, continued research and clinical observations proved that certain temperatures related to the human body were indeed indicative of normal and abnormal physiologic processes.

In the 1950s, military research into infrared monitoring systems for nighttime troop movements ushered in a new era in thermal diagnostics. Once declassified in the mid-1950s, infrared imaging technology was made available for medical purposes. The first diagnostic use of infrared imaging came in 1956 when Lawson discovered that the skin temperature over a cancer in the breast was higher than that of normal tissue [2–4]. He also showed that the venous blood draining the cancer is often warmer than its arterial supply.

The Department of Health Education and Welfare released a position paper in 1972 in which the director, Thomas Tiernery, wrote, "The medical consultants indicate that thermography, in its present state of development, is beyond the experimental state as a diagnostic procedure in the following 4 areas: (1) Pathology of the female breast …." On January 29, 1982, the Food and Drug Administration published its approval and classification of thermography as an adjunctive diagnostic screening procedure for the detection of breast cancer. Since the late 1970s, numerous medical centers and independent clinics have used thermography for a variety of diagnostic purposes.

Since Lawson's groundbreaking research, infrared imaging has been used for over 40 years as an adjunctive screening procedure in the evaluation of the breast. In this time, significant advances have been made in infrared detection systems and the application of sophisticated computerized image processing.

9.2 Fundamentals and Standards in Infrared Breast Imaging

Clinical infrared imaging is a procedure that detects, records, and produces an image of a patient's skin surface temperatures or thermal patterns. The image produced resembles the likeness of the anatomic area under study. The procedure uses equipment that can provide both qualitative and quantitative representations of these temperature patterns.

Infrared imaging does not entail the use of ionizing radiation, venous access, or other invasive procedures; therefore, the examination poses no harm to the patient. Classified as a functional imaging technology, infrared imaging of the breast provides information on the normal and abnormal physiologic functioning of the sensory and sympathetic nervous systems, vascular system, and local inflammatory processes.

9.2.1 Physics

All objects with a temperature above absolute zero (-273K) emit infrared radiation from their surface. The Stefan–Boltzmann Law defines the relation between radiated energy and temperature by stating that the total radiation emitted by an object is directly proportional to the object's area and emissivity and the fourth power of its absolute temperature. Since the emissivity of human skin is extremely high (within 1% of that of a blackbody), measurements of infrared radiation emitted by the skin can be converted directly into accurate temperature values. This makes infrared imaging an ideal procedure to evaluate surface temperatures of the body.

9.2.2 Equipment Considerations

Infrared rays are found in the electromagnetic spectrum within the wavelengths of 0.75 μm to 1 mm. Human skin emits infrared radiation mainly in the 2 to 20 μm wavelength range, with an average peak at 9 to 10 μm [5]. With the application of Plank's equation and Wein's Law, it is found that approximately 90% of the emitted infrared radiation in humans is in the longer wavelengths (6 to 14 μm).

There are many important technical aspects to consider when choosing an appropriate clinical infrared imaging system. (The majority of which is outside the scope of this chapter.) However, minimum equipment standards have been established from research studies, applied infrared physics, and human anatomic and physiologic parameters [6–7]. Absolute, spatial, and temperature resolution along with thermal stability and adequate computerized image processing are just a few of the critical specifications to take into account. Real-time image capture is a basic requirement in modern clinical imaging systems. Absolute resolution, or the number of distinct infrared detectors dedicated to forming the image (resolvable elements per line in a scanning system), must be adequate enough to produce a quality image. The ability of the system to resolve discrete areas on the surface of the skin is defined as spatial resolution. Standards for clinical systems require that the spatial resolution of the camera should be able to resolve 1 mm^2 at the surface of the skin when the patient is placed at 40 cm from the detector (2.5 mrad). The temperature resolution, or thermal sensitivity, of the camera should be 0.1°C. This level of temperature discernment is necessary to maintain adequate objective temperature measurements when performing quantitative analyses. Although these specifications are extremely important, the most fundamental consideration in the selection of clinical infrared imaging equipment is the wavelength sensitivity of the infrared detector. The decision on which area in the infrared spectrum to select a detector from depends on the object one wants to investigate and the environmental conditions in which the detection is taking place. Considering that the object in question is the human body, Plank's equation leads us to select a detector in the 6 to 14 μm region. Assessment of skin temperature by infrared measurement in the 3 to 5 μm region is less reliable due to the emissivity of human skin being farther from that of a blackbody in that region [8,9]. The environment under which the examination takes place is well controlled, but not free from possible sources of detection errors. Imaging room environmental artifacts such as reflectance can cause errors when shorter wavelength detectors (under 7 μm) are used [10]. Consequently, the optimum infrared detector to use in imaging the breast, and the body as a whole, would have sensitivity in the longer wavelengths spanning the 9 to 10 μm range [7–14].

The problems encountered with first generation infrared camera systems, such as incorrect detector sensitivity (shorter wavelengths), thermal drift, calibration, analog interface, and so forth have been solved for almost two decades. Modern clinical infrared imaging systems exceed the minimum specification standards mentioned above. However, no studies have been published demonstrating the need for a change in the standards. Modern computerized infrared imaging systems have the ability to discern minute variations in thermal emissions while producing extremely high-resolution images that can undergo digital manipulation by sophisticated computerized analytical processing.

9.2.3 Laboratory and Patient Preparation Protocols

In order to produce diagnostic quality infrared images, certain laboratory and patient preparation protocols must be strictly adhered to. Infrared imaging must be performed in a controlled environment. The primary reason for this is the nature of human physiology. Changes from a different external (noncontrolled room) environment, clothing, and so forth produce thermal artifacts. In order to properly prepare the patient for imaging, the patient should be instructed to refrain from sun exposure, stimulation or treatment of the breasts, cosmetics, lotions, antiperspirants, deodorants, exercise, and bathing before the examination.

The imaging room must be temperature- and humidity controlled and maintained between 18 and 23°C, and kept to within 1°C of change during the examination. This temperature range ensures that the patient is not placed in an environment in which their physiology is stressed into a state of shivering or perspiring. The room should also be free from drafts and infrared sources of heat (i.e., sunlight and incandescent lighting). In keeping with a physiologically neutral temperature environment, the floor should be carpeted or the patient must wear shoes in order to prevent increased physiologic stress.

Lastly, the patient must undergo 15 min of waist-up nude acclimation in order to reach a condition in which the body is at thermal equilibrium with the environment. At this point, further changes in the surface temperatures of the body occur very slowly and uniformly; thus, not affecting changes in homologous anatomic regions. Thermal artifacts from clothing or the outside environment are also removed at this time. The last 5 min of this acclimation period is usually spent with the patient placing their hands on top of their head in order to facilitate an improved anatomic presentation of the breasts for imaging. Depending on the patient's individual anatomy, certain positioning maneuvers may need to be implemented such that all of the pertinent surfaces of the breasts may be imaged. In summary, adherence to proper patient and laboratory protocols is absolutely necessary to produce a physiologically neutral image free from artifact and ready for interpretation.

9.2.4 Imaging

The actual process of imaging is undertaken with the intent to adequately detect the infrared emissions from the pertinent surface areas of the breasts. As with mammography, a minimum series of images is needed in order to facilitate adequate coverage. The series includes the bilateral frontal breast along with the right and left oblique views (a right and left single breast close-up view may also be included). The bilateral frontal view acts as a scout image to give a baseline impression of both breasts. The oblique views (approximately 45° to the detector) expose the lateral and medial quadrants of the breasts for analysis. The optional close-up views maximize the use of the detector allowing for the highest thermal and spatial resolution image of each breast. This series of images takes into consideration the infrared analyses of curved surfaces and adequately provides for an accurate analysis of all the pertinent surface areas of the breasts (see Figures 9.1 to 9.5).

Positioning of the patient prior to imaging facilitates acclimation of the surface areas and ease of imaging. Placing the patient in a seated or standing posture during the acclimation period is ideal to facilitate these needs. In the seated position, the patient places their arms on the arm rests away from the body to allow for proper acclimation. When positioning the patient in front of the camera, the use of a rotating chair or having the patient stand makes for uncomplicated positioning for the necessary views.

FIGURE 9.1 (See color insert at the back of the book.) Bilateral frontal.

Infrared Imaging of the Breast

FIGURE 9.2 (**See color insert.**) Right oblique.

FIGURE 9.3 (**See color insert.**) Left oblique.

FIGURE 9.4 (**See color insert.**) Right close-up.

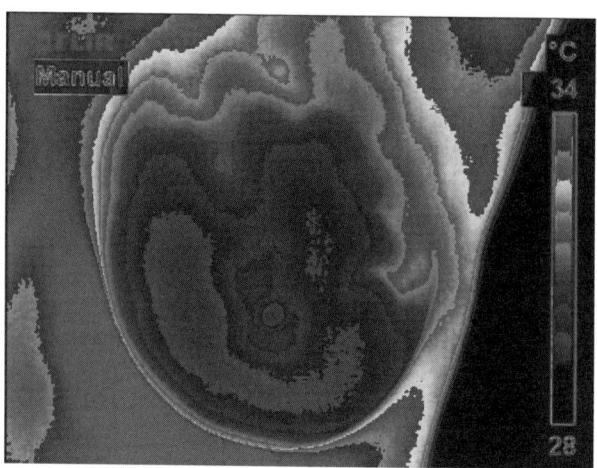

FIGURE 9.5 (See color insert.) Left close-up.

Because of differing anatomy from patient to patient, special views may be necessary to adequately detect the infrared emissions from the pertinent surface areas of the breasts. The most common problem encountered is inadequate viewing of the inferior quadrants due to nipple ptosis. This is easily remedied by adding "lift views." Once the baseline images are taken, the patient is asked to gently "lift" each breast from the superior most aspect of the Tail of Spence exposing the inferior quadrants for detection. Additional images are then taken in this position in order to maintain the surface areas covered in the standard views.

9.2.5 Special Tests

In the past, an optional set of views may have been added to the baseline images. Additional views would be taken after the patient placed their hands in ice cold water as a thermoregulatory challenge. It was hoped that this dynamic methodology would increase the sensitivity and specificity of the thermographic procedure.

In order to understand the hopes placed on this test, one needs to understand the underlying physiologic mechanisms of the procedure. The most common and accepted method of applied thermoregulatory challenge involves ice water immersion of the hands or feet (previous studies investigating the use of fans or alcohol spray noted concerns over the creation of thermal artifacts along with the methods causing a limited superficial effect). The mechanism is purely neurovascular and involves a primitive survival reflex initiated from peripheral neural receptors and conveyed to the central nervous system. To protect the body from hypothermia, the reflex invokes a sympathetically mediated blood vessel constriction in the periphery in an attempt to maintain the normal core temperature set point. This stress test is intended to increase the sensitivity of the thermogram by attempting to identify nonresponding blood vessels such as those involved in angiogenesis associated with neoplasm. Blood vessels produced by cancerous tumors are simple endothelial tubes devoid of a muscular layer and the neural regulation afforded to embryologic vessels. As such, these new vessels would fail to constrict in response to a sympathetic stimulus. In the normal breast, test results would produce an image of relative cooling with attenuation of vascular diameter. A breast harboring a malignancy would theoretically remain unchanged in temperature or demonstrate hyperthermia with vascular dilatation. However, to date it has not been found that the stress test offers any advantage over the baseline images [15].

For well over a decade, the largest infrared breast imaging centers worldwide, along with the leading experts and researchers in the field of infrared breast imaging, have discontinued the use of the cold challenge. Yet, in a 2004 detailed review of the literature combined with an investigational study, Amalu explored the validity of the thermoregulatory challenge test [15]. Results from 23 patients with

FIGURE 9.6 (See color insert.) TH1 (normal uniform nonvascular).

histologically confirmed breast cancers along with 500 noncancerous patients were presented demonstrating positive and negative responses to the challenge. From the combined literature review and study analysis it was found that the test did not alter the clinical decision-making process for following up suspicious thermograms, nor did it enhance the detection of occult cancers found in normal thermograms. In summary, it was found that there was no evidence to support the use of the cold challenge. The study noted insufficient evidence to warrant its use as a mandated test with all women undergoing infrared breast imaging. It also warned that it would be incorrect to consider a breast thermogram substandard, inaccurate, or incomplete if a thermoregulatory challenge was not included. In conclusion, Amalu stated that "Until further studies are performed and ample evidence can be presented to the contrary, a review of the available data indicates that infrared imaging of the breast can be performed excluding the cold challenge without any known loss of sensitivity or specificity in the detection of breast cancers."

9.2.6 Image Interpretation

Early methods of interpretation of infrared breast images was based solely on qualitative (subjective) criteria. The images were read for variations in vascular patterning with no regard to temperature variations between the breasts (Tricore method) [16]. This lead to wide variations in the outcomes of studies preformed with inexperienced interpreters. Research throughout the 1970s proved that when both qualitative and quantitative data were incorporated in the interpretations, an increase in sensitivity and specificity was realized. In the early 1980s, a standardized method of thermovascular analysis was proposed. The interpretation was composed of 20 discrete vascular and temperature attributes in the breast [17,18]. This method of analysis was based on previous research and large-scale studies comprising tens of thousands of patients. Using this methodology, thermograms would be graded into one of 5 TH (thermobiological) classifications. Based on the combined vascular patterning and temperatures across the two breasts, the images would be graded as TH1 (normal uniform nonvascular), TH2 (normal uniform vascular), TH3 (equivocal), TH4 (abnormal), or TH5 (severely abnormal) (see Figures 9.6 and 9.7). The use of this standardized interpretation method significantly increased infrared imaging's sensitivity, specificity, positive and negative predictive value, and inter-/intraexaminer interpretation reliability. Continued patient observations and research over the past two decades has caused changes in some of the thermovascular values; thus, keeping the interpretation system up-to-date. Variations in this methodology have also been adopted with great success. However, it is recognized that, as with any other imaging procedure, specialized training and experience produces the highest level of screening success.

FIGURE 9.7 (See color insert.) Right TH5 (severely abnormal).

9.2.7 Correlation between Pathology and Infrared Imaging

The empirical evidence that an underlying breast cancer alters regional skin surface temperatures was investigated early on. In 1963, Lawson and Chughtai, two McGill University surgeons, published an elegant intraoperative study demonstrating that the increase in regional skin surface temperature associated with breast cancer was related to venous convection [19]. This early quantitative experiment added credence to previous research suggesting that infrared findings were linked to increased vascularity.

Infrared imaging of the breast may also have critical prognostic significance since it may correlate with a variety of pathologic prognostic features such as tumor size, tumor grade, lymph node status, and markers of tumor growth [20]. Continued research is underway investigating the pathologic basis for these infrared findings. One possibility is increased blood flow due to vascular proliferation (assessed by quantifying the microvascular density [MVD]) as a result of tumor-associated angiogenesis. Although in one study [21], the MVD did not correlate with abnormal infrared findings. However, the imaging method used in that study consisted of contact plate technology (liquid crystal thermography [LCT]), which is not capable of modern computerized analysis. Consequently, LCT does not possess the discrimination and digital processing necessary to begin to correlate histological and discrete vascular changes [22].

In 1993, Head and Elliott reported that improved images from second generation infrared systems allowed more objective and quantitative analysis [20], and indicated that growth-rate-related prognostic indicators were strongly associated with the infrared image interpretation.

In a 1994 detailed review of the potential of infrared imaging [23], Anbar suggested that the previous empirical observation that small tumors were capable of producing notable infrared changes could be due to enhanced perfusion over a substantial area of the breast surface via regional tumor induced nitric oxide (NO) vasodilatation. NO is synthesized by nitric oxide synthase (NOS), found both as a constitutive form of NOS, especially in endothelial cells, and as an inducible form of NOS, especially in macrophages [24]. NOS has been demonstrated in breast carcinoma [25] using tissue immunohistochemistry, and is associated with a high tumor grade.

Nitric oxide is a molecule with potent vasodilating properties. It is a simple highly reactive free radical that readily oxidizes to form nitrite or nitrate ions. It diffuses easily through both hydrophilic and hydrophobic media. Thus, once produced, NO diffuses throughout the surrounding tissues, inside and outside the vascular system, and induces a variety of biochemical changes depending on the specific receptors involved. NO exerts its influence by binding to receptor sites in the endothelium of arteries or arterioles. This causes inhibition of sympathetic vasoconstriction. The end result is NO induced vasodilatation, which in turn may produce an asymmetrical thermovascular infrared image.

The largest body of evidence surrounding the physiologic mechanism by which infrared imaging detects precancerous and malignant states of the breast lies in the recruitment of existing blood vessels and the formation of new ones (angiogenesis). The process of angiogenesis begins with the release of angiogenesis factors (AF) from precancerous or cancerous cells. In the early stages of tumor growth, the majority of neoplasms exhibit a lower cellular metabolic demand. As such, the release of AF causes the existing vessels to resist constriction in order to maintain a steady supply of nutrients to the growing mass. As the tumor increases in size the need for nutrients becomes greater. AF begins to exert its influence by opening the dormant vessels in the breast. Once this blood supply becomes too little to maintain the growth of the neoplasm, AF causes the formation of new blood vessels. These new vessels are simple endothelial tubes connecting the tumor to existing nearby arteries and arterioles. This augmented blood supply produces the increase in heat and vascular asymmetry seen in infrared images.

The concept of angiogenesis, as an integral part of early breast cancer, was emphasized in 1996 by Guidi and Schnitt. Their observations suggested that it is an early event in the development of breast cancer and may occur before tumor cells acquire the ability to invade the surrounding stroma and even before there is morphologic evidence of an *in situ* carcinoma [26]. In 1996, in his highly reviewed textbook entitled *Atlas of Mammography—New Early Signs in Breast Cancer,* Gamagami studied angiogenesis by infrared imaging and reported that hypervascularity and hyperthermia could be shown in 86% of nonpalpable breast cancers. He also noted that in 15% of these cases infrared imaging helped to detect cancers that were not visible on mammography [27].

The greatest evidence supporting the underlying principle by which infrared imaging detects precancerous growths and cancerous tumors surrounds the well-documented recruitment of existing vascularity and angiogenesis that is necessary to maintain the increased metabolism of malignant cellular growth and multiplication. The biomedical engineering evidence of infrared imaging's value, both in model *in vitro* and clinically *in vivo* studies of various tissue growths, normal and neoplastic, has been established [28–34].

9.3 The Role of Infrared Imaging in the Detection of Cancer

In order to determine the value of infrared imaging, two viewpoints must be considered: first, the sensitivity of thermograms taken preoperatively in patients with known breast carcinoma; and second, the incidence of normal and abnormal thermograms in asymptomatic populations (specificity) and the presence or absence of malignancy in each of these groups.

In 1965, Gershon-Cohen, a radiologist and researcher from the Albert Einstein Medical Center, introduced infrared imaging to the United States [35]. Using a Barnes thermograph, he reported on 4000 cases with a sensitivity of 94% and a false-positive rate of 6%. This data was included in a review of the then current status of infrared imaging published in 1968 in California—*A Cancer Journal for Physicians* [36].

In prospective studies, Hoffman first reported on thermography in a gynecologic practice. He detected 23 carcinomas in 1924 patients (a detection rate of 12.5 per 1000), with an 8.4% false-negative (91.6% sensitivity) and a 7.4% false-positive (92.6% specificity) rate [37].

Stark and Way screened 4621 asymptomatic women, 35% of whom were under 35 years of age, and detected 24 cancers (detection rate of 7.6 per 1000), with a sensitivity and specificity of 98.3 and 93.5%, respectively [38].

In a study comprising 25,000 patients screened and 1878 histologically proven breast cancers, Amalric and Spitalier reported on their results with infrared imaging. From this group, a false-negative and false-positive rate of 9% (91% sensitivity and specificity) was found [39].

In a mobile unit examination of rural Wisconsin, Hobbins screened 37,506 women using thermography. He reported the detection of 5.7 cancers per 1000 women screened with a 12% false-negative and 14% false-positive rate. His findings also corroborated with others that thermography is the sole early initial signal in 10% of breast cancers [17,40].

Reporting his Radiology division's experience with 10,000 thermographic studies done concomitantly with mammography over a 3-year period, Isard reiterated a number of important concepts including the remarkable thermal and vascular stability of the infrared image from year to year in the otherwise healthy patient and the importance of recognizing any significant change [41]. In his experience, combining these modalities increased the sensitivity rate of detection by approximately 10%; thus, underlining the complementarity of these procedures since each one did not always suspect the same lesion. It was Isard's conclusion that, had there been a preliminary selection of his group of 4393 asymptomatic patients by infrared imaging, mammographic examination would have been restricted to the 1028 patients with abnormal infrared imaging, or 23% of this cohort. This would have resulted in a cancer detection rate of 24.1 per 1000 combined infrared and mammographic examinations as contrasted to the expected 7 per 1000 by mammographic screening alone. He concluded that since infrared imaging is an innocuous examination, it could be utilized to focus attention upon asymptomatic women who should be examined more intensely. Isard emphasized that, like mammography and other breast imaging techniques, infrared imaging does not diagnose cancer, but merely indicates the presence of an abnormality.

Spitalier and associates screened 61,000 women using thermography over a 10-year period. The false-negative and false-positive rate was found to be 11% (89% sensitivity and specificity). Thermography also detected 91% of the nonpalpable cancers (Grade T0: tumors less than 1 cm in size). The authors noted that of all the patients with cancer, thermography alone was the first alarm in 60% of the cases [42].

Two small-scale studies by Moskowitz (150 patients) [43] and Treatt (515 patients) [44] reported on the sensitivity and reliability of infrared imaging. Both used unknown experts to review the images of breast cancer patients. While Moskowitz excluded unreadable images, data from Threatt's study indicated that less than 30% of the images produced were considered good, the rest being substandard. Both of these studies produced poor results; however, this could be expected considering the lack of adherence to accepted imaging methods and protocols. The greatest error in these studies is found in the methods used to analyze the images. The type of image analysis consisted of the sole use of abnormal vascular pattern recognition. At the time these studies were performed, the accepted method of infrared image interpretation consisted of a combined vascular pattern and quantitative analysis of temperature variations across the breasts. Consequently, the data obtained from these studies is highly questionable. Their findings were also inconsistent with numerous previous large-scale multicenter trials. The authors suggested that for infrared imaging to be truly effective as a screening tool, there needed to be a more objective means of interpretation and proposed that this would be facilitated by computerized evaluation. This statement is interesting considering that recognized quantitative and qualitative reading protocols (including computer analysis) were being used at the time.

In a unique study comprising 39,802 women screened over a 3-year period, Haberman and associates used thermography and physical examination to determine if mammography was recommended. They reported an 85% sensitivity and 70% specificity for thermography. Haberman cautioned that the findings of thermographic specificity could not be extrapolated from this study as it was well-documented that long-term observation (8 to 10 years or more) is necessary to determine a true false-positive rate. The authors noted that 30% of the cancers found would not have been detected if it were not for thermography [45].

Gros and Gautherie reported on a large-scale study comprising 85,000 patients screened. Culmination of the data resulted in a 90% sensitivity and 88% specificity for thermography [46–49].

In a large-scale multicenter review of nearly 70,000 women screened, Jones reported a false-negative and false-positive rate of 13% (87% sensitivity) and 15% (85% sensitivity), respectively for thermography [50].

In a study performed in 1986, Usuki reported on the relation of thermographic findings in breast cancer diagnosis. He noted an 88% sensitivity for thermography in the detection of breast cancers [51].

Parisky and associates published a study from a multicenter 4-year clinical trial using infrared imaging to evaluate mammographically suspicious lesions. Data from a blinded subject set was obtained in 769 women with 875 biopsied lesions resulting in 187 malignant and 688 benign findings. The index of suspicion resulted in a 97% sensitivity in the detection of breast cancers [52].

In a study comparing clinical examination, mammography, and thermography in the diagnosis of breast cancer, three groups of patients were used: 4716 patients with confirmed carcinoma, 3305 patients with histologically diagnosed benign breast disease, and 8757 general patients (16,778 total participants). This paper also compared clinical examination and mammography to other well-known studies in the literature including the National Cancer Institute (NCI) sponsored Breast Cancer Detection and Demonstration Projects (BCDDPs). In this study, clinical examination had an average sensitivity of 75% in detecting all tumors and 50% in cancers less than 2 cm in size. This rate is exceptionally good when compared to many other studies at between 35 and 66% sensitivity. Mammography was found to have an average of 80% sensitivity and 73% specificity. Thermography had an average sensitivity of 88% (85% in tumors less than 1 cm in size) and a specificity of 85%. An abnormal thermogram was found to have a 94% predictive value. From the findings in this study, the authors suggested that "none of the techniques available for screening for breast carcinoma and evaluating patients with breast-related symptoms is sufficiently accurate to be used alone. For the best results, a multimodal approach should be used [53]."

In a series of 4000 confirmed breast cancers, Thomassin and associates observed 130 subclinical carcinomas ranging in diameter of 3 to 5 mm. Both mammography and thermography were used alone and in combination. Of the 130 cancers, 10% were detected by mammography, 50% by thermography, and 40% by both techniques. Thus, there was a thermal alarm in 90% of the patients and the only sign in 50% of the cases [54].

In a simple review of over 15 large-scale studies from 1967 to 1998, infrared imaging of the breast has showed an average sensitivity and specificity of 90%. With continued technological advances in infrared imaging in the past decade, some studies are showing even higher sensitivity and specificity values. However, until further large-scale studies are performed, these findings remain in question.

9.4 Infrared Imaging as a Risk Indicator

As early as 1976, at the *Third International Symposium on Detection and Prevention of Cancer* held in New York, thermal imaging was established by consensus as the highest risk marker for the possibility of the presence of an undetected breast cancer. It had also been shown to predict such a subsequent occurrence [55–57]. The Wisconsin Breast Cancer Detection Foundation presented a summary of its findings in this area, which has remained undisputed [58]. This, combined with other reports, has confirmed that an abnormal infrared image is the highest risk indicator for the future development of breast cancer and is ten times as significant as a first-order family history of the disease [48].

In a study of 10,000 women screened, Gautherie found that, when applied to asymptomatic women, thermography was very useful in assessing the risk of cancer by dividing patients into low- and high-risk categories. This was based on an objective evaluation of each patient's thermograms using an improved reading protocol that incorporated 20 thermopathological factors [59].

A screening of 61,000 women using thermography was performed by Spitalier over a 10-year period. The authors concluded that "in patients having no clinical or radiographic suspicion of malignancy, a persistently abnormal breast thermogram represents the highest known risk factor for the future development of breast cancer [42]."

From a patient base of 58,000 women screened with thermography, Gros and associates followed 1527 patients with initially healthy breasts and abnormal thermograms for 12 years. Of this group, 44% developed malignancies within 5 years. The study concluded that "an abnormal thermogram is the single most important marker of high-risk category for the future development of breast cancer [49]."

Spitalier and associates followed 1416 patients with isolated abnormal breast thermograms. It was found that a persistently abnormal thermogram, as an isolated phenomenon, is associated with an actuarial breast cancer, a risk of 26% at 5 years. Within this study, 165 patients with nonpalpable cancers were observed. In 53% of these patients, thermography was the only test which was positive at the time of initial evaluation. It was concluded that:

1. A persistently abnormal thermogram, even in the absence of any other sign of malignancy, is associated with a high risk of developing cancer.

2. This isolated abnormality also carries with it a high risk of developing interval cancer, and as such the patient should be examined more frequently than the customary 12 months.
3. Most patients diagnosed as having minimal breast cancer have abnormal thermograms as the first warning sign [60,61].

In a study by Gautherie and associates, the effectiveness of thermography in terms of survival benefit was discussed. The authors analyzed the survival rates of 106 patients in whom the diagnosis of breast cancer was established as a result of the follow-up of thermographic abnormalities found on the initial examination when the breasts were apparently healthy (negative physical and mammographic findings). The control group consisted of 372 breast cancer patients. The patients in both groups were subjected to identical treatment and followed for 5 years. A 61% increase in survival was noted in the patients who were followed-up due to initial thermographic abnormalities. The authors summarized the study by stating that "the findings clearly establish that the early identification of women at high risk of breast cancer based on the objective thermal assessment of breast health results in a dramatic survival benefit [62,63]."

Infrared imaging provides a reflection of functional tumor-induced angiogenesis and metabolic activity rather than structurally based parameters (i.e., tumor size, architectural distortion, and microcalcifications). Recent advances in cancer research have determined that the biological activity of a neoplasm is far more significant an indicator of aggressiveness than the size of the tumor. As a direct reflection of the biological activity in the breast, infrared imaging has been found to provide a significant biological risk marker for cancer.

9.5 Infrared Imaging as a Prognostic Indicator

Studies exploring the biology of cancers have shown that the amount of thermovascular activity in the breast is directly proportional to the aggressiveness of the tumor. As such, infrared imaging provides the clinician with an invaluable tool in prognosis and treatment monitoring.

In a study of 209 breast cancers, Dilhuydy and associates found a positive correlation between the degree of infrared abnormalities and the existence of positive axillary lymph nodes. It was reported that the amount of thermovascular activity seen in the breast was directly related to the prognosis. The study concluded that infrared imaging provides a highly significant factor in prognosis and that it should be included in the pretherapeutic assessment of a breast cancer [64].

Amalric and Spitalier reported on 25,000 patients screened and 1878 histologically proven breast cancers investigated with infrared imaging. The study noted that the amount of infrared activity in the breast was directly proportional to the survival of the patient. The "hot" cancers showed a significantly poorer prognosis with a 24% survival rate at 3 years. A much better prognosis with an 80% survival rate at 3 years was seen in the more biologically inactive or "cooler" cancers. The study also noted a positive association between the amount of thermal activity in the breast and the presence of positive axillary nodes [65].

Reporting on a study of breast cancer doubling times and infrared imaging, Fournier noted significant changes in the thermovascular appearance of the images. The shorter the tumor doubling time, the more thermographic pathological signs were evident. It was concluded that infrared imaging served as a warning signal for the faster-growing breast cancers [66].

A retrospective analysis of 100 normal patients, 100 living cancer patients, and 126 deceased cancer patients was published by Head. Infrared imaging was found to be abnormal in 28% of the normal patients, compared to 65% of the living cancer patients and 88% of the deceased cancer patients. Known prognostic indicators related to tumor growth rate were compared to the results of the infrared images. The concentration of tumor ferritin, the proportion of cells in DNA synthesis and proliferating, and the expression of the proliferation-associated tumor antigen Ki-67 were all found to be associated with an abnormal infrared image. It was concluded that "the strong relationships of thermographic results with these three growth rate-related prognostic indicators suggest that breast cancer patients with abnormal thermograms have faster-growing tumors that are more likely to have metastasized and to recur with a shorter disease-free interval [20]."

In a paper by Gros and Gautherie, the use of infrared imaging in the prognosis of treated breast cancers was investigated. The authors considered infrared imaging to be absolutely necessary for assessing pretherapeutic prognosis or carrying out the follow-up of breast cancers treated by exclusive radiotherapy. They noted that before treatment, infrared imaging yields evidence of the cancer growth rate (aggressiveness) and contributes to the therapeutic choice. It also indicates the success of radio-sterilization or the suspicion of a possible recurrence or radio-resistance. The authors also noted a weaker 5-year survival with infrared images that showed an increase in thermal signals [67].

In a recent study by Keyserlingk, 20 women with core-biopsy proven locally advanced breast cancer underwent infrared imaging before and after chemohormonotherapy. All 20 patients were found to have abnormal thermovascular signs prior to treatment. Upon completion of the final round of chemotherapy, each patient underwent curative-intent surgery. Prior to surgery, all 20 patients showed improvement in their initial infrared scores. The amount of improvement in the infrared images was found to be directly related to the decrease in tumor size. A complete normalization of prechemotherapy infrared scores was seen in five patients. In these patients, there was no histological evidence of cancer remaining in the breast. In summary, the authors stated that "Further research will determine whether lingering infrared detected angiogenesis following treatment reflects tumor aggressiveness and ultimately prognosis, as well as early tumor resistance, thus providing an additional early signal for the need of a therapeutic adjustment [68]."

9.6 Breast Cancer Detection and Demonstration Project

The BCDDP is the most frequently quoted reason for the decreased interest in infrared imaging. The BCDDP was a large-scale study performed from 1973 through 1979, which collected data from many centers around the United States. Three methods of breast cancer detection were studied: physical examination, mammography, and infrared imaging.

Just before the onset of the BCDDP, two important papers appeared in the literature. In 1972, Gerald D. Dodd of the University of Texas Department of Diagnostic Radiology presented an update on infrared imaging in breast cancer diagnosis at the *Seventh National Cancer Conference* sponsored by the National Cancer Society and the NCI [69]. In his presentation, he suggested that infrared imaging would be best employed as a screening agent for mammography. He proposed that in any general survey of the female population aged 40 and over, 15 to 20% of these subjects would have positive infrared imaging and would require mammograms. Of these, approximately 5% would be recommended for biopsy. He concluded that infrared imaging would serve to eliminate 80 to 85% of the potential mammograms. Dodd also reiterated that the procedure was not competitive with mammography and, reporting the Texas Medical School's experience with infrared imaging, noted that it was capable of detecting approximately 85% of all breast cancers. Dodd's ideas would later help to fuel the premise and attitudes incorporated into the BCDDP.

Three years later, J.D. Wallace presented to another Cancer Conference, sponsored by the American College of Radiology, the American Cancer Society and the Cancer Control Program of the NCI, an update on infrared imaging of the breast [70]. The author's analysis suggested that the incidence of breast cancer detection per 1000 patients screened could increase from 2.72 when using mammography to 19 when using infrared imaging. He then underlined that infrared imaging poses no radiation burden on the patient, requires no physical contact, and, being an innocuous technique, could concentrate the sought population by a significant factor selecting those patients that required further investigation. He concluded that "the resulting infrared image contains only a small amount of information as compared to the mammogram, so that the reading of the infrared image is a substantially simpler task."

Unfortunately, this rather simplistic and cavalier attitude toward the generation and interpretation of infrared images was prevalent when it was hastily added and then prematurely dismissed from the BCDDP, which was just getting underway. Exaggerated expectations led to the ill-founded premise that infrared imaging might replace mammography rather than complement it. A detailed review of the Report of the Working Group of the BCDDP, published in 1979, is essential to understand the subsequent evolution of infrared imaging [71].

The work scope of this project was issued by the NCI on the March 26, 1973 with six objectives, the second being to determine if a negative infrared image was sufficient to preclude the use of clinical examination and mammography in the detection of breast cancer. The Working Group, reporting on results of the first 4 years of this project, gave a short history regarding infrared imaging in breast cancer detection. They wrote that, as of the 1960s, there was intense interest in determining the suitability of infrared imaging for large-scale applications, and mass screening was one possibility. The need for technological improvement was recognized and the authors stated that efforts had been made to refine the technique. One of the important objectives behind these efforts had been to achieve a sufficiently high sensitivity and specificity for infrared imaging in order to make it useful as a prescreening device in selecting patients for referral for mammographic examination. It was thought that, if successful, the incorporation of this technology would result in a relatively small proportion of women having mammography (a technique that had caused concern at that time because of the carcinogenic effects of radiation). The Working Group indicated that the sensitivity and specificity of infrared imaging readings, with clinical data emanating from interinstitutional studies, were close to the corresponding results for physical examination and mammography. They noted that these three modalities selected different subgroups of breast cancers, and for this reason further evaluation of infrared imaging as a screening device in a controlled clinical trial was recommended.

9.6.1 Poor Study Design

While the Working Group describes in detail the importance of quality control of mammography, the entire protocol for infrared imaging was summarized in one paragraph and simply indicated that infrared imaging was conducted by a BCDDP-trained technician. The detailed extensive results from this report, consisting of over 50 tables, included only one that referred to infrared imaging showing that it had detected only 41% of the breast cancers during the first screening while the residual were either normal or unknown. There is no breakdown as far as these two latter groups were concerned. Since 28% of the first screening and 32% of the second screening were picked up by mammography alone, infrared imaging was dropped from any further evaluation and consideration. The report stated that it was impossible to determine whether abnormal infrared images could be predictive of interval cancers (cancers developing between screenings) since they did not collect this data.

By the same token, the Working Group was unable to conclude, with their limited experience, whether the findings were related to the then available technology of infrared imaging or with its application. They did, however, conclude that the decision to dismiss infrared imaging should not be taken as a determination of the future of this technique, rather that the procedure continued to be of interest because it does not entail the risk of radiation exposure. In the Working Group's final recommendation, they state that "infrared imaging does not appear to be suitable as a substitute for mammography for routine screening in the BCDDP." The report admitted that several individual programs of the BCDDP had results that were more favorable than what was reported for the BCDDP as a whole. They encouraged investment in the development and testing of infrared imaging under carefully controlled study conditions and suggested that high priority be given to these studies. They noted that a few suitable sites appeared to be available within the BCDDP participants and proposed that developmental studies should be solicited from sites with sufficient experience.

9.6.2 Untrained Personnel and Protocol Violations

JoAnn Haberman, who was a participant in this project [72], provided further insight into the relatively simplistic regard assigned to infrared imaging during this program. The author reiterated that expertise in mammography was an absolute requirement for the awarding of a contract to establish a screening center. However, the situation was just the opposite with regard to infrared imaging—no experience was required at all. When the 27 demonstration project centers opened their doors, only five had any preexisting expertise in infrared imaging. Of the remaining screening centers, there was no experience at all in this technology. Finally, more than 18 months after the project had begun, the NCI-established centers where radiologists and their technicians could obtain sufficient training in infrared imaging. Unfortunately, only 11 of the demonstration project directors considered this training of sufficient importance to send their technologists to learn proper infrared technique. The imaging sites also disregarded environmental controls. Many of the project sites were mobile imaging vans that had poor heating and cooling capabilities, and often kept their doors open in the front and rear to permit an easy flow of patients. This, combined with a lack of adherence to protocols and preimaging patient acclimation, lead to unreadable images.

In summary, with regard to infrared imaging, the BCDDP was plagued with problems and seriously flawed in five critical areas:

1. The study was initiated with an incorrect premise that infrared imaging might replace mammography. A functional imaging procedure that detects metabolic thermovascular aberrations cannot replace a test that looks for specific areas of structural changes in the breast.
2. Completely untrained technicians were used to perform the scans.
3. The study used radiologists who had no experience or knowledge in reading infrared images.
4. Proper laboratory environmental controls were completely ignored. In fact, many of the research sites were mobile trailers with extreme variations in internal temperatures.
5. No standardized reading protocol had yet been established for infrared imaging. It was not until the early 1980s that established and standardized reading protocols were adopted.

Considering these facts, the BCDDP could not have properly evaluated infrared imaging. Since the termination of the BCDDP, a considerable amount of published research has demonstrated the true value of this technology.

9.7 Mammography and Infrared Imaging

From a scientific standpoint, mammography and infrared imaging are completely different screening tests. As a structural imaging procedure, mammography cannot be compared to a functional imaging technology such as infrared imaging. While mammography attempts to detect architectural tissue shadows, infrared imaging observes for changes in the subtle metabolic milieu of the breast. Even though mammography and infrared imaging examine completely different aspects of the breast, research has been performed that allows for a statistical comparison of the two technologies. Since a review of the research on infrared imaging has been covered, data on the current state of mammography is presented.

In a study by Rosenberg, 183,134 screening mammograms were reviewed for changes in sensitivity due to age, breast density, ethnicity, and estrogen replacement therapy. Out of these screening mammograms 807 cancers were discovered at screening. The results showed that the sensitivity for mammography was 54% in women younger than 40 years, 77% in women aged 40 to 49, 78% in women aged 50 to 64, and 81% in women older than 64 years. Sensitivity was 68% in women with dense breasts and 74% in estrogen replacement therapy users [73].

Investigating the cumulative risk of a false-positive result in mammographic screening, Elmore and associates performed a 10-year retrospective study of 2400 women aged 40 to 69 years of age. A total of 9762 mammograms were investigated. It was found that a woman had an estimated 49.1% cumulative risk of having a false-positive result after ten mammograms. Even though no breast cancer was present, over one third of the women screened were required to have additional evaluations [74].

In a review of the literature, Head investigated the sensitivity, specificity, positive predictive value, and negative predictive values for mammography and infrared imaging. The average reported performance for mammography was 86% sensitivity, 79% specificity, 28% positive predictive value, and 92% negative predictive value. For infrared imaging the averaged performance was: 86% sensitivity, 89% specificity, 23% positive predictive value, and 99.4% negative predictive value [75].

Pisano, along with a large investigational group, provided a detailed report on the Digital Mammographic Imaging Screening Trial (DMIST). The study investigated the diagnostic performance of digital vs.

film mammography in breast cancer screening. Both digital and film mammograms were taken on 42,760 asymptomatic women presenting for screening mammography. Data was gathered from 33 sites in the United States and Canada. Digital mammography was found to be more accurate in women under age 50 and in women whose breasts were radiographically dense. The sensitivity for both film and digital mammography was found to be 69% [76].

Keyserlingk and associates published a retrospective study reviewing the relative ability of clinical examinations, mammography, and infrared imaging to detect 100 new cases of ductal carcinoma *in situ*, stage I and II breast cancers. Results from the study found that the sensitivity for clinical examination alone was 61%, mammography alone was 66%, and infrared imaging alone was 83%. When suspicious and equivocal mammograms were combined the sensitivity was increased to 85%. A sensitivity of 95% was found when suspicious and equivocal mammograms were combined with abnormal infrared images. However, when clinical examination, mammography, and infrared images were combined a sensitivity of 98% was reached [77].

From a review of the cumulative literature database, it can be found that the average sensitivity and specificity for mammography is, at best, 80 and 79%, respectively, for women over the age of 50 [78–80]. A significant decrease in sensitivity and specificity is seen in women below this age. This same research also shows that mammography routinely misses interval cancers (cancers that form between screening exams) [80] that may be detected by infrared imaging. Taking into consideration all the available data, mammography leaves much to be desired as the current gold standard for breast cancer screening. As a stand alone screening procedure, it is suggested that mammography may not be the best choice. In the same light, infrared imaging should also not be used alone as a screening test. The two technologies are of a complimentary nature. Neither used alone are sufficient, but when combined each builds on the deficiencies of the other. In reviewing the literature it seems evident that a multimodal approach to breast cancer screening would serve women best. A combination of clinical examination, mammography, and infrared imaging would provide the greatest potential for breast conservation and survival.

9.8 Current Status of Breast Cancer Detection

Current first-line breast cancer detection strategy still depends essentially on clinical examination and mammography. The limitations of the former, with its reported sensitivity rate often below 65% [77,82] is well-recognized, and even the proposed value of self-breast examination is being contested [83]. While mammography is accepted as the most cost-effective imaging modality, its contribution continues to be challenged with persistent false-negative rates ranging up to 30% [73,76,84,85]; with decreasing sensitivity in younger patients and those on estrogen replacement therapy [73,85]. In addition, there is recent data suggesting that denser and lesser informative mammography images are precisely those associated with an increased cancer risk [86]. Echoing some of the shortcomings of the BCDDP concerning their study design and infrared imaging, Moskowitz indicated that mammography is also not a procedure to be performed by the inexperienced technician or radiologist [88].

With the current emphasis on earlier detection, there is now renewed interest in the parallel development of complimentary imaging techniques that can also exploit the precocious metabolic, immunological, and vascular changes associated with early tumor growth. While promising, techniques such as scintimammography [89], Doppler ultrasound [90], and magnetic resonance imaging (MRI) [91], are associated with a number of disadvantages that include exam duration, limited accessibility, need of intravenous access, patient discomfort, restricted imaging area, difficult interpretation, and limited availability of the technology. Like ultrasound, they are more suited to use as second-line options to pursue the already abnormal screening evaluations. While practical, this stepwise approach currently results in the nonrecognition, and thus delayed utilization of second-line technology in approximately 10% of established breast cancers [88]. This is consistent with a study published by Keyserlingk [77].

As an addition to the breast health screening process, infrared imaging has a significant role to play. Owing to infrared imaging's unique ability to image the metabolic aspects of the breast, extremely early warning signals (up to 10 years before any other detection method) have been observed in long-term studies. It is for this reason that an abnormal infrared image is the single most important marker of high risk for the existence of or future development of breast cancer. This, combined with the proven sensitivity, specificity, and prognostic value of the technology, places infrared imaging as one of the major front-line methods of breast cancer screening.

9.9 Future Advancements in Infrared Imaging

Modern high-resolution uncooled focal plane array cameras coupled with high-speed computers running sophisticated image analysis software are commonplace in today's top infrared imaging centers. However, research in this field continues to produce technological advancements in image acquisition and digital processing.

Research is currently under way investigating the possible subtle alterations in the blood supply to the breast during the earliest stages of malignancy. Evidence suggests that there may be a normal vasomotor oscillation frequency in the arterial structures of the human body. It is theorized that there may be disturbances in this normal oscillatory rate when a malignancy is forming. Research using infrared detection systems capturing 200 frames per second with a sensitivity of 0.009 of a degree centigrade may be able to monitor alterations in this vasomotor frequency band.

Another unique methodology is investigating the possibility of using infrared emission data to extrapolate depth and location of a metabolic heat source within the body. In the case of cancer, the increased tissue metabolism resulting from rapid cellular multiplication and growth generates heat. With this new approach in infrared detection, it is theorized that an analysis based on an analogy to electrical circuit theory—termed the thermal-electric analog—may possibly be used to determine the depth and location of the heat source.

The most promising of all the advances in medical infrared imaging are the adaptations being used from military developments in the technology. Hardware advances in narrow-band filtering hold promise in providing multispectral and hyperspectral images. One of the most intriguing applications of multispectral/hyperspectral imaging may include real-time intraoperative cytology. Investigations are also underway utilizing smart processing, also known as artificial intelligence. This comes in the form of postimage processing of the raw data from the infrared sensor array. Some of the leading-edge processing currently under study includes automated target recognition (ATR), artificial neural networks (ANN), and threshold algorithms, to mention only a few. The uses of ATR and threshold algorithms are dependent on a reliable normative database. The images are processed based on what the system has learned as normal and compares the new image to that database. Unlike ATR and threshold algorithms, ANN uses data summation to produce pattern recognition. This is extremely important when it comes to the complex thermovascular patterns seen in infrared breast imaging. Ultimately, these advancements will lead to a decrease in operator dependence and a substantial increase in both objectivity and accuracy.

New breast cancer treatments are also exploring methods of targeting the angiogenic process. Owing to a tumor's dependence on a constant blood supply to maintain growth, antiangiogenesis therapy is becoming one of the most promising therapeutic strategies and has been found to be pivotal in the new paradigm for consideration of breast cancer development and treatment [92]. The future may see infrared imaging and antiangiogenesis therapy combined as the state-of-the-art in the biological assessment and treatment of breast cancer.

These and other new methodologies in medical infrared imaging are being investigated and may prove to be significant advancements. However, a great deal of research will need to be performed before new technologies can be adopted for medical use.

9.10 Conclusion

The large patient populations and long survey periods in many of the above clinical studies yields a high significance to the various statistical data obtained. This is especially true for the contribution of infrared imaging to early cancer diagnosis, as an invaluable marker of high-risk populations, and in therapeutic decision making.

Currently available high-resolution digital infrared imaging technology benefits greatly from enhanced image production, computerized image processing and analysis, and standardized image interpretation protocols. Over 40 years of research and 800 indexed papers encompassing well over 300,000 women participants has demonstrated infrared imaging's abilities in the early detection of breast cancer. Infrared imaging has distinguished itself as the earliest detection technology for breast cancer. It has the ability to signal an alarm that a cancer may be forming up to 10 years before any other procedure can detect it. In seven out of ten cases, infrared imaging will detect signs of a cancer before it is seen on a mammogram. Clinical trials have also shown that infrared imaging significantly augments the long-term survival rates of its recipients by as much as 61%. And when used as part of a multimodal approach (clinical examination, mammography, and infrared imaging), 95% of all early stage cancers will be detected. Ongoing research into the thermal characteristics of breast pathologies will continue to investigate the relationships between neoangiogenesis, chemical mediators, and the neoplastic process.

It is unfortunate, but many clinicians still hesitate to consider infrared imaging as a useful tool in spite of the considerable research database, steady improvements in both infrared technology and image analysis, and continued efforts on the part of the infrared imaging societies. This attitude may be due in part to the average clinician's unfamiliarity with the physical and biological basis of infrared imaging. The other methods of cancer investigations refer directly to topics of medical teaching. For instance, radiography and ultrasonography refer to structural anatomy. Infrared imaging, however, is based on thermodynamics and thermokinetics, which are unfamiliar to most clinicians; though man is experiencing heat production and exchange in every situation he undergoes or creates.

Considering the contribution that infrared imaging has demonstrated thus far in the field of early breast cancer detection, all possibilities should be considered for promoting further technical, biological, and clinical research along with the incorporation of the technology into common clinical use.

References

[1] Adams, F., *The Genuine Works of Hippocrates*. Williams and Wilkins, Baltimore, MD, 1939.
[2] Lawson, R.N., Implications of surface temperatures in the diagnosis of breast cancer. *Can. Med. Assoc. J.*, 75, 309, 1956.
[3] Lawson, R.N., Thermography—a new tool in the investigation of breast lesions. *Can. Serv. Med.*, 13, 517, 1957.
[4] Lawson, R.N., A new infrared imaging device. *Can. Med. Assoc. J.*, 79, 402, 1958.
[5] Archer, F. and Gros, C., Classification thermographique des cancers mammaries. *Bull. Cancer*, 58, 351, 1971.
[6] Amalu, W., et al., Standards and protocols in clinical thermographic imaging. *International Academy of Clinical Thermology*, September 2002.
[7] Kurbitz, G., Design criteria for radiometric thermal-imaging devices. In *Thermological Methods*, VCH mbH, pp. 94–100, 1985.
[8] Houdas, Y. and Ring, E.F.J., Models of thermoregulation. In *Human Temperature: Its Measurement and Regulation*. Plenum Press, New York, pp. 136–141, 1982.
[9] Flesch, U., Physics of skin-surface temperature. In *Thermological Methods*, VCH mbH, pp. 21–33, 1985.
[10] Anbar, M., *Quantitative Dynamic Telethermometry in Medical Diagnosis and Management*. CRC Press, Boca Raton, FL, p. 106, 1994.
[11] Anbar, M., Potential artifacts in infrared thermographic measurements. *Thermology*, 3, 273, 1991.
[12] Friedrich, K. (Optic research laboratory, Carl Zeiss—West Germany), Assessment criteria for infrared thermography systems. *Acta Thermographica*, 5, 68–72.
[13] Engel, J.M., Thermography in locomotor diseases. *Acta Thermographica*, 5, 11–13.

[14] Cuthbertson, G.M., The development of IR imaging in the United Kingdom. In *The Thermal Image in Medicine and Biology*. Uhlen-Verlag, Wien, pp. 21–32, 1995.

[15] Amalu, W., Nondestructive testing of the human breast: the validity of dynamic stress testing in medical infrared breast imaging. *Proceedings of the 26th Annual International Conference of the IEEE Engineering in Medicine and Biology Society*. 1174–1177, 2004.

[16] Gautherie, M., Kotewicz, A., and Gueblez, P., Accurate and objective evaluation of breast thermograms: basic principles and new advances with special reference to an improved computer-assisted scoring system. In *Thermal Assessment of Breast Health*, MTP Press Ltd., pp. 72–97, 1983.

[17] Hobbins, W.B., Abnormal thermogram—significance in breast cancer. *Interamer. J. Rad.*, 12, 337, 1987.

[18] Gautherie, M., New protocol for the evaluation of breast thermograms. In *Thermological Methods*, VCH mbH, pp. 227–235, 1985.

[19] Lawson, R.N. and Chughtai, M.S., Breast cancer and body temperatures. *Can. Med. Assoc. J.*, 88, 68, 1963.

[20] Head, J.F., Wang, F., and Elliott, R.L., Breast thermography is a noninvasive prognostic procedure that predicts tumor growth rate in breast cancer patients. *Ann. NY Acad. Sci.*, 698, 153, 1993.

[21] Sterns, E.E., Zee, B., Sen Gupta, J., and Saunders, F.W., Thermography: its relation to pathologic characteristics, vascularity, proliferative rate and survival of patients with invasive ductal carcinoma of the breast. *Cancer*, 77, 1324, 1996.

[22] Head, J.F. and Elliott, R.L., Breast thermography. *Cancer*, 79, 186, 1995.

[23] Anbar, M., *Quantitative Dynamic Telethermometry in Medical Diagnosis and Management*. CRC Press, Boca Raton, FL, pp. 84–94, 1994.

[24] Rodenberg, D.A., Chaet, M.S., Bass, R.C., et al. Nitric oxide: an overview. *Am. J. Surg.*, 170, 292, 1995.

[25] Thomsen, L.L., Miles, D.W., Happerfield, L., et al. Nitric oxide synthase activity in human breast cancer. *Br. J. Cancer*, 72, 41, July 1995.

[26] Guidi, A.J. and Schnitt, S.J., Angiogenesis in pre-invasive lesions of the breast. *Breast J.*, 2, 364, 1996.

[27] Gamagami, P., Indirect signs of breast cancer: Angiogenesis study. In *Atlas of Mammography*. Blackwell Science, Cambridge, MA, pp. 231–26, 1996.

[28] Love, T., Thermography as an indicator of blood perfusion. *Proc. NY Acad. Sci. J.*, 335, 429, 1980.

[29] Chato, J., Measurement of thermal properties of growing tumors. *Proc. NY Acad. Sci.*, 335, 67, 1980.

[30] Draper, J., Skin temperature distribution over veins and tumors. *Phys. Med. Biol.*, 16, 645, 1971.

[31] Jain, R. and Gullino, P., Thermal characteristics of tumors: applications in detection and treatment. *Ann. NY Acad. Sci.*, 335, 1, 1980.

[32] Gautherie, M., Thermopathology of breast cancer; measurement and analysis of *in-vivo* temperature and blood flow. *Ann. NY Acad. Sci.*, 365, 383, 1980.

[33] Gautherie, M., Thermobiological assessment of benign and malignant breast diseases. *Am. J. Obstet. Gynecol*, 147, 861, 1983.

[34] Gamigami, P., *Atlas of Mammography: New Early Signs in Breast Cancer*. Blackwell Science, Cambridge, MA, 1996.

[35] Gershen-Cohen, J., Haberman, J., and Brueschke, E., Medical thermography: a summary of current status. *Radiol. Clin. North Am.*, 3, 403, 1965.

[36] Haberman, J., The present status of mammary thermography. *Can Cancer J. Clin.*, 18, 314, 1968.

[37] Hoffman, R., Thermography in the detection of breast malignancy. *Am. J. Obstet. Gynecol.*, 98, 681, 1967.

[38] Stark, A. and Way, S., The screening of well women for the early detection of breast cancer using clinical examination with thermography and mammography. *Cancer*, 33, 1671, 1974.

[39] Amalric, D., et al., Value and interest of dynamic telethermography in detection of breast cancer. *Acta Thermographica*, 1, 89–96, 1976.

[40] Hobbins, W., Mass breast cancer screening. *Proceedings, Third International Symposium on Detection and Prevention of Breast Cancer*. New York City, NY, 637, 1976.

[41] Isard, H.J., Becker, W., Shilo, R., et al., Breast thermography after four years and 10,000 studies. *Am. J. Roentgenol.*, 115, 811, 1972.

[42] Spitalier, H., Giraud, D., Amalric, R., et al., Does infrared thermography truly have a role in present-day breast cancer management? In *Biomedical Thermology*. Alan R. Liss, Inc., New York, NY, pp. 269–278, 1982.

[43] Moskowitz, M., Milbrath, J., Gartside, P., et al., Lack of efficacy of thermography as a screening tool for minimal and stage I breast cancer. *N. Engl. J. Med.*, 295, 249, 1976.

[44] Threatt, B., Norbeck, J.M., Ullman, N.S., et al., Thermography and breast cancer: an analysis of a blind reading. *Ann. NY Acad. Sci.*, 335, 501, 1980.

[45] Haberman, J., Francis, J., and Love, T., Screening a rural population for breast cancer using thermography and physical examination techniques. *Ann. NY Acad. Sci.*, 335, 492, 1980.

[46] Sciarra, J., Breast cancer: strategies for early detection. In *Thermal Assessment of Breast Health (Proceedings of the International Conference on Thermal Assessment of Breast Health)*. MTP Press Ltd., pp. 117–129, 1983.

[47] Gautherie, M., Thermobiological assessment of benign and malignant breast diseases. *Am. J. Obstet. Gynecol.*, 147, 861, 1983.

[48] Louis, K., Walter, J., and Gautherie, M., Long-term assessment of breast cancer risk by thermal imaging. In *Biomedical Thermology*. Alan R. Liss, Inc., 279–301, 1982.

[49] Gros, C. and Gautherie, M., Breast thermography and cancer risk prediction. *Cancer*, 45, 51, 1980.

[50] Jones, C.H., Thermography of the female breast. In Parsons, C.A. (Ed.), *Diagnosis of Breast Disease*, University Park Press, Baltimore, MD, 214–234, 1983.

[51] Useki, H., Evaluation of the thermographic diagnosis of breast disease: relation of thermographic findings and pathologic findings of cancer growth. *Nippon Gan Chiryo Gakkai Shi*, 23, 2687, 1988.

[52] Parisky, Y.R., Sardi, A., et al., Efficacy of computerized infrared imaging analysis to evaluate mammographically suspicious lesions. *Am. J. Roentgenol.*, 180, 263, 2003.

[53] Nyirjesy, I., Ayme, Y., et al., Clinical evaluation, mammography, and thermography in the diagnosis of breast carcinoma. *Thermology*, 1, 170, 1986.

[54] Thomassin, L., Giraud, D., et al., Detection of subclinical breast cancers by infrared thermography. In *Recent Advances in Medical Thermology (Proceedings of the Third International Congress of Thermology)*. Plenum Press, New York, NY, 575–579, 1984.

[55] Amalric, R., Gautherie, M., Hobbins, W., and Stark, A., The future of women with an isolated abnormal infrared thermogram. *La Nouvelle Presse Med.*, 10, 3153, 1981.

[56] Gautherie, M. and Gros, C., Contribution of infrared thermography to early diagnosis, pre-therapeutic prognosis, and post-irradiation follow-up of breast carcinomas. Laboratory of Electroradiology, Faculty of Medicine, Louis Pasteur University, Strasbourg, France, 1976.

[57] Hobbins, W., Significance of an "isolated" abnormal thermogram. *La Nouvelle Presse Med.*, 10, 3155, 1981.

[58] Hobbins, W., Thermography, highest risk marker in breast cancer. *Proc. Gynecol. Soc. Study Breast Dis.*, 267–282, 1977.

[59] Gautherie, M., Improved system for the objective evaluation of breast thermograms. In *Biomedical Thermology*. Alan R. Liss, Inc., New York, 897–905, 1982.

[60] Amalric, R., Giraud, D., et al., Combined diagnosis of small breast cancer. *Acta Thermographica*, 1984.

[61] Spitalier, J., Amalric, D., et al., The Importance of infrared thermography in the early suspicion and detection of minimal breast cancer. In *Thermal Assessment of Breast Health*. MTP Press Ltd., 173–179, 1983.

[62] Gautherie, M., et al., Thermobiological assessment of benign and malignant breast diseases. *Am. J. Obstet. Gynecol.*, 147, 861, 1983.

[63] Jay, E. and Karpman, H., Computerized breast thermography. In *Thermal Assessment of Breast Health*. MTP Press Ltd., 98–109, 1983.

[64] Dilhuydy, M.H., et al., The importance of thermography in the prognostic evaluation of breast cancers. *Acta Thermographica*, 130–136.

[65] Amalric, D., et al., Value and interest of dynamic telethermography in detection of breast cancer. *Acta Thermographica*, 89–96.

[66] Fournier, V.D., Kubli, F., et al., Infrared thermography and breast cancer doubling time. *Acta Thermographica*, 107–111.

[67] Gros, D., Gautherie, M., and Warter, F., Thermographic prognosis of treated breast cancers. *Acta Thermographica*, 11–14.

[68] Keyserlingk, J.R., Ahlgren P.D., et al., Preliminary evaluation of high resolution functional infrared imaging to monitor pre-operative chemohormonotherapy-induced changes in neo-angiogenesis in patients with locally advanced breast cancer. Ville Marie Oncology Center/St. Mary's Hospital, Montreal, Canada. In submission for publication, 2003.

[69] Dodd, G.D., Thermography in breast cancer diagnosis. In *Abstracts for the Seventh National Cancer Conference Proceedings*. Lippincott Philadelphia, Los Angeles, CA, 267, 1972.

[70] Wallace, J.D., Thermographic examination of the breast: an assessment of its present capabilities. In Gallagher, H.S. (Ed.), *Early Breast Cancer: Detection and Treatment*, American College of Radiology, Wiley, NY, 13–19, 1975.

[71] Report of the Working Group to Review the National Cancer Institute Breast Cancer Detection Demonstration Projects. *J. Natl. Cancer Inst.*, 62, 641, 1979.

[72] Haberman, J., An overview of breast thermography in the United States. In Margaret Abernathy and Sumio Uematsu (Eds.), *Medical Thermography*, American Academy of Thermology, Washington, DC, 218–223, 1986.

[73] Rosenberg, R.D., Hunt, W.C., et al., Effects of age, breast density, ethnicity, and estrogen replacement therapy on screening mammographic sensitivity and cancer stage at diagnosis: Review of 183,134 screening mammograms in Albuquerque, New Mexico. *Radiology*, 209, 511, 1998.

[74] Elmore, J., et al., Ten-year risk of false positive screening mammograms and clinical breast examinations. *N. Engl. J. Med.*, 338, 1089, 1998.

[75] Head, J.F., Lipari, C.A., and Elliot, R.L., Comparison of mammography, and breast infrared imaging: sensitivity, specificity, false negatives, false positives, positive predictive value and negative predictive value. *IEEE*, 1999.

[76] Pisano, E.D., Gatsonis, C., et al., Diagnostic performance of digital versus film mammography for breast-cancer screening. *N. Engl. J. Med.*, 353, October, 2005.

[77] Keyserlignk, J.R., Ahlgren, P.D., et al., Infrared imaging of the breast; initial reappraisal using high-resolution digital technology in 100 successive cases of stage 1 and 2 breast cancer. *Breast J.*, 4, 4, July/August 1998.

[78] Schell, M.J., Bird, R.D., and Desrochers, D.A., Reassessment of breast cancers missed during routine screening mammography. *Am. J. Roentgenol.*, 177, 535, 2001.

[79] Poplack, S.P., Tosteson, A.N., Grove, M., et al., The practice of mammography in 53,803 women from the New Hampshire mammography network. *Radiology*, 217, 832, 2000.

[80] Pullon, S. and McLeod, D., The early detection and diagnosis of breast cancer: a literature review. General Practice Department, Wellington School of Medicine, December 1996.

[81] Gilliland, F.D., Joste, N., Stauber, P.M., et al., Biologic characteristics of interval and screen-detected breast cancers. *J. Natl. Cancer Inst.*, 92, 743, 2000.

[82] Sickles, E.A., Mammographic features of "early" breast cancer. *Am. J. Roentgenol.*, 143, 461, 1984.

[83] Thomas, D.B., Gao, D.L., Self, S.G., et al., Randomized trial of breast self-examination in Shanghai: methodology and preliminary results. *J. Natl. Cancer Inst.*, 5, 355, 1997.

[84] Moskowitz, M., Screening for breast cancer. How effective are our tests? *CA Cancer J. Clin.*, 33, 26, 1983.

[85] Elmore, J.G., Wells, C.F., Carol, M.P., et al., Variability in radiologists interpretation of mammograms. *N. Engl. J. Med.*, 331, 1493, 1994.

[86] Laya, M.B., Effect on estrogen replacement therapy on the specificity and sensitivity of screening mammography. *J. Natl. Cancer Inst.*, 88, 643, 1996.
[87] Boyd, N.F., Byng, J.W., Jong, R.A., et al., Quantitative classification of mammographic densities and breast cancer risk. *J. Natl. Cancer Inst.*, 87, 670, 1995.
[88] Moskowitz, M., Breast imaging. In Donegan, W.L. and Spratt, J.S. (Eds.), *Cancer of the Breast*, Saunders, New York, 206–239, 1995.
[89] Khalkhali, I., Cutrone, J.A., et al., Scintimammography: the complementary role of Tc-99m sestamibi prone breast imaging for the diagnosis of breast carcinoma. *Radiology*, 196, 421, 1995.
[90] Kedar, R.P., Cosgrove, D.O., et al., Breast carcinoma: measurement of tumor response in primary medical therapy with color doppler flow imaging. *Radiology*, 190, 825, 1994.
[91] Weinreb, J.C. and Newstead, G., MR imaging of the breast. *Radiology*, 196, 593, 1995.
[92] Love, S.M. and Barsky, S.H., Breast cancer: an interactive paradigm. *Breast J.*, 3, 171, 1996.

10
Functional Infrared Imaging of the Breast: Historical Perspectives, Current Application, and Future Considerations

John R. Keyserlingk
P.D. Ahlgren
E. Yu
Normand Belliveau
Mariam Yassa
Ville Marie Medical and Women's Health Center

10.1 Historical Perspectives 10-2
   Pre-Breast Cancer Detection Demonstration Projects Era • The Breast Cancer Detection Demonstration Projects Era • Post-Breast Cancer Detection Demonstration Projects Era
10.2 The Ville Marie Multi-Disciplinary Breast Center Experience with High-Resolution Digital Infrared Imaging to Detect and Monitor Breast Cancer 10-7
   Infrared Imaging as Part of a First-Line Multi-Imaging Strategy to Promote Early Detection of Breast Cancer • Preliminary Evaluation of Digital High-Resolution Functional Infrared Imaging to Monitor Pre-Operative Chemohormonotherapy-Induced Changes in Neo-Angiogenesis in Patients with Advanced Breast Cancer • Results
10.3 Future Considerations Concerning Infrared Imaging 10-24
References 10-28

There is general consensus that earlier detection of breast cancer should result in improved survival. For the last two decades, first-line breast imaging has relied primarily on mammography. Despite better equipment and regulation, particularly with the recent introduction of digital mammography, variability in interpretation and tissue density can affect mammography accuracy. To promote earlier diagnosis, a number of adjuvant functional imaging techniques have recently been introduced, including Doppler ultrasound and gadolinium-enhanced magnetic resonance imaging (MRI) that can detect cancer-induced regional neovascularity. While valuable modalities, problems relating to complexity, accessibility, cost, and in most cases the need for intravenous access make them unsuitable as components of a first-line imaging strategy.

In order to re-assess the potential contribution of infrared (IR) imaging as a first-line component of a multi-imaging strategy, using currently available technology, we will first review the history of its introduction and early clinical application, including the results of the Breast Cancer Demonstration Projects (BCDDP). We will then review the Ville Marie Multi-Disciplinary Breast Center's more recent experience with currently available high-resolution computerized IR technology to assess IR imaging both as a complement to clinical exam and mammography in the early detection of breast cancer and also as a tool to monitor the effects of pre-operative chemohormonotherapy in advanced breast cancer. Our goal is to show that high-resolution IR imaging provides additional safe, practical, cost effective, and objective information in both of these instances when produced by strict protocol and interpreted by sufficiently trained breast physicians. Finally, we will comment on its further evolution.

10.1 Historical Perspectives

10.1.1 Pre-Breast Cancer Detection Demonstration Projects Era

In 1961 in the *Lancet*, Williams and Handley [1] using a rudimentary hand-held thermopile, reported that 54 of 57 of their breast cancer patients were detectable by IR imaging, and "among these were cases in which the clinical diagnosis was in much doubt." The authors reported that the majority of these cancers had a temperature increase of 1 to 2°C, and that the IR imaging permitted excellent discrimination between benign and malignant processes. Their protocol at the Middlesex Hospital consisted of having the patient strip to the waist and be exposed to the ambient temperature for 15 min.

The authors demonstrated a precocious understanding of the significance of IR imaging by introducing the concept that increased cooling to 18°C further enhanced the temperature discrepancy between cancer and the normal breast. In a follow-up article the subsequent year, Handley [2] demonstrated a close correlation between the increased thermal pattern and increased recurrence rate. While only four of 35 cancer patients with a 1 to 2°C discrepancy recurred, five of the six patients with over 3°C rise developed recurrent cancer, suggesting already that the prognosis could be gauged by the amount of rise of temperature in the overlying skin.

In 1963, Lawson and Chughtai [3], two McGill University surgeons, published an elegant intra-operative study demonstrating that the increase in regional temperature associated with breast cancer was related to venous convection. This quantitative experiment added credence to Handley's suggestion that IR findings were related to both increased venous flow and increased metabolism.

In 1965, Gershon-Cohen [4], a radiologist and researcher from the Albert Einstein Medical Center, introduced IR imaging to the United States. Using a Barnes thermograph that required 15 min to produce a single IR image, he reported 4000 cases with a remarkable true positive rate of 94% and a false positive rate of 6%. This data was included in a review of the then current status of infrared imaging published in 1968 in *CA—A Cancer Journal for Physicians* [5]. The author, JoAnn Haberman, a radiologist from Temple University School of Medicine, reported the local experience with IR imaging, which produced a true positive rate of 84% compared with a concomitant true positive rate of 80% for mammography. In addition, she compiled 16,409 IR imaging cases from the literature between 1964 and 1968 revealing an overall true positive rate of 87% and a false positive rate of 13%.

A similar contemporary review compiled by Jones, consisting of nearly 70,000 cases, revealed an identical true positive rate of 85% and an identical false positive rate of 13%. Furthermore, Jones [6] reported on over 20,000 IR imagings from the Royal Marsden Hospital between 1967 and 1972, and noted that approximately 70% of Stage I and Stage II cancers and up to 90% of Stage III and Stage IV cancers had abnormal IR features. These reports resulted in an unbridled enthusiasm for IR imaging as a front-line detection modality for breast cancer.

Sensing a potential misuse of this promising but unregulated imaging modality, Isard made some sobering comments in 1972 [7] in a publication of the *American Journal of Roentengology*, where he emphasized that, like other imaging techniques, IR imaging does not diagnose cancer but merely indicates the presence of an abnormality. Reporting his Radiology division's experience with 10,000 IR studies done concomitantly with mammography between 1967 and 1970, he reiterated a number of important concepts, including the remarkable stability of the IR image from year to year in the otherwise healthy patient, and the importance of recognizing any significant change. Infrared imaging detected 60% of occult cancers in his experience, vs. 80% with mammography. The combination of both these modalities increased the sensitivity by approximately 10%, thus underlining the complimentarity of both of these processes, since each one did not always suspect the same lesion.

It was Isard's conclusion that, had there been a preliminary selection of his group of 4393 asymptomatic patients by IR imaging, mammography examination would have been restricted to the 1028 patients with abnormal IR imaging (23% of this cohort). This would have resulted in a cancer detection rate of 24.1 per 1000 mammographic examinations, as contrasted to the expected 7 per 1000 by mammographic screening. He concluded that since IR imaging is an innocuous examination, it could be utilized to focus attention upon asymptomatic women who should be examined more intensely.

In 1972, Gerald D. Dodd [8] of the Department of Diagnostic Radiology of the University of Texas presented an update on IR imaging in breast cancer diagnosis at the Seventh National Cancer Conference sponsored by the National Cancer Society, and the National Cancer Institute. He also suggested that IR imaging would be best employed as a screening agent for mammography and proposed that in any general survey of the female population age 40 and over, 15–20% would have positive IR imaging and would require mammograms. Of these, approximately 5% would be recommended for biopsy. He concluded that IR imaging would serve to eliminate 80–85% of the potential mammograms. Reporting the Texas Medical School's experience with IR imaging, he reiterated that IR was capable of detecting approximately 85% of all breast cancers. The false positive rate of 15–20% did not concern the author, who stated that these were false positives only in the sense that there was no corroborative evidence of breast cancer at the time of the examination and that they could serve to identify a high-risk population.

Feig et al. [9], reported the respective abilities of clinical exam, mammography, and IR imaging to detect breast cancer in 16,000 self-selected women. While only 39% of the initial series of overall established cancer patients had an abnormal IR imaging, this increased to 75% in his later cohort, reflecting an improved methodology. Of particular interest was the ability of IR imaging to detect 54% of the smallest tumors, four times that of clinical examination. This potential important finding was not elaborated, but it could reflect IR's ability to detect vascular changes that are sometimes more apparent at the initiation of tumor genesis. The authors suggested that the potential of IR imaging to select high-risk groups for follow-up screening merited further investigation.

Wallace [10] presented an update on IR imaging of the breast to another contemporary Cancer Conference sponsored by the American College of Radiology, the American Cancer Society, and the Cancer Control Programme of the National Cancer Institute. The analysis suggested that the incidence of breast cancer detection per 1000 screenees could increase from 2.72 when using mammography to 19 when using IR imaging. He then underlined that IR imaging poses no radiation burden on the patient, requires no physical contact, and, being an innocuous technique, could concentrate the sought population by a significant factor, selecting those patients that required further investigation. He concluded that "the resulting IR image contains only a small amount of information as compared to the mammogram, so that the reading of the IR image is a substantially simpler task."

Unfortunately, this rather simplistic and cavalier attitude toward the acquisition and interpretation of IR imaging was widely prevalent when it was hastily added to the BCDDP, which was just getting underway. Rather than assess, in a controlled manner, its potential as a complementary first-line detection modality, it was hastily introduced into the BCDDP as a potential replacement for mammography and clinical exam.

10.1.2 The Breast Cancer Detection Demonstration Projects Era

A detailed review of the Report of the Working Group of the BCDDP is essential to understand the subsequent evolution of IR imaging [11]. The scope of this project was issued by the National Cancer

Institute (NCI) on March 26, 1973, with six objectives, the second being to determine if a negative IR imaging was sufficient to preclude the use of clinical examination and mammography in the detection of breast cancer. The Working Group, reporting on results of the first 4 years of this project, gave a short history regarding IR imaging in breast cancer detection. They reported that as of the 1960s, there was intense interest in determining the suitability of IR imaging for large-scale applications, and mass screening was one possibility. The need for technological improvement was recognized and the authors stated that efforts had been made to refine the technique. One of the important objectives behind these efforts had been to achieve a sufficiently high sensitivity and specificity for IR imaging under screening conditions to make it useful as a prescreening device in selecting patients who would then be referred for mammographic examination. It was thought that if successful, this technology would result in a relatively small proportion of women having mammography, a technique that caused concern because of the carcinogenic effects of radiation. The Working Group indicated that the sensitivity and specificity of IR imaging readings from clinical data emanating from interinstitutional studies were close to the corresponding results for physical examination and for mammography. While they noted that these three modalities selected different subgroups of breast cancers, further evaluation of IR imaging as a potential stand-alone screening device in a controlled clinical trial was recommended.

The authors of the BCDDP Working Group generated a detailed review of mammography and efforts to improve its quality control in image quality and reduction in radiation. They recalled that in the 1960s, the Cancer Control Board of the U.S. Public Health Service had financed a national mammography training programme for radiologists and their technologists. Weekly courses in mammography were taught at approximately ten institutions throughout the country with material supplied by the American College of Radiology. In 1975, shortly after the beginning of this project, the NCI had already funded seven institutions in the United States in a 3-year effort aimed at reorienting radiologists and their technologists in more advanced mammographic techniques and interpretation for the detection of early breast cancer.

In the interim, the American College of Radiology and many interested mammographers and technologists had presented local postgraduate refresher courses and workshops on mammography. Every year for the previous 16 years, the American College of Radiology had supported, planned and coordinated week-long conferences and workshops aimed at optimizing mammography to promote the earlier detection and treatment of breast cancer. It was recognized that the well-known primary and secondary mammographic signs of a malignant condition, such as ill-defined mass, skin thickening, skin retraction, marked fibrosis and architectural distortion, obliteration of the retromammary space, and enlarged visible axillary lymph nodes, could detect an established breast cancer. However, the authors emphasized that more subtle radiographic signs that occur in minimal, clinically occult, and early cancers, such as localized punctate calcifications, focal areas of duct prominence, and minor architectural distortion, could lead to an earlier diagnosis even when the carcinoma was not infiltrating, which was a rare finding when previous mammographic techniques were used.

The authors reiterated that the reproduction of early mammography signs required a constant high-quality technique for fine image detail, careful comparison of the two breasts during interpretation, and the search for areas of bilateral, parenchymal asymmetry that could reflect underlying cancer. The BCDDP Working Group report stated that mammographies were conducted by trained technicians and that, while some projects utilized radiological technicians for the initial interpretation, most used either a radiologist or a combination of technician and radiologist. Quality control for mammography consisted of reviews by the project radiologists and site visits by consultants to identify problems in procedures and the quality of the films.

On the other hand, the entire protocol for IR imaging within this study was summarized in one paragraph, and it indicated that IR imaging was conducted by a BCDDP trained technician. Initial interpretation was made mostly by technicians; some projects used technicians plus radiologists and a few used radiologists and/or physicians with other specialties for all readings. Quality control relied on review of procedures and interpretations by the project physicians. Positive physical exams and mammographies were reported in various degrees of certainty about malignancy or as suspicious-benign; IR imaging was reported simply as normal or abnormal. While the protocol for the BCDDP required that the three clinical components of this study (physical examination, IR imaging, and mammography) be conducted separately, and initial findings and recommendations be reported independently, it was not possible for the Working Group to assess the extent to which this protocol was adhered to or to evaluate the quality of the examinations.

The detailed extensive results from this Working Group report consisted of over 50 tables. There was, however, only one table that referred to IR imaging, showing that it had detected 41% of the breast cancers during the first screening, while the residuals were either normal or unknown. There is no breakdown as far as these two latter groups were concerned. Since 28% of the first screening and 32% of the second screening were picked up by mammography alone, IR imaging was dropped from any further evaluation and consideration. The report stated that it was impossible to determine whether abnormal IR imaging could be predictive of interval (developing between screenings) cancers, since these data were not collected.

By the same token, the Working Group was unable to conclude, with their limited experience, whether the findings were related to the then existing technology of IR imaging or with its application. They did, however, indicate that the decision to dismiss IR imaging should not be taken as a determination of the future of this technique, rather that the procedure continued to be of interest because it does not entail the risk of radiation exposure. In the Working Group's final recommendation, they state that "infrared imaging does not appear to be suitable as a substitute for mammography for routine screening in the BCDDP" but could not comment on its role as a complementary modality. The report admitted that several individual programs of the BCDDP had results that were more favorable than for the BCDDP as a whole. They also insisted that high priority be given to development and testing of IR imaging under carefully controlled study conditions. They noted that a few suitable sites appeared to be available among the BCDDP and proposed that developmental studies should be solicited from the sites with sufficient experience.

Further insight into the inadequate quality control assigned to IR imaging during this program was provided by Haberman, a participant in that project [12]. The author reiterated that, while proven expertise in mammography was an absolute requirement for the awarding of a contract to establish a Screening Center, the situation was just the opposite as regards to IR imaging. As no experience was required, when the 27 demonstration projects opened their doors, only five of the centers had pre-existing expertise in IR imaging. Of the remaining screening centers, there was no experience at all in this technology. Finally, more than 18 months after the BCDDP project had begun operating, the NCI, recognizing this problem, established centers where radiologists and their technicians could obtain further training in IR imaging. Unfortunately, only 11 of the demonstration project directors considered this training of sufficient importance to send their technologists. In some centers, it was reported that there was no effort to cool the patient prior to examination. In other centers, there was complete lack of standardization, and a casual attitude prevailed with reference to interpretation of results. While quality control of this imaging technology could be considered lacking, it was nevertheless subjected to the same stringent statistical analysis as was mammography and clinical breast examination.

10.1.3 Post-Breast Cancer Detection Demonstration Projects Era

Two small-scale studies carried out in the 1970s by Moskowitz [13] and Threatt [14] reported on the sensitivity and reliability of IR imaging. Both used "experts" to review the images of breast cancer patients. While Moskowitz excluded unreadable images, data from Threatt's study indicated that less than 30% of the images produced were considered good, with the rest being substandard. Both these studies produced poor results, inconsistent with numerous previous multicenter trials, particularly that of Stark [15] who, 16 years earlier, reported an 81% detection rate for preclinical cancers.

Threatt noted that IR imaging demonstrated an increasing accuracy as cancers increased in size or aggressiveness, as did the other testing modalities (i.e., physical examination and mammography). The author also suggested that computerized pattern recognition would help solve the reproducibility problems sometimes associated with this technology and that further investigation was warranted. Moskowitz also suggested that for IR imaging to be truly effective as a screening tool, there needed to be more objective means of interpretation. He proposed that this would be much facilitated by computerized evaluation.

In a frequently cited article, Sterns and Cardis [16] reviewed their group's limited experience with IR in 1982. While there were only 11 cancer cases in this trial, they were concerned about a sensitivity of 60% and a false positive rate of IR of 12%. While there was no mention of training, they concluded, based on a surprisingly low false positive rate of clinical exam of only 1.4%, that IR could not be recommended for breast diagnosis or as an indication for mammography.

Thirteen years later, reviewing the then status of breast imaging, Moskowitz [17] challenged the findings of the recent Canadian National Breast Screening Study (NBSS) that questioned the value of mammography, much in the same way that the Working Group of the BCDDP questioned IR imaging 20 years previously. Using arguments that could have qualified the disappointing results of the IR imaging used in the BCDDP study, the author explained the poor results of mammography in the NBSS on the basis of inadequate technical quality. He concluded that only 68% of the women received satisfactory breast imaging.

In addition to the usual causes of poor technical quality, failure to use the medial lateral oblique view resulted in exclusion of the tail of Spence and of much of the upper outer quadrant in many of the subjects screened. There was also a low interobserver agreement in the reading of mammographies, which resulted in a potential diagnostic delay. His review stated that of all noncontrast, nondigital radiological procedures, mammography required the greatest attention to meticulous detail for the training of technologists, selection of the film, contrast monitoring of processing, choosing of equipment, and positioning of the patient. For mammography to be of value, it required dedicated equipment, a dedicated room, dedicated film, and the need to be performed and interpreted by dedicated people. Echoing some of the criticisms that could be pertinent to the BCDDP's use of IR imaging, he indicated that mammography is not a procedure to be performed by the untutored. In rejecting any lack of quality control of IR imaging during the BCDDP studies by stating that "most of the investigators in the BCDDP did undergo a period of training." The author once again suggested that the potential of IR imaging would only increase if there was better standardization of technology and better-designed clinical trials.

Despite its initial promise, this challenge was not taken up by the medical community, who systematically lost interest in this technique, primarily due to the nebulous BCDDP experience. Nevertheless, during the 1980s, a number of isolated reports continued to appear, most emphasizing the risk factors associated with abnormal IR imaging. In *Cancer* in 1980, Gautherie and Gros [18] reported their experience with a group of 1245 women who had a mildly abnormal infrared image along with either normal or benign disease by conventional means, including physical exam, mammography, ultrasonography, and fine needle aspiration or biopsy. They noted that within 5 years, more than one-third of this group had histologically confirmed cancers. They concluded that IR imaging is useful not only as a predictor of breast cancer risk but also to identify the more rapidly growing neoplasms.

The following year, Amalric et al. [19], expanded on this concept by reporting that 10 to 15% of patients undergoing IR imaging will be found to be mildly abnormal when the remainder of the examination is essentially unremarkable. They noted that among these "false positive" cases, up to 38% will eventually develop breast cancer when followed closely. In 1981, Mariel [20] carried out a study in France on 655 patients and noted an 82% sensitivity. Two years later, Isard [21] discussed the unique characteristics and respective roles of IR imaging and ultrasonography and concluded that, when used in conjunction with mammography in a multi-imaging strategy, their potential advantages included enhanced diagnostic accuracy, reduction of unnecessary surgery, and improved prognostic ability. The author emphasized that neither of these techniques should be used as a sole screening modalitiy for breast cancer in asymptomatic women, but rather as a complementary modality to mammography.

In 1984, Nyirjesy [22] reported in *Obstetrics and Gynecology* a 76% sensitivity for IR imaging of 8767 patients. The same year, Bothmann [23] reported a sensitivity of 68% from a study carried out in Germany on 2702 patients. In 1986, Useki [24] published the results of a Japanese study indicating an 88% sensitivity.

Despite newly available IR technology, due in large part to military research and development, as well as compelling statistics of over 70,000 documented cases showing the contribution of functional IR imaging in a hitherto structurally based strategy to detect breast cancer, few North American centers have shown an interest, and fewer still have published their experience. This is surprising in view of the current consensus regarding the importance of vascular-related events associated with tumor initiation and growth that finally provide a plausible explanation for the IR findings associated with the early development of smaller tumors. The questionable results of the BCDDP and a few small-scale studies are still being referred to by a dwindling authorship that even mention the existence of this imaging modality. This has resulted in a generation of imagers that have neither knowledge of nor training in IR imaging. However, there are a few isolated centers that have continued to develop an expertise in this modality and have published their results.

In 1993, Head et al. [25] reported that improved images of the second generation of IR systems allowed more objective and quantitative visual analysis. They also reported that growth-rate-related prognostic indicators were strongly associated with the IR results [26]. In 1996, Gamagami [27] studied angiogenesis by IR imaging and reported that hypervascularity and hyperthermia could be shown in 86% of nonpalpable breast cancers. He also noted that in 15% of these cases, this technique helped to detect cancers that were not visible on mammography.

The concept of angiogenesis, suggested by Gamagami as an integral part of early breast cancer, was reiterated in 1996 by Guidi and Schnitt [28], whose observations suggested that angiogenesis is an early event in the development of breast cancer. They noted that it may occur before tumor cells acquire the ability to invade the surrounding stroma and even before there is morphologic evidence of an *in situ* carcinoma.

In contemporary publications, Anbar [29,30], using an elegant biochemical and immunological cascade, suggested that the empirical observation that small tumors capable of producing notable IR changes could be due to enhanced perfusion over a substantial area of breast surface via tumor-induced nitric oxide vasodilatation. He introduced the importance of dynamic area teletherometry to validate IR's full potential.

Parisky and his colleagues working out of six radiology centers [31] published an interesting report in Radiology in 2003 relating to the efficacy of computerized infrared imaging analysis of mammographically suspicious lesions. They reported a 97% sensitivity, a 14% specificity, and a 95% negative predictive value when IR was used to help determine the risk factors relating to mammographically noted abnormal lesions in 875 patients undergoing biopsy. They concluded that infrared imaging offers a safe, noninvasive procedure that would be valuable as an adjunct to mammography determining whether a lesion is benign or malignant.

10.2 The Ville Marie Multi-Disciplinary Breast Center Experience with High-Resolution Digital Infrared Imaging to Detect and Monitor Breast Cancer

10.2.1 Infrared Imaging as Part of a First-Line Multi-Imaging Strategy to Promote Early Detection of Breast Cancer

There is still a general consensus that the crucial strategy for the first-line detection of breast cancer depends essentially on clinical examination and mammography. Limitation of the former, with its reported sensitivity rate below 65% is well recognized [32], and even the proposed value of breast self-examination is now being contested [33]. With the current emphasis on earlier detection, there is an increasing reliance on better imaging. Mammography is still considered as our most reliable and cost-effective imaging modality [17]. However, variable inter-reader interpretation [34] and tissue density, now proposed as a risk factor itself [35] and seen in both younger patients and those on hormonal replacement [36], prompted us to reassess currently available IR technology spearheaded by military research and development, as a first-line component of a multi-imaging breast cancer detection strategy (Figure 10.1).

This modality is capable of quantifying minute temperature variations and qualifying abnormal vascular patterns, probably associated with regional angiogenesis, neovascularization (Figure 10.2), and nitric oxide-induced regional vasodilatation [29], frequently associated with tumor initiation and progression, and potentially an early predictor of tumor growth rate [26,28]. We evaluated a new fully integrated high-resolution computerized IR imaging station to complement mammography units. To validate its

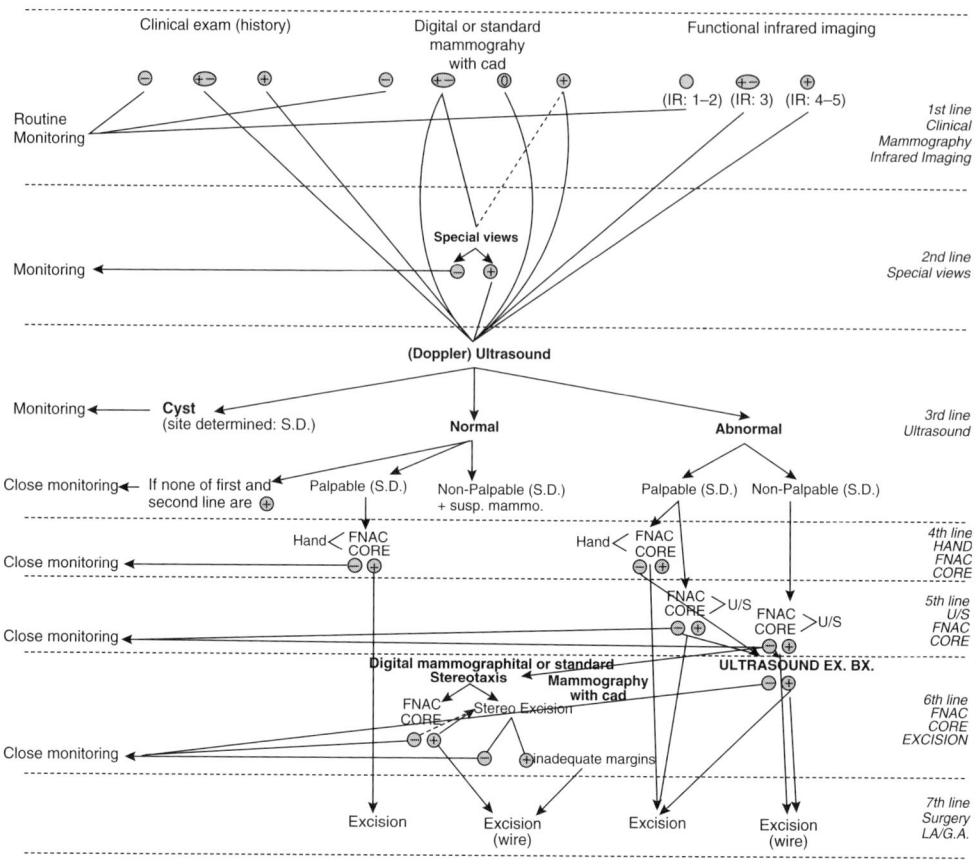

FIGURE 10.1 Ville Marie breast center: clinical and multi-imaging breast cancer detection strategy.

reported ability to help detect early tumor-related regional metabolic and vascular changes [27], we limited our initial review to a series of 100 successive cases of breast cancer who filled the following three criteria: (a) minimal evaluation included a clinical exam, mammography, and IR imaging; (b) definitive surgical management constituted the preliminary therapeutic modality carried out at one of our affiliated institutions; and (c) the final staging consisted of either noninvasive cancer ($n = 4$), Stage I ($n = 42$), or Stage II ($n = 54$) invasive breast cancer.

While 94% of these patients were referred to our Multidisciplinary Breast Center for the first time, 65% from family physicians and 29% from specialists, the remaining 6% had their diagnosis of breast cancer at a follow-up visit. Age at diagnosis ranged from 31 to 84 years, with a mean age of 53. The mean histologic tumor size was 2.5 cm. Lymphatic, vascular, or neural invasion was noted in 18% of patients; and concomitant noninvasive cancer was present, along with the invasive component, in 64%. One-third of the 89 patients had axillary lymph node dissection, one-third had involved nodes, and 38% of the tumors were histologic Grade III.

While most of these patients underwent standard four-view mammography, with additional views when indicated, using a GE DMR apparatus at our center, in 17 cases we relied on recent and adequate quality outside films. Mammograms were interpreted by our examining physician and radiologist, both having access to the clinical findings. Lesions were considered suspicious if either of them noted findings indicative of carcinoma. The remainder were considered either contributory but equivocal or nonspecific. A nonspecific mammography required concordance with our examining physician, radiologist, and the authors.

Functional Infrared Imaging of the Breast

FIGURE 10.2 (See color insert at the back of the book.) (a) Tumor angiogenesis. (b) High nuclear grade ductal carcinoma *in situ* with numerous blood vessels (angiogenesis) (Tabar). (c) Invasive ductal carcinoma with central necrosis and angiogenesis (Tabar).

Our integrated IR station at that time consisted of a scanning-mirror optical system containing a mercury–cadmium–telleride detector (Bales Scientific, CA) with a spatial resolution of 600 optical lines, a central processing unit providing multitasking capabilities, and a high-resolution color monitor capable of displaying 1024 × 768 resolution points and up to 110 colors or shades of gray per image. IR imaging took place in a draft-free thermally controlled room, maintained at between 18 and 20°C, after a 5 min equilibration period during which the patient sat disrobed with her hands locked over her head. We requested that the patients refrain from alcohol, coffee, smoking, exercise, deodorant, and lotions 3 h prior to testing.

Four images (an anterior, an under-surface, and two lateral views), were generated simultaneously on the video screen. The examining physician would digitally adjust them to minimize noise and enhance

TABLE 10.1 Ville Marie Infrared (IR) Grading Scale

Abnormal signs

1. Significant vascular asymmetry[a]
2. Vascular anarchy consisting of unusual tortuous or serpiginous vessels that form clusters, loops, abnormal arborization, or aberrant patterns
3. A 1°C focal increase in temperature (ΔT) when compared to the contralateral site and when associated with the area of clinical abnormality[a]
4. A 2°C focal ΔT versus the contralateral site[a]
5. A 3°C focal ΔT versus the rest of the ipsilateral breast when not present on the contralateral site[a]
6. Global breast ΔT of 1.5°C versus the contralateral breast[a]

Infrared scale

IR1 = Absence of any vascular pattern to mild vascular symmetry
IR2 = Significant but symmetrical vascular pattern to moderate vascular asymmetry, particularly if stable
IR3 = One abnormal sign
IR4 = Two abnormal signs
IR5 = Three abnormal signs

[a] Unless stable on serial imaging or due to known non-cancer causes (e.g., abcess or receent benign surgery).
Infrared Imaging takes place in a draft free, thermally controlled room maintained between 18 and 20°C, after a 5 min equilibration period during which the patient is disrobed with her hands locked over her head. Patients are asked to refrain from alcohol, coffee, smoking, exercise, deodorant, and lotions 3 h prior to testing.

detection of more subtle abnormalities prior to exact on-screen computerized temperature reading and IR grading. Images were then electronically stored on retrievable laser discs. Our original Ville Marie grading scale relies on pertinent clinical information, comparing IR images of both breasts with previous images. An abnormal IR image required the presence of at least one abnormal sign (Table 10.1). To assess the false-positive rate, we reviewed, using similar criteria, our last 100 consecutive patients who underwent an open breast biopsy that produced a benign histology. We used the Carefile Data Analysis Program to evaluate the detection rate of variable combinations of clinical exam, mammography, and IR imaging.

Of this series, 61% presented with a suspicious palpable abnormality, while the remainder had either an equivocal (34%) or a nonspecific clinical exam (5%). Similarly, mammography was considered suspicious for cancer in 66%, while 19% were contributory but equivocal, and 15% were considered nonspecific. Infrared imaging revealed minor variations (IR-1 or IR-2) in 17% of our patients while the remaining 83% had at least one (34%), two (37%), or three (12%) abnormal IR signs. Of the 39 patients with either a nonspecific or equivocal clinical exam, 31 had at least one abnormal IR sign, with this modality providing pertinent indication of a potential abnormality in 14 of these patients who, in addition, had an equivocal or nonspecific mammography.

Among the 15 patients with a nonspecific mammography, there were 10 patients (mean age of 48; 5 years younger than the full sample) who had an abnormal IR image. This abnormal finding constituted a particularly important indicator in six of these patients who also had only equivocal clinical findings. While 61% of our series presented with a suspicious clinical exam, the additional information provided by the 66 suspicious mammographies resulted in an 83% detection rate. The combination of only suspicious mammograms and abnormal IR imaging increased the sensitivity to 93%, with a further increase to 98% when suspicious clinical exams were also considered (Figure 10.3).

The mean histologically measured tumor size for those cases undetected by mammography was 1.66 cm. while those undetected by IR imaging averaged 1.28 cm. In a concurrent series of 100 consecutive eligible patients who had an open biopsy that produced benign histology, 19% had an abnormal IR image while 30% had an abnormal pre-operative mammography that was the only indication for surgery in 16 cases.

Functional Infrared Imaging of the Breast

FIGURE 10.3 Relative contribution of clinical exam, mammography, and IR imaging to detect breast cancer in the Ville Marie Breast Center series. In this series, adding infrared imaging to both suspicious and equivocal mammographies increased the detection rate. (1) Suspicious clinical exam; (2) suspicious mammography; (3) suspicious clinical exam or suspicious mammography; (4) abnormal infrared imaging; (5) suspicious or equivocal mammography; (6) abnormal infrared imaging or suspicious mammography; (7) abnormal infrared imaging or equivocal or suspicious mammography; and (8) abnormal infrared imaging or suspicious mammography or suspicious clinical exam.

The 83% sensitivity of IR imaging in this series is higher than the 70% rate for similar Stage I and II patients tested from the Royal Marsden Hospital two decades earlier [6]. Although our results might reflect an increased index of suspicion associated with a referred population, this factor should apply equally to both clinical exam and mammography, maintaining the validity of our evaluation. Additional factors could include our standard protocol, our physicians' prior experience with IR imaging, their involvement in both image production and interpretation, as well as their access to much improved image acquisition and precision (Figure 10.4).

While most previous IR cameras had 8-bit (one part in 256) resolution, current cameras are capable of one part in 4096 resolution, providing enough dynamic range to capture all images with 0.05°C discrimination without the need for range switching. With the advancement of video display and enhanced gray and colors, multiple high-resolution views can be compared simultaneously on the same monitor. Faster computers now allow processing functions such as image subtraction and digital filtering techniques for image enhancement. New algorithms provide soft tissue imaging by characterizing dynamic heat-flow patterns. These and other innovations have made vast improvements in the medical IR technology available today.

The detection rate in a series where half the tumors were under 2 cm, would suggest that tumor-induced thermal patterns detected by currently available IR technology are more dependent on early vascular and metabolic changes. These changes possibly are induced by regional nitric oxide diffusion and ferritin interaction, rather than strictly on tumor size [29]. This hypothesis agrees with the concept that angiogenesis may precede any morphological changes [28]. Although both initial clinical exam and mammography are crucial in signaling the need for further investigation, equivocal and nonspecific findings can still result in a combined delayed detection rate of 10% [17].

When eliminating the dubious contribution of our 34 equivocal clinical exams and 19 equivocal mammograms, which is disconcerting to both physician and patient, the alternative information provided by IR imaging increased the index of concern of the remaining suspicious mammograms by 27% and the combination of suspicious clinical exams or suspicious mammograms by 15% (Figure 10.3). An imaging-only strategy, consisting of both suspicious and equivocal mammography and abnormal IR imaging, also detected 95% of these tumors, even without the input of the clinical exam. Infrared imaging's most tangible contribution in this series was to signal an abnormality in a younger cohort of breast cancer patients who had noncontributory mammograms and also nonspecific clinical exams who conceivably would not have been passed on for second-line evaluation.

FIGURE 10.4 (See color insert.) (a) A 46-year-old patient: Lump in the upper central area of the right breast. *Infrared imaging* (A): Significant vascular asymmetry (SVA) in the upper central area of the right breast (IR-3). *Mammography* (B): Corresponding speculated opacity. *Surgical histology*: 2 cm infiltrating ductal carcinoma with negative sentinel nodes. (b) A 44-year-old patient. *Infrared imaging* (A): Revealed a significant vascular asymmetry in the upper central and inner quadrants of the right breast with a ΔT of 1.8°C (IR-4.8). *Corresponding mammography* (B): Reveals a spiculated lesion in the upper central portion of the right breast. *Surgical histology*: 0.7 cm infiltrating ductal carcinoma. Patient underwent adjuvant brachytherapy.

While 17% of these tumors were undetected by IR imaging, either due to insufficient production or detection of metabolic or vascular changes, the 19% false positive rate in histologically proven benign conditions, in part a reflection of our current grading system, suggests sufficient specificity for this modality to be used in an adjuvant setting.

Our validation of prior data would also suggest that IR imaging, based more on process than structural changes and requiring neither contact, compression, radiation, nor venous access, can provide pertinent and practical complementary information to both clinical exam and mammography, our current first-line detection modalities. Quality-controlled abnormal IR imaging heightened our index of suspicion

FIGURE 10.4 (Continued) **(See color insert.)** (c) A 52-year-old patient presented with a mild fullness in the lower outer quadrant of the right breast. *Infrared imaging* (A): Left breast (B): right breast reveals extensive significant vascular asymmetry with a ΔT of 1.35°C (IR-5.3). A 2 cm cancer was found in the lower outer area of the right breast. (d) A 37-year-old patient. *Infrared image* (A): Significant vascular asymmetry in the upper inner quadrant of the left breast with a ΔT of 1.75°C (IR-4) (mod IR-4.75). *Mammography* (B): Corresponding spiculated lesion. *Ultrasound* (C): 6 mm lesion. *Surgical histology*: 0.7 cm infiltrating ductal carcinoma.

A   B

FIGURE 10.4 (Continued) (**See color insert.**) (e) An 82-year-old patient. *Infrared imaging anterior view:* Significant vascular asymmetry and a ΔT of 1.90°C (IR-4) in the left subareolar area. *Corresponding mammography:* (not included) asymmetrical density in the left areolar area. *Surgical histology:* Left subareolar 1 cm infiltrating ductal carcinoma. (f) A 34-year-old patient with a palpable fullness in the supra-areolar area of the right breast. *Infrared imaging* (A): Extensive significant vascular asymmetry and a ΔT of 1.3°C in the right supra areolar area (IR-4) (mod IR-5.3). *Mammography* (B): Scattered and clustered central microcalcifications. *Surgical histology:* After total right mastectomy and TRAM flap: multifocal DCIS and infiltrating ductal CA centered over a 3 cm area of the supra areolar area.

in cases where clinical or mammographic findings were equivocal or nonspecific, thus signaling further investigation rather than observation or close monitoring (Figure 10.5) and to minimize possibility of further delay (Figure 10.6).

10.2.2 Preliminary Evaluation of Digital High-Resolution Functional Infrared Imaging to Monitor Pre-Operative Chemohormonotherapy-Induced Changes in Neo-Angiogenesis in Patients with Advanced Breast Cancer

Approximately 10% of our current breast cancer patients present with sufficient tumor load to be classified as having locally advanced breast cancer (LABC). This heterogeneous subset of patients, usually diagnosed

Functional Infrared Imaging of the Breast

FIGURE 10.5 (See color insert.) (a) A 48-year-old patient *Infrared imaging* (A): Significant vascular asymmetry and a ΔT of 0.8°C (IR-3) in the lower inner quadrant of the left breast. *Corresponding mammography* (B): A nonspecific density. *Surgical histology*: 1.6 cm left lower inner quadrant infiltrating ductal carcinoma. (b) A 40-year-old patient. *Infrared imaging* (A): left breast (B) right breast: focal hot spot in the right subareolar area on a background of increased vascular activity with a ΔT of 1.1°C (IR-4). *Corresponding mammography* (C): Reveals dense tissue bilaterally. *Surgical histology*: reveals a 1 cm right infiltrating ductal carcinoma and positive lymph nodes.

with either stage T3 or T4 lesions without evidence of metastasis, and thus judged as potential surgical candidates, constitutes a formidable therapeutic challenge. Pre-operative or neo-adjuvant chemotherapy (PCT), hormonotherapy or both, preferably delivered within a clinical trial, is the current favored treatment strategy.

FIGURE 10.5 (Continued) (**See color insert.**) (c) A 51-year-old patient. *Infrared imaging* (A): Significant vascular asymmetry and a ΔT of 2.2°C (IR-5) in the upper central area of the left breast. *Corresponding mammography* (B): Mild scattered densities. *Surgical histology*: 2.5 cm infiltrating ductal carcinoma in the upper central area of the left breast. (d) A 44-year-old patient. *Infrared imaging* (A): Significant vascular asymmetry and a ΔT of 1.58°C (IR-4) in the upper inner quadrant of the left breast. *Corresponding mammography* (B): A nonspecific corresponding density. *Surgical histology*: A 0.9 cm left upper inner quadrant infiltrating ductal carcinoma.

Pre-operative chemotherapy offers a number of advantages, including ensuring improved drug access to the primary tumor site by avoiding surgical scarring, the possibility of complete or partial tumor reduction that could down-size the extent of surgery and also the ability to better plan breast reconstruction when the initial tumor load suggests the need for a possible total mastectomy. In addition, there is sufficient data to suggest that the absence of any residual tumor cells in the surgical pathology specimen following PTC confers the best prognosis, while those patients achieving at least a partial clinical response as measured by at least a 50% reduction in the tumor's largest diameter often can aspire to a better survival than nonresponders [37]. While current clinical parameters do not always reflect actual PCT-induced tumor changes, there is sufficient correlation to make measuring the early clinical response to PTC an important element in assessing the efficacy of any chosen regimen. Unfortunately, the currently available conventional

Functional Infrared Imaging of the Breast

FIGURE 10.5 (Continued) (**See color insert.**) (e) A 45-year-old patient with a nodule in central area of left breast. *Infrared imaging* (A): Extensive significant vascular asymmetry (SVA) in the central inner area of the left breast with a ΔT of 0.75°C (IR-3) (mod IR-4.75). *Mammography* (B): Non-contributory. *Surgical histology*: 1.5 cm infiltrating ductal carcinoma with necrosis in the central inner area and 3 + axillary nodes. (f) A 51-year-old patient. *Infrared imaging* (A): Extensive significant vascular asymmetry and a ΔT of 2.2° (IR-5) (mod IR-6.2) in the upper central area of the left breast. *Corresponding mammography* (B) scattered densities. *Surgical histology*: 2.5 cm infiltrating ductal carcinoma in the upper central area of the left breast.

monitoring tools, such as palpation combined with structural/anatomic imaging such as mammography and ultrasound have a limited ability to precisely measure the initial tumor load, and even less to reflect the effect of PCT [34].

These relatively rudimentary tools are dependent on often-imprecise anatomical and structural parameters. A more effective selection of often quite aggressive therapeutic agents and ideal duration of their use could be enhanced by the introduction of a convenient, safe, and accessible modality that could provide an alternative and serial measurement of their therapeutic efficacy.

There is thus currently a flurry of interest to assess the potential of different functional imaging modalities that could possibly monitor tumor changes looking at metabolic and vascular features to fill the void. Detecting early metabolic changes associated early tumor initiation and growth using positron emission

FIGURE 10.5 (Continued) (**See color insert.**) (g) A 74-year-old patient. *Infrared imaging* (A): significant vascular asymmetry in the upper central portion of the right breast with a ΔT of 2.8°C (IR-5) (Mod VM IR: 6.8). *Corresponding mammography* (B): Bilateral extensive density. *Surgical histology*: 1 cm right central quadrant infiltrating ductal carcinoma.

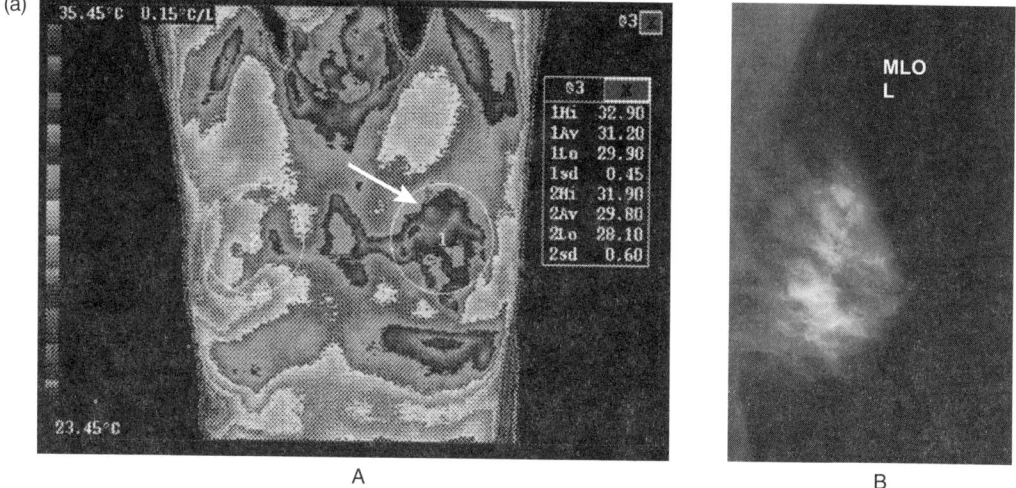

FIGURE 10.6 (**See color insert.**) (a) A 66-year-old patient. Initially seen 2 years prior to diagnosis of left breast cancer for probable fibrocystic disorder (FCD) and scattered cysts, mostly on the left side. *Initial infrared imaging* (A): Extensive significant vascular asymmetry left breast and a near global ΔT of 1.4°C (IR-4) (Mod IR: 5.4). *Initial mammography* (B): Scattered opacities and ultrasound and cytologies were consistent with FCD. Two years later a 1.7 cm cancer was found in the central portion of the left breast.

tomography [38,39], MRI, and Sestamibi scanning are all potential candidates to help monitor PCT-related effects. Unfortunately, they are all hampered by limited access for serial use, duration of the exam, costs, and the need of intravenous access. High-resolution digital infrared imaging, on the other hand, a convenient functional imaging modality free of these inconveniences and requiring neither radiation, nuclear material, contact, nor compression, can be used repeatedly without safety issues. There is ample data indicating its ability to effectively and reliably detect, in a multi-imaging strategy, neoangiogenesis

Functional Infrared Imaging of the Breast

FIGURE 10.6 (Continued) (**See color insert.**) (b) A 49-year-old patient. *Infrared imaging* 1997 (A): Significant vascular asymmetry in the upper central aspect of the left breast (IR-3) *Corresponding mammography* 1997 (B): Dense tissue (contd. 6B2) (c) Patient presents 2 years later with a lump in the upper central portion of the left breast. *Corresponding infrared imaging* (C): Still reveals significant vascular asymmetry and a ΔT of 0.7°C (IR-3) (Mod VM IR″: 3.7). *Corresponding mammography* (D): Now reveals an opacity in the upper aspect of the left breast. *Surgical histology*: 1 cm infiltrating ductal carcinoma.

related to early tumor growth [40]. The premise of our review is that this same phenomenon should even be more obvious when using IR as a monitoring tool in patients with tumors associated with extensive vascular activity as seen in LABC.

To evaluate the ability of our high-resolution digital IR imaging station and a modified Ville Marie scoring system to monitor the functional impact of PCT, 20 successive patients with LABC underwent prospective IR imaging, both prior to and after completion of PCT, usually lasting between 3 and 6 months, which was then followed by curative-intent surgery [41]. Ages ranged between 32 and 82 with a mean of 55. Half of the patients were under 50. Patients presented with T2, T3, or inflammatory carcinoma were all free of any distant disease, thus remaining post-PCT surgical candidates. IR was done at the initial clinical evaluation and prior to core biopsy, often ultrasound guided to ensure optimal specimen harvesting,

TABLE 10.2 Modified Ville Marie Infrared Scoring Scale

IR-1	Absence of any vascular pattern to mild vascular symmetry
IR-2	Symmetrical vascular pattern to moderate vascular asymmetry, particularly if stable or due to known non-cancer causes (eg.: infection, abscess, recent or prior surgery or anatomical asymmetry). Local clinically related vascular assymetry
IR-3	Regional significant vascular asymmetry (SVA)
IR-4	Extensive SVA, involving at least one-third of the breast area

Add the temperature difference (ΔT) in degrees centigrade between the involved area and the corresponding area of the non-involved contralateral breast to calculate final IR score

which was used to document invasive carcinoma. Both sets of IR images were acquired according to our published protocol [38] using the same integrated infrared station described in our previous section.

We used a modification of the original Ville Marie IR scale (Table 10.2) where IR-1 reflects the absence of any significant vascular pattern to minimal vascular symmetry; IR-2 encompasses symmetrical to moderately asymmetrical vascular patterns, including focal clinically related significant vascular asymmetry; IR-3 implies a regional significant vascular asymmetry (SVA) while an extensive SVA, occupying more than a third of the involved breast, constitutes an IR-4. Mean temperature difference (ΔT) in degrees centigrade between the area of focal, regional or extensive SVA and the corresponding area of the noninvolved breast is then added, resulting in the final IR score.

Conventional clinical response to PCT was done by measuring the maximum tumor diameter in centimeters, both before beginning and after completion of PCT.

Induction PCT in 10 patients, 8 on a clinical trial (NSABP B-27 or B-57) consisted of 4 cycles of adriamycin (A) 60 mg/m^2 and cyclophosphamide (C) 600 mg/m^2, with or without additional taxotere (T) 100 mg/m^2, or 6 cycles of AT every 21 days. Eight other patients received AC with additional 5 FU (1000 mg/m^2) and methotrexate (300 mg/m^2). Tamoxifen, given to select patients along with the chemotherapy, was used as sole induction therapy in two elderly patients.

Values in both clinical size and IR scoring both before and after chemotherapy were compared using a paired t-test.

10.2.3 Results

All 20 patients in this series with LABC presented with an abnormal IR image (IR $\geq$ 3). The pre-induction PCT mean IR score was 5.5 (range: 4.4 to 6.9). Infrared imaging revealed a decrease in the IR score in all 20 patients following PCT, ranging from 1 to 5 with a mean of 3.1 ($p < .05$). This decrease following PCT reflected the change in the clinical maximum tumor dimension, which decreased from a mean of 5.2 cm prior to PCT to 2.2 cm ($p < .05$) following PCT in the two-thirds of our series who presented with a measurable tumor. Four of the complete pathological responders in this series saw their IR score revert to normal (<3) following PCT (Figure 10.7) while a fifth had a post-PCT IR score of 3.6. An additional seven patients had a final post-PCT IR score that reflected the final tumor size as measured at surgery (Figure 10.8).

Locally advanced breast cancer is considered an aggressive process that is typically associated with extensive neo-angiogenesis required to sustain rapid and continued tumor growth [27]. Functional IR imaging provided a vivid real-time visual reflection of this invasive process in all our patients. The dramatic IR findings associated with LABC, often occupying more than a third of the breast, are further emphasized by the comparative absence of any significant vascular findings in the uninvolved breast. These images thus provided a new parameter and baseline to complement the traditional structurally based imaging, particularly for the seven patients with clinically nonmeasurable LABC.

The significant reduction in the mean IR score following PCT is primarily an indication of its effect on neo-angiogenesis. While this reduction can sometimes correspond to tumor size, as it did in half of

Functional Infrared Imaging of the Breast

FIGURE 10.7 (See color insert.) (a) A 52-year-old patient. *Infrared imaging* (A): Extensive vascular asymmetry (SVA) in the right breast with a ΔT of 1.2°C (IR-5.2). The patient was started on pre-operative chemotherapy (PCT). *Post-PCT infrared imaging* (B): Resolution of previously noted SVA (IR-2). *Surgical histology*: no residual carcinoma in the resected right breast specimen. (b) A 32-year-old patient. *Infrared imaging* (A): Extensive significant vascular asymmetry and tortuous vascular pattern and a ΔT of 1.3°C (IR-5.3) in the right breast. *Corresponding mammography* (B): Scattered densities. Patient was started on pre-operative chemotherapy (PCT). *Post-PCT infrared image* (C—left breast; D—right breast): Notable resolution of SVA, with a whole breast ΔT of 0.7°C (IR-2). *Surgical histology*: No residual right carcinoma and chemotherapy induced changes.

FIGURE 10.7 (Continued) (**See color insert.**) (c) A 47-year-old patient. *Infrared imaging* (A): Extensive significant vascular asymmetry in the inner half of the left breast with a ΔT of 2°C (IR-6.0). The patient was started on pre-operative chemotherapy (PCT). *Post-PCT infrared imaging* (B): no residual asymmetry (IR-1). *Surgical histology*: No viable residual carcinoma, with chemotherapy induced dense fibrosis surrounding nonviable tumor cells. (d) A 56-year-old patient. *Pre-chemotherapy infrared imaging* (A): Significant vascular asymmetry overlying the central portion of the left breast with a ΔT of 1.35°C (IR-4.35). The patient was given pre-operative chemotherapy (PCT). *Post-PCT infrared* (C): mild bilateral vascular symmetry (IR-). *Surgical histology*: no residual tumor.

this series, IR's main contribution concerns functional parameters that can both precede and linger after structural tumor-induced changes occur. Because IR-detected regional angiogenesis responded slightly slower to PCT than did the anatomical parameters in nine patients underscores the fundamental difference between functional imaging such as IR and structural dependent parameters such as clinical tumor dimensions currently used to assess PCT response. IR has the advantage of not being dependent on a minimal tumor size but rather on the tumor's very early necessity to develop an extensive network to survive and proliferate. This would be the basis of IR's ability to sometimes detect tumor growth earlier than can structurally based modalities. The slight discrepancy between the resolving IR score and the anatomical findings in nine of our patients could suggest that this extensive vascular network, most evident in LABC, requires more time to dismantle in some patients. It could reflect the variable volume of angiogenesis, the inability of PCT to affect it, and thus possibly constitute a prognostic factor. This feature could also result from a deficiency in our proposed scoring scale.

Functional Infrared Imaging of the Breast

A   B

FIGURE 10.7 (Continued) **(See color insert.)** (e) A 54-year-old patient. *Infrared image* (A): extensive significant vascular asymmetry right breast with a r*T* of 2.8°C (IR-6.8). Received pre-operative chemotherapy (PCT). *Post-PCT infrared* (B): Mild local residual vascular asymmetry with a r*T* of 1.65°C (IR-3.65). *Surgical pathology*: No residual viable carcinoma.

FIGURE 10.8 **(See color insert.)** Pre- and post-PCT IR Score and histological maximum tumor dimension (MTD).

Further study and follow-up are needed to better evaluate whether the sequential utilization of this practical imaging modality can provide additional pertinent information regarding the efficacy of our current and new therapeutic strategies, particularly in view of the increasing number with anti-angiogenesis properties, and whether lingering IR-reflected neo-angiogenesis following PCT ultimately reflects on prognosis.

FIGURE 10.9 (**See color insert.**) (a) A stable vascular distribution in the lower inner quadrant of the left breast over a 12-month period. *Infrared imaging* of the breast usually remains remarkably stable in the absence of any on going developing significant pathology. It is important in grading these images to determine if the findings are to be considered evolving and important or stable and possibly relating to the patient's vascular anatomy. (b) An identical vascular distribution of the left breast over a 12-month period. (c) A stable vascular distribution in both breasts over a 12-month period.

10.3 Future Considerations Concerning Infrared Imaging

Mammography, our current standard first-line imaging modality only reflects an abnormality that could then prompt the alert clinician to intervene rather than to observe. This decision is crucial since it is at this first level that sensitivity and specificity are most vulnerable. There is a clear consensus that we have not yet developed the ideal breast cancer imaging technique and this is reflected in the flurry of

Functional Infrared Imaging of the Breast

FIGURE 10.10 (See color insert.) (a) A 50-year-old patient. *Infrared imaging* (A): Significant vascular asymmetry and a ΔT of 3.4°C (IR-5) in the right breast. *Corresponding mammography* (B): Increased density and microcalcifications in the right breast. Surgical histology: extensive right multifocal infiltrating ductal carcinoma requiring a total mastectomy. (b) A 50-year-old patient. *Infrared imaging* (A): Significant vascular asymmetry with a near global ΔT of 2.35°C in the left breast (IR-5). *Mammography* (not available) diffuse density. *Surgical histology:* Left multi-focal infiltrating ductal carcinoma requiring a total mastectomy.

new modalities that have recently appeared. While progress in imaging and better training have resulted in the gradual decrease in the average size of breast tumors over the previous decade, the continued search for improved imaging must continue to further reduce the false negative rate and promote earlier detection.

Digital mammography is already recognized as a major imaging facilitator with the capability to do tomosynthesis and substraction, along with state of the art 3D and 4D ultrasound. However, there is now new emphasis on developing functional imaging that can exploit early vascular and metabolic changes associated with tumor initiation that often predate morphological changes that most of our current structural imaging modalities still depend on; thus, the enthusiasm in the development of sestamibi scanning, doppler ultrasound, and MRI of the breast [42,43]. Unfortunately, as promising as these modalities are, they are often too cumbersome, costly, inaccessible, or require intravenous access to be used as first-line detection modalities alongside clinical exam and mammography.

FIGURE 10.11 (See color insert.) (a) Four years post right partial mastectomy, the patient is recurrence free. Current *Infrared imaging* (A): shows no activity and *Mammography* (B): shows scar tissue. (b) *Infrared image*, 5 years following a left partial mastectomy and radiotherapy for carcinoma revealing slight asymmetry of volume, but no abnormal vascular abnormality and resolution of radiation-induced changes. The patient is disease free.

On the other hand, integrating IR imaging, a safe and practical modality into the first-line strategy, can increase the sensitivity at this crucial stage by also providing an early warning signal of an abnormality that in some cases is not evident in the other components. Combining IR imaging and mammography in an "IR-Assisted Mammography Strategy" is particularly appealing in the current era of increased emphasis on detection by imaging with less reliance on palpation as tumor size further decreases.

Intercenter standardization of a protocol concerning patient preparation, temperature controlled environment, digital image production, enhanced grading, and archiving, as well as data collection and sharing are all important factors that are beginning to be addressed. New technology could permit real-time image acquisition that could be submitted to computerized assisted image reading which will further enhance the physician's ability to detect subtle abnormalities.

Physician training is an essential quality control component for this imaging modality to contribute its full potential. A thorough knowledge of all aspects of benign and malignant breast pathology and concomitant access to prior IR imaging that should normally remain stable (Figure 10.9) are all contributory features. This modality needs to benefit from the same quality control previously applied to mammography and should not, at this time, be used as stand alone. It should benefit from the same

Functional Infrared Imaging of the Breast

interaction between clinical knowledge and other imaging tools as is the case in current breast cancer detection in the clinical environment. This is especially important since there are no current IR regulations, as it poses no health threat and does not use radiation, and could thus fall victim to untrained personnel who could misuse it on unsuspecting patients as was previously the case.

Its future promise, however, resides primarily in its ability to qualify and quantify vascular and metabolic changes related to early tumor genesis. The proposals that a higher temperature difference (ΔT) and increased vascular asymmetry are prognostic factors of tumor aggressivity need to be validated by further research (Figure 10.10). The same applies to the probability that the reduction of IR changes seen with pre-operative chemohormonotherapy reflect reduction in neo-angiogenesis and thus treatment efficacy. These remain, at the very least, extremely interesting and promising areas for future research, particularly

FIGURE 10.12 (See color insert.) A 52-year-old patient, 5 years following right partial mastectomy, radiation, and chemotherapy for right breast cancer. Recent follow-up Infrared Imaging (A) now reveals significant vascular asymmetry (SVA) in the right breast with a ΔT of 1.5°C in the area of the previous surgery (IR-4). *Corresponding mammography* (B): Density and scar issue vs. possible recurrence. *Surgical histology:* 4 cm, recurrent right carcinoma in the area of the previous resection.

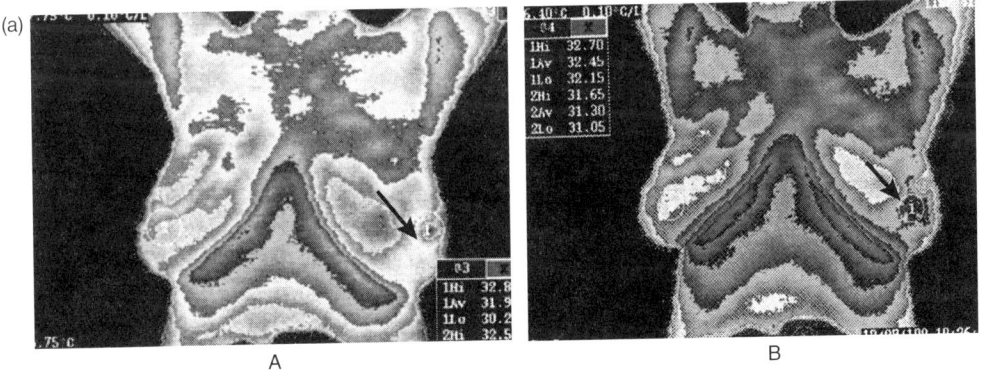

FIGURE 10.13 (See color insert.) (a) A 45-year-old patient with small nodular process just inferior and medial to the left nipple areolar complex. *Infrared imaging* (A), without digital enhancement, was carried out and circles were placed on the nipple area rather than just below and medial to it. The nonenhanced IR image was thus initially misinterpreted as normal with a ΔT of 0.25°C. The same image was recalled and *repeated* (B), now with appropriate digital enhancement and once again, documented the presence of increased vascular activity just inferior and medial to the left nipple areolar complex with a ΔT of 1.15°C (IR-4.15). A 1.5 cm. cancer was found just below the left nipple.

FIGURE 10.13 (Continued) (**See color insert.**) (b) A 37-year-old patient with lump in the upper inner quadrant of the left breast. Mammography confirms spiculated mass. *Infrared imaging* (A): Reported as "normal." Infrared imaging was repeated after appropriate *digital adjustment* (B): Now reveals obvious significant vascular asymmetry in the same area and a ΔT of 1.75°C (Ir-4) (mod IR-4.75). Using a different IR camera on the *same patient* (C) confirms same finding. *Surgical histology*: 1.5 cm infiltrating ductal CA.

in view of the current interest in new angiogenesis-related therapeutic strategies. Its contribution to monitoring post-operative patients (Figure 10.11) which is problematic with both mammography and ultrasound [44] and its ability to recognize recurrent cancer (Figure 10.12) are other areas for further clinical trials. Adequate physician training and strict attention to image acquisition are essential to avoid false negative interpretation (Figure 10.13).

As is the case for all current imaging modalities, the fact that this modality does not detect all tumors should not detract from its contribution as a functional adjuvant addition to our current first-line imaging strategy that is still based essentially on mammography alone, a structural modality that has reached its full potential. There is already sufficient data regarding IR's sensitivity and specificity that has been more recently validated and on going data collection will be important to justify its continued use in the ever evolving breast imaging field. Infrared imaging will soon replace current imaging modalities as an alternative, which would be both uninvasive and yet more informative first-line tool. In the meantime, to ignore its contribution to the very complex process of promoting earlier breast cancer detection could be questioned. A good first-line imaging modality must be safe, convenient, and able to help detect primarily the more aggressive tumors where early intervention can have a greater impact on survival.

References

[1] Lloyd-Williams K. and Handley R.S. Infra-red thermometry in the diagnosis of breast disease. *Lancet* 2, 1371–1381, 1961.

[2] Handley R.S. The temperature of breast tumors as a possible guide to prognosis. *Acta Unio. Int. Contra. Cancrum.* 18, 822, 1962.
[3] Lawson R.N. and Chughtai M.S. Breast cancer and body temperatures. *Can. Med. Assoc. J.* 88, 68–70, 1963.
[4] Gershen-Cohen J., Haberman J., and Brueschke E.E. Medical thermography: a summary of current status. *Radiol. Clin. North. Am.* 3, 403–431, 1965.
[5] Haberman J. The present status of mammary thermography. *Ca—Can. J. Clin.* 18, 314–321, 1968.
[6] Jones C.H. Thermography of the female breast. In Parsons C.A. (ed.), *Diagnosis of Breast Disease*, University Park Press, Baltimore, pp. 214–234, 1983.
[7] Isard H.J., Becker W., Shilo R. et al. Breast thermography after four years and 10,000 studies. *Am. J. Roentgenol.* 115, 811–821, 1972.
[8] Dodd G.D. Thermography in breast cancer diagnosis. In *Proceedings of the 7th National Cancer Conference.* Los Angeles, CA, September 27–29, Lippincott, Philadelphia, Toronto, p. 267, 1972.
[9] Feig S.A., Shaber G.S., Schwartz G.F. et al. Thermography, mammography, and clinical examination in breast cancer screening. *Radiology* 122, 123–127, 1977.
[10] Wallace J.D. Thermographic examination of the breast: an assessment of its present capabilities. In Gallagher H.S. (ed.), *Early Breast Cancer: Detection and Treatment.* American College of Radiology, Wiley, New York, pp. 13–19, 1975.
[11] Report of the working group to review the national cancer institute breast cancer detection demonstration projects. *J. Natl Cancer Inst.* 62, 641–709, 1979.
[12] Haberman J. An overview of breast thermography in the United States. In Margaret Abernathy and Sumio Uematsu (eds), *Medical Thermography.* American Academy of Thermology, Washington, pp. 218–223, 1986.
[13] Moskowitz M., Milbrath J., Gartside P. et al. Lack of efficacy of thermography as a screening tool for minimal and stage I breast cancer. *N. Engl. J. Med.* 295, 249–252, 1976.
[14] Threatt B., Norbeck J.M., Ullman N.S. et al. Thermography and breast cancer: an analysis of a blind reading. *Ann. N.Y. Acad. Sci.* 335, 501–519, 1980.
[15] Stark A. The use of thermovision in the detection of early breast cancer. *Cancer* 33, 1664–1670, 1964.
[16] Sterns E. and Cardis C. Thermography in breast diagnosis. *Cancer* 50, 323–325, 1982.
[17] Moskowitz M. Breast imaging. In Donegan W.L. and Spratt J.S. (eds), *Cancer of the Breast.* Saunders, New York, pp. 206–239, 1995.
[18] Gautherie M. and Gros C.M. Breast thermography and cancer risk prediction. *Cancer* 45, 51–56, 1980.
[19] Amalric R., Gautherie M., Hobbins W.B. et al. Avenir des femmes à thermogramme infra-rouge mammaire anormal isolé. *La. Nouvelle. Presse Médicale* 38, 3153–3155, 1981.
[20] Mariel L., Sarrazin D., Daban A. et al. The value of mammary thermography. A report on 655 cases. *Sem. Hop.* 57, 699–701, 1981.
[21] Isard H.J. Other imaging techniques. *Cancer* 53, 658–664, 1984.
[22] Nyirjesy I. and Billingsley F.S. Detection of breast carcinoma in a gynecological practice. *Obstet. Gynecol.* 64, 747–751, 1984.
[23] Bothmann G.A. and Kubli F. Plate thermography in the assessment of changes in the female breast. 2. Clinical and thermographic results. *Fortschr. Med.* 102, 390–393, 1984.
[24] Useki H. Evaluation of the thermographic diagnosis of breast disease: relation of thermographic findings and pathologic findings of cancer growth. *Nippon. Gan. Chiryo. Gakkai. Shi.* 23, 2687–2695, 1988.
[25] Head J.F., Wang F., and Elliott R.L. Breast thermography is a noninvasive prognostic procedure that predicts tumor growth rate in breast cancer patients. *Ann. N.Y. Acad. Sci.* 698, 153–158, 1993.
[26] Head J.F. and Elliott R.L. Breast thermography. *Cancer* 79, 186–188, 1995.

[27] Gamagami P. Indirect signs of breast cancer: angiogreneis study. In *Atlas of Mammography*. Blackwell Science, Cambridge, MA, pp. 231–226, 1996.
[28] Guidi A.J. and Schnitt S.J. Angiogenesis in preinvasive lesions of the breast. *Breast J.* 2, 364–369, 1996.
[29] Anbar M. Hyperthermia of the cancerous breast: analysis of mechanism. *Cancer Lett.* 84, 23–29, 1994.
[30] Anbar M. Breast cancer. In *Quantitative Dynamic Telethermometry in Medical Diagnosis and Management*. CRC Press, Ann Arbor, MI, pp. 84–94, 1994.
[31] Parisky H.R., Sard A. et al. Efficacy of computerized infrared imagng analysis to evaluate mammographically suspicious lesions. *Am. J. Radiol.* 180, 263–272, 2003.
[32] Sickles E.A. Mammographic features of "early" breast cancer. *Am. J. Roentgenol.* 143, 461, 1984.
[33] Thomas D.B., Gao D.L., Self S.G. et al. Randomized trial of breast self-examination in Shanghai: methodology and preliminary results. *J. Natl Cancer Inst.* 5, 355–365, 1997.
[34] Elmore J.G., Wells C.F., Carol M.P.H. et al. Variability in radiologists interpretation of mammograms. *N. Engl. J. Med.* 331, 99–104, 1993.
[35] Boyd N.F., Byng J.W., Jong R.A. et al. Quantitative classification of mammographic densities and breast cancer risk. *J. Natl Cancer Inst.* 87, 670–675, 1995.
[36] Laya M.B. Effect on estrogen replacement therapy on the specificity and sensibility of screening mammography. *J. Natl Cancer Inst.* 88, 643–649, 1996.
[37] Singletary S.E., McNeese M.D., and Hortobagyi G.N. Feasibility of breast-conservation surgery after induction chemotherapy for locally advanced breast carcinoma. *Cancer* 69, 2849–2852, 1992.
[38] Jansson T., Westlin J.E., Ahlstrom H. et al. Position emission tomography studies in patients with locally advanced and/or metastatic breast cancer: a method for early therapy evaluation? *J. Clin. Oncol.* 13, 1470–1477, 1995.
[39] Hendry J. Combined positron emission tomography and computerized tomography. Whole body imaging superior to MRI in most tumor staging. *JAMA* 290, 3199–3206, 2003.
[40] Keyserlingk J.R., Ahlgren P.D., Yu E., and Belliveau N. Infrared imaging of the breast: initial reappraisal using high-resolution digital technology in 100 successive cases of stage I and II breast cancer. *Breast J.* 4, 245–251, 1998.
[41] Keyserlingk J.R., Yassa, M., Ahlgren, P., and Belliveau N. Tozzi. Ville Marie Oncology Center and St. Mary's Hospital, Montreal, Canada D. *Preliminary Evaluation of Digital Functional Infrared Imaging to Reflect Preoperative Chemohormonotherapy-Induced Changes in Neoangiogenesis in Patients with Locally Advanced Breast Cancer*. European Oncology Society, Milan, Italy, September 2001.
[42] Berg et al. Tumor type and breast profile determine value of mammography, ultrasound and MR. *Radiology* 233, 830–849, 2004.
[43] Oestreicher et al. Breast exam and mammography. *Am. J. Radiol.* 151, 87–96, 2004.
[44] Mendelson, Berg et al. Ultrasound in the operated breast; presented at the *2004 RSNA*. Chicago, November 2005.

11
Detecting Breast Cancer from Thermal Infrared Images by Asymmetry Analysis

Hairong Qi
University of Tennessee

Phani Teja Kuruganti
Oak Ridge National Laboratory

Wesley E. Snyder
North Carolina State University

11.1 Introduction.. 11-1
   Measuring the Temperature of Human Body • Metabolic Activity of Human Body and Cancer Cells • Early Detection of Breast Cancer
11.2 Asymmetric Analysis in Breast Cancer Detection 11-4
   Automatic Segmentation • Asymmetry Identification by Unsupervised Learning • Asymmetry Identification Using Supervised Learning Based on Feature Extraction
11.3 Conclusions 11-12
References 11-13

One of the popular methods for breast cancer detection is to make comparisons between contralateral images. When the images are relatively symmetrical, small asymmetries may indicate a suspicious region. In thermal infrared (IR) imaging, asymmetry analysis normally needs human intervention because of the difficulties in automatic segmentation. In order to provide a more objective diagnostic result, we describe an automatic approach to asymmetry analysis in thermograms. It includes automatic segmentation and supervised pattern classification. Experiments have been conducted based on images provided by Elliott Mastology Center (Inframetrics 600M camera) and Bioyear, Inc. (Microbolometer uncooled camera).

11.1 Introduction

The application of IR imaging in breast cancer study starts as early as 1961 when Williams and Handley first published their results in the *Lancet* [1]. However, the premature use of the technology and its poorly controlled introduction into breast cancer detection in the 1970s have led to its early demise [2]. IR-based diagnosis was criticized as generating a higher false-positive rate than mammography, and thus was not recommended as a standard modality for breast cancer detection. Therefore, despite its deployment in many areas of industry and military, IR usage in medicine has declined [3]. Three decades later, several papers and studies have been published to reappraise the use of IR in medicine [2,3] for the following three reasons: (1) we have greatly improved IR technology. New generations of IR cameras have been developed with much enhanced accuracy; (2) we have much better capabilities in image processing. Advanced techniques including image enhancement, restoration, and segmentation have been effectively used in processing IR images; and (3) we have a deeper understanding of the patho-physiology of heat generation.

The main objective of this work is to evaluate the viability of IR imaging as a noninvasive imaging modality for early detection of breast cancer so that it can be performed both on the symptomatic and the asymptomatic patient and can thus be used as a complement to traditional mammography. This report summarizes how the identification of the asymmetry can be automated using image segmentation, feature extraction, and pattern recognition techniques. We investigate different features that contribute the most toward the detection of asymmetry. This kind of approach helps reduce the false-positive rate of the diagnosis and increase chances of disease cure and survival.

11.1.1 Measuring the Temperature of Human Body

Temperature is a long established indicator of health. The Greek physician, Hippocrates, wrote in 400 B.C. "In whatever part of the body excess of heat or cold is felt, the disease is there to be discovered" [4]. The ancient Greeks immersed the body in wet mud and the area that dried more quickly, indicating a warmer region, was considered the diseased tissue. The use of hands to measure the heat emanating from the body remained well into the sixteenth and the seventeenth centuries. It wasn't until Galileo, who made a thermoscope from a glass tube, that some form of temperature sensing device was developed, but it did not have a scale. It is Fahrenheit and later Celsius who have fixed the temperature scale and proposed the present day clinical thermometer. The use of liquid crystals is another method of displaying skin temperature. Cholesteric esters can have the property of changing colors with temperature and this was established by Lehmann in 1877. It was involved in use of elaborative panels that encapsulated the crystals and were applied to the surface of the skin, but due to large area of contact, they affected the temperature of the skin. All the methods discussed above are contact based.

Major advances over the past 30 years have been with IR thermal imaging. The astronomer, Sir William Herschel, in Bath, England discovered the existence of IR radiation by trying to measure the heat of the separate colors of the rainbow spectrum cast on a table in the darkened room. He found that the highest temperature was found beyond the red end of the spectrum. He reported this to the Royal society as Dark Heat in 1800, which eventually has been turned the IR portion of the spectrum. IR radiation occupies the region between visible and microwaves. All objects in the universe emit radiations in the IR region of the spectra as a function of their temperature. As an object gets hotter, it gives off more intense IR radiation, and it radiates at a shorter wavelength [3]. At moderate temperatures (above 200°F), the intensity of the radiation gets high enough that the human body can detect that radiation as heat. At sufficiently high temperatures (above 1200°F), the intensity gets high enough and the wavelength gets short enough that the radiation crosses over the threshold to the red end of the visible light spectrum. The human eye cannot detect IR rays, but they can be detected by using the thermal IR cameras and detectors.

11.1.2 Metabolic Activity of Human Body and Cancer Cells

Metabolic process in a cell can be briefly defined as the sum total of all the enzymatic reactions occurring in the cell. It can be further elaborated as a highly coordinated, purposeful activity in which many sets of interrelated multienzyme systems participate, exchanging both matter and energy between the cell and its environment. Metabolism has four specific functions: (1) to obtain chemical energy from the fuel molecules; (2) to convert exogenous nutrients into the building blocks or precursor of macromolecular cell components; (3) to assemble such building blocks into proteins, nucleic acids, lipids, and other cell components; and (4) to form and degrade biomolecules required in specialized functions of the cell.

Metabolism can be divided into two major phases, Catabolism and Anabolism. Catabolism is the degradative phase of metabolism in which relatively large and complex nutrient molecules (carbohydrates, lipids, and proteins) are degraded to yield smaller, simpler molecules such as lactic acid, acetic acid, CO_2, ammonia, or urea. Catabolism is accompanied by conservation of some of the energy of the nutrient in the form of phosphate bond energy of adenosine triphosphate (ATP). Conversely, anabolism is the building up phase of metabolism, the enzymatic biosynthesis of such molecular components of cells as the nucleic acids, proteins, lipids, and carbohydrates from their simple building block precursors. Biosynthesis of organic molecules from simple precursors requires input of chemical energy, which is furnished by ATP generated during catabolism. Each of these pathways is promoted by a sequence of specific enzymes catalyzing consecutive reactions. The energy produced by the metabolic pathways is utilized by the cell for its division. Cells undergo mitotic cell division, a process in which a single cell divides into many cells and forms tissues, leading further into the development and growth of the multicellular organs. When cells divide, each resultant part is a complete relatively small cell. Immediately after division the newly formed cells grow rapidly soon reaching the size of the original cell. In humans, growth occurs through mitotic cell division with subsequent enlargement and differentiation of the reproduced cells into organs. Cancer cells also grow similarly but lose the ability to differentiate into organs. So, a cancer may be defined as an actively dividing undifferentiated mass of cells called the "tumor."

Cancer cells result from permanent genetic change in a normal cell triggered by some external physical agents such as chemical agents, x-rays, UV rays, etc. They tend to grow aggressively and do not obey normal pattern of tissue formation. Cancer cells have a distinctive type of metabolism. Although they possess all the enzymes required for most of the central pathways of metabolism, cancer cells of nearly all types show an anomaly in the glucose degradation pathway (viz. Glycolysis). The rate of oxygen consumption is somewhat below the values given by normal cells. However the malignant cells tend to utilize anywhere from 5 to 10 times as much glucose as normal tissue and convert most of it into lactate instead of pyruvate (lactate is a low energy compound whereas pyruvate is a high energy compound). The net effect is that in addition to the generation of ATP in mitochondria from respiration, there is a very large formation of ATP in extramitochondrial compartment from glycolysis. The most important effect of this metabolic imbalance in cancer cells is the utilization of a large amount of blood glucose and release of large amounts of lactate into blood. The lactate so formed is recycled in the liver to produce blood glucose again. Since the formation of blood glucose by the liver requires 6 molecules of ATP whereas breakdown of glucose to lactate produces only 2 ATP molecules, the cancer cells are looked upon as metabolic parasites dependent on the liver for a substantial part of their energy. Large masses of cancer cells thus can be a considerable metabolic drain on the host organism. In addition to this, the high metabolic rate of cancer cells causes an increase in local temperature as compared to normal cells. Local metabolic activity ceases when blood supply is stopped since glycolysis is an oxygen dependent pathway and oxygen is transported to the tissues by the hemoglobin present in the blood; thus, blood supply to these cells is important for them to proliferate. The growth of a solid tumor is limited by the blood supply. If it were not invaded by capillaries a tumor would be dependent on the diffusion of nutrients from its surroundings and could not enlarge beyond a diameter of a few millimeters. Thus, in order to grow further the tumor cells stimulate the blood vessels to form a capillary network that invades the tumor mass. This phenomenon is popularly called "angiogenesis," which is a process of vascularization of a tissue involving the development of new capillary blood vessels.

Vascularization is a growth of blood vessels into a tissue with the result that the oxygen and nutrient supply is improved. Vascularization of tumors is usually a prelude to more rapid growth and often to metastasis (advanced stage of cancer). Vascularization seems to be triggered by angiogenesis factors that stimulate endothelial cell proliferation and migration. In the context of this paper the high metabolic rate in the cancer cells and the high density of packaging makes them a key source of heat concentration (since the heat dissipation is low) thus enabling thermal IR imaging as a viable technique to visualize the abnormality.

11.1.3 Early Detection of Breast Cancer

There is a crucial need for early breast cancer detection. Research has shown that if detected earlier (tumor size less than 10 mm), the breast cancer patient has an 85% chance of cure as opposed to 10% if the cancer is detected late [5].

Different kinds of diagnostic imaging techniques exist in the field of breast cancer detection. The most popularly used method presently is x-ray mammography. The drawback of this technique is that it is invasive and experts believe that electromagnetic radiation can also be a triggering factor for cancerous growth. Because of this, periodic inspection might have a negative effect on the patient's health. Research shows that the mammogram sensitivity is higher for older women (age group 60 to 69 years) at 85% compared with younger women (<50 years) at 64% [5]. A new study in a British medical journal (The LANCET [6]) has asserted that there is no reliable evidence that screening with mammography for breast cancer reduces mortality. They show that screening actually leads to more aggressive treatment, increasing the number of mastectomies by about 20%, and the number of mastectomies and tumorectomies by about 30%.

In contrast to this IR imaging uses a noninvasive imaging technique as the diagnostic tool. The main source of IR rays is heat emitted from different bodies whose temperature is above absolute zero. Thus a thermogram of a patient provides the heat distribution in the body. The cancerous cells, due to high metabolic rates and angiogenesis, are at a higher temperature than the normal cells around it. Thus the cancer cells can be imaged as hotspots in the IR images. The thermogram provides more dynamic information of the tumor since the tumor can be small in size but can be fast growing making it appear as a high temperature spot in the thermogram [7,8]. However, this is not the case in mammography, in which unless the tumor is beyond certain size, it cannot be imaged as x-rays essentially pass through it unaffected. This qualifies IR imaging as an effective diagnostic tool for early detection of breast cancer. Keyserlingk et al. [2] reported that the average tumor size undetected by thermal imaging is 1.28 cm and 1.66 cm by mammography. It is also reported that thermography can provide results that can be correct even 8 to 10 years before mammography can detect a mass in the patient's body [9,10].

11.2 Asymmetric Analysis in Breast Cancer Detection

Radiologists routinely make comparisons between contralateral images. When the images are relatively symmetrical, small asymmetries may indicate a suspicious region. This is the underlying philosophy in the use of asymmetry analysis for mass detection in breast cancer study [11]. Unfortunately, due to various reasons like fatigue, carelessness, or simply because of the limitation of human visual system, these small asymmetries might not be easy to detect. Therefore, it is important to design an automatic approach to eliminate human factors.

There have been a few papers addressing techniques for asymmetry analysis of mammograms [11–16]. Head et al. [17,18] recently analyzed the asymmetric abnormalities in infrared images. In their approach, the thermograms are segmented first by an operator. Then breast quadrants are derived automatically based on unique point of reference, that is, the chin, the lowest, rightmost, and leftmost points of the breast.

This chapter describes an automatic approach to asymmetry analysis in thermograms. It includes automatic segmentation and pattern classification. Hough transform is used to extract the four feature curves that can uniquely segment the left and right breasts. The feature curves include the left and the right body boundary curves, and the two parabolic curves indicating the lower boundaries of the breasts. Upon segmentation, different pattern recognition techniques are applied to identify the asymmetry.

Both segmentation and classification results are shown on images provided by Elliott Mastology Center (Inframetrics 600M camera) and Bioyear, Inc. (Microbolometer uncooled camera).

11.2.1 Automatic Segmentation

There are several ways to perform segmentation, including *threshold-based* techniques, *edge-based* techniques, and *region-based* techniques. Threshold-based techniques assign pixels above (or below) a specified threshold to be in the same region. Edge-based techniques assume that the boundary formed by adjacent regions (or segments) has high edge strength. Through edge detection, we can identify the boundary that surrounds a region. Region-based methods start with elemental regions and split or merge them [19].

11.2.1.1 Edge Image Generation

In this research work, we choose to use the edge-based segmentation technique as we have identified four dominant curves in the edge image, which we call "feature curves," including the left and right body boundaries, and the two lower boundaries of the breasts (Figure 11.3) or the two shadow boundaries that are below the breasts (Figure 11.2) whichever is stronger.

Edges are areas in the image where the brightness changes suddenly. One way to find edges is to calculate the amplitude of the first derivative (Equation 11.1) that generates the so-called gradient magnitude image where $\partial f/\partial x$ is the derivative of the image f along the x direction, and $\partial f/\partial y$ is the derivative along the y direction (the x and y directions are orthogonal to each other) and to threshold the amplitude image.

$$\text{Gradient magnitude} = \sqrt{\left(\frac{\partial f}{\partial x}\right)^2 + \left(\frac{\partial f}{\partial y}\right)^2} \tag{11.1}$$

Another way is to calculate the second derivative and to locate the zero-crossing points, as the second derivative at edge pixels would appear as a point where the derivatives of its left and right pixels change signs.

Although effective, both derivative images are very sensitive to noise. In order to eliminate or reduce the effect of noise, a Gaussian smoothing low-pass filter is applied before taking the derivatives. The smoothing process, on the other hand, also results in thicker edges. The Canny edge detector [20] solves this problem by taking two extra steps, the *nonmaximum suppression* (NMS) step and the *hysteresis thresholding* step, in order to locate the true edge pixels (only one pixel wide along the gradient direction).

For each edge pixel in the gradient magnitude image, the NMS step looks one pixel in the direction of the gradient, and another pixel in the reverse direction. If the magnitude of the current pixel is not the maximum of the three, then this pixel is not a true edge pixel. NMS helps locate the true edge pixels properly. However, the new edges still suffer from extra edge points problem due to noise and missing edge points.

The hysteresis thresholding improves the quality of edge image by using a dual-threshold approach, in which two thresholds, τ_1 and τ_2 (τ_2 is significantly larger than τ_1), are applied on the NMS-processed edge image to produce two binary edge images, denoted as T_1 and T_2, respectively. Since T_1 was created using a lower threshold, it will contain more extra edge pixels than T_2. Edge pixels in T_2 are therefore considered to be parts of true edges. When some discontinuities in edges occur in the T_2 image, the pixels at the same location of the T_1 image is looked up that could be continuations of the edge. If such pixels are found, they are included in the true edge image. This process continues until the continuation of pixels in T_1 connects with an edge pixel in T_2 or no connected T_1 points are found. (See Figures 11.2 and 11.3 for examples of the edge image derived from Canny edge detector.)

11.2.1.2 Hough Transform for Edge Linking

From Figures 11.2 and 11.3, we find that the edge images still cannot be used directly for segmentation as the edge detector picks up all the intensity changes, which would complicate the segmentation. On the other hand, many edges show gaps among edge pixels that would result in segments that are not closed. We have identified four feature boundaries that could enclose the breast. The body boundaries are easy to detect. Difficulties lie in the detection of the lower boundaries of the breasts or the shadow. We observe that the breast boundaries are generally parabolic in shape. Therefore, the Hough transform [21] is used to detect the parabola.

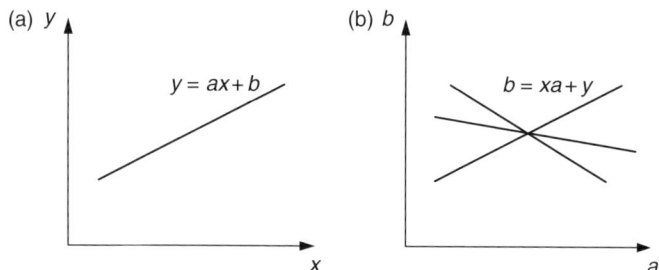

FIGURE 11.1 Illustration of the Hough transform. (a) The original image domain and (b) the parametric domain.

The Hough transform is one type of parametric transforms, in which the object in an image is expressed as a mathematical function of some parameters and the object can be represented in another transformation domain by these parameters. Take a straight edge in an image as an example, in the original image representation domain (or the $x-y$ domain), we can use $y = ax + b$ to describe this edge with a slope of a and an intercept of b, as shown in Figure 11.1a. In order to derive the two parameters, a and b, we can convert the problem to a parametric domain (or the $a-b$ domain) from the original $x-y$ space, and treat x and y as parameters. We find that for each point (x, y) on the edge, there are infinite number of possible corresponding (a, b)s and they form a line in the $a-b$ space, $b = xa + y$. We can imagine that for all the points on the edge, if each of which corresponds to a straight line in the $a-b$ space, then in theory, these lines must intersect at one and only one point (Figure 11.1b), which indicates the true slope and intercept of the edge.

Similarly, the problem of deriving the parameters that describe the parabola can be formulated in a three-dimensional (3D) parametric space of x_0-y_0-p as there are three unknown parameters:

$$y - y_0 = p(x - x_0)^2 \tag{11.2}$$

Each point on the parabola in the $x-y$ space corresponds to a parabola in the x_0-y_0-p space. All the points on the parabola in the $x-y$ space intersect at one point in the x_0-y_0-p space. In order to locate this intersection point in the parametric space, the idea of *accumulator array* is used in which the number of times that a certain pixel in the parametric space is "hit" by a transformed curve (line, parabola, etc.) is treated as the intensity of the pixel. Therefore, the value of the parameters can be derived based on the coordinates of the brightest pixel in the parametric space. The readers are referred to Reference 19 for details on how to implement this accumulator array.

The coordinates of the two brightest spot in the parametric space are used to describe the parabolic functions that form the lower boundaries of the breasts, as shown in Figures 11.2 and 11.3.

11.2.1.3 Segmentation Based on Feature Boundaries

Segmentation is based on three key points, the two armpits (P_L, P_R) derived from the left and right body boundaries by picking up the point where the largest curvature occurs and the intersection (O) of the two parabolic curves derived from the lower boundaries of the breasts/shadow of the breasts. The vertical line that goes through point O and is perpendicular to line $P_L P_R$ is the one used to separate the left and right breasts.

11.2.1.4 Experimental Results

The first set of testing images are obtained using the Inframetrics 600M camera, with a thermal sensitivity of $0.05°$K. The images are collected at Elliott Mastology Center. Results from two testing images (*lr*, *nb*) are shown in Figure 11.2, that includes the intermediate results from edge detection, feature curve extraction,

FIGURE 11.2 Segmentation results of two images. Left: results from lr. Right: results from nb. From top to bottom: original image, edge image, four feature curves, and segments (©2005 IEEE).

FIGURE 11.3 Hough transform based image segmentation. Top: image of a patient with cancer. Bottom: image of a patient without cancer. From left to right: the original TIR image, the edge image using Canny edge detector, and the segmentation based on Hough transform (©2005 IEEE).

and segmentation. From the figure, we can see that Hough transform can derive the parabola at the accurate location.

Another set of images are obtained using Microbolometer uncooled camera, with a thermal sensitivity of $0.05°K$. Some examples of the segmented images are shown in Figure 11.3.

FIGURE 11.4 The left figure show the intensity distribution of a cancerous image and the right figure shows the same for a noncancerous image. The cancerous image is more asymmetrical than the noncancerous one.

Figure 11.4 shows the 3D histogram of the thermal distribution described in the intensity component of the cancerous (*ca*) and noncancerous (*nm*) images. From the graphs, we observe that the *ca* image is more asymmetrical than the *nm* image.

11.2.2 Asymmetry Identification by Unsupervised Learning

Pixel values in a thermogram represent the thermal radiation resulting from the heat emanating from the human body. Different tissues, organs, and vessels have different amount of radiation. Therefore, by observing the heat pattern, or in another word, the pattern of the pixel value, we should be able to discover the abnormalities if there are any.

Usually, in pattern classification algorithms, a set of training data are given to derive the decision rule. All the samples in the training set have been correctly classified. The decision rule is then applied to the testing data set where samples have not been classified yet. This classification technique is also called supervised learning. In unsupervised learning, however, data sets are not divided into training sets or testing sets. No a priori knowledge is known about which class each sample belongs to.

In asymmetry analysis, none of the pixels in the segment knows its class in advance, thus there will be no training set or testing set. Therefore, this is an unsupervised learning problem. We use *k*-means algorithm to do the initial clustering. *k*-means algorithm is described as follows:

1. Begin with an arbitrary set of cluster centers and assign samples to nearest clusters
2. Compute the sample mean of each cluster
3. Reassign each sample to the cluster with the nearest mean
4. If the classification of all samples has not changed, then stop, else go to step 2

After each sample is relabeled to a certain cluster, the cluster mean can then be calculated. The segmented image can also be displayed in labeled format. From the difference of mean distribution, we can tell if there is any asymmetric abnormalities.

Figure 11.5 provides the histogram of pixel value from each segment that generated in Figure 11.2 with 10-bin setup. We can tell just from the shape of the histogram that *lr* is more asymmetric than *nb*. However, the histogram only reveals global information. Figure 11.6 displays the classification results for each segment in its labeled format. Here, we choose to use four clusters. The figure also shows the mean difference of each cluster in each segmented image. From Figure 11.6, we can clearly see the much bigger difference shown in the mean distribution or image *lr*, which can also be observed from the labeled image.

Detecting Breast Cancer from Thermal Infrared Images

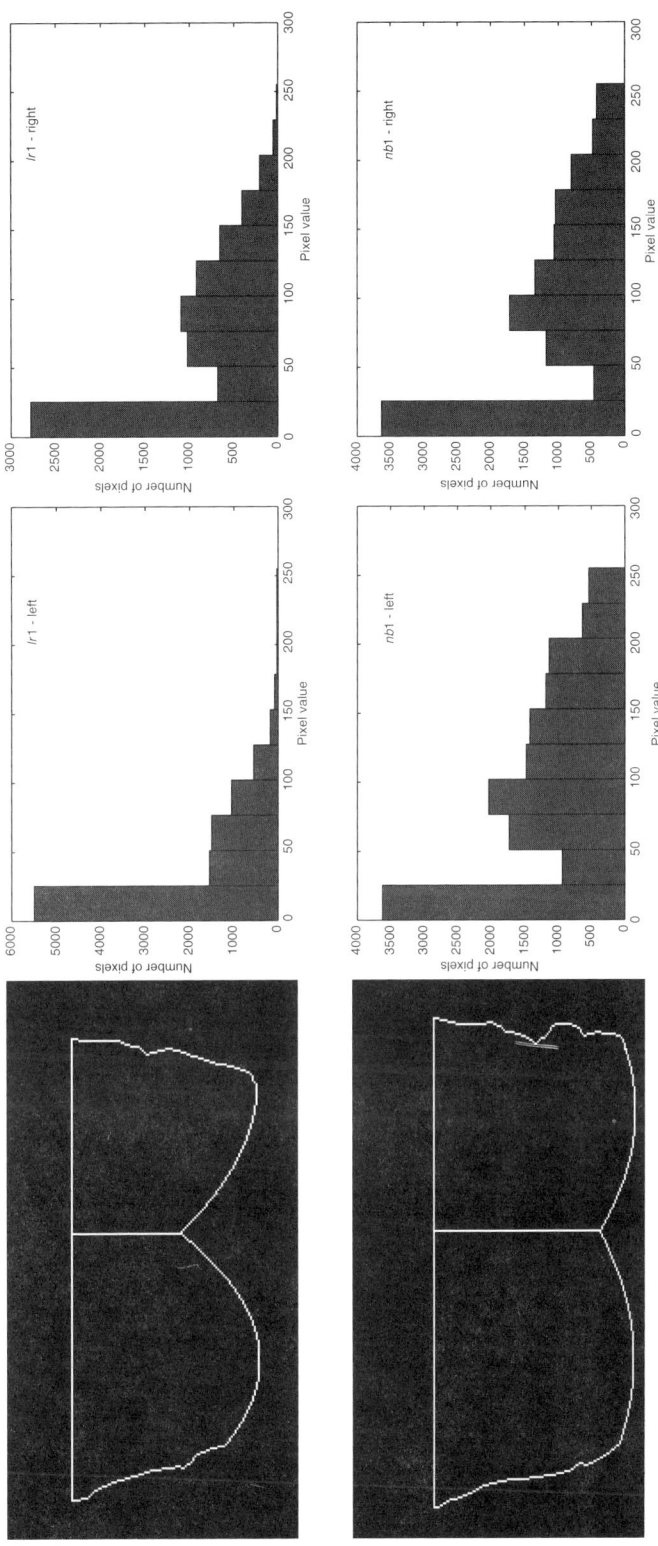

FIGURE 11.5 Histogram of the left and right segments. Top: results from *lr*. Bottom: results from *nb*. From left to right: the segments, histogram of the left segment, histogram of the right segment (©2005 IEEE).

FIGURE 11.6 Labeled image and the profile of mean for each cluster. (a) Results from *lr*, (b) labeled image, (c) results from *nb*, and (d) average pixel value profile of each cluster (©2005 IEEE).

11.2.3 Asymmetry Identification Using Supervised Learning Based on Feature Extraction

Feature extraction is performed on the segmented images. The aim of this research is to identify the effectiveness of the features in contributing toward the asymmetry analysis.

As discussed earlier, TIR imaging is a functional imaging technique representing thermal information as a function of intensity. The TIR image is a pseudo-colored image with different colors assigned to different temperature ranges.

The distribution of different intensities can now be quantified by calculating some high-order statistics as feature elements. We design the following features to form the feature space:

- *Moments of the intensity image*: The intensity component of the image directly corresponds to the thermal energy distribution in the respective areas. The histogram describing the intensity distributions essentially describes the texture of the image. The moments of the histogram give statistical information about the texture of the image. Figure 11.5 shows the intensity distribution of images of a cancerous patient and non-cancerous patient. The four moments, mean, variance, skewness, and kurtosis are taken as

$$\text{Mean } \mu = \frac{1}{N} \sum_{j=1}^{N} p_j \quad (11.3)$$

$$\text{Variance } \sigma^2 = \frac{1}{N-1} \sum_{j=1}^{N} (p_j - \mu)^2 \quad (11.4)$$

$$\text{Skewness} = \frac{1}{N} \sum_{j=1}^{N} \left[\frac{p_j - \mu}{\sigma} \right]^3 \quad (11.5)$$

$$\text{Kurtosis} = \frac{1}{N} \sum_{j=1}^{N} \left(\frac{p_j - \mu}{\sigma} \right)^4 \quad (11.6)$$

where p_j is the probability density of the jth bin in the histogram, and N is the total number of bins.
- *The peak pixel intensity of the correlated image*: The correlated image between the left and right (reflected) breasts is also a good indication of asymmetry. We use the peak intensity of the correlated image as a feature element since the higher the correlation value, the more symmetric the two breast segments.
- *Entropy*: Entropy measures the uncertainty of the information contained in the segmented images. The more equal the intensity distribution, the less information. Therefore, the segment with hot spots should have a lower Entropy.

$$\text{Entropy } H(X) = -\sum_{j=1}^{N} p_j \log p_j \quad (11.7)$$

- *Joint Entropy*: The higher the joint entropy between the left and right breast segments, the more symmetric they are supposedly to be, and the less possible of the existence of tumor.

$$\text{Joint Entropy } H(X, Y) = \sum_{i=1}^{N_X} \sum_{j=1}^{N_Y} p_{ij} \log(p_{ij}) \quad (11.8)$$

TABLE 11.1 Moments of the Histogram

	Cancerous		Noncancerous	
Moments	Left	Right	Left	Right
Mean	0.0010	0.0008	0.0012	0.0010
Variance (10^{-6})	2.0808	1.1487	3.3771	2.7640
Skewness (10^{-6})	2.6821	1.1507	4.8489	4.5321
Kurtosis (10^{-8})	1.0481	0.3459	2.1655	2.3641

TABLE 11.2 Entropy and Correlation Values

Feature	Cancerous	Noncancerous
Correlation	$\times 10^8$	2.35719×10^8
Joint Entropy	9.0100	17.5136
Entropy		
Left	1.52956	1.70684
Right	1.3033	1.4428

where p_{ij} is the joint probability density, N_X and N_Y are the number of bins of the intensity histogram of images X and Y respectively.

From the set of features derived from the testing images, the existence of asymmetry is decided by calculating the ratio of the feature from the left segment to the feature from the right segment. The closer the value to one, the more correlated the features or the less asymmetric the segments. Classic pattern classification techniques like the maximum posterior probability and the kNN classification [22] can be used for the automatic classification of the images. Table 11.1 describes the typical moments for the cancerous and noncancerous images.

The typical values of the cancerous images and noncancerous images are tabulated in Table 11.2. The asymmetry can be clearly stated with a close observation of the given feature values. We used 6 normal patient thermograms and 18 cancer patient thermograms. With a larger database, a training feature set can be derived and supervised learning algorithms like discriminant function or kNN classification can be implemented for a fast, effective, and automated classification.

Figure 11.7 evaluates the effectiveness of the features used. The first data point along the x-axis indicates *entropy*, the second to the fifth points indicate the four statistical moments (*means, variance, skewness,* and *kurtosis*). The y-axis shows the *closeness* metric we defined as

$$\text{Bilateral ratio closeness to 1} = \left| \frac{\text{feature value from left segment}}{\text{feature value from right segment}} - 1 \right| \quad (11.9)$$

From the figure, we observe that the high-order statistics are the most effective features to measure the asymmetry, while low-order statistics (*mean*) and *entropy* do not assist asymmetry detection.

11.3 Conclusions

This paper develops a computer-aided approach for automating asymmetry analysis of thermograms. This kind of approach will help the diagnostics as a useful second opinion. The use of TIR images for breast cancer detection and the advantages of thermograms over traditional mammograms are studied. From the experimental results, it can be observed that the Hough transform can be effectively used for breast segmentation. We propose two pattern classification algorithms, the unsupervised learning

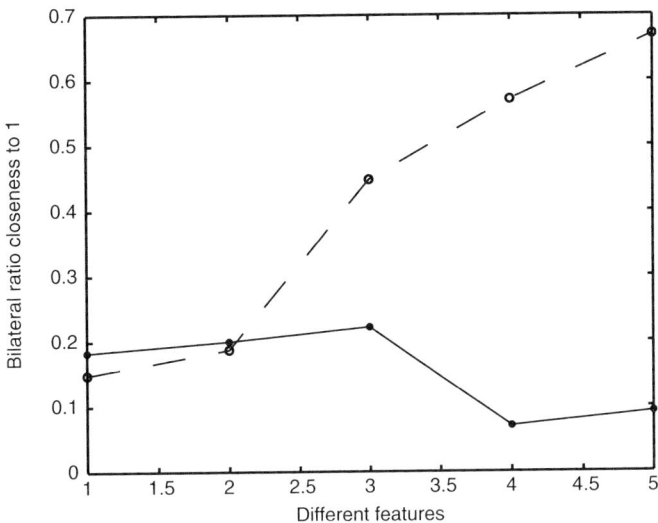

FIGURE 11.7 Performance evaluation of different feature elements. Solid line: non-cancerous image; Dash line: cancerous image. The five data points along the x-axis indicate (from left to right): entropy, mean, variance, skewness, and kurtosis (©2005 IEEE).

using k-means and the supervised learning using kNN based on feature extraction. Experimental results show that feature extraction is a valuable approach to extract the signatures of asymmetry, especially the joint entropy. With a larger database, supervised pattern classification techniques can be used to attain more accurate classification. These kind of diagnostic aids, especially in a disease like breast cancer where the reason for the occurrence is not totally known, will reduce the false-positive diagnosis rate and increase the survival rate among the patients since the early diagnosis of the disease is more curable than in a later stage.

References

[1] Llyod-Williams, K. and Handley, R.S., Infrared thermometry in the diagnosis of breast disease. *Lancet*, 2, 1378–1381, 1961.
[2] Keyserlingk, J.R., Ahlgren, P.D., Yu, E., Belliveau, N., and Yassa, M., Functional infrared imaging of the breast, *IEEE Engineering in Medicine and Biology*, 19, 30–41, 2000.
[3] Jones B.F., A reappraisal of the use of infrared thermal image analysis in medicine. *IEEE Transactions on Medical Imaging*, 17, 1019–1027, 1998.
[4] Thermology, http://www.thermology.com/history.htm
[5] Ng, E.Y.K. and Sudarshan, N.M., Numerical computation as a tool to aid thermographic interpretation. *Journal of Medical Engineering and Technology*, 25, 53–60, 2001.
[6] Oslen, O. and Gotzsche, P.C., Cochrane review on screening for breast cancer with mammography. *Lancet*, 9290, 1340–1342, 2001.
[7] Hay, G.A., *Medical Image: Formation, Perception and Measurement*. The Institute of Physics, John Wiley & Sons, 1976.
[8] Watmough, D.J., The role of thermographic imaging in breast screening, discussion by C.R. Hill. In *Medical Images: Formation, Perception and Measurement, 7th L H Gray Conference: Medical Images*, pp. 142–158, 1976.
[9] Gautheire, M., *Atlas of Breast Thermography with Specific Guidelines for Examination and Interpretation*. Milan, Italy, PAPUSA, 1989.

[10] Ng, E.Y.K., Ung, L.N., Ng, F.C., and Sim, L.S.J., Statistical analysis of healthy and malignant breast thermography, *Journal of Medical Engineering and Technology*, 25, 253–263, 2001.

[11] Good, W.F., Zheng, B., Chang, Y. et al., Generalized procrustean image deformation for subtractiuon of mammograms. In *Proceeding of SPIE Medical Imaging—Image Processing*, Vol. 3661, pp. 1562–1573, San Diego, CA, SPIE, 1999.

[12] Shen, L., Shen, Y.P., Rangayyan, R.M., and Desautels J., Measures of asymmetry in mammograms based upon shape spectrum. In *Proceedings of the Annual Conference on EMB*, Vol. 15, pp. 48–49, San Diego, CA, 1993.

[13] Yin, F.F., Giger, M.L., Doi, K. et al., Computerized detection of masses in digital mammograms: analysis of bilateral subtraction images. *Medical Physics*, 18, 955–963, 1991.

[14] Yin, F.F., Giger, M.L., Doi, K. et al., Computerized detection of masses in digital mammograms: automated alignment of breast images and its effect on bilateral-substraction technique. *Medical Physics*, 21, 445–452, 1994.

[15] Yin, F.F., Giger, Vyborny C.J. et al., Comparison of bilateral-subtraction and single-image processing techniques in the computerized detection of mammographic masses. *Investigative Radiology*, 6, 473–481, 1993.

[16] Zheng, B., Chang, Y.H., and Gur, D., Computerized detection of masses from digitized mammograms: comparison of single-image segmentation and bilateral image subtraction. *Academic Radiology*, 2, 1056–1061, 1995.

[17] Head J.F., Lipari, C.C., and Elliott R.L., Computerized image analysis of digitized infrared images of the breasts from a scanning infrared imaging system. In *Proceedings of the 1998 Conference on Infrared Technology and Applications XXIV, Part I*, Vol. 3436, pp. 290–294, San Diego, CA, SPIE, 1998.

[18] Lipari C.A. and Head J.F., Advanced infrared image processing for breast cancer risk assessment. In *Proceedings for 19th International Conference of IEEE/EMBS*, pp. 673–676, Chicago, IL, Oct. 30–Nov. 2. IEEE, 1997.

[19] Snyder, W.E. and Qi, H., *Machine Vision*, Cambridge University Press, 2004.

[20] Canny, J., A computational approach to edge detection. *IEEE Transactions on Pattern Analysis and Machine Intelligence*, 6, 679–698, 1995.

[21] Jafri M.Z. and Deravi, F., Efficient algorithm for the detection of parabolic curves. In *Vision Geometry III*, Vol. 2356, pp. 53–62, SPIE, 1998.

[22] Duda, R.O., Hart, P.E., and Strok, D.G., *Pattern Classification*. John Wiley & Sons, 2nd ed., 2001.

12
Advanced Thermal Image Processing

Boguslaw Wiecek
M. Strzelecki
T. Jakubowska
M. Wysocki
C. Drews-Peszynski
Technical University of Lodz

12.1 Histogram-Based First Order Thermal Signatures 12-3
12.2 Second Order Statistical Parameters 12-5
12.3 Wavelet Transformation 12-8
12.4 Classification 12-9
12.5 Conclusion 12-12
References 12-12

Thermal imaging can be useful as an early diagnostic technique that can detect many diseases, such as for example, breast cancer, malignant tumors, etc. There are many different methods that describe image features. A large group of methods is based on statistical parameters calculations. Parameters like mean value, standard deviation, skewness, kurtosis, etc. can be used to compare thermal images. We consider both the first and second order statistical parameters [1,2]. The first order statistical parameters methods use image's histogram (Figure 12.1) to compute signatures, while the second order statistical parameters are defined for so-called co-occurrence matrix of the image [2,11].

In medical applications, one of the principal features of the thermal image is its symmetry of temperature patterns. Thermal images are usually asymmetrical in pathological cases. Any significant asymmetry can indicate a physiologic abnormality (Figure 12.2). This may be pathological (including cancer, fibrocystic disease, an infection, or a vascular disease) or it might indicate an anatomical variant [4–6].

The next group of methods is based on image transformations, such as linear filtering, Fourier or wavelet analysis. All these methods allow to regenerate an image which is processed or converted, and signatures are defined in different domain, for example, frequency or scale domains. Well-known Karhunen-Loeve transform is implemented in form of principle component analysis (PCA). PCA is a technique that is usually used for reducing the dimensionality of multivariate data, preserving most of the variance [7–9].

Thermal image classification is a powerful tool for many medical diagnostic protocols, for example, during breast cancer screening [3,10,11]. Figures 12.3 and 12.4 show thermal images of a healthy breast and that with malignant tumor, respectively. Among the variety of different image features, statistical thermal signatures (first and second order) have been already effectively used for classification of images represented by raw data [1,2,10,12]. In another approach, the features obtained from wavelet transformation can also be used for successful classification.

FIGURE 12.1 (**See color insert at the back of the book.**) ROI of thermal image and its histogram.

FIGURE 12.2 (**See color insert.**) Nonsymmetrical temperature distribution for pneumonia with corresponding x-ray image.

FIGURE 12.3 (**See color insert.**) Thermal image of the healthy breast.

Advanced Thermal Image Processing

FIGURE 12.4 (See color insert.) Thermal image of the breast with malignant tumor (left side).

It is possible to define many features for an image, and obviously, the selection and reduction are needed. Two approaches are applied, based on Fischer coefficient as well as by using minimization of classification error probability (POE) and average correlation coefficients (ACC), calculated for chosen features [13]. It can reduce the number of features to a few ones. Features preprocessing which generates new parameters after linear or nonlinear transformations can be the next step in the procedure. It allows to get less correlated and of the lower order data. Two approaches are used, that is, PCA and linear discriminant analysis (LDA) [1,3,8]. Finally, classification can be performed using different artificial neural network (ANN), with or without additional hidden layers, and with different number of neurons. Alternatively, nearest neighbor classification (NNC) can also be employed for such image processing.

12.1 Histogram-Based First Order Thermal Signatures

An image is assumed to be a rectangular matrix of discretised data (pixels) pix $[m, n]$, where $m = 0, 1, \ldots, M$, $n = 0, 1, \ldots, N$. Each pixel takes a value from the range $i \in \langle 0, L-1 \rangle$. The histogram describes the frequency of existence of pixels of the same intensity in whole image or in the region of interest (ROI). Formally, the histogram represents the distribution of the probability function of the existence of the given intensity in an image and it is expressed using Kronecker delta function as:

$$H(i) = \sum_{n}^{N-1} \sum_{m}^{M-1} \delta(p[m, x], i), \quad \text{for } i = 0, 1, \ldots, L-1 \quad (12.1)$$

where

$$\delta(p[m, n], i) = \begin{cases} 1, & \text{for } p[m, n] = i \\ 0, & \text{for } p[m, n] \neq i \end{cases} \quad (12.2)$$

Histogram is used for defining first order statistical features of the image, such as mean value μ_H, variance σ_H, skewness, kurtosis, energy, and entropy. The definitions of these parameters are given below:

$$\mu_H = \sum_{i=0}^{L-1} i p(i)$$

$$\sigma_H = \sum_{i=0}^{L-1} (i - \mu_H)^2 p(i)$$

$$\text{Skewness} = \frac{\sum_{i=0}^{L-1} (i - \mu_H)^3 p(i)}{\sigma_H^3}$$

$$\text{Kurtosis} = \frac{\sum_{i=0}^{L-1} (i - \mu_H)^4 p(i)}{\sigma_H^4} - 3 \tag{12.3}$$

$$\text{Energy} = \sum_{i=0}^{L-1} p^2(i)$$

$$\text{Entropy} = -\sum_{i=0}^{L-1} \log_2(p(i)) p(i)$$

Histogram gives global information on an image. By converting histogram we can obtain some very useful image improvement, such as contrast enhancement [1,14]. The first order statistical parameters can be used to separate physiological and pathological breast thermal images. The results for breast cancer screening are presented below.

Thirty-two healthy patients and ten patients with malignant tumors were analyzed using thermography. There were four images registered for every patient that represented each breast in direct and lateral direction to the camera. Histograms were created for these images and on the basis of statistical parameters, the following features were calculated: mean temperature, standard deviation, variance, skewness, and kurtosis. Afterward, differences of parameter values for left and right breast were calculated. The degree of symmetry on the basis of these differences was then estimated (see Figures 12.5 and 12.6).

FIGURE 12.5 Histograms of healthy breast thermographs.

FIGURE 12.6 Histograms of breast thermographs with malignant tumor.

The mean temperature in the healthy group was estimated at the level $30.2 \pm 1.8°C$ in the direct position and $29.7 \pm 1.9°C$ in the lateral one. The mean temperature was higher in 8 cases out of 10 in malignant tumor group. Moreover, 6 cases out of 32 in the healthy group with mean temperatures exceeded normal level. Therefore, we have found that it is necessary to analyze symmetry between left and right breast. Comparison of mean temperature was not sufficient to separate physiological and pathological images. Among analyzed parameters, skewness was the most promising for successful classification of thermal images. Absolute differences of skewness for left and right side was equal to $0.4 \pm 0.3°C$ in frontal position and $0.6 \pm 0.4°C$ in lateral one for the healthy group. These differences were higher for images in lateral position in all cases in the pathological group in comparison to the healthy patients' images.

The image in Figure 12.4 confirm the evidence of asymmetry between left and right side for healthy and malignant tumor cases.

Analyzing the first order statistical parameter let us conclude that it is quite hard to use them for the image classification and detecting tumors. In some cases, only mean temperature and the skewness let us to separate and classify thermal images of breasts with and without malignant tumors. Frontal and lateral positions were used during this investigation, but no significant difference of the obtained result was noticed.

It is concluded that the first order parameters do not give the satisfactory results, and due to some physiological changes of the breast, we could observe that these parameters do not allow separating patients with and without tumors. That was the main reason, that the second order statistical parameters are used for the further investigations.

12.2 Second Order Statistical Parameters

More advanced statistical information on thermal images can be derived from second order parameters. They are defined on so-called co-occurrence matrix. Such a matrix represents the joint probability of two pixels having i-th and j-th intensity at the different distances d, in the different directions. Co-occurrence matrix gives more information on intensity distribution over the whole image, and in this sense, it can effectively be used to separate and classify thermal images.

Let us assume that each pixel has eight neighbors lying in four directions: horizontal, vertical, diagonal and antidiagonal. Let us consider only the nearest neighbors, so the distance $d = 1$ (see Figure 12.7).

As an example let us take an image 4×4 with 4 intensity levels given as (see Figure 12.8).

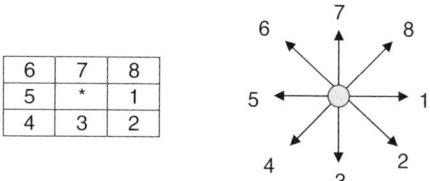

FIGURE 12.7 Eight neighboring pixels in four direct horizontal, vertical, diagonal, and antidiagonal.

FIGURE 12.8 Example of 4 × 4 image with 4 discrete intensity levels.

FIGURE 12.9 Difference variance vs. variance obtained from co-occurrence matrix for horizontal direction.

For horizontal direction the co-occurrence matrix takes a form:

$$m_{\text{horizontal}} = \begin{bmatrix} 2 & 1 & 0 & 0 \\ 1 & 4 & 2 & 2 \\ 0 & 2 & 4 & 2 \\ 0 & 2 & 2 & 0 \end{bmatrix} \quad (12.4)$$

The co-occurrence matrix is always square and diagonal with the dimension equal to the number of intensity levels in the image. After normalization, we get the matrix of the probabilities $p(i, j)$. Normalization is done by dividing the all elements by number of possible couple pixels for a given direction of analysis. For horizontal and vertical directions this number is equal to $2N(M - 1)$ and $2M(N - 1)$, while for diagonal directions it is $2(M - 1)(N - 1)$, respectively.

Second order parameters are presented by Equations 12.4 and 12.6. As an example of comparing thermal images μ_x, μ_y, σ_x, σ_y are mean values and standard deviations for the elements of co-occurrence matrices that were calculated for horizontal and vertical directions, respectively, and the results are presented in Figures 12.9 and 12.10.

Advanced Thermal Image Processing

FIGURE 12.10 Difference variance vs. variance obtained from co-occurrence matrix for diagonal direction.

Second order statistical parameters can be used to discriminate the physiological and pathological cases, for example, breast cancers. Most of them successfully discriminate healthy and malignant tumor cases. The protocol of the investigation assumes the symmetry analysis in the following way. At first, the square ROI were chosen for analysis. Then, co-occurrence matrixes were calculated for left and right breasts to evaluate second order statistical parameters for different directions. Only the neighboring pixels are considered in these investigations ($d = 1$). Finally, the differences of the values of these parameters for left and right sides were used for the image classification. Figures 12.9 and 12.10 illustrate that the differences of second order parameters for left and right sides are typically greater for pathological cases. Taking two parameters such as difference variance and variance allows successfully separating almost all healthy and malignant tumor cases.

$$\text{Energy} = \sum_{i=0}^{L-1}\sum_{j=0}^{L-1} p^2(i,j)$$

$$\text{Variance} = \sum_{i=0}^{L-1}\sum_{j=0}^{L-1} (i-j)^2 p(i,j) \tag{12.5}$$

$$\text{Difference variance} = \text{Var}(p_{x-y})$$

where

$$p_{x-y}(l) = \sum_{i=0}^{L-1}\sum_{j=0}^{L-1} p(i,j), \quad \text{for } |i-j| = l, \ l = 0, 1, \ldots, G-2$$

$$\text{Correlation} = \frac{\sum_{i=0}^{L-1}\sum_{j=0}^{L-1}(ij)p(i,j) - \mu_x \mu_y}{\sigma_x \sigma_y} \tag{12.6}$$

$$\text{Inverse difference} = \sum_{i=0}^{L-1}\sum_{j=0}^{L-1} \frac{p(i,j)}{1+(i-j)^2}$$

$$\text{Entropy} = -\sum_{i=0}^{L-1}\sum_{j=0}^{L-1} p(i,j) \log_2[p(i,j)]$$

12.3 Wavelet Transformation

Wavelet transformation is actually used in many domains, such as telecommunication and signal processing for compression and to extract quantitative features from the signal. In image processing it can be employed to get new features, representing both global and detail information. Wavelet transformation is based on image filtering represented by rows and columns using low and high pass linear filters (Figure 12.11). After filtering, decimation is used to reduce the number of pixels. The procedure can be repeated until 1×1 images are obtained. Practically, the processing is stopped earlier, after 2 to 4 steps, and then the features are derived from the filtered subimages.

As an example, the investigations of 10 patients with recognized breast tumors, as well as 30 healthy patients are presented. All healthy and pathological cases were confirmed by other diagnostic methods, such as mammography, USG, biopsy, and so on. We have used thermographic camera to take two images for each breast: frontal and side ones. Each patient was relaxing before the experiment for 15 min in a room where temperature were stabilized at $20°C$.

Then the numerical procedure was used to calculate features of the images. Figure 12.12 presents the pathological case where left breast has evidently higher temperature and the temperature distribution is very asymmetric.

One of the possible transformations uses wavelets realized by filtering as it has already been mentioned. The result of such processing is presented in Figure 12.13. As it is seen, the different filters are showing different details of the image, that is, high pass filters allows to present gradient of the temperature, while

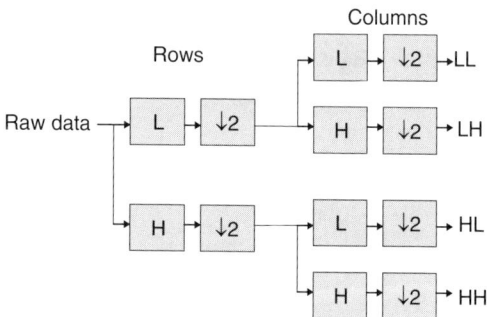

FIGURE 12.11 Wavelet transformation of an image.

FIGURE 12.12 (See color insert.) Example of thermal image with the tumor.

FIGURE 12.13 Result of wavelet transformation.

the low pass ones display the global temperature distribution and the energy of the signal understood as the level of temperature.

As a powerful tool, wavelet transformation gives the possibility of generating new features from different subimages, in different scales and subbands. Filtering can be easily parameterized in the sense of varying cutoff frequency, what provides the additional flexibility in the algorithm. It denotes, that a lot of different features can be produced by this method. Obviously, the selection of these features is necessary to obtain only these ones, which are the most discriminative and weakly correlated [11].

12.4 Classification

Artificial neural network are typically used for classification. The selected image features are used as inputs. It means that the number of input nodes is equal to number of the features. The number of neurons in the first hidden layer can be equal or lower than the number of features in the classification, as shown in Figure 12.14. ANN can have user-defined next hidden layers, which allow additional nonlinear processing of the input features. As ANN is the nonlinear system, such technique allows to additional decorrelating and data reduction, what in consequence improves the classification. Such approach is known as nonlinear discriminant analysis (NDA) [3,11].

It is well known that the training of ANN is the very important step in the entire protocol. It is an multivariable optimization problem typically based on back-propagation technique. In general case it can lead to wrong solutions if the there is no single minimum of the error function. That is why we need enough data during learning phase, and sometimes it is better or necessary to repeat training of ANN with different initial values of the neuron weight coefficients.

Classification can start from the raw data analysis. As seen in Figure 12.15, two classes of images containing (1) nonhealthy and (2) healthy cases are chosen. In this example, selection of features reduces the number of features to two, derived from the co-occurrence matrix (sum of squares and inverse difference moment) [1,10,12]. The third one is based on wavelet transformation—energy E_{HL} for the scale no.1 and high and low frequency subbands. Raw data analysis (Figure 12.15) does not give satisfactory feature separation and classification. It is hard to separate clusters of features corresponding to physiological and pathological images. The distance in between them in the multivariate space is not large enough, which means that the probability of erroneous classification is still quite high.

The next results were obtained by LDA (Figure 12.16), in which the most discriminative features (MDF) are generated [10,13]. LDA creates typically new set with smaller number of features. LDA is the linear

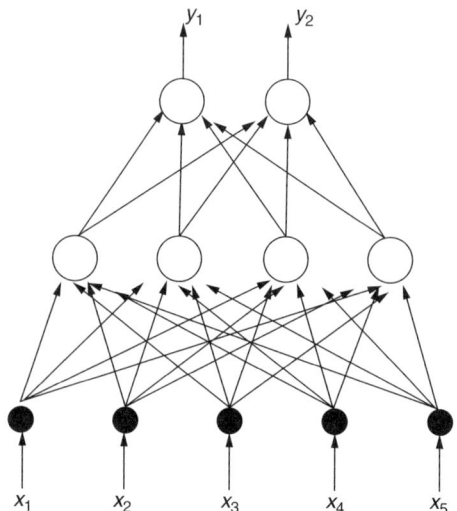

FIGURE 12.14 Neural network example with input, single hidden, and output layers.

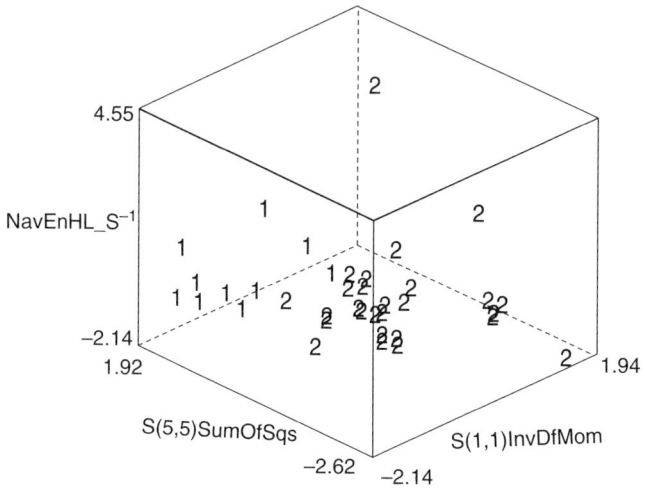

FIGURE 12.15 Raw data analysis result.

transformation, and produces linearly separated features, which means that in general case it is also not possible to separate them fully. This case is illustrated in Figure 12.16.

Nonlinear transformation of the features obtained by ANN with additional hidden layer is the most promising technique. The output of this additional hidden layer creates the new smaller set of features, which are typically much better separable. It can be simple verified by the larger value of Fisher coefficient. In our investigation, seven original features were selected using POE and ACC selection criteria. The first and second hidden layers contained only one and two neurons, respectively. It denotes that the original features were reduced to two new ones. The expectation that this approach allows better separation and classification is now confirmed [2].

The results of NDA are presented in Figures 12.17 and 12.18. Two new features are far away from each other on the feature space, both for frontal and side images. It is even not very surprising that the value of Fisher coefficient $F = 2.7$ for original features is now increased to $F = 443.4$. ANN together with

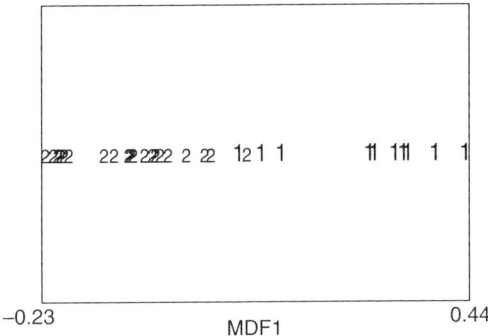

FIGURE 12.16 Nonacceptable separation of cluster using LDA.

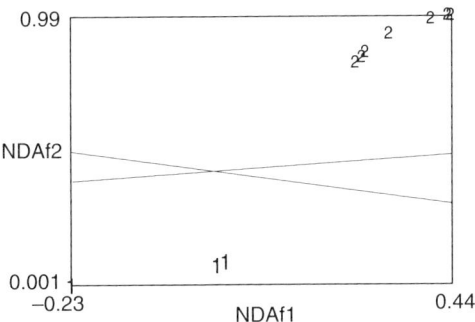

FIGURE 12.17 NDA classification results for side thermal images of the breast.

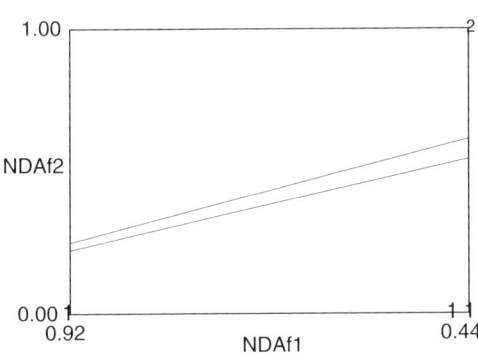

FIGURE 12.18 NDA classification results for frontal thermal images of the breast.

NDA have one more advantage. Besides data reduction and decorrelating, it also allows implementing classification realized by the last output layer of ANN.

We faced one problem in the presented research. The number of pathological cases was small, only ten. As it has been already mentioned it is difficult to get well diagnosed patients, especially in the young age [4–6]. The research is still in progress, and we actually enlarging our image database day-by-day. This research is a preliminary one, and shows the possibility of using advanced image processing tools. The effectiveness of the screening procedure can be verified later, when we will have enough input data.

Because of the above limits, the classification was carried out in the following simplified way: First we have chosen equal number of physiological and pathological images, that is, 10 + 10. Every image from

TABLE 12.1 Errors of Classification

	Frontal positions		Side positions	
	False negative	False positive	False negative	False positive
Raw data	2/10	3/30	1/10	2/30
PCA	2/10	3/30	1/10	2/30
LDA	1/10	2/30	1/10	1/30
NDA	2/10	2/30	0/10	2/30

each class (healthy and nonhealthy) was extracted, and the training of ANN was performed for all the rest. Then this one not being used before during learning was employed now for classification.

The results are presented in Table 12.1. First three rows in this table present nearest neighbor (NN) classification of the image features. The first results were obtained by using feature calculated on a image and NN classification after feature selection. In the subsequent experiments, preprocessing of original features using PCA and LDA was employed.

Finally, calculation using NDA was performed with an additional hidden layer that consisted of two neurons for generating two new more discriminative features. The results in Table 12.1 confirm the effectiveness of using both NN and ANN classifiers. Although it was not evidently proved that NDA results are better in the classification, we definitely conclude that ANN is a powerful tool for thermal image processing during breast cancer screening. Reducing false/positive errors of classification is the most important task for the future research.

12.5 Conclusion

This chapter presents the preliminary results of the feature analysis for thermal images for different medical applications, mainly used in breast oncology. Thermography as the additional and adjacent method can be very helpful for early screening that helps to recognize tumors. At first, we consider first and second order statistical parameters. Although we do not have many pathological cases for investigations yet, the first results are very promising. The second order parameters are more sensitive to the overall structure of an image. Actually, the study is being extended by choosing second order parameters for multivariate data classification. The presented approach includes the PCA to reduce the dimensionality of the problem and by selecting the eigen vectors it is possible to generate data, which represents the tumors more evidently.

Breast cancer screening is a challenge today for medical engineering. Breast temperature depends not only due to some pathological changes, but it also varies in normal physiological situations, it is even a consequence of emotional state of a patient. It was a main reason that we are looking for more advanced methods of thermal image processing, that could give satisfactory results.

One of the possible alternative for such processing is ANN classification based on multidimensional feature domain, with use of modern transformations, such as wavelets. The preliminary investigations are quite successful, and can be improved by increasing the number of samples taken for processing.

Future research will concentrate around selection of features and adjusting wavelet transformation parameters to get the best classification. We assume that the more satisfactory results can be obtained by using features based on asymmetry between left and right sides of a patient. It could help for one-side cancerous lesion classification, what is the most typical pathological case and frequently happens today.

References

[1] P. Cichy, Texture analysis of digital images, doctoral thesis, *Technical University of Lodz, Institute of Electronics*, Lodz, 2000, in Polish.

[2] A. Materka, M. Strzelecki, R. Lerski, and L. Schad, Evaluation of texture features of test objects for magnetic resonance imaging, *Infotech Oulu Workshop on Texture Analysis in Machine Vision*, June 1999, Oulu, Finland.

[3] P. Debiec, M. Strzelecki, and A. Materka, Evaluation of texture generation methods based on CNN and GMRF image texture models, *Proceedings of the International Conference on Signals and Electronic Systems*, 17–20 October 2000, Ustron, pp. 187–192.

[4] E.Y.K. Ng, L.N. Ung, F.C. Ng, and L.S.J. Sim, Statistical analysis of healthy and malignant breast thermography, *Journal of Medical Engineering and Technology*, 25, 253–263, 2001.

[5] B.F.J. Manly, *Multivariate Statistical Method: A Primer*. London, Chapman & Hall, 1994.

[6] Michael Bennett, Breast cancer screening using high-resolution digital thermography, *Total Health*, 22, 44, 1985.

[7] I.T. Jolliffe, *Principal Component Analysis*. New York, Springer-Verlag, 1986.

[8] B.F.J. Manly, *Multivariate Statistical Method: A Primer*. New York, London, Chapman & Hall, 1994.

[9] D.R. Causton, *A Biologist's Advanced Mathematics*. London, Allen and Unwin, 1987.

[10] Schürman J. *Pattern Classification*. New York, John Wiley & Sons, 1996.

[11] M. Kociolek, A. Materka, M. Strzelecki, and P. Szczypinski, Discrete wavelet transform-derived features for digital image texture analysis, *Proceedings of the International Conference on Signals and Electronic Systems ICSES'2001*, Lodz, 18–21 September 2001, pp. 111–116.

[12] T. Jakubowska, B. Wiecek, M. Wysocki, and C. Drews-Peszynski, Thermal signatures for breast cancer screening comparative study, *Proceedings of the IEEE EMBS Conference*, Cancun, Mexico, 17–21 September, 2003.

[13] P. Debiec, M. Strzelecki, and A. Materka, Evaluation of texture generation methods based on CNN and GMRF image texture models, *International Conference on Signals and Electronic Systems ICSES'2000*, Ustron, October 2000, pp. 187–192.

[14] B. Wiecek and S. Zwolenik, Thermal wave method—limits and potentialities of active thermography in biology and medicine, *2nd Joint EMBS-BMES Conference, 24th Annual International Conference of the IEEE Engineering in Medicine and Biology Society*, BMES-EMS 2002, Houston, 23–26 October, 2002.

13
Physiology-Based Face Recognition in the Thermal Infrared Spectrum

13.1 Introduction... **13**-1
13.2 Feature Extraction **13**-3
     Face Segmentation • Segmentation of Superficial Blood Vessels • Extraction of TMPs
13.3 Matching **13**-9
     Estimation of Facial Pose • Matching of TMPs
13.4 Experimental Results **13**-11
     Low Permanence Problem • Frontal Pose and Arbitrary Pose Experiments
13.5 Conclusions and Future Work **13**-14
References **13**-14

Pradeep Buddharaju
Ioannis Pavlidis
University of Houston

13.1 Introduction

Biometrics has received a lot of attention during the past few years both from the academic and business communities. It has emerged as a preferred alternative to traditional forms of identification, like card IDs, which are not embedded into one's physical characteristics. Research into several biometric modalities including face, fingerprint, iris, and retina recognition has produced varying degrees of success [1]. Face recognition stands as the most appealing modality, since it is the natural mode of identification among humans and is totally unobtrusive. At the same time, however, it is one of the most challenging modalities [2]. Research into face recognition has been biased toward the visible spectrum for a variety of reasons. Among those is the availability and low cost of visible band cameras and the undeniable fact that face recognition is one of the primary activities of the human visual system. Machine recognition of human faces, however, has proven more problematic than the seemingly effortless face recognition performed by humans. The major culprit is light variability, which is prevalent in the visible spectrum owing to the reflective nature of incident light in this band. Secondary problems are associated with the difficulty of detecting facial disguises [3].

As a solution to the aforementioned problems, researchers have started investigating the use of thermal infrared (IR) for face recognition purposes [4–6]. However, many of these research efforts in thermal face recognition use the thermal IR band only as a way to see in the dark or reduce the deleterious effect of light variability [7,8]. Methodologically, they do not differ very much from face recognition algorithms in the visible band, which can be classified as appearance- [9,10] and feature-based approaches [11,12]. Recently, attempts have been made to fuse the visible and IR modalities to increase the performance of face recognition [13–16].

In this chapter, we present a novel approach to the problem of thermal facial recognition that realizes the full potential of the thermal IR band. It consists of a statistical face segmentation and a physiological feature extraction algorithm tailored to thermal phenomenology. The use of vein structure for human identification has been studied during recent years using traits such as hand vein patterns [17,18] and finger vein patterns [19,20]. Prokoski and Riedel [21] anticipated the possibility of extracting the vascular network from thermal facial images and using it as a feature space for face recognition. However, they did not present an algorithmic approach for achieving this. To the best of our knowledge, this is the first attempt to develop a face recognition system using physiological information on the face. An early stage of this research was reported briefly in the *Proceedings of the 2005 IEEE Conference on Advanced Video and Signal based Surveillance* [22]. Our goal is to promote a different way of thinking in the area of face recognition in thermal IR, which can be approached in a distinct manner when compared with other modalities.

Figure 13.1 shows the architecture of the proposed system. The goal of face recognition is to match a query face image against a database of facial images to establish the identity of an individual. Our system operates in the following two phases to achieve this goal:

1. *Off-line phase*: The thermal facial images are captured by an IR camera. For each subject to be stored in the database, we record five different poses. A two-step segmentation algorithm is applied

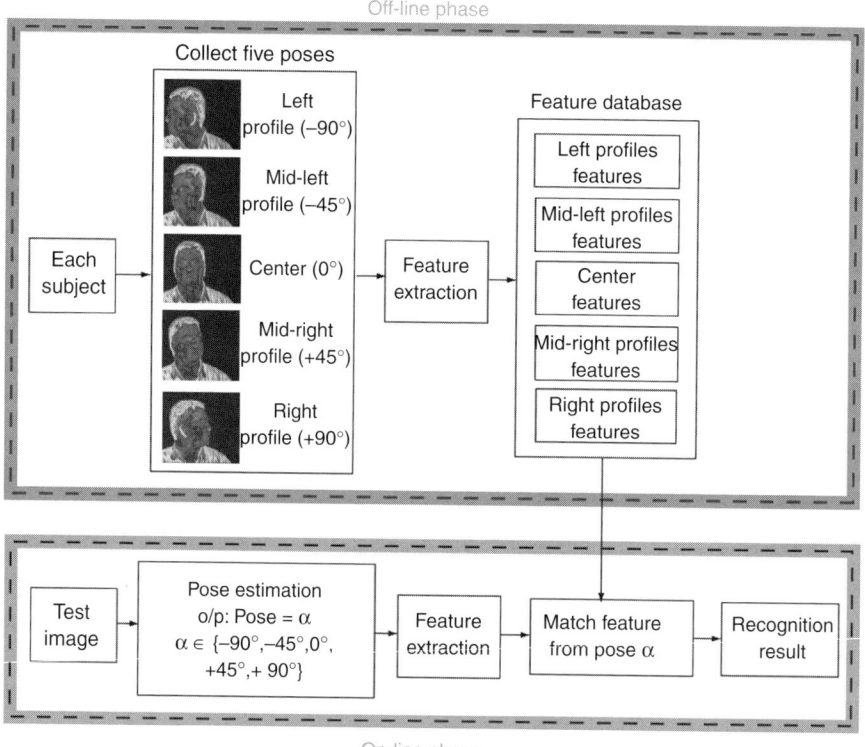

FIGURE 13.1 (See color insert at the back of the book.) Architecture of our face recognition system.

on each pose image to extract the vascular network from the face. Thermal Minutia Points (TMPs) are detected on the branching points of the vascular network and are stored in the database (see Figure 13.1).
2. *On-line phase*: Given a query image, TMPs of its vascular network are extracted and are matched against those of the corresponding pose images stored in the database (see Figure 13.1).

In the following sections, we will describe our face recognition system in detail. In Section 13.2, we present the feature extraction algorithm. In Section 13.3, we discuss our approach for vascular network matching. In Section 13.4, we present the experimental results and attempt a critical evaluation. We conclude this chapter in Section 13.5.

13.2 Feature Extraction

A thermal IR camera with good sensitivity provides the ability to directly image superficial blood vessels on the human face [23]. The pattern of the underlying blood vessels (see Figure 13.2) is characteristic to each individual, and the extraction of this vascular network can provide the basis for a feature vector. Figure 13.3 outlines the architecture of our feature extraction algorithm.

13.2.1 Face Segmentation

Owing to its physiology, a human face consists of "hot" parts that correspond to tissue areas that are rich in vasculature and "cold" parts that correspond to tissue areas with sparse vasculature. This casts the human face as a bimodal temperature distribution entity, which can be modeled using a mixture of two normal distributions. Similarly, the background can be described by a bimodal temperature distribution with walls being the "cold" objects and the upper part of the subject's body dressed in cloths being the "hot" object. Figure 13.4b shows the temperature distributions of the facial skin and the background from

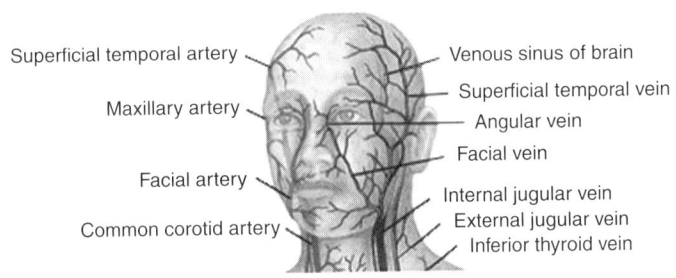

FIGURE 13.2 Superficial blood vessels on the face.

FIGURE 13.3 Architecture of feature extraction algorithm.

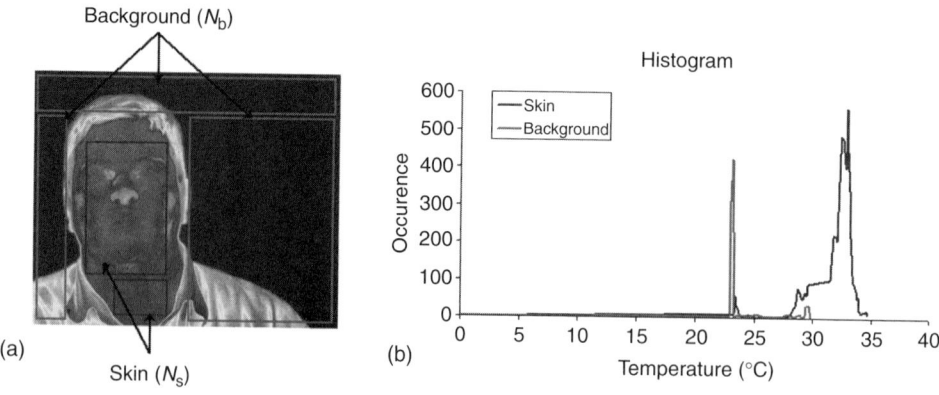

FIGURE 13.4 (See color insert.) Skin and background: (a) selection of samples for EM algorithm and (b) corresponding bimodal temperature distributions.

a typical IR facial image. We approach the problem of delineating facial tissue from background using a Bayesian framework [22,24] since we have *a priori* knowledge of the bimodal nature of the scene.

We call θ the parameter of interest, which takes two possible values (skin s or background b) with some probability. For each pixel x in the image at time t, we draw our inference of whether it represents skin (i.e., $\theta = s$) or background (i.e., $\theta = b$) based on the posterior distribution $p^{(t)}(\theta|x_t)$ given by

$$p^{(t)}(\theta|x_t) = \begin{cases} p^{(t)}(s|x_t), & \text{when } \theta = s \\ p^{(t)}(b|x_t) = 1 - p^{(t)}(s|x_t), & \text{when } \theta = b \end{cases} \quad (13.1)$$

We develop the statistics only for skin, and then the statistics for the background can easily be inferred from Equation 13.1.

According to the Bayes' theorem,

$$p^{(t)}(s|x_t) = \frac{\pi^{(t)}(s)f(x_t|s)}{\pi^{(t)}(s)f(x_t|s) + \pi^{(t)}(b)f(x_t|b)} \quad (13.2)$$

Here, $\pi^{(t)}(s)$ is the prior skin distribution and $f(x_t|s)$ is the likelihood for pixel x representing skin at time t. In the first frame ($t = 1$), the prior distributions for skin and background are considered equiprobable:

$$\pi^{(1)}(s) = \tfrac{1}{2} = \pi^{(1)}(b) \quad (13.3)$$

For $t > 1$, the prior skin distribution $\pi^{(t)}(s)$ at time t is equal to the posterior skin distribution at time $t-1$:

$$\pi^{(t)}(s) = p^{(t-1)}(s|x_{t-1}) \quad (13.4)$$

The likelihood $f(x_t|s)$ of pixel x representing skin at time $t \geq 1$ is given by

$$f(x_t|s) = \sum_{i=1}^{2} w_{s_i}^{(t)} N(\mu_{s_i}^{(t)}, \sigma_{s_i}^{2(t)}) \quad (13.5)$$

where the mixture parameters w_{s_i} (weight), μ_{s_i} (mean), $\sigma_{s_i}^2$ (variance): $i = 1, 2$ and $w_{s_2} = 1 - w_{s_1}$ of the bimodal skin distribution can be initialized and updated using the EM algorithm. For that, we select N representative facial frames (off-line) from a variety of subjects that we call the training set. Then, we

(a) (b)

FIGURE 13.5 (See color insert.) Segmentation of facial skin region: (a) original thermal facial image and (b) result of Bayesian segmentation.

manually segment, for each of the N frames, skin (and background) areas, which yields N_s skin (and N_b background) pixels as shown in Figure 13.4a.

To estimate the mixture parameters for the skin, we initially provide the EM algorithm with some crude estimates of the parameters of interest: $w_{s_0}, \mu_{s_0}, \sigma_{s_0}^2$. Then, we apply the following loop for $k = 0, 1, \ldots$:

$$z_{ij}^{(k)} = \frac{w_{s_i}^{(k)}(\sigma_{s_i}^{(k)})^{-1}\exp\left\{-\frac{1}{2(\sigma_{s_i}^{(k)})^2}(x_j - \mu_{s_i}^{(k)})^2\right\}}{\sum_{t=1}^{2} w_{s_t}^{(k)}(\sigma_{s_t}^{(k)})^{-1}\exp\left\{-\frac{1}{2(\sigma_{s_t}^{(k)})^2}(x_j - \mu_{s_t}^{(k)})^2\right\}}$$

$$w_{s_i}^{(k+1)} = \frac{\sum_{j=1}^{N_s} z_{ij}^{(k)}}{N_s}$$

$$\mu_{s_i}^{(k+1)} = \frac{\sum_{j=1}^{N_s} z_{ij}^{(k)} x_j}{N_s w_{s_i}^{(k+1)}}$$

$$(\sigma_{s_i}^{(k+1)})^2 = \frac{\sum_{j=1}^{N_s} z_{ij}^{(k)}(x_j - \mu_{s_i}^{(k+1)})^2}{N_s w_{s_i}^{(k+1)}}$$

where $i = 1, 2$ and $j = 1, \ldots, N_s$. Then, we set $k = k + 1$ and repeat the loop. The condition for terminating the loop is

$$\left|w_{s_i}^{(k+1)} - w_{s_i}^{(k)}\right| < \epsilon, \quad i = 1, 2 \qquad (13.6)$$

We apply a similar EM process for determining the initial parameters of the background distributions. Once a data point x_t becomes available, we decide that it represents skin if the posterior distribution for the skin, $p^{(t)}(s|x_t) > 0.5$ and that it represents background if the posterior distribution for the background, $p^{(t)}(b|x_t) > 0.5$. Figure 13.5b depicts the visualization of Bayesian segmentation on the subject shown in Figure 13.5a. Part of the subject's nose has been erroneously classified as background and a couple of cloth patches from the subject's shirt have been erroneously marked as facial skin. This is due to occasional overlapping between portions of the skin and background distributions. The isolated nature of these mislabeled patches makes them easily correctable through postprocessing. We apply our three-step postprocessing algorithm on the binary segmented image. Using foreground (and background) correction, we find the mislabeled pixels in the foreground (and background) and remove them. Following is the algorithm for achieving this:

1. Label all the regions in the foreground and background using a simple floodfill or connected component labeling algorithm [25]. Let the foreground regions be $R_f(i), i = 1, \ldots, N_f$ where N_f represents the number of foreground regions, and let the background regions be $R_b(j), j = 1, \ldots, N_b$, where N_b represents the number of background regions.

2. Compute the number of pixels in each of the foreground and background regions. Find the maximum foreground (R_f^{max}) and background (R_b^{max}) areas:

$$R_f^{max} = \max\{R_f(i), i = 1, \ldots, N_f\}$$
$$R_b^{max} = \max\{R_b(i), i = 1, \ldots, N_b\}$$

3. Change all foreground regions that satisfy the condition $R_f(i) < R_f^{max}/4$ to background. Similarly, change all background regions that satisfy the condition $R_b(i) < R_b^{max}/4$ to foreground. We found experimentally that outliers tend to have an area smaller than one-fourth of the maximum area, and hence can be corrected with the above conditions. Figure 13.6 shows the result of our postprocessing algorithm.

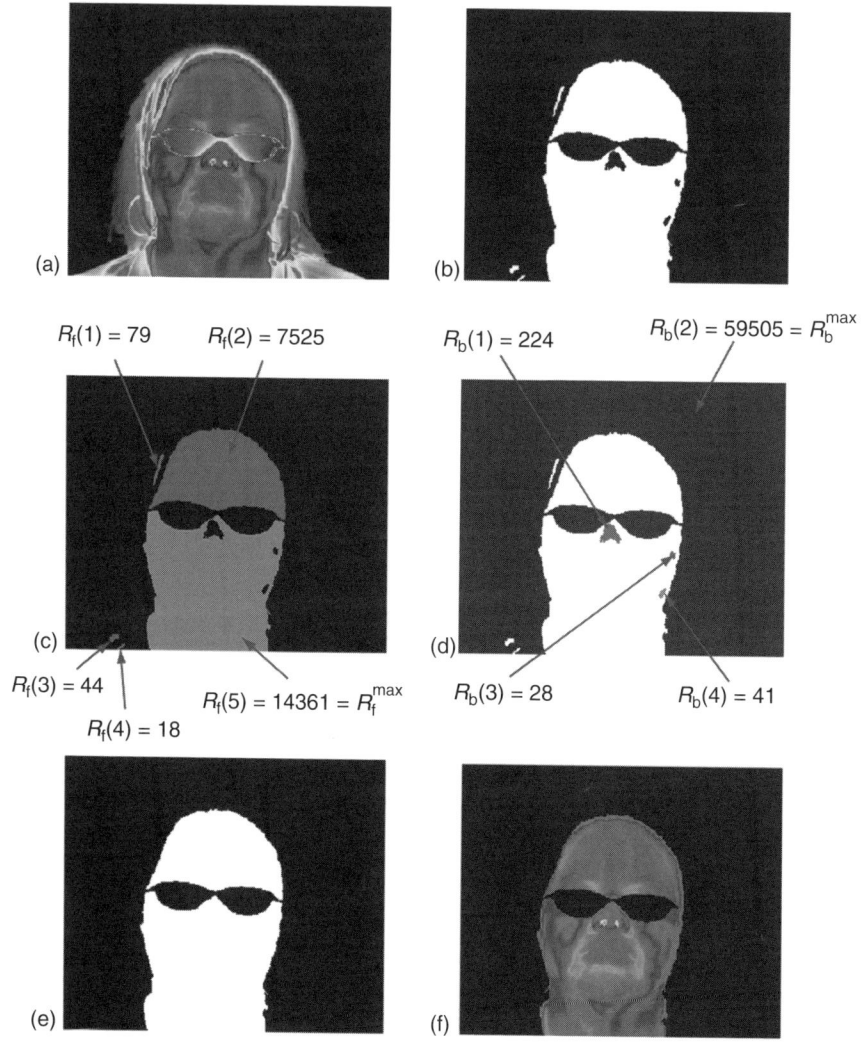

FIGURE 13.6 (See color insert.) Segmentation of facial skin region: (a) original thermal facial image; (b) binary segmented image; (c) foreground regions each represented in different color; (d) background regions each represented in different color; (e) binary mask after foreground and background corrections; and (f) final segmentation result after postprocessing.

13.2.2 Segmentation of Superficial Blood Vessels

Once a face is delineated from the rest of the scene, the segmentation of superficial blood vessels from the facial tissue is carried out in the following two steps [23,24]:

1. The image is processed to reduce noise and enhance edges
2. Morphological operations are applied to localize the superficial vasculature

In thermal imagery of human tissue the major blood vessels have weak sigmoid edges, which can be handled effectively using anisotropic diffusion. The anisotropic diffusion filter is formulated as a process that enhances object boundaries by performing intraregion as opposed to inter-region smoothing. The mathematical equation for the process is

$$\frac{\partial I(\bar{x}, t)}{\partial t} = \nabla(c(\bar{x}, t)\nabla I(\bar{x}, t)) \quad (13.7)$$

In our case $I(\bar{x}, t)$ is the thermal IR image, $\bar{x}$ refers to the spatial dimensions, and t to time. $c(\bar{x}, t)$ is called the diffusion function. The discrete version of the anisotropic diffusion filter of Equation 13.7 is as follows:

$$I_{t+1}(x, y) = I_t + \frac{1}{4} * [c_{N,t}(x, y)\nabla I_{N,t}(x, y) + c_{S,t}(x, y)\nabla I_{S,t}(x, y) \\ + c_{E,t}(x, y)\nabla I_{E,t}(x, y) + c_{W,t}(x, y)\nabla I_{W,t}(x, y)] \quad (13.8)$$

The four diffusion coefficients and four gradients in Equation 13.8 correspond to four directions (i.e., north, south, east, and west) with respect to the location (x, y). Each diffusion coefficient and the corresponding gradient are calculated in the same manner. For example, the coefficient along the north direction is calculated as follows:

$$c_{N,t}(x, y) = \exp\left(\frac{-\nabla I_{N,t}^2(x, y)}{k^2}\right) \quad (13.9)$$

where $I_{N,t} = I_t(x, y + 1) - I_t(x, y)$.

Image morphology is then applied on the diffused image to extract the blood vessels that are at a relatively low contrast compared with that of the surrounding tissue. We employ for this purpose a top-hat segmentation method, which is a combination of erosion and dilation operations. Top-hat segmentation takes two forms. First form is the white top-hat segmentation that enhances the bright objects in the image, while the second one is the black top-hat segmentation that enhances dark objects. In our case, we are interested in the white top-hat segmentation because it helps with enhancing the bright ("hot") ridge-like structures corresponding to the blood vessels. In this method the original image is first opened and then this opened image is subtracted from the original image as shown below:

$$I_{\text{open}} = (I \ominus S) \oplus S \\ I_{\text{top}} = I - I_{\text{open}} \quad (13.10)$$

where I, I_{open}, I_{top} are the original, opened, and white top-hat segmented images respectively, S is the structuring element, and $\ominus, \oplus$ are morphological erosion and dilation operations, respectively. Figure 13.7a depicts the result of applying anisotropic diffusion to the segmented facial tissue shown in Figure 13.4b, and Figure 13.7b shows the corresponding blood vessels extracted using white top-hat segmentation.

FIGURE 13.7 (See color insert.) Vascular network extraction: (a) original segmented image; (b) anisotropically diffused image; and (c) blood vessels extracted using white top-hat segmentation.

13.2.3 Extraction of TMPs

The extracted blood vessels exhibit different contour shapes between subjects. We call the branching points of the blood vessels Thermal Minutia Points (TMPs). TMPs can be extracted from the blood vessel network in ways similar to those used for fingerprint minutia extraction. A number of methods have been proposed [26] for robust and efficient extraction of minutia from fingerprint images. Most of these approaches describe each minutia point by at least three attributes, including its type, its location in the fingerprint image, and the local vessel orientation. We adopt a similar approach for extracting TMPs from vascular networks, which is outlined in the following steps:

1. The local orientation of the vascular network is estimated
2. The vascular network is skeletonized
3. The TMPs are extracted from the thinned vascular network
4. The spurious TMPs are removed

Local orientation $\Psi(x, y)$ is the angle formed at (x, y) between the blood vessel and the horizontal axis. Estimating the orientation field at each pixel provides the basis for capturing the overall pattern of the vascular network. We use the approach proposed in Reference 27 for computing the orientation image because it provides pixel-wise accuracy.

Next, the vascular network is thinned to one-pixel thickness [28]. Each pixel in the thinned map contains a value of 1 if it is on the vessel and 0 if it is not. Considering eight-neighborhood $(N_0, N_1, \ldots, N_7)$ around each pixel, a pixel (x, y) represents a TMP if $(\sum_{i=0}^{7} N_i) > 2$ (see Figure 13.8).

Physiology-Based Face Recognition in the Thermal Infrared Spectrum

FIGURE 13.8 (See color insert.) TMP extracted from the thinned vascular network.

FIGURE 13.9 (See color insert.) Spurious TMPs: (a) clustered TMPs and (b) spike formed due to a trivially short branch.

It is desirable that the TMP extraction algorithm does not leave any spurious TMPs since this will adversely affect the matching performance. Removal of clustered TMPs (see Figure 13.9a) and spikes (see Figure 13.9b) helps to reduce the number of spurious TMPs in the thinned vascular network.

The vascular network of a typical facial image contains around 50 to 80 genuine TMPs whose location (x, y) and orientation (Ψ) are stored in the database. Figure 13.10 shows the results of each stage of the feature extraction algorithm on a thermal facial image.

13.3 Matching

Each subject's record in the database consists of five (5) different poses to account for pose variation during the testing phase. Since facial images from the same person look quite different across multiple views, it is very important that the search space includes facial images with pose similar to the pose of the test image. Given a test image, we first estimate its pose. Then, the task is simply to match the TMP network extracted from the test image against the TMP database corresponding to the estimated pose.

13.3.1 Estimation of Facial Pose

To the best of our knowledge, it is the first time that the issue of pose estimation in thermal facial imagery is addressed. However, as it is the case with face recognition in general, a number of efforts have been made to address the issue of facial pose estimation in visible band imagery [29,30]. We capitalize upon the algorithm proposed in Reference 29 for estimating head pose across multiple views. We apply principal component analysis (PCA) on the thermal facial images in the training set to reduce the dimensionality of the training examples. Figure 13.11 illustrates sample face images in the database across multiple views. Then, we train the Support Vector Machine (SVM) classifier with the PCA vectors of face samples. Given a test image, SVM can classify it against one of the five poses (center, mid-left profile, left profile, mid-right profile, and right profile) under consideration.

FIGURE 13.10 (See color insert.) Visualization of the various stages of the vascular feature extraction algorithm: (a) a typical thermal facial image; (b) facial tissue delineated from the background; (c) network of vascular contours extracted from the thermal facial image; (d) skeletonized vessel map; (e) extracted TMPs from branching points; and (f) cleaned TMP set.

13.3.2 Matching of TMPs

Numerous methods have been proposed for matching fingerprint minutiae, most of which try to simulate the way forensic experts compare fingerprints [26]. Popular techniques are alignment-based point pattern matching, local structure matching, and global structure matching. Local minutiae matching algorithms are fast, simple, and more tolerant to distortions. Global minutiae matching algorithms feature high distinctiveness. A few hybrid approaches [31,32] have been proposed where the advantages of both local and global methods are exploited. We use such a method [31] to perform TMP matching.

For each TMP $M(x_i, y_i, \Psi_i)$ that is extracted from the vascular network, we consider its N nearest-neighbor TMPs $M(x_n, y_n, \Psi_n)$, $n = 1, \ldots, N$. Then, the TMP $M(x_i, y_i, \Psi_i)$ can be defined by a new feature vector:

$$L_M = \{\{d_1, \varphi_1, \vartheta_1\}, \{d_2, \varphi_2, \vartheta_2\}, \ldots, \{d_N, \varphi_N, \vartheta_N\}, \Psi_i\} \tag{13.11}$$

where

$$\begin{aligned} d_n &= \sqrt{(x_n - x_i)^2 + (y_n - y_i)^2} \\ \varphi_n &= \text{diff}(\Psi_n, \Psi_i), \quad n = 1, 2, \ldots, N \\ \vartheta_n &= \text{diff}\left(\arctan\left(\frac{y_n - y_i}{x_n - x_i}\right), \Psi_i\right) \end{aligned} \tag{13.12}$$

The function diff () calculates the difference of two angles and scales the result within the range $[0, 2\pi)$ [32]. Given a test image $\mathbf{I}_t$, the feature vector of each of its TMP is compared with the feature vector of each

Physiology-Based Face Recognition in the Thermal Infrared Spectrum

FIGURE 13.11 (**See color insert.**) Samples from our training set featuring five (5) different poses per subject. From left to right the views depicted are left profile, mid-left profile, center, mid-right profile, and right profile.

TMP of a database image. Two TMPs M and M' are marked to be a matched pair if the absolute difference between corresponding features is less than specific threshold values $\{\delta_d, \delta_\varphi, \delta_\vartheta, \delta_\psi\}$. The threshold values should be chosen in such a way that they accommodate linear deformations and translations. The final matching score between the test image and a database image is given by

$$\text{Score} = \frac{\text{NUM}_{\text{match}}}{\max(\text{NUM}_{\text{test}}, \text{NUM}_{\text{database}})} \qquad (13.13)$$

where $\text{NUM}_{\text{match}}$ represents number of matched TMP pairs, and NUM_{test}, $\text{NUM}_{\text{database}}$ represent number of TMPs in test and database images, respectively. If the highest matching score between the test and database images is greater than a specific threshold, the corresponding database image is classified as a match. If not, the test image is classified to be not in the database.

13.4 Experimental Results

We collected a large database of thermal facial images in our laboratory from volunteers representing different sex, race, and age groups. The images were captured using a high-quality mid-wave IR Phoenix camera produced by Indigo Systems. Following are the specifications of the camera:

Detector: InSb 640 × 512 element FPA
Spectral range: 3.0–5.0 μm
NETD (sensitivity): 0.01°C
Focal length: 50 mm

FIGURE 13.12 (**See color insert.**) (a) Thermal facial image of a subject acquired on October 17, 2003; (b) corresponding vascular network; (c) thermal facial image of the same subject acquired on April 29, 2004; and (d) corresponding vascular network.

We used a subset of the dataset for evaluating the performance of proposed face recognition algorithm. The dataset consists of 7590 thermal facial images from 138 different subjects (55 images per subject) with varying pose and facial expressions. Five images from each subject (each image representing one of the five training poses) were used for training, TMPs of which were extracted and stored in the database. The remaining 50 images per subject at arbitrary poses were used for testing.

13.4.1 Low Permanence Problem

A major challenge associated with thermal face recognition is the recognition performance over time [33]. Facial thermograms may change depending on the physical condition and environmental conditions. This makes the task of acquiring similar features for the same person over time difficult. A few approaches that use direct temperature data for recognition reported degraded performance over time [10]. However, our approach attempts to solve this problem by using facial anatomical information as feature space, which is unique to each person and at the same time is invariable to physical and environmental conditions as shown in Figure 13.12. The vascular network extracted from the same person with a time gap of about 6 months exhibits a similar pattern.

13.4.2 Frontal Pose and Arbitrary Pose Experiments

Many face recognition algorithms that perform well on the frontal image dataset often have problems when tested on images with arbitrary poses [2]. Our face recognition algorithm overcomes this problem by using multiple pose images for training, which allows pose invariance in the test image. We found experimentally that the five poses we used for training our face recognition algorithm are sufficient to accommodate all yaw rotations (including tilt rotations to a certain extent) without confusing our matching algorithm significantly. As shown in Figure 13.13, when an image that is close to the mid-left profile is queried, pose estimation picked the corresponding mid-left profile image from the training dataset for matching. The small variation in pose that still exists between the query and database images might cause minor position and angle differences in corresponding TMPs extracted from those images. This can be compensated by choosing appropriate values for thresholds $\{\delta_d, \delta_\varphi, \delta_\vartheta, \delta_\Psi\}$, discussed in Section 13.3.2.

We conducted two set of experiments in order to evaluate the performance of our face recognition system. The first experiment is the frontal pose experiment where the test set contains images with poses

FIGURE 13.13 (See color insert.) (a) Test image and (b) corresponding vascular network. (c) Mid-left profile image picked from training database by pose estimation and (d) corresponding vascular network.

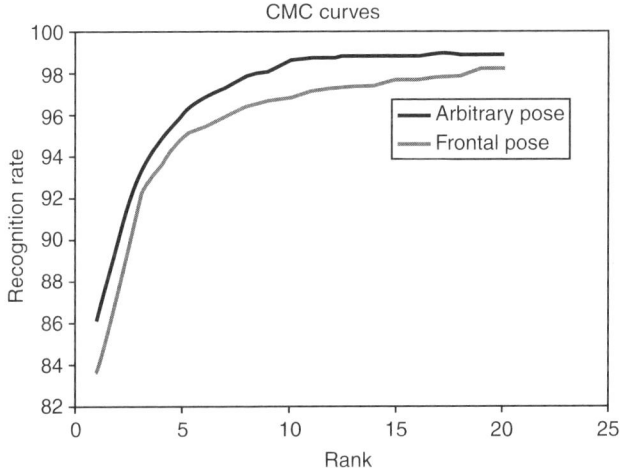

FIGURE 13.14 CMC curves of our method for the frontal and arbitrary pose experiments.

between mid-left and mid-right profiles. This test set is matched against only frontal images of the training database. This is the typical experimental procedure used for testing most of the current face recognition algorithms. The second experiment is the arbitrary pose experiment where test set contains all possible poses between left and right profiles. This test set is matched against the entire training set containing five pose images per subject. Figures 13.14 and 13.15 show comparative results of these two experiments. We noticed that the arbitrary pose experiment showed better results when compared to the frontal pose experiment in both cases.

Figure 13.14 shows the cumulative math characteristic (CMC) curves of the two experiments, and Figure 13.15 shows the ROC curves based on various threshold values for the matching score discussed in Section 13.3.2. The results demonstrate the promise as well as some problems with our proposed approach. Specifically, CMC shows that rank 1 recognition is over 86% and rank 5 recognition is over 96%. This performance puts a brand new approach very close to the performance of mature visible band recognition methods. In contrast, ROC reveals a weakness of the current method, as it requires false acceptance rate

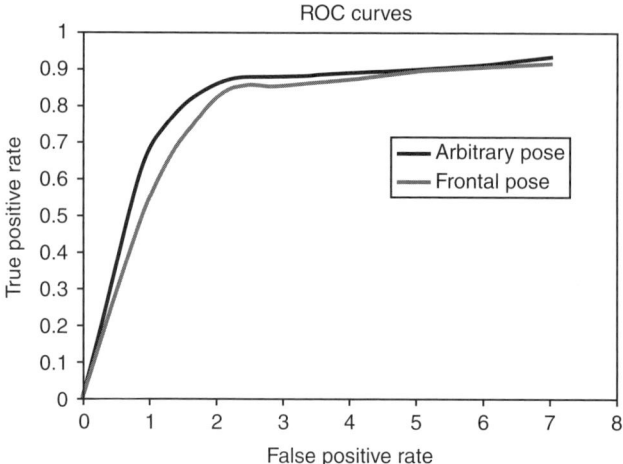

FIGURE 13.15 ROC curves of our method for the frontal and arbitrary pose experiments.

over 20% to reach positive acceptance rate above the 86% range. To address this problem we believe we need to estimate and eliminate the incorrect TMPs and non-linear deformations in the extracted vascular network.

13.5 Conclusions and Future Work

We have outlined a novel approach to the problem of face recognition in thermal IR — one of the fastest growing biometrics. The cornerstone of the approach is the use of unique and time invariant physiological information as feature space. We collect five different poses for each subject to be stored in the training database. We have shown that these five poses are capable of accommodating all yaw rotations in the test image. The facial tissue is first separated from the background using a Bayesian segmentation method. The vascular network on the surface of the skin is then extracted based on a white top-hat segmentation preceded by anisotropic diffusion. TMPs are extracted from the vascular network and are used as features for matching the test to database images. The experimental results demonstrate that our approach is very promising.

The method although young, performed well in a nontrivial database. Our ongoing work is directed toward improving the sophistication of the method regarding nonlinear deformations of the vascular network and testing it comparatively in larger databases.

References

[1] Jain, A., Bolle, R., and Pankanti, S., *Biometrics: Personal Identification in Networked Society*, 1st edn., Kluwer Academic Publishers, Norwell, MA, USA, 1999.

[2] Zhao, W., Chellappa, R., Phillips, P. J., and Rosenfeld, A., Face recognition: a literature survey. *ACM Computing Surveys (CSUR)*, 35, 399, 2003.

[3] Pavlidis, I. and Symosek, P., The imaging issue in an automatic face/disguise detection system. In *Proceedings of IEEE Workshop on Computer Vision Beyond the Visible Spectrum: Methods and Applications*, Hilton Head Island, SC, USA, 2000, p. 15.

[4] Prokoski, F., History, current status, and future of infrared identification. In *Proceedings of IEEE Workshop on Computer Vision Beyond the Visible Spectrum: Methods and Applications*, Hilton Head Island, SC, USA, 2000, p. 5.

[5] Socolinsky, D.A. and Selinger, A., A comparative analysis of face recognition performance with visible and thermal infrared imagery. In *Proceedings of 16th International Conference on Pattern Recognition*, 4, Quebec, Canada, 2002, p. 217.

[6] Wilder, J., Phillips, P.J., Jiang, C., and Wiener, S., Comparison of visible and infrared imagery for face recognition. In *Proceedings of the Second International Conference on Automatic Face and Gesture Recognition*, Killington, VT, 1996, p. 182.

[7] Socolinsky, D.A., Wolff, L.B., Neuheisel, J.D., and Eveland, C.K., Illumination invariant face recognition using thermal infrared imagery. In *Proceedings of the IEEE Computer Society Conference on Computer Vision and Pattern Recognition (CVPR 2001)*, 1, Kauai, H1, USA, 2001, p. 527.

[8] Selinger, A. and Socolinsky, D.A., Face recognition in the dark. In *Proceedings of the Joint IEEE Workshop on Object Tracking and Classification Beyond the Visible Spectrum*, Washington, DC, 2004.

[9] Cutler, R., Face recognition using infrared images and eigenfaces, cs.umd.edu/rgc/face/face.htm, 1996.

[10] Chen, X., Flynn, P.J., and Bowyer, K.W., PCA-based face recognition in infrared imagery: baseline and comparative studies. In *Proceedings of the IEEE International Workshop on Analysis and Modeling of Faces and Gestures*, Nice, France, 2003, p. 127.

[11] Srivastava, A. and Liu, X., Statistical hypothesis pruning for recognizing faces from infrared images, *Journal of Image and Vision Computing*, 21, 651, 2003.

[12] Buddharaju, P., Pavlidis, I., and Kakadiaris, I., Face recognition in the thermal infrared spectrum. In *Proceedings of the Joint IEEE Workshop on Object Tracking and Classification Beyond the Visible Spectrum*, Washington, DC, 2004.

[13] Heo, J., Kong, S.G., Abidi, B.R., and Abidi, M.A., Fusion of visual and thermal signatures with eyeglass removal for robust face recognition. In *Proceedings of the Joint IEEE Workshop on Object Tracking and Classification Beyond the Visible Spectrum*, Washington, DC, 2004.

[14] Gyaourova, A., Bebis, G., and Pavlidis, I., Fusion of infrared and visible images for face recognition. In *Proceedings of the eighth European Conference on Computer Vision*, Prague, Czech Republic, 2004.

[15] Socolinsky, D.A. and Selinger, A., Thermal face recognition in an operational scenario. In *Proceedings of the IEEE Computer Society Conference on Computer Vision and Pattern Recognition*, 2, Washington DC, 2004, p. 1012.

[16] Wang, J.G., Sung, E., and Venkateswarlu, R., Registration of infrared and visible-spectrum imagery for face recognition. In *Proceedings of the Sixth IEEE International Conference on Automatic Face and Gesture Recognition*, Seoul, Korea, 2004, p. 638.

[17] Lin, C.L. and Fan, K.C., Biometric verification using thermal images of palm-dorsa vein patterns, *IEEE Transactions on Circuits and Systems for Video Technology*, 14, 199, 2004.

[18] Im, S.K., Choi, H.S., and Kim, S.W., A direction-based vascular pattern extraction algorithm for hand vascular pattern verification, *ETRI Journal*, 25, 101, 2003.

[19] Shimooka, T. and Shimizu, K., Artificial immune system for personal identification with finger vein pattern. In *Proceedings of the eighth International Conference on Knowledge-Based Intelligent Information and Engineering Systems*, Lecture Notes in Computer Science, Wellington, New Zealand, 3214, 2004, p. 511.

[20] Miura, N., Nagasaka, A., and Miyatake, T., Feature extraction of finger vein patterns based on iterative line tracking and its application to personal identification, *Systems and Computers in Japan*, 35, 61, 2004.

[21] Prokoski, F.J. and Riedel, R., *BIOMETRICS: Personal Identification in Networked Society*, Infrared Identification of Faces and Body Parts, Kluwer Academic Publishers, Norwell, MA, USA, 1998, chapter 9.

[22] Buddharaju, P., Pavlidis, I.T., and Tsiamyrtzis, P., Physiology-based face recognition. In *Proceedings of the IEEE Advanced Video and Signal based Surveillance*, Como, Italy, 2005.

[23] Manohar, C., Extraction of superficial vasculature in thermal imaging, Master's thesis, University of Houston, Houston, TX, 2004.

[24] Pavlidis, I., Tsiamyrtzis, P., Manohar, C., and Buddharaju, P., *Biomedical Engineering Handbook*, Biometrics: Face Recognition in Thermal Infrared, CRC Press, Boca Raton, FL, 2006, chapter 22.

[25] Di Stefano, L. and Bulgarelli, A., Simple and efficient connected components labeling algorithm. In *Proceedings of the International Conference on Image Analysis and Processing*, Venice, Italy, 1999, p. 322.

[26] Maltoni, D., Maio, D., Jain, A.K., and Prabhakar, S., *Handbook of Fingerprint Recognition*, Springer-Verlag, 2003.

[27] Oliveira, M.A. and Leite, N.J., Reconnection of fingerprint ridges based on morphological operators and multiscale directional information, In *17th Brazilian Symposium on Computer Graphics and Image Processing*, Curitiba, PR, Brazil, 2004, p. 122.

[28] Jang, B.K. and Chin, R.T., One-pass parallel thinning: analysis, properties, and quantitative evaluation, *IEEE Transactions on Pattern Analysis and Machine Intelligence*, 14, 1129, 1992.

[29] Yang, Z., Ai, H., Wu, B., Lao, S., and Cai, L., Face pose estimation and its application in video shot selection. In *Proceedings of the 17th International Conference on Pattern Recognition*, 1, Cambridge, UK, 2004, p. 322.

[30] Li, Y., Gong, S., Sherrah, J., and Liddell, H., Support vector machine based multi-view face detection and recognition, *Image and Vision Computing*, 22, 413, 2004.

[31] Yang, S. and Verbauwhede, I.M., A secure fingerprint matching technique. In *Proceedings of the 2003 ACM SIGMM Workshop on Biometrics Methods and Applications*, Berkley, CA, 2003, p. 89.

[32] Jiang, X. and Yau, W.Y., Fingerprint minutiae matching based on the local and global structures. In *Proceedings of the 15th International Conference on Pattern Recognition*, 2, Barcelona, Catalonia, Spain, 2000, p. 1038.

[33] Socolinsky, D.A. and Selinger, A., Thermal face recognition over time. In *Proceedings of the 17th International Conference on Pattern Recognition*, 4, Cambridge, UK, 2004, p. 23.

14

Infrared Imaging for Functional Monitoring of Disease Processes

Moinuddin Hassan
Victor Chernomordik
Abby Vogel
David Hattery
Israel Gannot
Richard F. Little
Amir H. Gandjbakhche
National Institute of Child Health and Human Development

Robert Yarchoan
National Cancer Institute

14.1 NIR Quantitative Imaging of Deep Tissue Structure.. 14-2
  Optical Properties of Biological Tissue • Measurable Quantities and Experimental Techniques • Models of Photon Migration in Tissue • RWT Applied to Quantitative Spectroscopy of the Breast • Quantitative Fluorescence Imaging and Spectroscopy • Future Directions
14.2 Infrared Thermal Monitoring of Disease Processes: Clinical Study 14-16
  Emissivity Corrected Temperature • Temperature Calibration • Clinical Study
Acknowledgments... 14-23
References 14-23

Noninvasive imaging techniques are emerging into the forefront of medical diagnostics and treatment monitoring. Both near-infrared imaging (NIR) and mid-infrared imaging techniques have provided invaluable information in the clinical setting. Most *in vivo* biomedical applications of functional imaging use light in the NIR spectrum. The main advantage of the interaction of NIR light with tissue is increased penetration: light with wavelengths between 700 and 1100 nm passes through skin and other tissues better than visible light does.

In the infrared (IR) thermal waveband, information about blood circulation, local metabolism, sweat gland malfunction, inflammation, and healing can be extracted. Originally used to detect breast carcinoma, IR imaging was subsequently reported to have clinical utility in a multitude of neuromusculoskeletal, vascular, and rheomatolgoic disorders. There is an especially strong interest in developing optical technologies that have the capability of performing *in situ* tissue diagnosis without the need for sample excision and processing. At present, excisional biopsy followed by histology is considered to be the "gold standard" for the diagnosis of early neoplastic changes and carcinoma. In some cases, cytology, rather than excisional biopsy, is performed. These techniques are powerful diagnostic tools because they provide high-resolution spatial and morphological information of the cellular and subcellular structures of tissues. The use of staining and processing can enhance visual contrast and specificity of histopathology. Both of these diagnostic procedures, however, require physical removal of specimens followed by tissue processing in a laboratory. The current status of modern IR imaging is that of a first-line supplement to both clinical examination and current imaging methods. Using IR imaging to detect breast pathology is based on the principle that both metabolic and vascular activity in the tissue surrounding a new and developing tumor is usually higher than in normal tissue. Early cancer growth is dependent on increasing blood circulation by creating new blood vessels (angiogenesis). This process results in regional variations that can often be detected by IR imaging.

The spectroscopic power of light, along with the revolution in molecular characterization of disease processes have given rise to new methods and instrumentation for the early or noninvasive diagnosis of various medical conditions, including arteriosclerosis, heart arrhythmia, cancer, and many other diseases. NIR imaging has been used to functionally monitor disease processes including cancer and lymph node detection and optical biopsies. Spectroscopic imaging modalities have been shown to improve the diagnosis of tumors and add new knowledge about the physiological properties of the tumor and surrounding tissues. Particular emphasis should be placed on identifying markers that predict the risk of precancerous lesions progressing to invasive cancers, thereby providing new opportunities for cancer prevention. This might be accomplished through the use of markers as contrast agents for imaging using conventional techniques or through refinements of newer technologies such as magnetic resonance imaging (MRI) or position emission tomography (PET) scanning.

IR imaging techniques have the potential for performing *in vivo* diagnosis on tissue without the need for sample excision and processing. Another advantage of diagnosis through IR imaging is that the resulting information can be available in real time. In addition, since removal of tissue is not required for diagnosis, a more complete examination of the organ of interest can be achieved than with excisional biopsy or cytology.

Section 14.1 discusses NIR imaging and its applications in imaging biological tissues. Mid-IR thermal imaging techniques, calibration, and a current clinical trial of Kaposi's sarcoma (KS) are described in Section 14.2.

14.1 NIR Quantitative Imaging of Deep Tissue Structure

In vivo optical imaging has traditionally been limited to superficial tissue surfaces, directly or endoscopically accessible, and to tissues with a biological window (e.g., along the optical axis of the eye). These methods are based on geometric optics. Most tissues scatter light so strongly, however, that for geometric optics-based equipment to work special techniques are needed to remove multiply scattered light (such as pinholes in confocal imaging or interferometry in optical coherence microscopies). Even with these special designs, high-resolution optical imaging fails at depths of more than 1 mm below the tissue surface.

Collimated visible or IR light impinging on thick tissue is scattered many times in a distance of approximately 1 mm, so the analysis of light–tissue interactions requires theories based on the diffusive nature of light propagation. In contrast to x-ray and PET, a complex underlying theoretical picture is needed to describe photon paths as a function of scattering and absorption properties of the tissue.

Approximately a decade ago, a new field called "photon migration" was born that seeks to characterize the statistical physics of photon motion through turbid tissues. The goal is to image macroscopic structures in three dimension (3D) at greater depths within tissues and to provide reliable pathlength estimation for noninvasive spectral analysis of tissue changes. Although geometrical optics fails to describe light propagation under these conditions, the statistical physics of strong, multiply scattered light provides powerful approaches to macroscopic imaging and subsurface detection and characterization. Techniques using visible and NIR light offer a variety of functional imaging modalities, in addition to density imaging, while avoiding ionizing radiation hazards.

In Section 14.1, the optical properties of biological tissue are discussed. Section 14.2 is devoted to different measurement methods. Theoretical models for spectroscopy and imaging are discussed in Section 14.3. In Sections 14.4 and 14.5, two studies on breast imaging and the use of exogenous fluorescent markers are presented as examples of NIR spectroscopy. Finally, the future direction of the field is discussed in Section 14.6.

FIGURE 14.1 (See color insert at the back of the book.) Absorption spectra of the three major components of tissue in the NIR region; oxy- and deoxy-hemoglobin, and water.

14.1.1 Optical Properties of Biological Tissue

The difficulty of tissue optics is to define optical coefficients of tissue physiology and quantify their changes to differentiate structures and functional status *in vivo*. Light–tissue interactions dictate the way that these parameters are defined. The two main approaches are the wave and particle descriptions of light propagation. Wave propagation uses Maxwell's equations and therefore quantifies the spatially varying permittivity as a measurable quantity. For simplistic and historic reasons, the particle interpretation of light has been used more often (see Section 14.3). In photon transport theory, one considers the behavior of discrete photons as they move through the tissue. This motion is characterized by absorption and scattering and, when interfaces (e.g., layers) are involved, refraction. The absorption coefficient, $\mu_a [\text{mm}^{-1}]$, represents the inverse mean pathlength of a photon before absorption. The distance in a medium where intensity is attenuated by a factor of $1/e$ (Beer's Lambert Law) is considered to be $1/\mu_a$. Absorption in tissue is strongly wavelength dependent and is due to chromophores and water. Among the chromophores in tissue, the dominant component is the hemoglobin in blood. In Figure 14.1, hemoglobin absorption is divided into oxygenated and deoxygenated hemoglobin. As seen in this figure, in the visible range (600 to 700 nm), the blood absorption is relatively high compared to absorption in the NIR. By contrast, water absorption is low in the visible and NIR regions and increases rapidly above approximately 950 nm. Thus, for greatest penetration of light in tissue, wavelengths in the 650 to 950 nm spectra are used most often. This region of the light spectrum is called the "therapeutic window." One should note that different spectra of chromophores allow one to separate the contribution of varying functional species in tissue (e.g., quantification of oxy- and deoxy-hemoglobin to study tissue oxygenation). Similarly, scattering is characterized by a coefficient, μ_s, which is the inverse mean free path of photons between scattering events. The average size of the scattered photons in tissue, proportional to the wavelength of light, places the scattering in the Mie region. In the Mie region, a scattering event does not result in isotropic scattering angles [1,2]. Instead, the scattering in tissue is biased in the forward direction.

For example, by studying the development of neonatal skin, Saidi et al. [3] were able to show that the principal sources of anisotropic scattering in muscle are collagen fibers. The fibers were determined to have a mean diameter of 2.2 μm. In addition to the Mie scattering from the fibers, there is isotropic Rayleigh scattering due to the presence of much smaller scatterers such as organelles in cells.

Anisotropic scattering is quantified in a coefficient, g:

$$g \equiv \langle \cos(\theta) \rangle \equiv \frac{\int_0^\pi p(\theta) \cos(\theta) \sin(\theta)\, d\theta}{\int_0^\pi p(\theta) \sin(\theta)\, d\theta} \tag{14.1}$$

where g is defined as the mean cosine of the scattering angle and $(p\theta)$ is the probability of a particular scattering angle. For isotropic scattering, $g = 0$. For complete forward scattering, $g = 1$, and for complete back scattering, $g = -1$. In tissue, g is typically 0.7 to 0.98 [3–5].

Likewise, different tissue types have differing scattering properties that are wavelength dependent. The scattering coefficients of many soft tissues have been measured at a variety of optical wavelengths, and are within the range of 10 to 100 mm^{-1}. Compared to absorption, however, scattering changes, as a function of wavelength, are more gradual and have smaller extremes. Abnormal tissues such as tumors, fibro-adenomas and cysts all have scattering properties that are different from normal tissue [6,7]. Thus, the scattering coefficient of an inclusion may also be an important clue to disease diagnosis.

Theories of photon migration are often based on isotropic scattering. Therefore, one must find the appropriate scaling relationships that will allow for an isotropic scattering model. For the case of diffusion-like models [8], it has been shown that one may use an isotropic scattering model with a corrected scattering coefficient, μ'_s, and obtain equivalent results where:

$$\mu'_s = \mu_s(1 - g) \tag{14.2}$$

The corrected scattering coefficient is smaller than the actual scattering that corresponds to a greater distance between isotropic scattering events than would occur with anisotropic scattering. For this reason, μ'_s is typically called the transport-corrected scattering coefficient.

There are instances when the spectroscopic signatures will not be sufficient to detect disease. This can occur when the specific disease results in only very small changes to the tissue's scattering and absorption properties, or when the scattering and absorption properties are not unique to the disease. Although it is not clear what the limits of detectability are in relation to diseased tissue properties, it is clear that there will be cases for which optical techniques based on elastic absorption are inadequate. In such cases, another source of optical contrast, such as fluorescence, will be required to detect and locate the disease. The presence of fluorescent molecules in tissue can provide useful contrast mechanisms. Concentration of these endogenous fluorophores in the body can be related to functional and metabolic activities, and therefore to the disease processes. For example, the concentrations of fluorescent molecules such as collagen and NADH have been used to differentiate between normal and abnormal tissue [9].

Advances in the molecular biology of disease processes, new immunohistopathological techniques, and the development of fluorescently labeled cell surface markers have led to a revolution in specific molecular diagnosis of disease by histopathology, as well as in research on molecular origins of disease processes (e.g., using fluorescence microscopy in cell biology). As a result, an exceptional level of specificity is now possible due to the advances in the design of exogenous markers. Molecules can now be tailor-made to bind only to specific receptor sites in the body. These receptor sites may be antibodies or other biologically interesting molecules. Fluorophores may be bound to these engineered molecules and injected into the body, where they will preferentially concentrate at specific sites of interest [10,11].

Furthermore, fluorescence may be used as a probe to measure environmental conditions in a particular locality by capitalizing on changes in fluorophore lifetime [12,13]. Each fluorophore has a characteristic lifetime that quantifies the probability of a specific time delay between fluorophore excitation and emission. In practice, this lifetime may be modified by specific environmental factors such as temperature, pH, and concentrations of substances such as oxygen. In these cases, it is possible to quantify local concentrations of specific substances or specific environmental conditions by measuring the lifetime of fluorophores at the site. Whereas conventional fluorescence imaging is very sensitive to nonuniform fluorophore transport and distribution (e.g., blood does not transport molecules equally to all parts of the body), fluorescence lifetime imaging is insensitive to transport nonuniformity as long as a detectable quantity of fluorophores is present in the site of interest. Throughout the following sections, experimental techniques and differing models used to quantify these sources of optical contrast are presented.

14.1.2 Measurable Quantities and Experimental Techniques

Three classes of measurable quantities prove to be of interest to transform results of remote sensing measurements in tissue into useful physical information. The first is the spatial distribution of light or the intensity profile generated by photons reemitted through a surface and measured as a function of the radial distance from the source and the detector when the medium is continually irradiated by a point source (e.g., a laser). This type of measurement is called continuous wave (CW). The intensity, nominally, does not vary in time. The second class is the temporal response to a very short pulse (~picosecond) of photons impinging on the surface of the tissue. This technique is called time-resolved and the temporal response is known as the time-of-flight (TOF). The third class is the frequency-domain technique in which an intensity-modulated laser beam illuminates the tissue. In this case, the measured outputs are the AC modulation amplitude and the phase shift of the detected signal. These techniques can be implemented in geometries with different arrangements of source(s) and detector(s):

1. In reflection mode, source(s) and detector(s) are placed at the same side of the tissue.
2. In transmission mode, source(s) and detector(s) are located on opposite sides of the tissue. In the latter, the source(s) and detector(s) can move in tandem while scanning the tissue surface and detectors with lateral offsets can also be used.
3. Tomographic sampling often uses multiple sources and detectors placed around the circumference of the target tissue.

For CW measurements, the instrumentation is simple and requires only a set of light sources and detectors. In this technique, the only measurable quantity is the intensity of light, and, owing to multiple scattering, strong pathlength dispersion occurs, which results in a loss of localization and resolution. Hence, this technique is widely used for spectroscopic measurements of bulk tissue properties in which the tissue is considered to be homogeneous [14,15]. However, CW techniques for imaging abnormal targets that use only the coherent portion of light, and thereby reject photons with long pathlengths, have also been investigated. Using the transillumination geometry, collimated detection is used to isolate nonscattered photons [16–18]. Spatial filtering has been proposed that employs a lens to produce the Fourier spectrum of the spatial distribution of light from which the high-order frequencies are removed. The resulting image is formed using only the photons with angles close to normal [19]. Polarization discrimination has been used to select those photons that undergo few scattering events and therefore preserve a fraction of their initial polarization state, as opposed to those photons that experience multiple scattering resulting in complete randomization of their initial polarization state [20]. Several investigators have used heterodyne detection that involves measuring the beat frequency generated by the spatial and temporal combination of a light beam and a frequency-modulated reference beam. Constructive interference occurs only for the coherent portion of the light [20–22]. However, the potential of direct imaging using CW techniques in very thick tissue (e.g., breast) has not been established. On the other hand, use of models of photon migration implemented in inverse method based on backprojection techniques has shown promising results. For example, Phillips Medical has used 256 optical fibers placed at the periphery of a white conical-shaped vessel. The area of interest—in this case the breast—is suspended in the vessel and surrounded by a matching fluid. Three CW laser diodes sequentially illuminate the breast using one fiber. The detection is done simultaneously by 255 fibers. It is now clear that CW imaging cannot provide direct images with clinically acceptable resolution in thick tissue. Attempts are under way to devise inverse algorithms to separate the effects of scattering and absorption and therefore use this technique for quantitative spectroscopy as proposed by Phillips [23]. However, until now, clinical application of CW techniques in imaging has been limited by the mixture of scattering and absorption of light in the detected signal. To overcome this problem, time-dependent measurement techniques have been investigated.

Time-domain techniques involve the temporal resolution of photons traveling inside the tissue. The basic idea is that photons with smaller pathlengths are those that arrive earlier to the detector. In order to discriminate between unscattered- or less-scattered light and the majority of the photons, which experience a large number of multiple scattering, subnanosecond resolutions are needed. This short time gating of an imaging system requires the use of a variety of techniques involving ultrafast phenomena and/or fast detection systems. Ultrafast shuttering is performed using the Kerr effect. The birefringence in the Kerr cell, placed between two crossed polarizers, is induced using very short pulses. Transmitted light through the Kerr cell is recorded, and temporal resolution of a few picoseconds is achieved [19]. When an impulse of light (~picoseconds or hundreds of femtoseconds) is launched at the tissue surface, the whole temporal distribution of photon intensity can be recorded by a streak camera. The streak camera can achieve temporal resolution on the order of few picoseconds up to several nanosececonds detection time. This detection system has been widely used to assess the performance of breast imaging and neonatal brain activity [24,25]. The time of flight recorded by the streak camera is the convolution of the pulsed laser source (in practice with a finite width) and the actual Temporal Point Spread Function (TPSF) of the diffuse photons. Instead of using very short pulse lasers (e.g., Ti-Sapphire lasers), the advent of pulse diode lasers with relatively larger pulse width (100 to 400 ps) has reduced the cost of time-domain imaging much lower. However, deconvolutions of the incoming pulse and the detected TPSF have been a greater issue. Along with diode laser sources, several groups have also used time-correlated single photon counting with photomultipliers for recording the TPSF [26,27]. Fast time gating is also obtained by using Stimulated Raman Scattering. This phenomenon is a nonlinear Raman interaction in some materials such as hydrogen gas involving the amplification of photons with Stokes shift by a higher energy pump beam. The system operates by amplifying only the earliest arriving photons [28]. Less widely used techniques such as second-harmonic generation [29], parametric amplification [30], and a variety of others have been proposed for time-domain (see an excellent review in Reference 31).

For frequency-domain measurements, the requirement is to measure the DC amplitude, the AC amplitude, and the phase shift of the photon density wave. For this purpose, a CW light source is modulated with a given frequency (~100 MHz). Lock-in amplifiers and/or phase-sensitive CCD camera have been used to record the amplitude and phase [32,33]. Multiple sources at different wavelengths can be modulated with a single frequency or multiple frequencies [6,34]. In the latter case, a network analyzer is used to produce modulation swept from several hundreds of MHz to up to 1 GHz.

14.1.3 Models of Photon Migration in Tissue

Photon migration theories in biomedical optics have been borrowed from other fields such as astrophysics, atmospheric science, and specifically from nuclear reactor engineering [35,36]. The common properties of these physical media and biological tissues are their characterization by elements of randomness in both space and time. Because of many difficulties surrounding the development of a theory based on a detailed picture of the microscopic processes involved in the interaction of light and matter, investigations are often based on statistical theories. These can take a variety of forms, ranging from quite detailed multiple-scattering theories [36] to transport theory [37]. However, the most widely used theory is the time-dependent diffusion approximation to the transport equation:

$$\vec{\nabla} \cdot (D\vec{\nabla}\Phi(\vec{r},t)) - \mu_a \Phi(\vec{r},t) = \frac{1}{c}\frac{\partial \Phi(\vec{r},t)}{\partial t} - S(\vec{r},t) \tag{14.3}$$

where $\vec{r}$ and t are spatial and temporal variables, c is the speed of light in tissue, and D is the diffusion coefficient related to the absorption and scattering coefficients as follows:

$$D = \frac{1}{3[\mu a + \mu's]} \tag{14.4}$$

The quantity $\Phi(\vec{r},t)$ is called the fluence, defined as the power incident on an infinitesimal volume element divided by its area. Note that the equation does not incorporate any angular dependence, therefore assuming an isotropic scattering. However, for the use of the diffusion theory for anisotropic scattering, the diffusion coefficient is expressed in terms of the transport-corrected scattering coefficient. $S(\vec{r},t)$ is the source term. The gradient of fluence, $J(\vec{r}, t)$, at the tissue surface is the measured flux of photons by the detector:

$$J(\vec{r}, t) = -D\vec{\nabla}\Phi(\vec{r}, t) \qquad (14.5)$$

For CW measurements, the time dependence of the flux vanishes, and the source term can be seen as the power impinging in its area. For time-resolved measurement, the source term is a Dirac delta function describing a very short photon impulse. Equation 14.3 has been solved analytically for different types of measurements such as reflection and transmission mode assuming that the optical properties remain invariant through the tissue. To incorporate the finite boundaries, the method of images has been used. In the simplest case, the boundary has been assumed to be perfectly absorbing, which does not take into account the difference between indices of refraction at the tissue–air interface. For semi-infinite and transillumination geometries, a set of theoretical expressions has been obtained for time-resolved measurements [38].

The diffusion approximation equation in the frequency domain is the Fourier transformation of the time-domain with respect to time. Fourier transformation applied to the time-dependent diffusion equation leads to a new equation:

$$\vec{\nabla} \cdot (D\vec{\nabla}\Phi(\vec{r}, \omega)) - \left[\mu_a + \frac{i\omega}{c}\right]\Phi(\vec{r}, \omega) + S(\vec{r}, \omega) = 0 \qquad (14.6)$$

Here the time variable is replaced by the frequency ω. This frequency is the modulation angular frequency of the source. In this model, the fluence can be seen as a complex number describing the amplitude and phase of the photon density wave, dumped with a DC component:

$$\Phi(\vec{r}, \omega) = \Phi_{AC}(\vec{r}, \omega) + \Phi_{DC}(\vec{r}, 0) = I_{AC} \exp(i\theta) + \Phi_{DC}(\vec{r}, 0) \qquad (14.7)$$

In the right-hand side of Equation 14.7, the quantity θ is the phase shift of the diffusing wave. For a nonabsorbing medium, its wavelength is

$$\lambda = 2\pi \sqrt{\frac{2c}{3\mu'_s \omega}} \qquad (14.8)$$

Likewise in the time-domain, Equation 14.3 has an analytical solution for the case that the tissue is considered homogeneous. The analytical solution permits one to deduce the optical properties in a spectroscopic setting.

For imaging, where the goal is to distinguish between structures in tissue, the diffusion coefficient and the absorption coefficient in Equations 14.3 and 14.6 become spatial dependent and are replaced by $D(r)$ and $\mu_a(r)$. For the cases that an abnormal region is embedded in otherwise homogeneous tissue, perturbation methods based on Born approximation or Rytov approximation have been used (see excellent review in Reference 39). However, for the cases that the goal is to reconstruct the spectroscopic signatures inside the tissue, no analytical solution exists. For these cases inverse algorithms are devised to map the spatially varying optical properties. Numerical methods such as finite-element or finite-difference methods have been used to reconstruct images of breast, brain, and muscle [40–42]. Furthermore, in those cases that structural heterogeneity exists, a priori information from other image modalities such as MRI. An example is given in Figure 14.2. Combining MRI and NIR imaging, rat cranium functional imaging during changes in inhaled oxygen concentration was studied [43]. Figure 14.2a,b correspond to the MRI image and the corresponding constructed finite element mesh. Figure 14.2c,d correspond to the oxygen map of the brain with and without incorporation of MRI geometry and constraints.

The use of MRI images has improved dramatically the resolution of the oxygen map. The use of optical functional imaging in conjunction with other imaging modalities has opened new possibilities in imaging and treating diseases at the bedside.

The second theoretical framework used in tissue optics is the Random Walk Theory (RWT) on a lattice developed at the National Institutes of Health [44,45] and historically precedes the use of the diffusion

FIGURE 14.2 (See color insert.) Functional imaging of rat cranium during changes in inhaled oxygen concentration. (a) MRI image; (b) creation of the mesh to distinguish different compartments in the brain; (c) map of hemoglobin concentration and oxygen saturation of the rat brain without structural constraints from MRI; and (d) same as (c) with structural constraints including tissue heterogeneity. In (c) and (d) the rows from top correspond to 13, 8, and 0% (after death) oxygen inhaled. (Courtesy of Dartmouth College.)

approximation theory. It has been shown that RWT may be used to derive an analytical solution for the distribution of photon pathlengths in turbid media such as tissue [44]. RWT models the diffusion-like motion of photons in turbid media in a probabilistic manner. Using RWT, an expression may be derived for the probability of a photon arriving at any point and time given a specific starting point and time.

Tissue may be modeled as a 3D cubic lattice containing a finite inclusion, or region of interest, as shown in Figure 14.3. The medium has an absorbing boundary corresponding to the tissue surface, and the lattice spacing is proportional to the mean photon scattering distance, $1/\mu'_s$. The behavior of photons in the RWT model is described by three-dimensionless parameters, ρ, n, μ, which are respectively the radial distance, the number of steps, and the probability of absorption per lattice step. In the RWT model, photons may move to one of the six nearest neighboring lattice points, each with probability 1/6. If the number of steps, n, taken by a photon traveling between two points on the lattice is known, then the length of the photon's path is also known.

RWT is useful in predicting the probability distribution of photon pathlengths over distances of at least five mean-photon scattering distances. The derivation of these probability distributions is described in review papers [44,45]. For simplicity in this derivation, the tissue–air interface is considered to be perfectly absorbing; a photon arriving at this interface is counted as arriving at a detector on the tissue surface. The

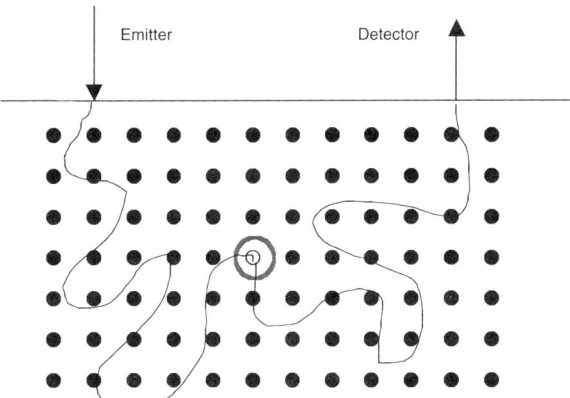

FIGURE 14.3 Two-dimensional random walk lattice showing representative photon paths from an emitter to a specific site and then to a detector.

derivation uses the Central Limit Theorem and a Gaussian distribution around lattice points to obtain a closed-form solution that is independent of the lattice structure.

The dimensionless RWT parameters, ρ, n, and μ, described above, may be transformed to actual parameters, in part, by using time, t, the speed of light in tissue, c, and distance traveled, r, as follows:

$$\rho \to \frac{r\mu'_s}{\sqrt{2}}, \quad n \to \mu'_s ct, \quad \mu \to \frac{\mu_a}{\mu'_s} \tag{14.9}$$

As stated previously, scattering in tissue is highly anisotropic. Therefore, one must find the appropriate scaling relationships that will allow the use of an isotropic scattering model such as RWT. Like diffusion theory, for RWT [46], it has been shown that one may use an isotropic scattering model with a corrected scattering coefficient, μ'_s, and obtain equivalent results. The corrected scattering coefficient is smaller than the actual scattering that corresponds to a greater distance between isotropic scattering events than would occur with anisotropic scattering. RWT has been used to show how one would transition from the use of μ_s to μ'_s as the distance under consideration increases [47].

As an example, for a homogeneous slab into which a photon has been inserted, the probability P of a photon arriving at a point ρ after n steps is [48]:

$$P(n,\rho) = \frac{\sqrt{3}}{2} \left[\frac{1}{2\pi (n-2)} \right]^{3/2} e^{\frac{-3\rho^2}{2(n-2)}} \sum_{k=-\infty}^{\infty} \left[e^{\frac{-3[(2k+1)L-2]^2}{2(n-2)}} - e^{\frac{-3[(2k+1)L]^2}{2(n-2)}} \right] e^{-n\mu} \tag{14.10}$$

where L is the thickness of the slab. The method of images has been used to take into account the two boundaries of the slab. Plotting Equation 14.10 yields a photon arrival curve as shown in Figure 14.4; Monte Carlo simulation data are overlaid. In the next two sections, the use of RWT for imaging will be presented.

14.1.4 RWT Applied to Quantitative Spectroscopy of the Breast

One important and yet extremely challenging area to apply diffuse optical imaging of deep tissues is the human breast (see review article of Hawrysz and Sevick-Muraca [49]). It is clear that any new imaging or spectroscopic modalities that can improve the diagnosis of breast tumors or can add new knowledge about the physiological properties of the breast and surrounding tissues will have a great significance in medicine.

Conventional transillumination using CW light was used for breast screening several decades ago [50]. However, because of the high-scattering properties of tissue, this method resulted in poor resolution. In the late 1980s, time-resolved imaging techniques were proposed to enhance spatial resolution by detecting

FIGURE 14.4 RWT prediction and Monte Carlo simulation results for transillumination of a 15-mm thick slab with scattering 1/mm and 109 photons.

photons with very short TOF within the tissue. In this technique, a very short pulse, of approximately picosecond duration, impinges on the tissue. Photons experience dispersion in their pathlengths, resulting in temporal dispersion in their TOF.

To evaluate the performance of time-resolved transillumination techniques, RWT on a lattice was used. The analysis of breast transillumination was based on the calculation of the point spread function (PSF) of time-resolved photons as they visit differing sites at different planes inside a finite slab. The PSF [51], defined as the probability that a photon inserted into the tissue visits a given site, is detected at the nth step (i.e., a given time), and has the following rather complicated analytical expression:

$$W_n(\mathbf{s}, \mathbf{r}, \mathbf{r}_0) = \sum_{l=0}^{n} p_l(\mathbf{r}, \mathbf{s}) p_{n-l}(\mathbf{s}, \mathbf{r}_0)$$

$$= \frac{9}{16\pi^{5/2} n^{3/2}} \sum_{k=-\infty}^{\infty} \sum_{m=-\infty}^{\infty} \{F_n[\alpha_+(k), \beta_+(m, \rho)] \quad (14.11)$$

$$+ F_n[\alpha_-(k), \beta_-(m, \rho)] - F_n[\alpha_+(k), \beta_-(m, \rho)] - F_n[\alpha_-(k), \beta_+(m, \rho)]\}$$

$$F_n(a, b) = \left(\frac{1}{a} + \frac{1}{b}\right) \exp\left[-\frac{(a+b)^2}{n}\right] \quad (14.12)$$

$$\alpha_\pm(k) = \left\{\frac{3}{2}\left[s_1^2 + (s_3 + 2kN \pm 1)^2\right]\right\}^{1/2} \quad (14.13)$$

$$\beta_\pm(k, \rho) = \left\{\frac{3}{2}\left[(\rho - s_1)^2 + (N - s_3 + 2kN \pm 1)^2\right]\right\}^{1/2} \quad (14.14)$$

where $N = (L\mu_s'/\sqrt{2}) + 1$ is dimensionless RWT thickness of the slabs, $\bar{s}(s_1, s_2, s_3)$ are the dimensionless coordinates (see Equation 14.9). Evaluation of time-resolved imaging showed that strong scattering properties of tissues prevent direct imaging of abnormalities [52]. Hence, devising theoretical constructs to separate the effects of the scattering from the absorption was proposed, thus allowing one to map the optical coefficients as spectroscopic signatures of an abnormal tissue embedded in thick, otherwise normal tissue. In this method, accurate quantification of the size and optical properties of the target becomes a critical requirement for the use of optical imaging at the bedside. RWT on a lattice has been used to analyze the time-dependent contrast observed in time-resolved transillumination experiments and deduce the size and optical properties of the target and the surrounding tissue from these contrasts. For the theoretical construction of contrast functions, two quantities are needed: first, the set of functions [51] defined previously and, second, the set of functions [53] defined as the probability that a photon is detected at the nth step (i.e., time) in a homogeneous medium (Equation 14.10) [48].

FIGURE 14.5 (a) Two-dimensional optical image of the breast with the tumor. (Courtesy of Physikalich-Techniche-Bundesanstalt, Berlin.) (b) contrast obtained from linear scan through the tumor plotted vs. the derivative of PSF. From the linear regression the scattering coefficient of the tumor is deduced.

To relate the contrast of the light intensity to the optical properties and location of abnormal targets in the tissue, one can take advantage of some features of the theoretical framework. One feature is that the early time response is most dependent on scattering perturbations, whereas the late time behavior is most dependent on absorptive perturbations, thus allowing one to separate the influence of scattering and absorption perturbations on the observed image contrast. Increased scattering in the abnormal target is modeled as a time delay. Moreover, it was shown that the scattering contrast is proportional to the time derivative of the PSF, dW_n/dn, divided by P_n [53]. The second interesting feature in RWT methodology assumes that the contrast from scattering inside the inclusion is proportional to the cross-section of the target (in the z direction) [51,53], instead of depending on its volume as modeled in the perturbation analysis [54].

Several research groups intend to implement their theoretical expressions into general inverse algorithms for optical tomography, that is, to reconstruct 3D maps of spatial distributions of tissue optical characteristics [49], and thereby quantify optical characteristics, positions, and sizes of abnormalities. Unlike these approaches, the method is a multistep analysis of the collected data. From images observed at differing flight times, one can construct the time-dependent contrast functions, fit theoretical expressions, and compute the optical properties of the background, and those of the abnormality along with its size. The outline of the data analysis is given in Reference 55.

By utilizing the method for different wavelengths, one can obtain diagnostic information (e.g., estimates of blood oxygenation of the tumor) for corresponding absorption coefficients that no other imaging modality can provide directly. Several research groups have already successfully used multiwavelength measurements using frequency-domain techniques, to calculate physiological parameters (oxygenation, lipid, and water) of breast tumors (diagnosed with other modalities) and normal tissue [56].

Researchers at Physikalich-Techniche-Bundesanstalt (PTB) of Berlin have designed a clinically practical optical imaging system, capable of implementing time-resolved *in vivo* measurements on the human breast [27]. The breast is slightly compressed between two plates. A scan of the whole breast takes but a few minutes and can be done in mediolateral and craniocaudal geometries. The first goal is to quantify the optical parameters at several wavelengths and thereby estimate blood oxygen saturation of the tumor and surrounding tissue under the usual assumption that the chromophores contributing to absorption are oxy- and deoxy-hemoglobin and water. As an example, two sets of data, obtained at two wavelengths ($\lambda = 670$ and 785 nm), for a patient (84 year old) with invasive ductal carcinoma, were analyzed. Though the images exhibit poor resolution, the tumor can be easily seen in the optical image shown in Figure 14.5a. In this figure, the image is obtained from reciprocal values of the total integrals of the distributions of times of flight of photons, normalized to a selected "bulk" area. The tumor center is located at $x = -5, y = 0.25$ mm.

TABLE 14.1 Optical Parameters of Tumor and Background Breast Tissue

Unknown coefficients	Reconstructed values (mm)$^{-1}$ $\lambda = 670$ nm	Reconstructed values (mm)$^{-1}$ $\lambda = 785$ nm
Absorption (background)	0.0029	0.0024
Scattering (background)	1.20	1.10
Absorption (tumor)	0.0071	0.0042
Scattering (tumor)	1.76	1.6

The best spatial resolution is observed, as expected, for shorter time delays allowing one to determine the position of the tumor center on the 2D image (transverse coordinates) with accuracy ~2.5 mm. After preliminary data processing that includes filtering and deconvolution of the raw time-resolved data, we created linear contrast scans passing through the tumor center and analyzed these scans, using the algorithm. It is striking that one observes similar linear dependence of the contrast amplitude on the derivative of PSF ($\lambda = 670$ nm), as expected in the model (see Figure 14.5b). The slope of this linear dependence was used to estimate the amplitude of the scattering perturbation [55].

Dimensions and values of optical characteristics of the tumor and surrounding tissues were then reconstructed for both wavelengths. Results show that the tumor had larger absorption and scattering than the background. Estimated parameters are presented in Table 14.1.

Both absorption and scattering coefficients of the tumor and background all proved to be larger at the red wavelength (670 nm). Comparison of the absorption in the red and NIR range is used to estimate blood oxygen saturation of the tumor and background tissue. Preliminary results of the analysis gave evidence that the tumor tissue is in a slightly deoxygenated state with higher blood volume, compared to surrounding tissue.

The spectroscopic power of optical imaging, along with the ability to quantify physiological parameters of human breast have opened a new opportunity for assessing metabolic and physiological activities of human breast during treatment.

14.1.5 Quantitative Fluorescence Imaging and Spectroscopy

As mentioned in Section 14.1.1, advances in the molecular biology of disease processes, new immunohistopathological techniques, and the development of specific fluorescently labeled cell surface markers have led a revolution in research on the molecular origins of disease processes. On the other hand, reliable, sensitive, and specific, noninvasive techniques are needed for *in vivo* determinations of abnormalities within tissue. If successfully developed, noninvasive "optical biopsies" may replace conventional surgical biopsies and provide the advantages of smaller sampling errors and reduction in cost and time for diagnosis, resulting in easier integration of diagnosis and therapy by following the progression of disease or its regression in response to therapy. Clinically practical fluorescence-imaging techniques must meet several requirements. First, the pathology under investigation must lie above a depth where the attenuation of the signal results in a poor signal-to-noise ratio and resolvability. Second, the specificity of the marker must be high enough that one can clearly distinguish between normal and abnormal lesions. Finally, one must have a robust image reconstruction algorithm that enables one to quantify the fluorophore concentration at a given depth.

The choices of projects in this area of research are dictated by the importance of the problem, and the impact of the solution on health care. Below, the rationale of two projects is described that the unit at the National Institutes of Health is pursuing.

Sjøgren's Syndrome (SS) has been chosen as an appropriate test case for developing a noninvasive optical biopsy based on 3D localization of exogenous specific fluorescent labels. SS is an autoimmune disease affecting minor salivary glands that are near (0.5 to 3.0 mm below) the oral mucosal surface [57]. Therefore, the target pathology is relatively accessible to noninvasive optical imaging. The hydraulic conductivity of the oral mucosa is relatively high, which along with the relatively superficial location of the minor salivary glands, makes topical application and significant labeling of diseased glands with large fluorescent molecules easy to accomplish. Fluorescent ligands (e.g., fluorescent antibodies specific to $CD4^+$ T-cell-activated lymphocytes infiltrating the salivary glands) are expected to bind specifically to the atypical cells in the tissue, providing high contrast and a quantitative relationship to their concentration (and therefore to the stage of the disease process). The major symptoms (dry eyes and dry mouth due to decreased tear and saliva secretion) are the result of progressive immune-mediated dysfunction of the lacrimal and salivary glands. Currently, diagnosis is made by excisional biopsies of the minor salivary glands in the lower lip. This examination though considered the best criterion for diagnosis, involves a surgical procedure under local anesthesia followed by postoperative discomfort (swelling and pain) and, frequently, a temporary loss of sensation at the lower lip biopsy site. Additionally, biopsy is inherently subject to sampling errors, and the preparation of histopathological slides is time consuming, complicated, expensive, and requires the skills of several professionals (dentist, pathologist, and laboratory technician). Thus, there is a clear need for a noninvasive diagnostic procedure that reflects the underlying gland pathology and has good specificity. A quantitative noninvasive assay would also allow repetition of the test to monitor disease progression and the effect of treatment. However, the quantification of fluorophore concentration within the tissue from surface images requires determining the intensities of different fluorophore sources, as a function of depth and transverse distance and predicting the 3D distribution of fluorophores within the tissue from a series of images [58].

The second project involves the lymphatic imaging-sentinel node detection. The stage of cancer at initial diagnosis often defines prognosis and determines treatment options. As part of the staging procedure of melanoma and breast cancer, multiple lymph nodes are surgically removed from the primary lymphatic draining site and examined histologically for the presence of malignant cells. Because it is not obvious which nodes should be removed at the time of resection of the primary tumor, standard practice involves dissection of as many lymph nodes as feasible. Since such extensive removal of lymphatic tissue frequently results in compromised lymphatic drainage in the examined axilla, alternatives have been sought to define the stage at the time of primary resection. A recent advance in lymph node interrogation has been the localization and removal of the "sentinel" node. Although there are multiple lymphatic channels available for trafficking from the primary tumor, the assumption was made that the anatomic location of the primary tumor in a given individual drains into lymphatic channels in an orderly and reproducible fashion. If that is in fact the case, then there is a pattern by which lymphatic drainage occurs. Thus, it would be expected that malignant cells from a primary tumor site would course from the nearest and possibly most superficial node into deeper and more distant lymphatic channels to ultimately arrive in the thoracic duct, whereupon malignant cells would gain access to venous circulation. The sentinel node is defined as the first drainage node in a network of nodes that drain the primary cancer. Considerable evidence has accrued validating the clinical utility of staging breast cancer by locating and removing the sentinel node at the time of resection of the primary tumor. Currently, the primary tumor is injected with a radionucleotide 1 day before removal of the primary tumor. Then, just before surgery, it is injected with visible dye. The surgeon localizes crudely the location of the sentinel node using a hand-held radionucleotide detector, followed by a search for visible concentrations of the injected dye. The method requires expensive equipment and also presents the patient and hospital personnel with the risk of exposure to ionizing radiation. As an alternative to the radionucleotide, we are investigating the use of IR-dependent fluorescent detection methods to determine the location of sentinel node(s).

For *in vivo* fluorescent imaging, a complicating factor is the strong attenuation of light as it passes through tissue. This attenuation deteriorates the signal-to-noise ratio of detected photons. Fortunately, development of fluorescent dyes (such as porphyrin and cyanine) that excite and reemit in the "biological window" at NIR wavelengths, where scattering and absorption coefficients are relatively low, have provided new possibilities for deep fluorescence imaging in tissue. The theoretical complication occurs at depths greater than 1 mm where photons in most tissues enter a diffusion-like state with a large dispersion in their pathlengths. Indeed, the fluorescent intensity of light detected from deep tissue structures depends not only on the location, size, concentration, and intrinsic characteristics (e.g., lifetime, quantum efficiency) of the fluorophores, but also on the scattering and absorption coefficients of the tissue at both the excitation and emission wavelengths. Hence, in order to extract intrinsic characteristics of fluorophores within tissue, it is necessary to describe the statistics of photon pathlengths that depend on all these differing parameters.

Obviously, the modeling of fluorescent light propagation depends on the kinds of experiments that one plans to perform. For example, for frequency-domain measurements, Patterson and Pogue [59] used the diffusion approximation of the transport equation to express their results in terms of a product of two Green's function propagators multiplied by a term that describes the probability of emission of a fluorescent photon at the site. One Green's function describes the movement of an incident photon to the fluorophore, and the other describes movement of the emitted photon to the detector. In this representation, the amount of light emitted at the site of the fluorophore is directly proportional to the total amount of light impinging on the fluorophore, with no account for the variability in the number of visits by a photon before an exciting transformation. Since a transformation on an early visit to the site precludes a transformation on all later visits, this results in an overestimation of the number of photons that have a fluorescence transformation at a particular site. This overestimation is important when fluorescent absorption properties are spatially inhomogeneous and largest at later arrival times. RWT has been used to allow for this spatial inhomogeneity by introducing the multiple-passage probabilities concept, thus rendering the model more physically plausible [60]. Another incentive to devise a general theory of diffuse fluorescence photon migration is the capability to quantify local changes in fluorescence lifetime. By selecting fluorophore probes with known lifetime dependence on specific environmental variables, lifetime imaging enables one to localize and quantify such metabolic parameters as temperature and pH, as well as changes in local molecular concentrations *in vivo*.

In the probabilistic RWT model, the description of a photon path may be divided into three parts: (1) the path from the photon source to a localized, fluorescing target; (2) the interaction of the photon with the fluorophore; and (3) the path of the fluorescently emitted photon to a detector. Each part of the photon path may be described by a probability: first, the probability that an incident photon will arrive at the fluorophore site; second, the probability that the photon has a reactive encounter with the fluorophore and the corresponding photon transit delay, which is dependent on the lifetime of the fluorophore and the probability of the fluorophore emitting a photon; and third, the probability that the photon emitted by the fluorophore travels from the reaction site to the detector. Each of these three sequences is governed by a stochastic process. The mathematical description of the three processes is extremely complicated. The complete solution for the probability of fluorescence photon arrival at the detector is [61]

$$\hat{\gamma}(r, s, r_0) = \frac{\eta \Phi \hat{p}'_\xi(r|s) \hat{p}_\xi(s|r_0)}{\langle \Delta n \rangle (1-\eta) [\exp(\xi) - 1] + \{\eta \langle \Delta n \rangle [\exp(\xi) - 1] + 1\} \left\{ 1 + \left[\frac{1}{8} \left(\frac{3}{\pi}\right)^{3/2} \sum_{j=1}^{\infty} \frac{\exp(-2j\xi)}{j^{3/2}} \right] \right\}}$$

(14.15)

where η is the probability of fluorescent absorption of an excitation wavelength photon; Φ is the quantum efficiency of the fluorophore, which is the probability that an excited fluorophore will emit a photon at the emission wavelength; $\langle \Delta n \rangle$ is the mean number of steps the photon would have taken had the photon not been exciting the fluorophore (which corresponds to the fluorophore lifetime in random walk parameters); and ξ is a transform variable corresponding to the discrete analog of the Laplace transform and may be considered analogous to frequency. The probability of a photon going from the excitation source to the fluorophore site is $\hat{p}_\xi(s|r_0)$, and the probability of a fluorescent photon going from the fluorophore site to the detector is $\hat{p}'_\xi(r|s)$; the prime indicates that the wavelength of the photon has changed and therefore the optical properties of the tissue may be different. In practice, this solution is difficult to work with, so some simplifying assumptions are desired. With some simplification the result in the frequency domain is

$$\hat{\gamma}(r, s, r_0) = \eta \Phi \left\{ \hat{p}'_\xi(r|s) \hat{p}_\xi(s|r_0) - \xi \langle \Delta n \rangle \hat{p}'_\xi(r|s) \hat{p}_\xi(s|r_0) \right\}$$

(14.16)

FIGURE 14.6 Intensity scan of a fluorophore 10.4 mm below the tissue surface.

The inverse Laplace transform of this equation gives the diffuse fluorescent intensity in the time-domain, and the integral of the latter over time leads to CW measurements. The accuracy of such cumbersome equations is tested in well-defined phantoms and fluorophores embedded in *ex vivo* tissue. In Figure 14.6, a line scan of fluorescent intensity collected from 500 μm^3 fluorescent dye (Molecular Probe, far red microspheres: 690 nm excitation; 720 nm emission), embedded in 10.4 mm porcine tissue with a lot of heterogeneity (e.g., fat) are presented. The dashed line is the corresponding RWT fit. The inverse algorithm written in C++ was able to construct the depth of the fluorophore with 100% accuracy. Knowing the heterogeneity of the tissue (seen in the intensity profile), this method presents huge potential to interrogate tissue structures deeply embedded in tissue, for which specific fluorescent labeling such as antibodies for cell surfaces exists.

14.1.6 Future Directions

A clinically useful optical imaging device requires multidisciplinary and multistep approaches. At the desk, one devises quantitative theories, and develops methodologies applicable to *in vivo* quantitative tissue spectroscopy and tomographic imaging in different imaging geometries (i.e., transmission or reflection), different types of measurements (e.g., steady-state or time-resolved). Effects of different optical sources of contrast such as endogenous or exogenous fluorescent labels, variations in absorption (e.g., hemoglobin or chromophore concentration), and scattering should be incorporated in the model. At the bench, one designs and conducts experiments on tissue-like phantoms and runs computer simulations to validate the theoretical findings. If successful, one tries to bring the imaging or spectroscopic device to the bedside. For this task, one must foster strong collaborations with physicians who can help in identifying physiological sites where optical techniques may be clinically practical and can offer new diagnostic knowledge and/or less morbidity over existing methods. An important intermediate step is the use of animal models for preclinical studies. Overall, this is a complicated path. However, the spectroscopic power of light, along with the revolution in molecular characterization of disease processes has created a huge potential for *in vivo* optical imaging and spectroscopy. Maybe the twenty-first century will be the second "*siecle des lumieres.*"

14.2 Infrared Thermal Monitoring of Disease Processes: Clinical Study

The relationship between a change in body temperature and health status has been of interest to physicians since Hippocrates stated "should one part of the body be hotter or colder than the rest, then disease is present in that part." Thermography provides a visual display of the surface temperature of the skin. Skin temperature recorded by an IR scanner is the resultant balance of thermal transport within the tissues and transport to the environment. In medical applications, thermal images of human skin contain a large amount of clinical information that can help in detecting numerous pathological conditions ranging from cancer to emotional disorders. For the clinical assessment of cancer, physicians need to determine the activity of the tumor and location, extent, and response to therapy. All of these factors make it possible for tumors to be examined using thermography. Advantages of using this method are that it is completely nonionizing, safe, and can be repeated as often as required without exposing the patient to risk. Unfortunately, the skin temperature distribution is misinterpreted in many cases, because a high skin temperature does not always indicate a tumor. Therefore, thermography requires extensive education about how to interpret the temperature distribution patterns as well as additional research to clarify of various diseases based on skin temperature.

Before applying the thermal technique in the clinical setting, it is important to consider how to avoid possible error in the results. Before the examination, the body should attain thermal equilibrium with its environment. A patient should be unclothed for at least 20 min in a controlled environment at a temperature of approximately $22°C$. Under such clinical conditions, thermograms will show only average temperature patterns over an interval of time. The evaluation of surface temperature by IR techniques requires wavelength and emissive properties of the surface (emissivity) to be examined over the range of wavelengths to which the detector is sensitive. In addition, a thermal camera should be calibrated with a known temperature reference source to standardize clinical data.

Before discussing a specific clinical application of thermography, an accurate technique for measuring emissivity is presented in Section 14.2.1. In Section 14.2.2, a procedure for temperature calibration of an IR detector is discussed. The clinical application of thermography with Kaposi's sarcoma (KS) is detailed in Section 14.2.3.

14.2.1 Emissivity Corrected Temperature

Emissivity is described as a radiative property of the skin. It is a measure of how well a body can radiate energy compared to a black body. Knowledge of emissivity is important when measuring skin temperature with an IR detector system at different ambient radiation temperatures. Currently, different spectral band infrared detector systems are used in clinical studies such as 3–5 and 8–14 μm. It is well known that the emissivity of the skin varies according to the spectral range. The skin emits IR radiation mainly between 2 and 20 μm with maximum emission at a wavelength around 10 μm [62]. Jones [63] showed with an InSb detector that only 2% of the radiation emitted from a thermal black body at $30°C$ was within the 3 to 5 μm spectral range; the wider spectral response of HgCdTe detector (8 to 14 μm) corresponded to 40 to 50% of this blackbody radiation.

Many investigators have reported on the values for emissivity of skin *in vivo*, measured in different spectral bands with different techniques. Hardy [64] and Stekettee [65] showed that the spectral emissivity of skin was independent of wavelength (λ) when $\lambda > 2$ μm. These results contradicted those obtained by Elam et al. [66]. Watmough and Oliver [67] pointed out that emissivity lies within 0.98 to 1 and was not less than 0.95 for a wavelength range of 2 to 5 μm. Patil and Williams [68] reported that the average emissivity of normal breast skin was $0.99 \pm 0.045, 0.972 \pm 0.041$, and 0.975 ± 0.043 within the ranges 4–6, 6–18, and 4–18 μm, respectively. Steketee [65] indicated that the average emissivity value of skin was 0.98 ± 0.01 within the range 3 to 14 μm. It is important to know the precise value of emissivity because an emissivity difference of 0.945 to 0.98 may cause an error of skin temperature of $0.6°C$ [64].

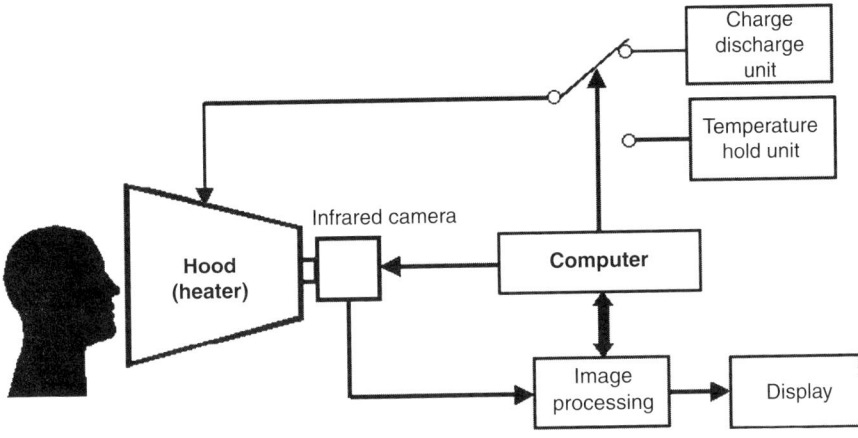

FIGURE 14.7 Schematic diagram of the emissivity measurement system [70].

TABLE 14.2 Emissivity Values

Average normal forearm skin of 12 subjects	
IR-camera (3–5 μm)	0.958 ± 0.002
Radiometer (8–14 μm)	0.973 ± 0.0003

There is considerable diversity in the reported values of skin emissivity even in the same spectral band. The inconsistencies among reported values could be due to unreliable and inadequate theories and techniques employed for measuring skin emissivity. Togawa [69] proposed a technique in which the emissivity was calculated by measuring the temperature upon a transient stepwise change in ambient radiation temperature [69,70] surrounding an object surface, as shown in Figure 14.7.

The average emissivity of skin for the 12 normal subjects measured by a radiometer and infrared camera are presented in Table 14.2. The emissivity values were found to be significantly different between 3–5 and 8–14 μm spectral bands ($p < .001$). An example of a set of images obtained during measurement using an IR-camera (3 to 5 μm bands) on the forearm of a healthy male subject is shown in Figure 14.8.

An accurate value of emissivity is important, because an incorrect value of emissivity can lead to a temperature error in radiometric thermometry especially when the ambient radiation temperature varies widely. The extent to which skin emissivity depends on the spectral range of the IR detectors is demonstrated in Table 14.2, which shows emissivity values measured at 0.958 ± 0.002 and 0.973 ± 0.003 by an IR detector with spectral bands of 3–5 and 8–14 μm, respectively. These results can give skin temperatures that differ by 0.2°C at a room temperature of 22°C. Therefore, it is necessary to consider the wavelength dependence of emissivity, when high precision temperature measurements are required.

Emissivity not only depends on wavelength but is also influenced by surface quality, moisture on the skin surface, and so forth. In the IR region of 3 to 50 μm, the emissivity of most nonmetallic substances is higher for a rough surface than a smooth one [71]. The presence of water also increases the value of emissivity [72]. These influences may account for the variation in results.

14.2.2 Temperature Calibration

In IR-thermography, any radiator is suitable as a temperature reference if its emissivity is known and constant within a given range of wavelengths. Currently, many different commercial blackbody calibrators are available to be used as temperature reference sources. A practical and simple blackbody radiator with a known temperature and measurement system is illustrated in Figure 14.9. The system consists of a hollow

FIGURE 14.8 (See color insert.) An example of images obtained from the forearm of a normal healthy male subject. (a) Original thermogram; (b) emissivity image; and (c) thermogram corrected by emissivity.

FIGURE 14.9 Schematic diagram of temperature calibration system.

copper cylinder, a temperature-controlled water bath and a precise temperature meter with probe. The height of the cylinder is 15 cm and the diameter is 7.5 cm. The cylinder is closed except for a hole in the center of the upper end that is 2 cm in diameter. To make the blackbody radiator, the inner surface of the cylinder is coated with black paint (3M Velvet Coating no. 2010) with emissivity of 0.93. Before the calibration, three-fourth of the cylinder is placed vertically in the water and the thermal camera is placed on the top of the cylinder in a vertical direction with a distance of focus length between the surface of the hole and the camera. The water temperature ranges from 18 to 45°C by 2°C increments. This range was selected since human temperature generally varies from 22 to 42°C in clinical studies. After setting the water temperature, the thermal camera measures the surface temperature of the hole while the temperature meter with probe measures the water temperature. The temperature of the camera is calibrated according to the temperature reading of the temperature meter.

14.2.3 Clinical Study

14.2.3.1 Kaposi's Sarcoma

The oncology community is testing a number of novel targeted approaches such as antiangiogenic, antivascular, immuno-, and gene therapies for use against a variety of cancers. To monitor such therapies, it is desirable to establish techniques to assess tumor vasculature and changes with therapy [73]. Currently, several imaging techniques such as dynamic contrast-enhanced MRI [74–76], PET [77–79], computed tomography (CT) [80–83], color Doppler ultrasound (US) [84,85], and fluorescence imaging [86,87] have been used in angiogenesis-related research. With regard to monitoring vasculature, it is desirable to develop and assess noninvasive and quantitative techniques that can not only monitor structural changes but can also assess the functional characteristics or the metabolic status of the tumor. There are currently no standard noninvasive techniques to assess parameters of angiogenesis in lesions of interest and to monitor changes in these parameters with therapy. For antiangiogenic therapies, factors associated with blood flow are of particular interest.

Kaposi's sarcoma (KS) is a highly vascular tumor that occurs frequently among people infected with acquired immunodeficiency syndrome (AIDS). During the first decade of the AIDS epidemic, 15 to 20% of AIDS patients developed this type of tumor [88]. Patients with KS often display skin and oral lesions and KS frequently involves lymph nodes and visceral organs [89]. KS is an angio-proliferative disease characterized by angiogenesis, endothelial spindle-cell growth (KS cell growth), inflammatory-cell infiltration, and edema [90]. A gamma herpesvirus called Kaposi's sarcoma associated herpesvirus (KSHV) or human herpesvirus type 8 (HHV-8) is an essential factor in the pathogenesis of KS [91]. Cutaneous KS lesions are easily accessible for noninvasive techniques that involve imaging of tumor vasculature, and they may thus represent a tumor model in which to assess certain parameters of angiogenesis [92,93].

Two potential noninvasive imaging techniques, IR thermal imaging (thermography) and laser Doppler imaging (LDI), have been used to monitor patients undergoing an experimental anti-KS therapy [94,95]. Thermography graphically depicts temperature gradients over a given body surface area at a given time. It is used to study biological thermoregulatory abnormalities that directly or indirectly influence skin temperature [96–100]. However, skin temperature is only an indirect measure of skin blood flow, and the superficial thermal signature of skin is also related to local metabolism. Thus, this approach is best used in conjunction with other techniques. LDI can more directly measure the net blood velocity of small blood vessels in tissue, which generally increases as blood supply increases during angiogenesis [101,102]. Thermal patterns were recorded using an IR camera with a uniform sensitivity in the wavelength range of 8–12 μm and LDI images were acquired by scanning the lesion area of the KS patients at two wavelengths, 690 and 780 nm.

An example of the images obtained from a typical KS lesion using different modalities is shown in Figure 14.10 [95]. As can be seen in the thermal image, the temperature of the lesion was approximately 2°C higher than that of the normal tissue adjacent to the lesion. Interestingly, in a number of lesions, the area of increased temperature extended beyond the lesion edges as assessed by visual inspection or palpation. This may reflect relatively deep involvement of the tumor in areas underlying normal skin. However, the thermal signature of the skin reflects not only superficial vascularity, but also deep tissue metabolic activity. In the LDI image of the same lesion, there was increased blood flow in the area of the lesion as compared with the surrounding tissue, with a maximum increase of over 600 AU (arbitrary units). Unlike the thermal image, the increased blood velocity extended only slightly beyond the area of this visible lesion, possibly because the tumor process leading to the increased temperature was too deep to be detected by LDI. Both of these techniques were used successfully to visualize KS lesions, and although each measure an independent parameter (temperature or blood velocity), there was a strong correlation in a group of 16 patients studied by both techniques (Figure 14.11). However, there were some differences in individual lesions since LDI measured blood flow distribution in the superficial layer of the

FIGURE 14.10 (See color insert.) Typical multimodality images obtained from a patient with KS lesion. The number '1' and '5' in the visual image were written on the skin to identify the lesions for tumor measurement. The solid line in the thermal and LDI demarks the border of the visible KS lesion. Shown is a representative patient from the study reported in Reference 95.

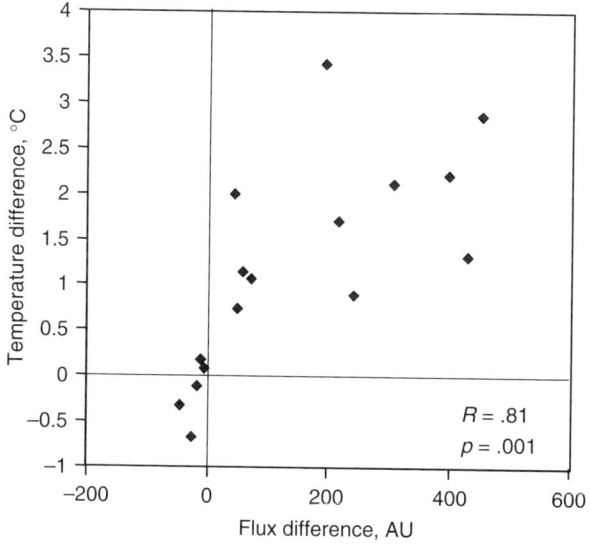

FIGURE 14.11 Relationship between the difference in temperature and flux assessed by LDI of the lesion and surrounding area of the lesion of each subject. A positive correlation was observed between these two methods ($R = .8, p < .001$). (Taken from Hassan et al., *TCRT*, 3, 451–457, 2004. With permission.)

FIGURE 14.12 (See color insert.) Typical example of lesion obtained from a subject with KS (a) before, and (b) after the treatment. Improvement after the treatment can be assessed by the thermal or LDI images after 18 weeks. Shown is a patient from the clinical trial reported in Reference 95.

skin of the lesion, whereas the thermal signature provided a combined response of superficial vascularity and metabolic activities of deep tissue.

In patients treated with an anti-KS therapy, there was a substantial decrease in temperature and blood velocity during the initial 18-week treatment period, as shown in Figure 14.12 [95]. The changes in these two parameters were generally greater than those assessed by either measurement of tumor size or palpation. In fact, there was no statistically significant decrease in tumor size overall. These results suggest that thermography and LDI may be relatively more sensitive in assessing the response of therapy in KS than conventional approaches. Assessing responses to KS therapy is now generally performed by visual measuring and palpating the numerous lesions and using rather complex response criteria. However, the current tools are rather cumbersome and often subject to observer variation, complicating the assessment of new therapies. The techniques described earlier, possibly combined with other techniques to assess vasculature and vessel function, have the potential of being more quantitative, sensitive, and reproducible than established techniques.

Recently, near-infrared spectroscopy (NIS), a noncontact and noninvasive method of monitoring changes in concentrations of blood volume and oxygenated- and deoxygenated hemoglobin, has been added to the clinical study to assess the pathogenesis of the status and changes of KS lesions during therapy. Such an approach can be used to provide early markers for tumor responses and to learn about the pathophysiology of the disease and its changes in response to treatment.

NIS is most closely related to visual assessment. With S. Demos at the Lawrence Livermore National Laboratory, a portable spectral imaging system was designed that captures images with a high-resolution CCD camera at six NIR wavelengths (700, 750, 800, 850, 900, and 1000 nm). A white light held approximately 15 cm from tissue illuminates the surface uniformly. Using optical filters, images are obtained at the six wavelengths, and the intensity images are used in a mathematical optical model of skin containing two layers: an epidermis and a much thicker, highly scattering dermis. Each layer contains major chromophores that determine absorption in the corresponding layer, and the layers together determine the total reflectance of the skin. Local variations in melanin, oxygenated hemoglobin (HbO_2), and blood volume can be reconstructed through a multivariate analysis.

For the mathematical optical skin model, the effect of the thin epidermis layer on the intensity of the diffusely reflected light is determined by the effective attenuation of light, A_{epi}:

$$A_{epi}(\lambda) = e^{-\mu_{a(epi)}(\lambda)t}, \quad (14.17)$$

where $\mu_{a(epi)}(\lambda)t$ is the epidermis absorption coefficient [mm^{-1}], λ is the wavelength [nm], and t is the thickness of the epidermis [mm]. The epidermis absorption coefficient is determined by the percentage of melanin, the absorption coefficient of melanin, and the absorption coefficient of normal tissue. Researchers have used different equations to calculate the melanin [103,104] and baseline skin [103–106] absorption coefficients. This model uses the equations of Meglinski and Matcher [107] and Jacques [103] for the melanin and baseline skin absorption coefficients, respectively. The influence of the much thicker, highly scattering dermis layer on the skin reflectance should be estimated by a stochastic model of photon migration (e.g., random walk theory). Fitting the known random walk expression for diffuse reflectivity of the turbid slab [45] yields a formula that depends on the reduced scattering coefficient and dermis absorption coefficient. The dermis absorption coefficient is based on the volume of blood in the tissue and hemoglobin oxygenation, that is, relative fractions of HbO_2 and deoxygenated hemoglobin (Hb). At wavelengths greater than 850 nm, the contribution of water and lipids should be taken into account. The absorption coefficient of blood was calculated by the volume fraction of HbO_2 times the absorption coefficient of HbO_2 plus the volume fraction of Hb times the absorption coefficient of Hb. In the dermis, large cylindrical collagen fibers are responsible for Mie scattering, while smaller scale collagen fibers and other microstructures are responsible for Rayleigh scattering [103]. The reduced scattering coefficient was calculated by combining Mie and Rayleigh components [108].

Each multispectral image was corrected for the light intensity, light source and camera. Then each was divided by a weight factor to bring the intensity of the images into the physiologically acceptable range. A best-fit procedure was used to reconstruct for the melanin volume, HbO_2 fraction, and blood volume fraction. For this preliminary study, the epidermis thickness was assumed to be constant at 60 μm [108] and the melanin content was based on Reference 109.

An example of multimodality images obtained from a KS patient before any anti-KS therapy is shown in Figure 14.13. Relatively high contrast of HbO_2 and tissue blood volume are observed in the tumor

FIGURE 14.13 (See color insert.) Set of comparative images of a KS patient. (a) Visual, (b) thermal, (c) laser Doppler, (d) HbO_2 fraction, and (e) tissue blood volume fraction images are provided [110].

region, which is expected for a metabolically active tumor. The normal tissue blood volume fraction is approximately 5%. This follows previous research that the volume fraction of blood in tissue is 0.2 to 5% [110].

The novel imaging modality could potentially be used as predictive tools for the outcome, and therefore also used for individualization of therapeutic strategies.

Acknowledgments

Special thanks go to Dr. Herbert Rinneberg (Physikalich-Techniche-Bundesanstalt, Berlin) and Dr. Brian Pogue (Dartmouth College) for providing optical images. The authors also wish to express their thanks to Dr. Tatsuo Togawa, a former professor of the Institutes of Biomaterials and Bioengineering, Tokyo Medical and Dental University, Tokyo, Japan, for his valuable suggestions and for allowing emissivity measurements to be performed in his lab. The authors also thank Stavros Demos at the Lawrence Livermore National Laboratory for helping to design and construct the multispectral imaging system used in the KS clinical trials.

References

[1] M. Born and E. Wolf, *Principles in Optics*, 7th ed. Cambridge: Cambridge University Press, 1999.
[2] A. T. Young, Rayleigh Scattering, *Physics Today*, 42, 1982.
[3] I. S. Saidi, S. L. Jacques, and F. K. Tittel, Mie and Rayleigh modeling of visible-light scattering in neonatal skin, *Applied Optics*, 34, 7410, 1995.
[4] M. J. C. Van Gemert, S. L. Jacques, H. J. C. M. Sterenberg, and W. M. Star, Skin optics, *IEEE Transactions*, 36, 1146, 1989.
[5] R. Marchesini, A. Bertoni, S. Andreola, E. Melloni, and A. Sicherolli, Extinction and absorption coefficients and scattering phase functions of human tissues *in vitro*, *Applied Optics*, 28, 2318, 1989.
[6] J. Fishkin, O. Coquoz, E. Anderson, M. Brenner, and B. Tromberg, Frequency-domain photon migration measurements of normal and malignant tissue optical properties in a human subject, *Applied Optics*, 36, 10, 1997.
[7] T. L. Troy, D. L. Page, and E. M. Sevick-Muraca, Optical properties or normal and diseased breast tissues: prognosis for optical mammography, *Journal of Biomedical Optics*, 1, 342, 1996.
[8] A. H. Gandjbakhche, R. F. Bonner, and R. Nossal, Scaling relationships for anisotropic random walks, *Journal of Statistical Physics*, 69, 35, 1992.
[9] G. A. Wagnieres, W. M. Star, and B. C. Wilson, *In vivo* fluorescence spectroscopy and imaging for oncological applications, *Photochemistry and Photobiology*, 68, 603, 1998.
[10] R. Weissleder, A clearer vision for *in vivo* imaging, *Nature Biotechnology*, 19, 316, 2001.
[11] V. F. Kamalov, I. A. Struganova, and K. Yoshihara, Temperature dependent radiative lifetime of J-aggregates, *Journal of Physical Chemistry*, 100, 8640, 1996.
[12] S. Mordon, J. M. Devoisselle, and V. Maunoury, *In vivo* pH measurement and imaging of a pH-sensitive fluorescent probe (5-6 carboxyfluorescein): instrumental and experimental studies, *Photochemistry and Photobiology*, 60, 274, 1994.
[13] C. L. Hutchinson, J. R. Lakowicz, and E. M. Sevick-Muraca, Fluorescence lifetime-based sensing in tissues: a computational study, *Biophysical Journal*, 68, 1574, 1995.
[14] F. F. Jobsis, Noninvasive infrared monitoring of cerebral and myocardial oxygen sufficiency and circulatory parameters, *Science*, 198, 1264, 1977.
[15] T. J. Farrell, M. S. Patterson, and B. Wilson, A diffusion theory model of spatially resolved, steady-state diffuse reflectance for the noninvasive determination of tissue optical properties *in vivo*, *Medical Physics*, 9, 879, 1992.
[16] P. C. Jackson, P. H. Stevens, J. H. Smith, D. Kear, H. Key, and P. N. T. Wells, Imaging mammalian tissues and organs using laser collimated transillumination, *Journal Biomedical Engineering*, 6, 70, 1987.

[17] G. Jarry, S. Ghesquiere, J. M. Maarek, F. Fraysse, S. Debray, M.-H. Bui, and D. Laurent, Imaging mammalian tissues and organs using laser collimated transillumination, *Journal of Biomedical Engineeing*, 6, 70, 1984.

[18] M. Kaneko, M. Hatakeyama, P. He et al., Construction of a laser transmission photo-scanner: pre-clinical investigation, *Radiation Medicine*, 7, 129, 1989.

[19] L. Wang, P. P. Ho, C. Liu, G. Zhang, and R. R. Alfano, Ballistic 2-D imaging through scattering walls using an ultrafast optical Kerr gate, *Science*, 253, 769, 1991.

[20] A. Schmitt, R. Corey, and P. Saulnier, Imaging through random media by use of low-coherence optical heterodyning, *Optics Letters*, 20, 404, 1995.

[21] H. Inaba, M. Toida, and T. Ichmua, Optical computer-assisted tomography realized by coherent detection imaging incorporating laser heterodyne method for biomedical applications, *SPIE Proceedings*, 1399, 108, 1990.

[22] H. Inaba, Coherent detection imaging for medical laser tomography, In G. Muller (ed.) *Medical Optical Tomography: Functional Imaging and Monitoring.*, 317, 1993.

[23] S. B. Colak, D. G. Papaioannou, G. W. T'Hoooft, M. B. van der Mark, H. Schomberg, J. C. J. Paasschens, J. B. M. Melissen, and N. A. A. J. van Austen, Tomographis image reconstruction from optical projections in light diffusing media, *Applied Optics*, 36, 180, 1997.

[24] J. C. Hebden, D. J. Hall, M. Firbank, and D. T. Delpry, Time-resolved optical imaging of a solid tissue-equivalent phantom, *Applied Optics*, 34, 8038, 1995.

[25] J. C. Hebden, Evaluating the spatial resolution performance of a time-resolved optical imaging system, *Medical Physics*, 19, 1081, 1992.

[26] R. Cubeddu, A. Pifferi, P. Taroni, A. Torriceli, and G. Valentini, Time-resolved imaging on a realistic tissue phantom: us' and ua images versus time-integrated images, *Applied Optics*, 35, 4533, 1996.

[27] D. Grosenick, H. Wabnitz, H. Rinneberg, K. T. Moesta, and P. Schleg, Development of a time-domain optical mammograph and first *in-vivo* application, *Applied Optics*, 38, 2927, 1999.

[28] M. Bashkansky, C. Adler, and J. Reinties, Coherently amplified Raman polarization gate for imaging through scattering media, *Optics Letters*, 19, 350, 1994.

[29] K. M. Yoo, Q. Xing, and R. R. Alfano, Imaging objects hidden in highly scattering media using femtosecond second-harmonic-generation cross-correlation time gating, *Optics Letters*, 16, 1019, 1991.

[30] G. W. Faris and M. Banks, Upconverting time gate for imaging through highly scattering media, *Optics Letters*, 19, 1813, 1994.

[31] J. C. Hebden, S. R. Arridge, and D. T. Delpry, Optical imaging in medicine I: experimental techniques, *Physics in Medicine and Biology*, 42, 825, 1997.

[32] J. R. Lakowitz and K. Brendt, Frequency domain measurements of photon migration in tissues, *Chemical Physics Letters*, 166, 246, 1990.

[33] M. A. Franceschini, K. T. Moesta, S. Fantini, G. Gaida, E. Gratton, H. Jess, W. W. Mantulin, M. Seeber, P. M. Schlag, and M. Kaschke, Frequency-domain techniques enhance optical mammography: initial clinical results, *Proceedings of the National Academy of Science, Medical Sciences*, 94, 6468, 1997.

[34] B. Tromberg, O. Coquoz, J. B. Fishkin, T. Pham, E. Anderson, J. Butler, M. Cahn, J. D. Gross, V. Venugopalan, and D. Pham, Non-invasive measurements of breast tissue optical properties using frequency-domain photon migration, *Philosophical Transactions of the Royal Society London Series*, B352, 661, 1997.

[35] J. J. Duderstadt and L. J. Hamilton, *Nuclear Reactor Analysis*. New York: Wiley, 1976.

[36] K. M. Case and P. F. Zweifel, *Linear Transport Theory*. Reading: Addison Wesley, 1967.

[37] A. Ishimaru, *Wave Propogation and Scattering in Random Media*. New York: Academic Press, 1978.

[38] M. S. Patterson, B. Chance, and B. Wilson, Time resolved reflectance and transmittance for the non-invasive measurement of tissue optical properties, *Applied Optics*, 28, 2331, 1989.

[39] S. R. Arridge and J. C. Hebden, Optical imaging in medicine: II. Modelling and reconstruction, *Physics Medicine and Biology*, 42, 841, 1997.

[40] S. R. Nioka, M. Miwa, S. Orel, M. Schnall, M. Haida, S. Zhao, and B. Chance, Optical imaging of human breast cancer, *Advances in Experimental Medicine and Biology*, 361, 171, 1994.

[41] S. Fantini, S. A. Walker, M. A. Franceschini, M. Kaschke, P. M. Schlag, and K. T. Moesta, Assessment of the size, position, and optical properties of breast tumors *in vivo* by noninvasive optical methods, *Applied Optics*, 37, 1982, 1998.

[42] M. Maris, E. Gratton, J. Maier, W. Mantulin, and B. Chance, Functional near-infrared imaging of deoxygenated haemoglobin during exercise of the finger extensor muscles using the frequency-domain techniques, *Bioimaging*, 2, 174, 1994.

[43] B. W. Pogue and K. D. Paulsen, High-resolution near-infrared tomographic imaging simulations of the rat cranium by use of a priori magnetic resonance imaging structural information, *Optics Letters*, 23, 1716, 1998.

[44] R. F. Bonner, R. Nossal, S. Havlin, and G. H. Weiss, Model for photon migration in turbid biological media, *Journal of Optical Society of American A*, 4, 423, 1987.

[45] A. H. Gandjbakhche and G. H. Weiss, Random walk and diffusion-like models of photon migration in turbid media, In E. Wolf (ed.), *Progress in Optics. Elsevier Science B.V.*, Vol. XXXIV, 333, 1995.

[46] A. H. Gandjbakhche, R. Nossal, and R. F. Bonner, Scaling relationships for theories of anisotropic random walks applied to tissue optics, *Applied Optics*, 32, 504, 1993.

[47] V. Chernomordik, R. Nossal, and A. H. Gandjbakhche, Point spread functions of photons in time-resolved transillumination experiments using simple scaling arguments, *Medical Physics*, 23, 1857, 1996.

[48] A. H. Gandjbakhche, G. H. Weiss, R. F. Bonner, and R. Nossal, Photon path-length distributions for transmission through optically turbid slabs, *Physical Review E*, 48, 810, 1993.

[49] D. J. Hawrysz and E. M. Sevick-Muraca, Developments toward diagnostic breast cancer imaging using near-infrared optical measurements and fluorescent contract agents, *Neoplasia*, 2, 388, 2000.

[50] M. Cutler, Transillumination as an aid in the diagnosis of breast lesions, *Surgery Gynecology and Obstetrics*, 48, 721, 1929.

[51] A. H. Gandjbakhche, V. Chernomordik, J. C. Hebden, and R. Nossal, Time-dependent contract functions for quantitative imaging in time-resolved transillumination experiments, *Applied Optics*, 37, 1973, 1998.

[52] A. H. Gandjbakhche, R. Nossal, and R. F. Bonner, Resolution limits for optical transillumination of abnormalities deeply embedded in tissues, *Medical Physics*, 21, 185, 1994.

[53] V. Chernomordik, D. Hattery, A. Pifferi, P. Taroni, A. Torricelli, G. Valentini, R. Cubeddu, and A. H. Gandjbakhche, A random walk methodology for quantification of the optical characteristics of abnormalities embedded within tissue-like phantoms, *Optics Letters*, 25, 951, 2000.

[54] M. Morin, S. Verreault, A. Mailloux, S. Frechette, Y. Chatingny, Y. Painchaud, and P. Beaudry, Inclusion characterization in a scattering slab with time-resolved transmittance measurements: perturbation analysis, *Applied Optics*, 39, 2840–2852, 2000.

[55] V. Chernomordik, D. W. Hattery, D. Grosenick, H. Wabnitz, H. Rinneberg, K. T. Moesta, P. M. Schlag, and A. Gandjbakhche, Quantification of optical properties of a breast tumor using random walk theory, *Journal of Biomedical Optics*, 7, 80–87, 2002.

[56] A. P. Gibson, J. C. Hebden, and S. R. Arridge, Recent advances in diffuse optical imaging, *Physics in Medicine and Biology*, 50, R1–R43, 2005.

[57] R. I. E. Fox, Sjogren syndrome, *Rhematic Disease Clinic of North America*, 1992.

[58] V. Chernomordik, D. Hattery, I. Gannot, and A. H. Gandjbakhche, Inverse method 3D reconstruction of localized *in-vivo* fluorescence. Application to Sjogren syndrome, *IEEE Journal of Selected Topics in Quantum Electronics*, 5, 930, 1999.

[59] M. S. Patterson and B. W. Pogue, Mathematical model for time-resolved and frequency-domain fluorescence spectroscopy in biological tissue, *Applied Optics*, 33, 1963, 1994.

[60] A. H. Gandjbakhche, R. F. Bonner, R. Nossal, and G. H. Weiss, Effects on multiple passage probabilities on fluorescence signals from biological media, *Applied Optics*, 36, 4613, 1997.

[61] D. Hattery, V. Chernomordik, M. Loew, I. Gannot, and A. H. Gandjbakhche, Analytical solutions for time-resolved fluorescence lifetime imaging in a turbid medium such as tissue, *Journal of the Optical Society of America A*, 18, 1523, 2001.

[62] E. Samuel, Thermography—some clinical applications, *Biomedical Engineering*, 4, 15–19, 1969.

[63] C. H. Jones, Physical aspects of thermography in relation to clinical techniques, *Bibl Radiology*, 1–8, 1975.

[64] J. Hardy, The radiation power of human skin in the infrared, *American Journal of Physiology*, 127, 454–462, 1939.

[65] J. Steketee, Spectral emissivity of skin and pericardium, *Physics in Medicine Biology*, 18, 686–694, 1973.

[66] R. Elam, D. Goodwin, and K. Willams, Optical properties of human epidermics, *Nature*, 198, 1001–1002, 1963.

[67] D. J. Watmough and R. Oliver, Emissivity of human skin in the waveband between 2 micron and 6 micron, *Nature*, 219, 622–624, 1968.

[68] K. D. Patil and K. L. Willaiam, Spectral study of human radiation. Non-ionizing Radiation, *Non-ionizing Radiation*, 1, 39–44, 1969.

[69] T. Togawa, Non-contact skin emissivity: measurement from reflectance using step change in ambient radiation temperature, *Clinical Physics and Physiological Measures*, 10, 39–48, 1989.

[70] M. Hassan and T. Togawa, Observation of skin thermal inertia distribution during reactive hyperaemia using a single-hood measurement system, *Physiological Measures*, 22, 187–200, 2001.

[71] W. H. McAdams, *Heat Transmission*, New York: Mc Graw Hill, p. 472, 1954.

[72] H. T. Hammel, J. D. Hardy, and D. Murgatroyd, Spectral transmittance and reflectance of excised human skin, *Journal of Applied Physiology*, 9, 257–264, 1956.

[73] D. M. McDonald and P. L. Choyke, Imaging of angiogenesis: from microscope to clinic, *Nature Medicine*, 9, 713–725, 2003.

[74] J. S. Taylor, P. S. Tofts, R. Port, J. L. Evelhoch, M. Knopp, W. E. Reddick, V. M. Runge, and N. Mayr, MR imaging of tumor microcirculation: promise for the new millennium, *Journal of Magnetic Resonance Imaging*, 10, 903–907, 1999.

[75] K. L. Verstraete, Y. De Deene, H. Roels, A. Dierick, D. Uyttendaele, and M. Kunnen, Benign and malignant musculoskeletal lesions: dynamic contrast-enhanced MR imaging—parametric "first-pass" images depict tissue vascularization and perfusion, *Radiology*, 192, 835–843, 1994.

[76] L. D. Buadu, J. Murakami, S. Murayama, N. Hashiguchi, S. Sakai, K. Masuda, S. Toyoshima, S. Kuroki, and S. Ohno, Breast lesions: correlation of contrast medium enhancement patterns on MR images with histopathologic findings and tumor angiogenesis, *Radiology*, 200, 639–649, 1996.

[77] A. Fredriksson and S. Stone-Elander, PET screening of anticancer drugs. A faster route to drug/target evaluations *in vivo*, *Methods in Molecular Medicine*, 85, 279-294, 2003.

[78] G. Jerusalem, R. Hustinx, Y. Beguin, and G. Fillet, The value of positron emission tomography (PET) imaging in disease staging and therapy assessment, *Annals Oncology*, 13, 227–234, 2002.

[79] H. C. Steinert, M. Hauser, F. Allemann, H. Engel, T. Berthold, G. K. von Schulthess, and W. Weder, Non-small cell lung cancer: nodal staging with FDG PET versus CT with correlative lymph node mapping and sampling, *Radiology*, 202, 441–446, 1997.

[80] S. D. Rockoff, The evolving role of computerized tomography in radiation oncology, *Cancer*, 39, 694–696, 1977.

[81] K. D. Hopper, K. Singapuri, and A. Finkel, Body CT and oncologic imaging, *Radiology*, 215, 27–40, 2000.

[82] K. A. Miles, M. Hayball, and A. K. Dixon, Colour perfusion imaging: a new application of computed tomography, *Lancet*, 337, 643–645, 1991.

[83] K. A. Miles, C. Charnsangavej, F. T. Lee, E. K. Fishman, K. Horton, and T. Y. Lee, Application of CT in the investigation of angiogenesis in oncology, *Academic Radiology*, 7, 840–850, 2000.

[84] N. Ferrara, Role of vascular endothelial growth factor in physiologic and pathologic angiogenesis: therapeutic implications, *Seminars in Oncology*, 29, 10–14, 2002.

[85] D. E. Goertz, D. A. Christopher, J. L. Yu, R. S. Kerbel, P. N. Burns, and F. S. Foster, High-frequency color flow imaging of the microcirculation, *Ultrasound in Medicine and Biology*, 26, 63–71, 2000.

[86] E. M. Gill, G. M. Palmer, and N. Ramanujam, Steady-state fluorescence imaging of neoplasia, *Methods in Enzymology*, 361, 452–481, 2003.

[87] K. Svanberg, I. Wang, S. Colleen, I. Idvall, C. Ingvar, R. Rydell, D. Jocham, H. Diddens, S. Bown, G. Gregory, S. Montan, S. Andersson-Engels, and S. Svanberg, Clinical multi-colour fluorescence imaging of malignant tumours—initial experience, *Acta Radiology*, 39, 2–9, 1998.

[88] V. Beral, T. A. Peterman, R. L. Berkelman, and H. W. Jaffe, Kaposi's sarcoma among persons with AIDS: a sexually transmitted infection? *Lancet*, 335, 123-128, 1990.

[89] B. A. Biggs, S. M. Crowe, C. R. Lucas, M. Ralston, I. L. Thompson, and K. J. Hardy, AIDS related Kaposi's sarcoma presenting as ulcerative colitis and complicated by toxic megacolon, *Gut*, 28, 1302-1306, 1987.

[90] E. Cornali, C. Zietz, R. Benelli, W. Weninger, L. Masiello, G. Breier, E. Tschachler, A. Albini, and M. Sturzl, Vascular endothelial growth factor regulates angiogenesis and vascular permeability in Kaposi's sarcoma, *American Journal of Pathology*, 149, 1851–1869, 1996.

[91] Y. Chang, E. Cesarman, M. S. Pessin, F. Lee, J. Culpepper, D. M. Knowles, and P. S. Moore, Identification of herpesvirus-like DNA sequences in AIDS-associated Kaposi's sarcoma, *Science*, 266, 1865–1869, 1994.

[92] R. Yarchoan, Therapy for Kaposi's sarcoma: recent advances and experimental approaches, *Journal of Acquired Immune Deficiency Syndrome*, 21 Suppl. 1, S66–S73, 1999.

[93] R. F. Little, K. M. Wyvill, J. M. Pluda, et al. Activity of thalidomide in AIDS-related Kaposi's sarcoma, *Journal of Clinical Oncology*, 18, 2593–2602, 2000.

[94] M. Hassan, D. Hattery, V. Chernomordik, K. Aleman, K. Wyvill, F. Merced, R. F. Little, R. Yarchoan, and A. Gandjbakhche, Non-invasive multi-modality technique to study angiogenesis associated with kaposi's sarcoma, *Proceedings of EMBS BMES*, 1139–1140, 2002.

[95] M. Hassan, R. F. Little, A. Vogel, K. Aleman, K. Wyvill, R. Yarchoan, and A. Gandjbakhche, Quantitative assessment of tumor vasculature and response to therapy in Kaposi's sarcoma using functional noninvasive imaging, *TCRT*, 3, In press, 2004.

[96] C. Maxwell-Cade, Principles and practice of clinical thermography, *Radiography*, 34, 23–34, 1968.

[97] J. F. Head and R. L. Elliott, Infrared imaging: making progress in fulfilling its medical promise, *IEEE Engineering in Medicine and Biology Magazine*, 21, 80–85, 2002.

[98] S. Bornmyr and H. Svensson, Thermography and laser-Doppler flowmetry for monitoring changes in finger skin blood flow upon cigarette smoking, *Clinical Physiology*, 11, 135–141, 1991.

[99] K. Usuki, T. Kanekura, K. Aradono, and T. Kanzaki, Effects of nicotine on peripheral cutaneous blood flow and skin temperature, *Journal of Dermatology Science*, 16, 173–181, 1998.

[100] M. Anbar, Clinical thermal imaging today, *IEEE Engineering in Medicine and Biology Magazine*, 17, 25–33, 1998.

[101] J. Sorensen, M. Bengtsson, E. L. Malmqvist, G. Nilsson, and F. Sjoberg, Laser Doppler perfusion imager (LDPI)—for the assessment of skin blood flow changes following sympathetic blocks, *Acta Anaesthesiologica Scandinavica*, 40, 1145–1148, 1996.

[102] A. Rivard, J. E. Fabre, M. Silver, D. Chen, T. Murohara, M. Kearney, M. Magner, T. Asahara, and J. M. Isner, Age-dependent impairment of angiogenesis, *Circulation*, 99, 111–120, 1999.

[103] S. L. Jacques, Skin optics, http://omlc.ogi.edu/news/jan98/skinoptics.html, 1998.

[104] R. Zhang, W. Verkruysse, B. Choi, J. A. Viator, B. Jung, L. O. Svaasand, G. Aguilar, and J. S. Nelson, Determination of human skin optical properties from spectrophotometric measurements based on optimization by genetic algorithms, *Journal of Biomedical Optics*, 10, 024030, 2005.

[105] L. F. A. Douven and G. W. Lucassen, Retrieval of optical properties of skin from measurement and modeling the diffuse reflectance, *Proceedings of SPIE*, 3914, 312–323, 2000.

[106] L. O. Svaasand, L. T. Norvang, E. J. Fiskerstrand, E. K. S. Stopps, M. W. Berns, and J. S. Nelson, Tissue parameters determining the visual appearance of normal skin and port-wine stains, *Lasers in Medical Science*, 10, 55–65, 1995.

[107] I. V. Meglinski and S. J. Matcher, Quantitative assessment of skin layers absorption and skin reflectance spectra simulation in the visible and near-infrared spectral regions, *Physiological Measures*, 23, 741–753, 2002.

[108] I. Nishidate, Y. Aizu, and H. Mishina, Estimation of absorbing components in a local layer embedded in the turbid media on the basis of visible and near-infrared (VIS-NIR) reflectance spectra, *Optical Review*, 10, 427–435, 2003.

[109] S. L. Jacques, Origins of tissue optical properties in the UVA, visible, and NIR regions, *R.R. Alfano and James G. Fujimoto* (eds.) *OSA TOPS on Advances in Optical Imaging and Photon Migration.*, Vol. 2, pp. 364–371, 1996.

[110] A. Vogel, M. Hassan, F. Amyot, V. Chernomordik, S. Demos, R. Little, R. Yarchoan, and A. H. Gandjbakhche, Using multi-modality imaging techniques to assess vascularity in AIDS-related Kaposi's Sarcoma, *Biomedical Optics*, 2006, Technical Digest, SG2, 2006.

15
Biomedical Applications of Functional Infrared Imaging

Arcangelo Merla
Gian Luca Romani
University of G. d'Annunzio

15.1	Introduction...	**15**-1
15.2	Diagnosis of Varicocele and Follow-Up of the Treatment...	**15**-2
15.3	Raynaud's Phenomenon and Scleroderma.............	**15**-4
15.4	Quantifying the Relevance and Stage of Disease with the τ Image Technique	**15**-7
15.5	Skin Temperature and Metabolism during Exercise...	**15**-11
15.6	Discussion and Conclusion	**15**-17
References		**15**-17

15.1 Introduction

Infrared imaging allows the representation of the surface thermal distribution of the human body. Several studies have been performed so far to assess the contribution that such information may provide to the clinicians. The skin temperature distribution of the human body depends on the complex relationships defining the heat exchange processes between skin tissue, inner tissue, local vasculature, and metabolic activity. All of these processes are mediated and regulated by the sympathetic and parasympathetic activity to maintain the thermal homeostasis. The presence of a disease can locally affect the heat balance or exchange processes, resulting in an increase or a decrease of the skin temperature. Such a temperature change can be better estimated with respect to the surrounding regions or the unaffected contra lateral region. But then, the dynamics of the local control of the skin temperature should also be influenced by the presence of the disease. Therefore, the characteristic parameters modeling the activity of the skin thermoregulatory system can be used as diagnostic parameters. The functional infrared (fIR) imaging—also named infrared functional imaging (IFRI imaging)—is the study for diagnostic purposes, based on the modeling of the bio-heat exchange processes, of the functional properties and alterations of the human thermoregulatory system. In this chapter, we will review some of the most important recent clinical applications of the fIR imaging of our group.

FIGURE 15.1 (See color insert at the back of the book.) (a) Second-grade right varicocele. The temperature distribution all over the scrotum clearly highlights significant differences between affected and unaffected testicles. (b) The same scrotum after varicocelectomy. The surgical treatment reduced the increased temperature on the affected hemiscrotum and restored the symmetry in the scrotal temperature distribution. (c) Third-grade left varicocele. (d) The same scrotum after varicocelectomy. The treatment was unsuccessful in repairing the venous reflux, as documented by the persisting asymmetric scrotal distribution.

15.2 Diagnosis of Varicocele and Follow-Up of the Treatment

Varicocele is a widely spread male disease caused by a dilatation of the pampiniform venous plexus and of the internal spermatic vein. Consequences of such a dilatation are an increase of the scrotal temperature and a possible impairment of the potential fertility [44,58,59]. In normal men, testicular temperature is 3 to 4°C lower than core body temperature [44]. Two thermoregulatory processes maintain this lower temperature: heat exchange with the environment through the scrotal skin and heat clearance by blood flow through the pampiniform plexus. Venous stasis due to the varicocele may increase the temperature of the affected testicle or pampiniform plexus. Thus, an abnormal temperature difference between the two hemiscrota may suggest the presence of varicocele [34,59], see Figure 15.1. Telethermography can reveal abnormal temperature differences between the two testicles and altered testicular thermal recovery after an induced cold stress. Affected testicles return to pre-stress equilibrium temperatures faster than do normal testicles [34]. fIR imaging has been used to determine whether altered scrotal thermoregulation is related to subclinical varicocele [42]. In a study conducted in 2001, Merla and Romani enrolled 60 volunteers, 18 to 27 years of age (average age, 21 ± 2 years), with no symptoms or clinical history of varicocele. After clinical examination, echo color Doppler imaging (the gold standard) and fIR imaging were performed. fIR imaging evaluation consisted of obtaining scrotal images, measuring the basal temperature at the level of the pampiniform plexus (T_p) and the testicles (T_t), and determining thermal recovery of the scrotum after cold thermal stress. The temperature curve of the hemiscrotum during rewarming showed an exponential pattern and was, therefore, fitted to an exponential curve. The time constant τ of the best exponential fit depends on the thermal properties of the scrotum and its blood perfusion [34,38]. Therefore, τ provides a quantitative parameter assessing how much the scrotal thermoregulation is affected by varicocele. Cooling was achieved by applying a dry patch to the scrotum that was 10°C colder than the basal scrotal temperature. The fIR measurements were performed accordingly usual standardization procedures [28]. The basal prestress temperature and the recovery time constant τ_p at the level of the pampiniform plexus and of the testicles (τ_t) were evaluated on each hemiscrotum. A basal testicular temperature greater than 32°C and basal pampiniform plexus temperature greater than 34°C were considered warning thresholds. Temperature differences among testicles (ΔT_t) or pampiniform plexus ΔT_p temperature greater than 1.0°C were also considered warning values, as were $\Delta \tau_t$ and $\Delta \tau_t$ values longer than 1.5 min. The fIR imaging evaluation classified properly the stages of disease, as confirmed by the echo color Doppler imaging and clinical examination in a blinded manner.

In 38 subjects, no warning basal temperatures or differences in rewarming temperatures were observed. These subjects were considered to be normal according to fIR imaging. Clinical examination and echo color Doppler imaging confirmed the absence of varicocele ($p < .01$, one-way ANOVA test).

In 22 subjects, one or more values were greater than the warning threshold for basal temperatures or differences in rewarming temperatures. Values for ΔT_p and the $\Delta \tau_p$ were higher than the warning thresholds in 8 of the 22 subjects, who were classified as having grade 1 varicocele. Five subjects had ΔT_t and $\Delta \tau_t$ values higher than the threshold. In nine subjects, three or more fIR imaging values were greater than the warning threshold values. The fIR imaging classification was grade 3 varicocele. Clinical examination and echo color Doppler imaging closely confirmed the fIR imaging evaluation of the stage of the varicocele. fIR imaging yielded no false-positive or false-negative results. All participants with positive results on fIR imaging also had positive results on clinical examination and echo color Doppler imaging. The sensitivity and specificity of fIR test were 100 and 93%, respectively. An abnormal change in the temperature of the testicles and pampiniform plexus may indicate varicocele, but the study demonstrated that impaired thermoregulation is associated with varicocele-induced alteration of blood flow. Time to recovery of prestress temperature in the testicles and pampiniform plexus appears to assist in classification of the disease. fIR imaging accurately detected 22 no symptomatic varicoceles.

The control of the scrotum temperature should improve after varicocelectomy as a complementary effect of the reduction of the blood reflux. Moreover, follow-up of the changes in scrotum thermoregulation after varicocelectomy may provide early indications on possible relapses of the disease.

To answer the above questions, Merla et al. [30] used fIR imaging to study changes in the scrotum thermoregulation of 20 patients (average age, 27 ± 5 years) that were judged eligible for varicocelectomy on the basis of the combined results of the clinical examination, echo color Doppler imaging, and spermiogram. No bilateral varicoceles were included in the study.

Patients underwent clinical examination, echo color Doppler imaging and instrument varicocele grading, and fIR evaluation before varicocelectomy and every 2 weeks thereafter, up to the 24th week. Out of the 20 patients 14 suffered from grade 2 left varicocele. All of them were characterized by basal temperatures and recovery time after cold stress according to Reference 30. Varicoceles were surgically treated via interruption of the internal spermatic vein using modified Palomo's technique. fIR imaging documented the changes in the thermoregulatory control of the scrotum after the treatment as following: 13 out of the 14 grade 2 varicocele patients exhibited normal basal T_t, T_p on the varicocele side of the scrotum, and normal temperature differences ΔT_t and ΔT_p starting from the fourth week after varicocelectomy. Their $\Delta \tau_t$ and $\Delta \tau_p$ values returned to normal range from the fourth to the sixth week. Four out of the six grade 3 varicocele patients exhibited normal basal T_t, T_p on the varicocele side of the scrotum, and normal temperature differences ΔT_t and ΔT_p starting from the sixth week after varicocelectomy. Their $\Delta \tau_t$ and $\Delta \tau_p$ values returned to normal range from the sixth to the eighth week. The other three patients did not return to normal values of the above specified parameters. In particular, $\Delta \tau_t$ and $\Delta \tau_p$ remained much longer than the threshold warning values [30] up to the last control (Figure 15.1). Echo color Doppler imaging and clinical examination assessed relapses of the disease. The study proved that the surgical treatment of the varicocele induces modification in the thermoregulatory properties of the scrotum, reducing the basal temperature of the affected testicle and pampiniform plexus, and slowing down its recovery time after thermal stress. Among the 17 with no relapse, 4 exhibited return to normal T_t, T_p, ΔT_t, and ΔT_p for the lateroanterior side of the scrotum, while the posterior side of the scrotum remained hyperthermal or characterized by ΔT_t and ΔT_p higher than the threshold warning value. This fact suggested that the surgical treatment via interruption of the internal spermatic vein using Palomo's technique may not be the most suitable method for those varicoceles. The time required for the scrotum to restore normal temperature distribution and control seems to be positively correlated to the volume and duration of the blood reflux lasting: the greater the blood reflux, the longer the time. The study demonstrated that IR imaging may provide early indication on the possible relapsing of the disease and may be used as a suitable complementary follow-up tool.

15.3 Raynaud's Phenomenon and Scleroderma

Raynaud's phenomenon (RP) is defined as a painful vasoconstriction—that may follow cold or emotional stress—of small arteries and arterioles of extremities, like fingers and toes. RP can be primary (PRP) or secondary (SSc) to scleroderma. The latter is usually associated with a connective tissues disease. RP precedes the systemic autoimmune disorders development, particularly scleroderma, by many years and it can evolve into secondary RP. The evaluation of vascular disease is crucial in order to distinguish between PRP and SSc. In PRP, episodic ischemia in response to cold exposure or to emotional stimuli is usually completely reversible: absence of tissue damage is the typical feature [2], but also mild structural changes are demonstrated [57]. In contrast, scleroderma RP shows irreversible tissue damage and severe structural changes in the finger vascular organization [27,48,50]. None of the physiological measurement techniques currently in use, except infrared imaging, are completely satisfactory in focusing primary or secondary RP [18]. The main limit of such techniques (nail fold capillary microscopy, cutaneous laser-Doppler flowmetry, and plethysmography) is the fact that they can proceed just into a partial investigation, usually assessing only one finger once. The measurement of skin temperature is an indirect method to estimate change in skin thermal properties and blood flow. Thermography protocols [8,10,18,21,46,49,54] usually include cold patch testing to evaluate the capability of the patient hands to rewarm. The pattern of the rewarming curves is usually used to depict the underlying structural diseases. Analysis of rewarming curves has been used in several studies to differentiate healthy subjects from PRP or SSc Raynaud's patients. Parameters usually considered so far are the lag time preceding the onset of rewarming or to reach a preset final temperature, the rate of the rewarming and the maximum temperature of recovery, and the degree of temperature variation between different areas of the hands.

Merla et al. [39] proposed to model the natural response of the fingertips to exposure to a cold environment to get a diagnostic parameter derived by the physiology of such a response. The thermal recovery following a cold stress is driven by thermal exchange with the environment, transport by the incoming blood flow, conduction from adjacent tissue layers, and metabolic processes. The finger temperature is determined by the net balance of the energy input/output. The more significant contributes come from the input power due to blood perfusion and the power lost to the environment [56,57]:

$$\frac{dQ}{dt} = -\frac{dQ_{env}}{dt} + \frac{dQ_{ctrl}}{dt} \tag{15.1}$$

Normal finger recovery after a cold stress is reported in Figure 15.2.

In absence of thermoregulatory control, fingers exchange heat only with the environment: in this case, their temperature T_{exp} follows an exponential pattern with time constant τ given by

$$\tau = \frac{\rho \cdot c \cdot V}{h \cdot A} \tag{15.2}$$

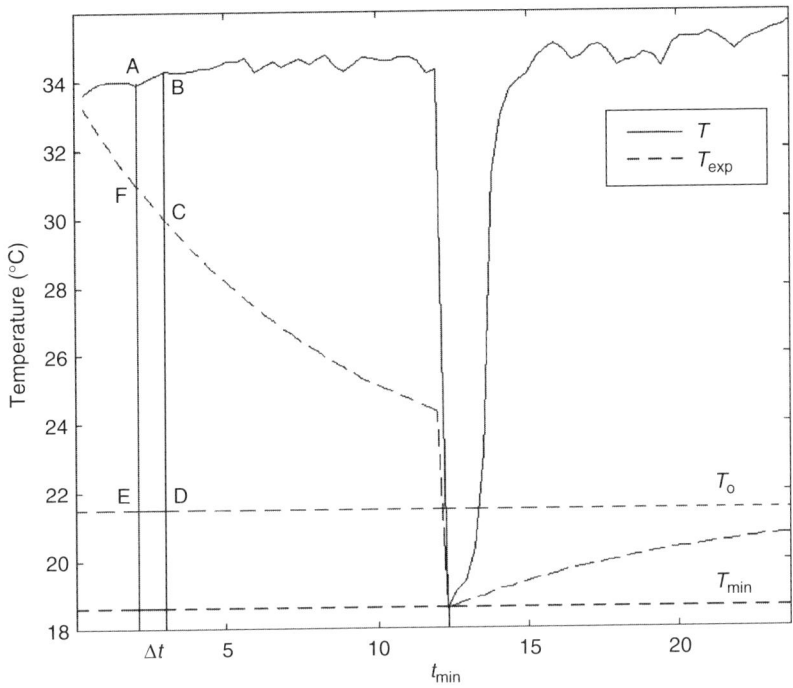

FIGURE 15.2 Experimental rewarming curves after cold stress in normal subjects. The continuous curve represents the recorded temperature finger. The outlined curve represents the exponential temperature pattern exhibited by the finger in absence of thermoregulatory control. In this case, the only heat source for the finger is the environment. (From Merla, A., et al., Infrared functional imaging applied to Raynaud's phenomenon, *IEEE Eng. Med. Biol. Mag.*, 21, 73, 2002, by permission of the editor.)

where ρ is the mass density, c the specific heat, V the finger volume, h is the combined heat transfer coefficient between the finger and the environment and A is the finger surface area. Thanks to the thermoregulatory control, the finger maintains its temperature T greater than T_{exp}. For a Δt time, the area of the trapezoid *ABCF* times $h \cdot A$ in Figure 15.2 computes the heat provided by the thermoregulatory system, namely ΔQ_{ctrl}. This amount summed to ΔQ_{env} yields Q, the global amount of heat stored in the finger.

Then, the area of the trapezoid *ABDE* is proportional to the amount Q of heat stored in the finger during a Δt interval. Therefore, Q can be computed integrating the area surrounded by the temperature curve T and the constant straight line T_o:

$$Q = -h \cdot A \cdot \int_{t_1}^{t_2} (T_o - T(\varsigma))d\varsigma \qquad (15.3)$$

where the minus sign takes into account that the heat stored by the finger is counted as positive. Q is intrinsically related to the finger thermal capacity, according to the expression

$$\Delta Q = \rho \cdot c \cdot V \cdot \Delta T \qquad (15.4)$$

Under the hypothesis of constant T_o, the numerical integration in (15.3) can be used to characterize the rewarming exhibited by a healthy or a suffering finger.

The Q parameter has been used in References 35 and 39 to discriminate and classify PRP, SSc, and healthy subjects on a set of 40 (20 PRP, 20 SSc) and 18 healthy volunteers. For each subject, the response to a mild cold challenge of hands in water was assessed by fIR imaging. Rewarming curves were recorded for each of the five fingers of both hands; the temperature integral Q was calculated along the 20 min following the cold stress. About 10 subjects, randomly selected within the 18 normal ones, repeated two times and in different days the test to evaluate the repeatability of the fIR imaging findings. The repeatability test confirmed that fIR imaging and Q computation is a robust tool to characterize the thermal recovery of the fingers.

The grand average Q values provided by the first measurement was $1060.0 \pm 130.5°C$ min, while for the second assessment it was $1012 \pm 135.1°C$ min ($p > .05$, one way ANOVA test). The grand average Q values for PRP, SSc, and healthy subjects groups are shown in Figure 15.3, whereas single values obtained for each finger of all of the subjects are reported in Figure 15.4. The results in References 35 and 39 highlight

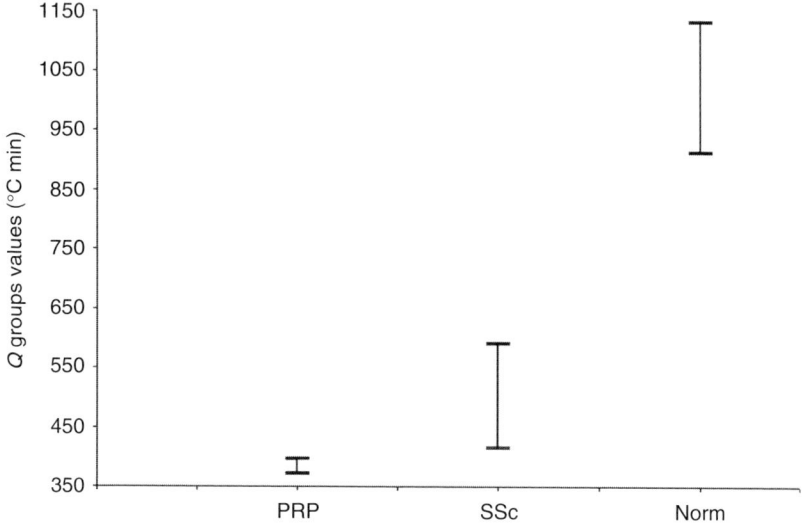

FIGURE 15.3 One-way ANOVA test applied to the Q parameter calculated for each group (PRP, SSc, and healthy). The Q parameter clearly discriminates the three groups. (From Merla, A., et al., Infrared functional imaging applied to Raynaud's phenomenon, *IEEE Eng. Med. Biol. Mag.*, 21, 73, 2002, by permission of the editor.)

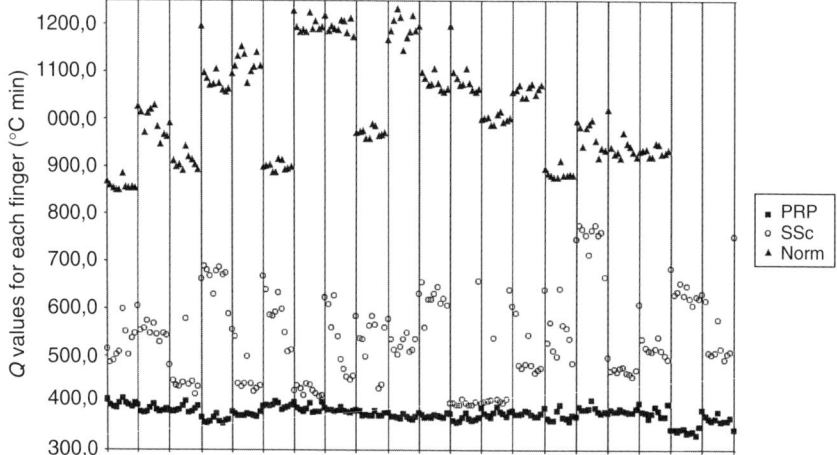

FIGURE 15.4 Q values calculated for each finger of each subjects. Vertical grid lines are placed to discriminate the ten fingers. PRP fingers are characterized by a strong intra and interindividual homogeneity. Greater mean Q values and greater intra and interindividual variations characterizes the SSc fingers. (From Merla, A., et al., Infrared functional imaging applied to Raynaud's phenomenon, *IEEE Eng. Med. Biol. Mag.*, 21, 73, 2002, by permission of the editor.)

that the PRP group features low intra- and interindividual variability, whereas the SSc group displays a large variability between healthy and unhealthy fingers. Q values for SSc finger are generally greater than PRP ones.

The temperature integral at different finger regions yields very similar results for all fingers of the PRP group, suggesting common thermal and BF properties. SSc patients showed different thermoregulatory responses in the different segments of finger. This feature is probably due to the local modification in the tissue induced by the scleroderma. Scleroderma patients also featured a significantly different behavior across the five fingers depending on the disease involvement.

In normal and PRP groups, all fingers show a homogeneous behavior and PRP fingers always exhibit a poorer recovery than normal ones. Additionally, in both groups, the rewarming always starts from the finger distal area differently from what happens in SSc patients. The sensitivity of the method in order to distinguish patients from normal is 100%. The specificity in distinguishing SSc from PRP is 95%.

Q clearly highlights the difference between PRP, SSc, and normal subjects. It provides useful information about the abnormalities of their thermoregulatory finger properties. The PRP patients exhibited common features in terms of rewarming. Such behavior can be explained in terms of an equally low and constant BF in all fingers and to differences in the amount of heat exchanged with the environment [48].

Conversely, no common behavior was found for the SSc patients, since their disease determines—for each finger—very different thermal and blood perfusion properties. Scleroderma seems to increase the tissue thermal capacity with a reduced ability to exchange. As calculated from the rewarming curves, Q parameter seems to be particularly effective to describe the thermal recovery capabilities of the finger. The method clearly highlighted the difference between PRP and SSc patients and provides useful information about the abnormalities of their thermal and thermoregulatory finger properties.

In consideration of the generally accepted theory that the different recovery curves of the patients is a reflection of the slow deterioration of the microcirculation, so that over time in the same patients, it is possible to observe changes in the thermal recovery curves, the method above described could be used for monitoring the clinical evolution of the disease. In addition, pharmacological treatment effects could be advantageously followed-up.

15.4 Quantifying the Relevance and Stage of Disease with the τ Image Technique

Infrared imaging can provide diagnostic information according different possible approaches. The approach generally followed consists of the detection of significant differences between the skin thermal distributions of the two hemisoma or in the pattern recognition of specific features with respect to average healthy population [5,9,11,15]. The underlying hypothesis is that the skin temperature distribution, at a given time, is considered at a steady-state. Of course this is a rough approximation of the reality because of the homeostasis. More valuable and quantitative information can be obtained from the study of the skin temperature dynamics in the unsteady state, where the processes involved and controlled by the thermoregulatory system can be modeled and described through their characteristic parameters. The presence of diseases interfering with the skin thermoregulatory system can be then inferred by the analysis of its functional alterations [28,38]. To enhance the functional content of the thermoregulatory response, one needs to pass through modeling of the thermal properties and dynamics of the skin thermoregulatory system. Such a modeling can bring more quantitative and detailed diagnostic parameters with respect to the particular disease being analyzed. Merla et al. [33,38,41] proposed a new imaging technique, based on this approach, for the clinical study of a variety of diseases. The theory behind the technique is based on the fact that the human thermoregulatory system maintains a reasonably constant body temperature against a wide range of environmental conditions. The body uses several physiologic processes to control the heat exchange with the environment. The mechanism controlling thermal emission and dermal microcirculation is driven by the sympathetic nervous system. A disease locally affecting

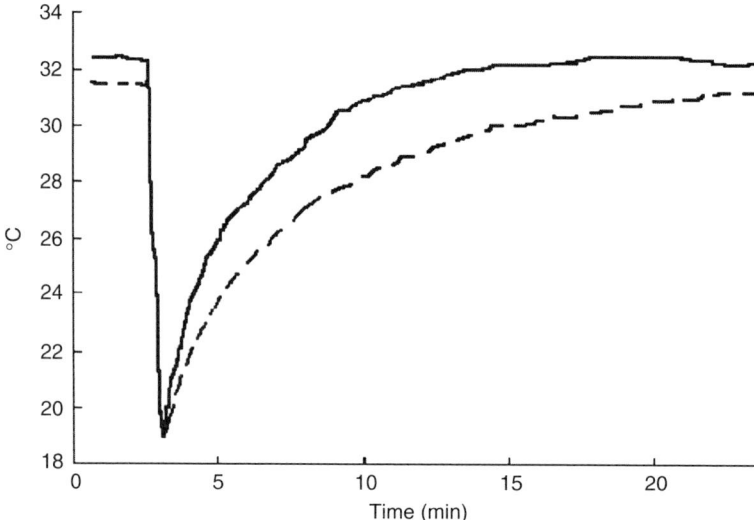

FIGURE 15.5 Muscular lesion on the left thigh abductor with hemorrhage shedding: thermal recovery curves following a cold thermal stress. The dotted line represents the recovery of a healthy area close to the damaged one. The continuous line represents the curve related to a muscular lesion region. Both recoveries exhibit exponential feature; the injured area exhibits a faster rewarming with a shorter time constant.

the thermoregulatory system (i.e., traumas, lesions, vein thrombosis, varicocele, dermatitis, RP and sclero-derma, etc.) may produce an altered sympathetic function and a change in the local metabolic rate. Local vasculature and microvasculature may be rearranged, resulting in a modification of the skin temperature distribution.

Starting from a general energy balance equation [3], it is straightforward to demonstrate that the recovery time from any kind of thermal stress for a given region of interest depends on its thermal properties. A given disease may alter the normal heat capacity and the tissue/blood ratio mass density of a region. An example is given in Figure 15.5 that shows the different thermoregulatory behaviors exhibited by two adjacent regions—one healthy and one affected by a muscular lesion—after local cooling applied to the skin.

A controlled thermal stress applied to the region of interest and the surrounding tissue permits to study and to model the response of the region itself. The most important terms involved in the energy balance during the recovery are the heat storage in the tissue, heat clearance by blood perfusion and convective heat exchange with the environment, as described by the following equation:

$$\frac{\partial T}{\partial t} \rho \cdot c \cdot V = h \cdot A(T_o - T) + \rho_{bl} \cdot c_{bl} \cdot w_{bl}(t) \cdot (T_{bl} - T) \tag{15.5}$$

where subscripts o and bl designate the properties of the environment and blood, respectively, while ρ is the density, c is the specific heat, V is the volume, T is the temperature, t is the time, h is the combined heat transfer coefficient between the skin and the environment, A is the surface area, and w is the blood perfusion rate.

The initial condition for (15.1) is

$$T = T_i, \quad \text{for } t = 0 \tag{15.6}$$

where T_i is the skin temperature and $t = 0$ is the time at the recovery starting.

Equation 15.1 can be easily integrated under the assumption of constant blood perfusion rate w_{bl} and blood temperature T_{bl}, yielding

$$T(t) = \frac{W \cdot (T_{bl} - T_o)}{W + H} + \left(T_i - T_o - \frac{W \cdot (T_{bl} - T_o)}{W + H}\right) \cdot e^{-(W+H) \cdot t} + T_o \quad (15.7)$$

where

$$H = \frac{h \cdot A}{\rho \cdot c \cdot V}; \quad W = \frac{\rho_{bl} \cdot c_{bl} \cdot w_{bl}}{\rho \cdot c \cdot V} \quad (15.8)$$

The time t_f to reach a certain preset (final) temperature T_f is then given by

$$t_f = -\frac{1}{W + H} \ln\left(\frac{(1 + H/W) \cdot (T_f - T_o) - W(T_{bl} - T_o)}{(1 + H/W) \cdot (T_i - T_o) - W(T_{bl} - T_o)}\right) \quad (15.9)$$

Equation 15.9, with the assumption of constant blood perfusion, relates the time to reach a pre-set temperature to the local thermal properties and to local blood perfusion.

The exponential solution described in Equation 15.7 suggests the usage of the time constant τ as a characterizing parameter for the description of the recovery process after any kind of controlled thermal stress, with τ mainly determined by the local blood flow and thermal capacity of the tissue. fIR imaging permits an easy evaluation of τ, which can be regarded as a parameter able to discriminate areas interested by the specific disease from healthy ones. Rather than a static imaging of the skin thermal distribution to pictorially describe the effect of the given disease, an image reporting pixel to pixel the τ recovery time can be used to characterize that disease [33,38,41]. Areas featuring an associated blood shedding, or an inflammatory state, or an increased blood reflux, often exhibit a faster recovery time with respect to the surroundings. Those areas exhibit then a smaller τ value. In contrast, in presence of localized calcifications, early ulcers or scleroderma, and impaired micro-vascular control, the involved areas show a slower recovery than the healthy surrounding areas and are therefore characterized by a longer τ time.

The reliability and value of the τ image technique rely on the good quality of the data and on their appropriate processing. While the interested reader can find a detailed description for proper materials and method for the τ image technique in Reference 38, it is worthwhile to report hereby the general algorithm for the method:

1. Subject marking (to permit movement correction of the thermal image series) and acclimation to the measurement room kept at controlled environmental conditions
2. Adequate calibration of the thermal imaging device
3. Recording of the baseline temperature dynamics for the region of interest
4. Execution of the thermal stress (usually performed through a cold or warm dry patch at controlled temperature and temperature exchange rate)
5. Recording of the thermal recovery until the complete restoration of the baseline features
6. Postprocessing movement correction of the thermal image series
7. Fitting of the pixel-by-pixel experimental recovery data to an exponential curve and extraction of the time constant τ for each pixel of the region of interest
8. Pixel-by-pixel color coding and mapping of the time constant τ values

The τ image technique has been first proposed as complementary diagnostic tool for the diagnosis of muscular lesions, RP and deep vein thrombosis [33,38,41,43]. In those studies, the technique correctly depicted the disease stages accordingly with the gold standard evaluation techniques. A mild cold stress has been used as a thermal stress. For the muscular lesions, according to the importance of the lesion, the lower values (2 to 4 min) of the recovery time τ were found in agreement with the location and the severity of the trauma (Figure 15.6). The dimensions of the lesions as estimated by ultrasonography

FIGURE 15.6 (See color insert.) Second-class muscular lesion on the left leg abductor—medial view. (a) Static thermography image. The color bar shows the pixel temperature color mapping. The light gray spots indicate the presence of the trauma. (b) Time constant τ image after mild cold stress. The color bar illustrates the recovery time, in minutes, for each pixel. The black spots are the markers used as position references. (From Merla, A., et al., Quantifying the relevance and stage of disease with the Tau imaging technique. *IEEE Eng. Biol. Mag.*, 21, 86, 2002, by permission of the editor.)

FIGURE 15.7 (See color insert.) Raynaud's Phenomenon Secondary to Scleroderma. (a) Static thermography image. The color bar shows the pixel temperature color mapping. (b) Time constant τ image after mild cold stress. The color bar illustrates the recovery time, in minutes, for each pixel. The regions associated with longer recovery times identify the main damaged finger regions. (From Merla, A., et al., Quantifying the relevance and stage of disease with the Tau imaging technique. *IEEE Eng. Biol. Mag.*, 21, 86, 2002, by permission of the editor.)

were proportionally related to those of their tracks on the τ image. In the diagnosis of RP secondary to scleroderma, greater values (18 to 20 min) of the recovery time τ corresponded to finger districts more affected by the disease (Figure 15.7). Clinical investigation and capillaroscopy confirmed the presence of scleroderma and the micro-vascular damage.

In the reported deep vein thrombosis cases, the authors found the lower values (1 to 3 min) of the recovery time τ in agreement with the location and the severity of the blood flow reflux according to the echo color Doppler findings (Figure 15.8).

The τ image technique provides useful diagnostic information and can be applied also as a follow up tool. It is an easy and noninvasive diagnostic procedure that can be successfully used in the diagnosis and monitoring of several diseases affecting the local thermoregulatory properties, both in a direct or indirect way. The τ image technique opens new possibilities for the applications of IR imaging in the clinical field. It is worth noting that a certain amount of information is already present—but embedded—in the traditional static image (e.g., Figure 15.6), but the interpretation is difficult and relies on the ability of the clinicians [12]. The method is based on the assumptions of a time constant blood perfusion and blood

FIGURE 15.8 (**See color insert.**) Bi-lateral vein thrombosis. (a) Static thermography image. The color bar shows the pixel temperature color mapping. (b) Time constant τ image after mild cold stress. The color bar illustrates the recovery time, in minutes, for each pixel. The areas associated with shorter recovery times identify the regions interested by the thrombosis. (From Merla, A., et al., Quantifying the relevance and stage of disease with the Tau imaging technique. *IEEE Eng. Biol. Mag.*, 21, 86, 2002, by permission of the editor.)

temperature. While such assumptions are not completely correct from the physiologic point of view, the experimental exponential-shaped recovery function allows such a simplification.

With respect to some diseases, such as the RP, the τ image technique may provide useful information to image the damage and quantitatively follow its time evolution.

15.5 Skin Temperature and Metabolism during Exercise

Skin layer constitutes the interface between human body and the surrounding environment. It plays a fundamental role in the thermoregulatory processes. Cutaneous temperature (Tc) is determined by complex interactions between cutaneous blood perfusion, heat exchanges with inner tissue layers, and the environment. Tc changes with exercise. An effective method to monitor and record Tc is provided by IR thermal imaging, which permits quantitatively to estimate Tc in a safe, noninvasive and touchless manner by measuring the thermal radiation emitted by the body. Studies based on the characterization of Tc during exercise recorded by means of IR thermal imaging are not numerous. In 1998, Zontak [61] used thermographic imaging of the hands to characterize the normal skin response to leg exercise on ten healthy active subjects. He found that graded load exercise results in a constant decrease of finger temperature. Steady-state exercise causes a similar initial temperature decrease followed by rewarming of hands. Vainer [60] recorded man's hips' thermograms after 1 h bicycling documenting the presence of irregular vascular segments.

In 2002, Merla et al. [37] studied thigh skin temperature during bicycle graded exercise by means of fIR. The exercise determined a progressive decrease of Tc during the exercise. On the contrary, the temperature increased during the after-exercise recovery. Cutaneous cooling and warming rates depended on the fitness level of the subjects, the latter being indirectly estimated through performance and anatomical parameters. Total body Tc decreased as the subjects started the exercise. Peripheral regions—like fingertips, legs, and forearms—exhibited the earliest response. As the intensity of the exercise increased, a further total body Tc diminution occurred. Tc increased after the interruption of the exercise. The earliest Tc augment involved the fingertips, face, and trunk. Then, the whole body Tc increased, featuring the presence of hot spots, sometimes tree-shaped, likely due to the presence of muscle perforator vessels [60] (see Figure 15.9). Since no specific attempt has been devoted in order to quantitatively assess whether Tc response to incremental exercise may depend on the level of the individual training, we searched for a possible correlation between the dynamics of the Tc and the actual oxygen consumption rate.

Ten male runners (Tr, having a regular training of six trainings per week) were randomly selected from a list of volunteers at the Sport Center of the University of Chieti-Pescara. Eight active untrained men (Untr,

FIGURE 15.9 (See color insert.) Total body Tc changes during incremental load exercise for a trained subject. (a) baseline Tc distribution; (b) Tc distribution immediately before reaching the age-predicted maximal HR value; (c) Tc distribution at the start of the recovery period (treadmill speed set at stage 1 value); (d) Tc distribution during postexercise period. The color bar reports the pseudo-colors associated the values of Tc.

TABLE 15.1 Modified Bruce's Scheme

Stage	Speed (Km/h)	Grade (%)	Time period (min)
1	3.0	12	2
2	5.0	12	2
3	7.0	12	2
4	9.0	12	2
5	11.0	12	2
6	13.0	12	2
7	15.0	12	2

not regularly performing exercise activity) were recruited as well. Mean age, weight, height, and surface area [6] were not significantly different between Tr and Untr groups (23.5±1.2 vs. 22.8±1.5 years, 70.2±3.8 vs. 72.5 ± 5.1 kg, 1.78 ± 0.05 vs. 1.76 ± 0.03 m, 1.85 ± 0.4 vs. 1.94 ± 0.3 m^2). All the participants were non-smokers, with no overt history of cardiovascular or pulmonary diseases. They presented normal ECG and arterial blood pressure at rest. No subject was taking drugs or medications with potential impact on cardiovascular or thermoregulatory functions. Subjects observed standard preparatory rules for thermal imaging measurements [1,28]. The subjects underwent to an incremental exercise on a computerized treadmill (Proform 330 RT, Milan, Italy) according to a modified Bruce's scheme (see Table 15.1). Incremental load exercise stopped when the subject's heart beat rate (HR) reached the age-predicted maximal value or the subject reached volitional exhaustion. At that time instant, the treadmill speed decreased to stage 1 speed (see Table 15.1) and maintained for two further minutes. Then the treadmill stopped once. Heart beat rate was continuously monitored by means of a standard ECG device (PowerLab ADInstruments, Sidney, Australia), the sampling frequency of which was set at 1000 Hz.

HR recording started 1 min before the exercise (rest data) and continued, after the exhaustion, until the complete restoration of baseline HR values.

Subjects performed the test in controlled environmental conditions: room temperature was set at 23 to 24°C; relative humidity maintained within the 50 ± 5% ranges, with no direct ventilation on the subject.

TABLE 15.2 $\dot{V}_{O_2 max}$, HR at the End of the Incremental Load Phase vs. Maximal HR, Maximal Speed Achieved, and Graded Load Phase Lasting for Tr and Untr Groups

	$\dot{V}_{O_2 max}$ (ml/min kg)	HR at the end of the incremental load phase vs. maximal HR (bpm)	maximal speed (km/hr)	Exercise duration (min:sec)
Untr ($n = 8$)	32.2 ± 5.1	$196 \pm 3 / 198 \pm 2$	9.7 ± 3.2	$8:15 \pm 0:45$
Tr ($n = 10$)	62.2 ± 2.4	$197 \pm 2 / 197 \pm 2$	14.3 ± 2.0	$12:20 \pm 0:20$
ANOVA	$p < .01$	$p > .05$	$p < .01$	$p < .01$

TABLE 15.3 Baseline Tav; Tav Variation at Volitional Exhaustion, and Tav at the End of the Recovery Period for Tr and Untr Groups

	Tav at rest (°C)	Tav variation at the volitional exhaustion (°C)	Tav at the end of recovery (°C)
Untr ($n = 8$)	28.0 ± 1.2	-1.2 ± 0.6	27.6 ± 1.4
Tr ($n = 10$)	28.7 ± 0.7	-2.3 ± 0.6	28.2 ± 1.2
ANOVA	$p > .05$	$p < .01$	$p > .05$

Oxygen consumption rate ($\dot{V}_{O_2}$) and respiratory exchange ratio were determined every second (K4, Cosmed srl, Rome, Italy). Gas analyzers were calibrated before and after each exercise using known concentration gases. The criteria for determining $\dot{V}_{O_2 max}$ were that the respiratory exchange ratio was >1.1, $\dot{V}_{O_2}$ leveled off despite increasing workload, and HR reached the age-predicted maximal value [47]. High-resolution thermal image series of the subjects' body during the exercise were obtained by means of a 14-bit digital infrared camera (AEG 256 PtSi, AEG Aim Heilbronn, Germany; 256×256 Focal Plane Array; 3 to 5 μm spectral range; 0.1 K Noise Equivalent Temperature Differences (NETD); 31 Hz sampling rate; optics: germanium lens, f 50, f/1.5).

Thermal response of the sensors matrix was blackbody calibrated. Residual shift/drift artifacts due to the sensors' response were removed through two-point off-line correction. Camera was set 3.5 to 4 m away from the subject. Such a setting allowed for imaging the desired projection of the whole subject's body at once. Thermal digital images of the frontal projection of the subjects' body were acquired every second. The acquired images were then re-aligned and corrected from motion artifacts through a three parameter rigid-body algorithm. We focused on monitoring thighs' Tc, since thigh skin is completely exposed and free from probes, electrodes, and any other measurement devices. The region of interest for which we computed the Tc profile over time included the anterior portion of the thigh, from the anterior projection of the trochanter to the insertion of the femoral quadriceps on the knee. For each image, average value of both thigh Tc was computed (Tav) and its time evolution during the exercise was obtained.

Comparisons between Tr and Untr data were tested by using one-way ANOVA. Where significant group differences occurred, appropriate *post hoc* pairwise comparisons were performed by using Sheffé's Test with a significance level of .05. Probability of making a type I error was set at $p < .05$.

Table 15.2 reports average values for Tr and Untr groups for $\dot{V}_{O_2 max}$, HR at the end of the incremental load phase vs. maximal HR, maximal working load (speed achieved at volitional exhaustion), and incremental load phase duration.

Table 15.3 reports baseline Tav average Values and Tav variation at volitional exhaustion and at the end of the recovery period for Tr and Untr groups.

Tav vs. time curves are plotted in Figure 15.10. Untr Tav decayed exponentially with the advancement of the exercise until the volitional exhaustion. Tr Tav decreased too along the incremental load phase of the exercise, but featuring two different exponential phases with a transition from the first to the second one around stage 4 to 5.

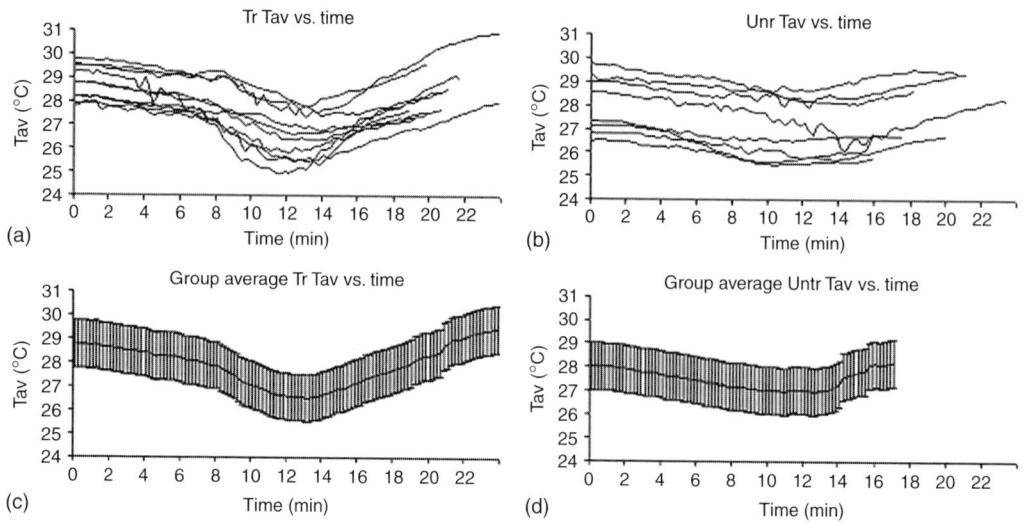

FIGURE 15.10 Tav vs. time curves. (a) Tr individuals; (b) Untr individuals; (c) Tr group (mean ± SE) ; (d) Untr group (mean ± SE). Tr individuals' Tav exhibits larger variation with respect Untr, both during the incremental load phase and the recovery period.

TABLE 15.4 A/τ During Incremental Load and Recovery Phases

	Graded load (°C/min)		Recovery (°C/min)
Untr ($n = 8$)	-0.23 ± 0.07		0.39 ± 0.13
Tr ($n = 10$)	Before slope change	After slope change	0.71 ± 0.3
	-0.21 ± 0.06	-0.98 ± 0.42	
ANOVA	$p > .05$	$p < .01$	$p < .01$

Once it reached the volitional exhaustion, Tav recovered exponentially to baseline values. Given the features shown by Tav, we fitted

1. Untr Tav vs. time curve with two single-exponential curves, one for the incremental load and one for the recovery phases, respectively.
2. Tr Tav vs. time curve during the graded load phase with two single-exponential functions, one to fit the curve before the slope change and one to fit it afterward. Tav recovery curve was fitted by a single-exponential function.

We used a standard Levenberg–Marquardt algorithm to obtain the best fit. The chosen fitting parameters were the Tav amplitude (A) and the time constant (τ). A/τ describes the rate of Tav variation along each exponential phase. Therefore, we used A/τ ratio to characterize the Tav dynamics. Table 15.4 shows A/τ values during the incremental load and the recovery phases of the exercise for Tr and Untr groups. Since Tr Tav dynamics during the incremental load phase was described by two different exponential curves, Table 15.4 reports two A/τ ratios for such a phase.

To verify whether Tav dynamics during the incremental load phase may depend on the actual oxygen consumption rate, we plotted Tav variations (with respect to the baseline) vs. $\dot{V}_{O_2}$ values on scatter-plots and searched for the best regression curve. Similarly, we produced scatter-plots of Tav variations (with respect to the minimum value achieved at the interruption of the incremental load phase) vs. $\dot{V}_{O_2}$ values and searched for the best regression curve for the recovery period from the exercise.

Figure 15.11 shows Tav variation vs. $\dot{V}_{O_2}$.

Regression curves were chosen accordingly to the best value of R^2. For Tr group, a second-order polynomial curve provided the best regression curve for both the incremental load and the recovery phases

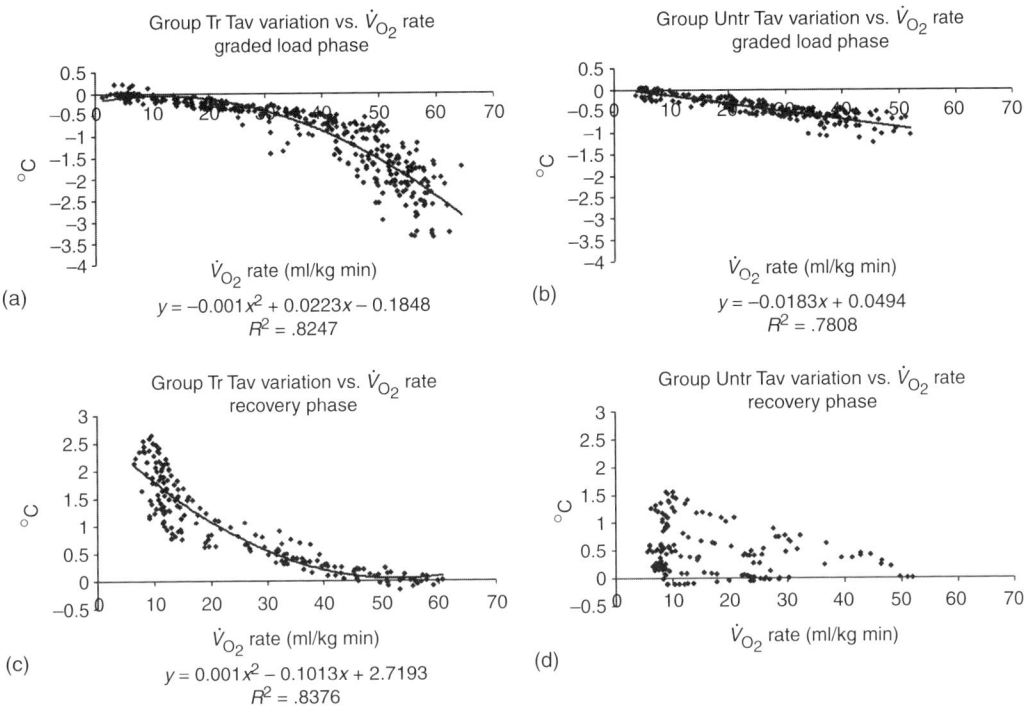

FIGURE 15.11 Tav variation vs. $\dot{V}_{O_2}$ for Tr and Untr groups. (a) Tr Tav variation (with respect to the baseline) vs. $\dot{V}_{O_2}$ during the incremental load phase; (b) Untr Tav variation (with respect to the baseline) vs. $\dot{V}_{O_2}$ during the incremental load phase; (c) Tr Tav variation (with respect to the minimum achieved temperature at the volitional exhaustion) vs. $\dot{V}_{O_2}$ during the recovery; (d) Untr Tav variation (with respect to the minimum achieved temperature at the volitional exhaustion) vs. $\dot{V}_{O_2}$ during the recovery. Tr Tav was significantly correlated to $\dot{V}_{O_2}$ both for the incremental load and the recovery phases ($y = -0.001x^2 + 0.023x - 0.1848$, $R^2 = .82$; $y = 0.001x^2 - 0.1013x + 2.7193$, $R^2 = .84$, respectively); Untr Tav was linearly correlated to $\dot{V}_{O_2}$ during the incremental load phase ($y = -0.0183x + 0.0494$, $R^2 = .78$), while no evident correlation was found during the recovery.

($y = -0.001x^2 + 0.023x - 0.1848$, $R^2 = .82$; $y = 0.001x^2 - 0.1013x + 2.7193$, $R^2 = .84$, respectively). A linear regression, instead, characterized Tav variation vs. $\dot{V}_{O_2}$ for the incremental load phase ($y = -0.0183x + 0.0494$, $R^2 = .78$) of the Untr group. No regression was found during the recovery phase for the Untr group.

Baseline Tr and Untr Tav did not differ from each other ($p > .05$). Also, final Tav at the end of the recovery time did not appear to be different in the two groups. Therefore, it seems that the individual level of training in a rest condition does not affect the cutaneous temperature. Both Tr and Untr Tav decreased during the incremental load phase of the exercise until reaching the volitional exhaustion. This finding is consistent with reports from previous similar studies [37,61]. Although Tav decreased in both groups during the incremental load phase, the dynamics of this temperature variation were similar only in the initial phase of the exercise. In fact, the temperature rate—measured through the A/τ ratio—were the same for both groups until stage 3 to 4. Prolonging the exercise over such stages determined a further marked temperature reduction for the Tr group, the rate of which was significantly higher than in the previous stages. No Untr individuals exhibited such a dynamics. It is worthwhile to note that the timeline for the load scheme was the same for both groups and that stage 3 to 4 did not correspond to the Untr exhaustion stage. Therefore, the differences in Tav dynamics in these stages seem to not depend on the actual exercise load and convective heat exchange. As a consequence of the temperature dynamics shown, the temperature at the volitional exhaustion (i.e., at the interruption of the incremental load phase) was markedly different between groups, with the Tr Tav values significantly lower than those for Untr. Temperature recovery rate was instead significantly higher for the Tr group.

Our data seem to indicate that baseline Tav values are indistinct between Tr and Untr, while Tav variation over time along the progression of the exercise highlights fundamental differences between the two groups. Since Tc, thus Tav, depends on the cutaneous blood flow [7], Tav variations reflected mostly cutaneous vasoconstriction and vasodilatation centrally controlled and sympathetically maintained [14,18]. Cutaneous vasoconstriction during the initial phase of muscular workout is due to an increase in catecholamine and vasoconstrictor hormones. Such a vasoconstriction serves to move the cutaneous blood to the muscular masses to guarantee adequate oxygenation and nutrient levels supply [22,23,24,25,26,29]. The additional Tav reduction exhibited by Tr may be an expression of their capability to further adapt regulatory systems involved in the exercise. Prolonged exercise causes metabolic heat production, thus resulting in a possible excessive muscular and core temperature increase. Heat removal is effectively performed shifting the blood from the muscle to the cutaneous layer, through cutaneous vasodilatation (i.e., Tav increasing) and muscle perforator vessels [61]. The latter process is effectively documented in the thermal images, resulting in the appearance of the tree-shaped hot spots during the recovery from the exercise (see Figure 15.9).

As reported by Fritzsche and Coyle [13], trained subjects have a higher cutaneous blood flow and produce more heat during exercise with respect to nontrained ones. But Tr and Untr maintain the same core temperature [4,14], and, therefore, Tr need to better dissipate extra heat. The higher Tav rates in Tr compared with that in Untr may represent a better capability of Tr to redistribute blood from the muscle to the cutaneous layers, thus allowing more effective peripheral thermal control. Results in present study seem to agree with Huonker' studies [20], which report that training may effect blood redistribution both to capillary and larger vessel.

Therefore, the first conclusion of the present study is that Tr and Untr individuals exhibit different cutaneous thermoregulation during incremental load exercise. In this study, we also attempted to verify whether Tav variation during exercise may be correlated to the actual $\dot{V}_{O_2}$. In particular, we separately searched possible correlations in the two main phases of the exercise: incremental load and recovery.

Tr Tav variation with respect to baseline results correlated with $\dot{V}_{O_2}$ ($R^2 = .82$) during the incremental load phase. Tr Tav variation with respect to the its minimum value at the volitional exhaustion correlated as well with $\dot{V}_{O_2}$ during the recovery ($R^2 = .84$). A second-order polynomial regression expressed the correlation between Tav variations and actual $\dot{V}_{O_2}$, and the absolute value of the second-order term coefficients were almost the same in both phases. A linear regression, instead, characterized Untr Tav variation vs. $\dot{V}_{O_2}$ in the incremental load phase ($R^2 = .78$), while no evident correlation appeared during the recovery phase.

To our knowledge, this is the first time that such correlations are reported. Saltin [52,53] reported tight correlation between muscle blood flow per muscle mass unit and muscular strength, measured by oxygen uptake. In this perspective, the results of our study may confirm that an higher muscular metabolic activity passes through a reorganization of the hemodynamic, and consequently thermoregulatory, balances aimed to facilitate blood recruitment and blood clearance according to the specific needs of the muscle involved in the exercise.

Moreover, our study suggests that these processes are differently expressed by Tr and Untr individuals. In fact, the presence of a second-order term coefficient in the regression curves indicates that the second-order derivative of Tav variations with respect to $\dot{V}_{O_2}$ is not null. Such a feature can be interpreted as an adjustment of the relationship between Tav variations and $\dot{V}_{O_2}$ functional to the workload, and it is not present in the linear relationship that regulates Tav variations vs. $\dot{V}_{O_2}$ in Untr regression curves (i.e., Tav variation and $\dot{V}_{O_2}$ rate are independent from workload).

Therefore, Tr individuals develop and maintain the capability to functionally adapt Tav control to the muscular metabolic needs and the workload while performing the exercise. The same capability is then reversed to adapt Tav control to the thermoregulatory processes induced by the metabolic heat production during the recovery from exercise. In both cases, Tav variations appear to be dependent on the actual oxygen consumption rate in a controlled manner.

On the other hand, Untr individuals seem to be not able to functionally adapt Tav variation and $\dot{V}_{O_2}$ rate to the actual workload. Moreover, the absence of a specific relationship between Tav variation and

$\dot{V}_{O_2}$ during the recovery phase seems to indicate the absence of a devoted control related to the actual oxygen intake.

Our data seem therefore to indicate that Tr individuals have an adaptation of the cutaneous thermoregulatory system, which is due to training. This adaptation is responsible for the modification of the Tav to sustain actual oxygen consumption rate, not present in Untr ones. Such a capability may be also depend on the muscle mass involved in the exercise, since such a muscle mass is one of the major factor elevating the sympathetic nervous activity governing peripheral vasomotion [45,55].

The present study does not consider several relevant parameters like body fat percentage or blood pressure variations during exercise. Also it does not take into account muscle mass or hematic parameters. Further studies are needed to assess how our results depend on these parameters. By the way, the study indicated that cutaneous thermoregulation—considered as a global process—during incremental exercise is differently exercised by trained and untrained individuals. Also it suggests that quantitative relationships may link cutaneous temperature control and oxygen consumption rate. Such findings rely on thermal imaging, which is a safe, noninvasive, and touchless imaging technique providing reliable information on cutaneous temperature.

15.6 Discussion and Conclusion

Functional Infrared imaging is a biomedical imaging technique that relies on high-resolution IR imaging and on the modeling of the heat exchange and control processes at the skin layer. fIR imaging is aimed to provide quantitative diagnostic parameters through the functional investigation of the thermoregulatory processes [31,36,40]. It is also aimed to provide further information about the studied disease to the physicians, like explanation of the possible physical reasons of some thermal behaviors and their relationships with the physiology of the involved processes. One of the great advantages of fIR imaging is the fact that is not invasive and it is a touchless imaging technique. fIR is not a static imaging investigation technique. Therefore, data for fIR imaging need to be processed adequately for movement. Adequate bioheat modeling is also required. The medical fields for possible applications of fIR imaging are numerous, ranging from those described in this chapter, to psychometrics, cutaneous blood flow modeling, peripheral nervous system activity, and some angiopathies. The applications described in this chapter show that fIR imaging provides highly effective diagnostic parameters. The method is highly sensitive, but also highly specific in discriminating different conditions of the same disease. For the studies reported hereby, fIR imaging is sensitive and specific as the corresponding golden standard techniques, at least. In some cases, fIR represents a useful follow up tool (like in varicocelectomy to promptly assess possible relapses) or even an elective diagnostic tool, as in RP. The τ image technique represents an innovative technique that provides useful and additional information to the golden standard techniques. Thanks to it, the whole functional processes associated with a disease can be depicted and summarized just in a single image.

References

[1] Aldemir, H. et al., A comparison of the immediate effects of moderate exercise in the late morning and late afternoon on core temperature and cutaneous thermoregulatory mechanisms, *Chronobiol. Int.*, 17, 197, 2000.

[2] Allen, E.V. and Brown, G.E., Raynaud's disease: a critical review of minimal requisites for diagnosis, *Am. J. Med. Sci.*, 183, 187, 1932.

[3] ASHRAE: Handbook Fundamentals SI Edition, ASHRAE, Atlanta, GA, 1985.

[4] Astrand, I. Aerobic work capacity in men and women with special reference to age. *Acta Physiol. Scand.*, 49, 1, 1960.

[5] Aweruch, M.S., Thermography: its current diagnostic status in muscular-skeletal medicine, *Med. J. Aust.*, 154, 441, 1991.

[6] Bois, D.D. and Bois, E.D., A formula to estimate the approximate surface area if height and weight be known, *Arch. Intern. Med.*, 863, 1916.
[7] Brengelmann, G.L., et al., Altered control of skin blood flow during exercise at high internal temperatures, *J. Appl. Fisiol.*, 43, 790, 1977.
[8] Clarks, S., et al., The distal-dorsal difference as a possible predictor of secondary Raynaud's phenomenon, *J. Rheumatol.*, 26, 1125, 1999.
[9] Cooke, E.D., et al., Reflex sympathetic dystrophy and repetitive strain injury: temperature and microcirculatory changes following mild cold stress, *J. Royal Soc. Med.*, 86, 690, 1993.
[10] Darton, K. and Black, C.M., Pyroelectric vidicon thermography and cold challenge quantify the severity of Raynaud's phenomenon, *Br. J. Rheumatol.*, 30, 190,1991.
[11] Di Benedetto, M., Regional hypothermia in response to minor injure, *Am. J. Phys. Med. Rehabil.*, 75, 270, 1996.
[12] Fauci, M., et al., Medical infrared imaging—differentiating facts from fiction, and the impact of high precision quantum well infrared photodetectors camera systems, and other factors, in its reemergence, *Infrared Phys. Technol.*, 42, 2001.
[13] Fritzsche, R.G. and Coyle, E.F., Cutaneous blood flow during exercise is higher in endurance-trained humans, *J. Appl. Physiol.*, 88, 738, 2000.
[14] Gant, N., Williams, C., King, J., and Hodge, B.J., Thermoregulatory responses to exercise: relative versus absolute intensity, *J. Sport. Sci.*, 22, 1083, 2004.
[15] Garagiola, U., Use of telethermography in the management of sports injuries, *Sport. Med.*, 10, 267, 1990.
[16] Garbey, M., Merla, A., and Pavlidis, I., Estimation of blood flow speed and vessel location from functional infrared imaging, *IFMBE Proc.*, 11, 4752, 2005.
[17] Sun, N., Garbey, M., Merla, A., and Pavlidis, I., Imaging the Cardiovascular pulse, *Proceedings of the 2005 IEEE Computer Society Conference on Computer Vision and Pattern Recognition*, 2, 416, 2005.
[18] Herrick, A.L. and Clark, S., Quantifying digital vascular disease in patients with primary Raynaud's phenomenon and systemic sclerosis, *Ann. Rheum. Dis.*, 57, 70, 1998.
[19] Hunold, S., Mietzsch, E., and Werner, J., Thermographic studies on patterns of cutaneous temperature after exercise, *Eur. J. Appl. Physiol. Occup. Physiol.*, 65, 550, 1992.
[20] Huonker, M., Halle, M., and Keul J., Structural and functional adaptations of the cardiovascular system by training, *Int. J. Sport. Med.*, 17, 164, 1996.
[21] Javanetti, S., et al., Thermography and nailfold capillaroscopy as noninvasive measures of circulation in children with Raynaud's phenomenon, *J. Rheumatol.*, 25, 997, 1998.
[22] Johnson, J.M., Exercise and the cutaneous circulation, *Exerc. Sport. Sci. Rev.*, 20, 59, 1992.
[23] Kenney, W.L. and Johnson, J.M., Control of skin blood flow during exercise, *Med. Sci. Sport. Exerc.*, 24, 303, 1992.
[24] Keul, J., et al., Adaptation to training and performance in elite athletes, *Res. Q. Exerc. Sport*, 67, 29, 1996.
[25] Kobayashi, Y., et al., Effects of endurance training on thermoregulation in females, *Med. Sci. Sport. Exerc.*, 12, 361, 1980.
[26] Kobayashi, Y., et al., Effects of heat acclimation of distance runners in a moderately hot environment, *Eur. J. Appl. Physiol. Occup. Physiol.*, 45, 189, 1980.
[27] Maricq, H.R., et al., Diagnostic potential of *in vivo* capillary microscopy in scleroderma and related disorders, *Arthr. Rheum.*, 23, 183, 1980.
[28] Merla, A. and Romani, G.L., Biomedical applications of functional infrared imaging, *Proceedings of the 2005 IEEE 27th EMBC Engineering in Medicine and Biology Conference*, IEEE Catalog Number: 05CH37611C, ISBN: 0-7803-8741-4, Shanghai, China, September 1–4, 2005.
[29] Merla, A., Di Donato, L., and Romani, G.L., Functional infrared imaging: analysis of skin temperature during exercise, *Proceedings of the 24th IEEE Engineering in Medicine and Biology Society Conference*, IEEE Catalog No: 02CH37392C, ISBN: 0-7803-7613-7, Houston, October 23–25, 2002.

[30] Merla, A., Ledda, A., Di Donato, L., and Romani, G.L., Assessment of the effects of the varicocelectomy on the thermoregulatory control of the scrotum, *Fertil. Steril.*, 81, 471, 2004.

[31] Merla, A., et al., Emotion detection through functional infrared imaging: preliminary results, *Biomedizinische Technik*, 48, 284, 2004.

[32] Merla, A., et al., Combined approach to the initial stage Raynaud's phenomenon diagnosis by means of dynamic digital telethermography, capilloroscopy and pletismography: preliminary findings, *Med. Biol. Eng. Comp.*, 37, 992, 1999.

[33] Merla, A., et al., Correlation of telethermographic and ultrasonographic reports in the therapeutic monitoring of second-class muscular lesions treated by hyperthermia, *Med. Biol. Eng. Comp.*, 37, 942, 1999.

[34] Merla, A., et al., Dynamic digital telethermography: a novel approach to the diagnosis of varicocele, *Med. Biol. Eng. Comp.*, 37, 1080, 1999.

[35] Merla, A., et al., Infrared functional imaging applied to Raynaud's phenomenon, *IEEE Eng. Med. Biol. Mag.*, 21, 73, 2002.

[36] Merla, A., et al., Infrared functional imaging applied to the study of emotional reactions: preliminary results, *Proceedings of the 4th International Non-Invasive Functional Source Imaging*, Chieti, Italy, September 9–13, 2003.

[37] Merla, A., et al., Infrared functional imaging: Analysis of skin temperature during exercise, *Proceedings of the 24th IEEE Engineering in Medicine and Biology Society Conference*, Houston, October 23–25, 2002.

[38] Merla, A., et al., Quantifying the relevance and stage of disease with the Tau image technique. *IEEE Eng. Med. Biol. Mag.*, 21, 86, 2002.

[39] Merla, A., et al., Raynaud's Phenomenon: infrared functional imaging applied to diagnosis and drugs effects, *Int. J. Immun. Pharm.*, 15, 41, 2002.

[40] Merla, A., et al., Recording of the sympathetic thermal response by means of infrared functional imaging, *Proceedings of the 25th Annual International Conference of the IEEE Engineering in Medicine and Biology Society*, Cancun, Mexico, September 17–21, 2003.

[41] Merla, A., et al., Time Recovery Image: a diagnostic image technique based on the Dynamic Digital Telethermography, *Thermol. Intern.*, 10, 142, 2000.

[42] Merla, A., et al., Use of infrared functional imaging to detect impaired thermoregulatory control in men with asymptomatic varicocele, *Fertil. Steril.*, 78, 199, 2002.

[43] Merla, A., et al., Tau image: a diagnostic imaging technique based on the dynamic digital telethermography, *Proceedings of the WC2000 Chicago World Congress on Medical Physics and Biomedical Engineering and 22th International Conference of IEEE Engineering in Medicine and Biology Society*, Digest of Papers CD, track 1,TU-FXH, Chicago, IL, July 2000.

[44] Mieusset, R. and Bujan, L., Testicular heating and its possible contributions to male infertility: a review, *Int. J. Andr.*, 18, 169, 1995.

[45] Nielsen, B., et al., Muscle blood flow and muscle metabolism during exercise and heat stress, *J. Appl. Physiol.*, 69, 1040, 1990.

[46] O'Reilly, D., et al., Measurement of cold challenge response in primary Raynaud's phenomenon and Raynaud's phenomenon associated with systemic sclerosis, *Ann. Rheum. Dis.*, 51, 1193, 1992.

[47] Okazaki, K., et al., Effects of exercise training on thermoregulatory responses and blood volume in older men. *J. Appl. Physiol.*, 93, 1630, 2002.

[48] Prescott, et al., Sequential dermal microvascular and perivascualr changes in the development of scleroderma, *J. Pathol.*, 166, 255, 1992.

[49] Ring, E.F.J., Cold Stress test for the hands, in *The Thermal Image in Medicine and Biology*, Uhlen Verlag Ed., Wien, 1995.

[50] Rodnan, G.P., Myerowitz, R.I., and Justh, G.O., Morphological changes in the digital arteries of patients with progressive systemic sclerosis and Raynaud phenomenon, *Medicine*, 59, 393, 1980.

[51] Roganski, A., Infrared detectors: an overview, *Infrared Phys. Technol.*, 43, 187, 2002.

[52] Saltin, B. and Hermansen, L., Esophageal, rectal, and muscle temperature during exercise, *J. Appl. Physiol.*, 21, 1757, 1966.

[53] Saltin, B., Radegran, G., Koskolou, M.D., and Roach, RC. Skeletal muscle blood flow in humans and its regulation during exercise, *Acta Physiol. Scand.*, 162, 421, 1998.

[54] Schuhfried, O., et al., Thermographic parameters in the diagnosis of Secondary Raynaud's Phenomenon, *Arch. Phys. Med. Rehabil.*, 81, 495, 2000.

[55] Secher, N.H., Mizuno, M., and Saltin, B. Adaptation of skeletal muscles to training. *Bull. Eur. Physiopathol. Respir.*, 20, 453, 1984.

[56] Shitzer, A., et al., Lumped parameter tissue temperature-blood perfusion model of a cold stressed finger, *J. Appl. Physiol.*, 80, 1829, 1996.

[57] Subcommittee for Scleroderma Criteria of the American Rheumatism Association Diagnostic and Therapeutic Criteria Committee, Preliminary criteria for the classification of systemic sclerosis (scleroderma), *Arthritis Rheum.*, 23, 581, 1980.

[58] Trum, J.W., The value of palpation, varicoscreen contact thermography and colour Doppler ultrasound in the diagnosis of varicocele, *Hum. Reprod.*, 11, 1232, 1996.

[59] Tucker, A., Infrared thermographic assessment of the human scrotum, *Fertil. Steril.*, 74, 802, 2000.

[60] Vainer, B.G., FPA-based infrared thermography as applied to the study of cutaneous and stimulated vascular response in humans. *Phy. Med. Biol.*, 50, R63–R94, 2005.

[61] Zontak, A., et al., Dynamic thermography: analysis of hand temperature during exercise, *Ann. Biomed. Eng.*, 26, 988, 1998.

16
Fever Mass Screening Tool for Infectious Diseases Outbreak: Integrated Artificial Intelligence with Bio-Statistical Approach in Thermogram Analysis

E.Y.K. Ng
E.C. Kee
Nanyang Technological University

Abstract		16-2
16.1	Preamble	16-2
16.2	Methodology	16-3
	Data Acquisition • Artificial Neural Networks • Radial Basis Function Network • Bio-Statistical Methods	
16.3	Designed Integrated Approach	16-12
	Case 1: Advanced Integrated Technique (PR + ANN RBFN + ROC) for Febrile and Nonfebrile Cases • Case 2: Conventional Bio-Statistical Technique (LR + ROC) for Febrile and Nonfebrile Cases	
16.4	Results and Discussion	16-14
	Case 1: Advanced Integrated Technique (PR + ANN RBFN + ROC) for Febrile and Nonfebrile Cases • Case 2: Conventional Bio-Statistical Technique (LR + ROC) for Febrile and Nonfebrile Cases • Comparison between the Advanced Integrated Technique and Conventional Bio-Statistical Technique	
16.5	Conclusion and Future Work	16-18
Acknowledgments		16-18
References		16-19

Abstract

Thermography is a noninvasive and environmental friendly imaging technique used widely in the medical and engineering arena. This chapter investigates the analysis of thermograms in the use of Artificial Neural Networks (ANN) in conjunction with bio-statistical methods. It is desired that through these approaches, highly accurate diagnosis using thermography techniques can be achieved.

The proposed method is a multipronged approach comprising of Parabolic Regression (PR), Radial Basis Function Network (RBFN), and Receiver Operating Characteristics (ROC) Analysis. It is a novel, integrative, and powerful technique that can be used to analyze complicated and massive numerical data such as the temperature data extracted from febrile thermograms during the severe acute respiratory syndrome (SARS) screening exercise 2003 (as an example).

The use of PR is to reveal the correlation between the variables and the actual health status of the subject, which is decided by the thermometer reading from the ear for fever screening. This is important as it helps to select the more appropriate variables to be used as inputs for building the neural network (NN). PR is used instead of linear regression (LR) because of its superiority in providing the correlation.

For ANN, RBFN is trained to produce the desired outcome, which is either positive or negative. When this is done, the RBFN will possess the ability to predict the outcome when there are new input variables. The advantages of using RBFN include fast training superior classification and decision-making abilities as compared to other networks like Back Propagation.

Next, ROC is used to evaluate the accuracy, sensitivity, and specificity of the outcome from the ANN. The results are very promising. For mass fever screening, the accuracy rate of the proposed technique scored a high 96%, with 95% sensitivity and 85.6% specificity. This is better than the method used by researchers during the SARS-2003 outbreak, which possesses 93% accuracy rate, 85.4% sensitivity, and 95% specificity. In short, the present tests suggested that the newly devised integrative approach is a success.

To sum up, through the combination use of ANN, bio-statistical, and ROC methods, advances are made in thermography application with regard to achieving a higher level of consistency. For elevated body temperature thermography, we have in place a reliable system for mass screening of fever cases. In other words, we possess the technology to differentiate febrile from nonfebrile cases in as short time as possible for a powerful and reliable first-defense mass blind screening tool in the event of infectious diseases outbreak.

All in all, this chapter provides an introduction of the ROC concept as used by Food and Drug Administration (FDA) to determine the added value of each imaging modality in a multimodality environment. Clinical data are presented to demonstrate the efficacy of infrared imaging in modern medical practice. Discussions include issues and areas that need to be further studied and resolved. New concepts and image processing techniques for enhancing the performance of this modality are addressed. This is important in view of the SARS outbreak in 2003 and the potentially lethal Avian flu or malaria. In the event of such a virus outbreak, we will be better prepared to handle the situation. To sum it up, thermography application is like an unpolished gemstone, waiting for us to unleash its full potential. The future focus in elevated body temperature thermography is testing other techniques like Adaptive Network-Based Fuzzy Inference System (ANFIS) to determine if the results can surpass ANN. Object Orientated Programming like Visual C++ can also be incorporated into ANN for coding purposes.

Keywords: Febrile; integrative thermograms; bio-statistical; AI, ROC

16.1 Preamble

A worldwide pandemic from mutated H5N1 bird flu virus could kill any number of people from 7 to 100 million if left unchecked,* according to worst case scenarios being studied by the World Health Organisation (WHO) and scientists. The mutated virus could sicken 20% of the world's population, with nearly 30 million people in need of hospital treatment and a quarter of these eventually dying.† As at 16

---

*The estimates are based mainly on the mortality rate—2% of the sick—of the 1918–1919 Spanish H1N1 flu virus pandemic, which killed up to 40 million people worldwide within 6 months. They also taken into account the rise in the world population, improved health care, and changing travel patterns.

†Forecasts in science magazine by WHO expert Dr. Klaus Stoehr [14].

Jan. 2007, bird flu has killed at least 161 people worldwide since it started ravaging Asian poultry stocks in late 2003, and millions of birds have been destroyed, causing estimated losses of between U.S.$10 and $15 billion for the poultry industry. But the ultimate impact of the virus depends on its virulence. As known, early detection of virus in which fever is one of the most important diagnostic symptoms, isolation of patients and proper medical care could help contain an epidemic and delay or stop it from becoming a pandemic. Monitoring personal temperature at hospital, airports, and border-crossing points are thus critical to prevent outbreak for such an endemic disaster [1–7], although the point prevalence of fever in such subjects would be very low. Traditional tools to measure the body temperature are through the mouth and ear canal. Oral and aural temperature measurements are accurate but are fairly invasive, time consuming, labor intensive, and skill dependent [8,9]. The ideal device for blind mass fever screening should be speedy, noninvasive, and be able to detect accurately those patients with fever [4]. Infrared thermography has been used to detect several inflammatory abnormalities and has the potential to serve as a tool for mass screening for fever [6].

Thermography is a passive, noncontact imaging method that is economic, quick, and does not inflict any pain on the patient. It is a relatively straightforward screening method that detects the variation of temperature on the surface of the human skin [10]. Thermography is widely used in the industrial and increasing application lately for medical arena. This includes the detection of elevated body temperature [8–10] and breast cancer [10–12]. Thermograms alone will not be sufficient for the medical practitioner to make an adjunct diagnosis. Analytical tools like bio-statistical methods and ANN will be utilized to analyze the thermograms [3].

Thermography application in elevated body temperature is a progressive and encouraging effort, as seen from the success in the way Singapore handled the SARS-2003 outbreak [7,13]. The Standards Technical References (2003* and 2004†) was discussed for the International Organization for Standardization (ISO) meeting in December 2005 at IEC-DIN Germany with the hope for acceptance of infrared imaging in medical community in infection control such as a possible bird flu epidemic. In our work, an integrated approach is used to analyze thermograms of elevated body temperature. Research in this area is necessary and timely because human bird flu is expected to be the next epidemic and according to experts, it will hit 20 to 30% of the world's population [14] in which fever is one of the most obvious symptoms [15]. Through the use of thermography, it is desired that the febrile subject is detected using the proposed approach. Figures 16.1 and 16.2 show two typical examples of normal and febrile thermograms.

RBFN is a pattern recognition program that has the ability to predict the outcome based on the various inputs fed into the program [16,17]. For elevated body temperature thermography, the program will predict if the subject is febrile or nonfebrile.

To enhance the performance of RBFN, a bio-statistical method PR—will be incorporated as data processing derived for thermal images to enhance the accuracy of the results. Selecting only useful and correlated inputs, which are used to predict the outcome, does this.

16.2 Methodology

16.2.1 Data Acquisition

The blind mass data were collected (502 without duplicate measurements, confirmed later 86 febrile, and 416 healthy cases with ear thermometer) from the designated SARS hospital (A&E Department, Tan Tock Seng Hospital [TTSH]) and the Civil Defense Force Academy [SCDF] in Singapore (indoor

---

*Standards Technical Reference for *"Thermal Imagers for Human Temperature Screening Part 1: Requirements and Test Methods,"* 2003. TR 15-1, Spring Singapore. ISBN 9971-67-963-9.

†Standards Technical Reference for *"Thermal Imagers for Human Temperature Screening Part 2: Users' implementation guidelines,"* 2004. TR 15-2, Spring Singapore. ISBN 9971-67-977-9.

FIGURE 16.1 Nonfebrile thermogram (aural temperature = 36.9°C).

FIGURE 16.2 Febrile thermogram (aural temperature = 38.4°C).

screening with ambient temperature of 25 ± 2°C, humidity ≈60%), in which thermal imagers are used as a first-line tool for the blind screening of hyperthermia. The subjects are considered febrile if his/her mean ear temperature is ≥37.7°C for adults (37.9°C for children) using Braun Thermoscan IRT 3520+. Results are drawn for the two important pieces of information: the best and yet practical region on the face to screen and guidance on optimal preset threshold temperature for the same handheld radiometric IR ThermaCAM S60 FLIR system [18]. The focal length from the subject to scanner was fixed at 2 m and the duration of time patients must be scanned was 3 s. Figure 16.3 illustrates an example of temperature profiles from a temperature operation using thermal imager with temperature reading. Visitors were directed to line up in a single file with the aid of barricades. Stand in position, remove spectacles and look at imager so that his/her face fills at least one-third vertical height of the display screen (Figures 16.4 and 16.5). The detector was a focal plane array, uncooled microbolometer 320 × 240 pixels with a thermal sensitivity of 0.06°C at 30°C, spectral range of 7.5 to 13 μm and measurement accuracy at ±2% of the real-time reading [18]. The average temperature of the skin surface was measured from the field of view of the thermal imager with an appropriate adjustment for skin emissivity. Human skin emissivity may vary from site to site ranging from 0.94 to 0.99 (0.98 was used here). Figures 16.6 and 16.7 present an example of the processed thermal images of both frontal and side (left) profiles from the same subject. The following spots were logged and analyzed from the subjects with frontal and side profiles: forehead;

Fever Mass Screening Tool for Infectious Diseases Outbreak

FIGURE 16.3 A typical thermal imager with direct threshold temperature setting. (Source: Zugo.)

FIGURE 16.4 A yellow square marked on the ground for visitors to stand in.

FIGURE 16.5 Face fills at least one-third vertical height for the field of view.

eye region; average cheeks; nose; mouth (closed); average temple; side face; ears and side temple (the last three are for side profile).

Reproducibility of both the instrument and physiological assumptions was established by comparing paired left–right readings of the temples and cheeks [19,20]. Comparing the ear core temperature of febrile

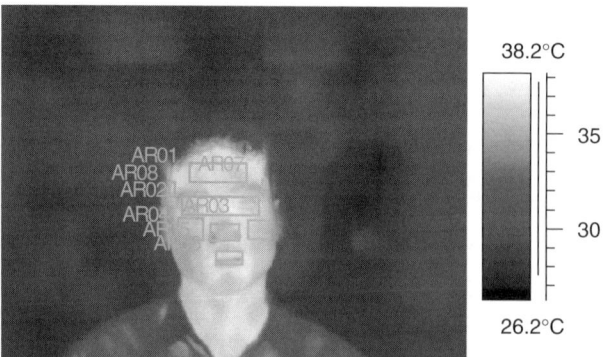

FIGURE 16.6 Processed thermal image of the frontal profile.

FIGURE 16.7 Processed thermal images of the side profile.

and nonfebrile data (Figures 16.8 to 16.11), it is noted that the mode of the nonfebrile data falls between 36.0 and 37.2°C. For febrile, it spread over a larger region, from 37.2 to 39.6°C.

16.2.2 Artificial Neural Networks

Artificial Neural Networks are a group of techniques for numerical learning [16]. They are made up of many nonlinear computational elements called neurons. These neurons, also known as network nodes, are linked to one another. Through this weighted interconnection, they formed the main architect of the NN. To draw an analogy, ANN is similar to the neurological system in humans and animals, which are made up of real NN. One important point to note is that ANN is much less complex than biological NN (BNN). As a result, it is not realistic to expect ANN to emulate BNN, which is responsible for the behavior of humans and animals. However, ANN has the capability to assist us in some tasks. This includes nonlinear estimation, classification, clustering and content-addressable memory.

Two or more inputs are connected to a node in an ANN [16]. Each of them has a weighted linkage attached to it (Figure 16.12). Based on the input values, a node has the ability to perform simple calculation. Both inputs and outputs are real numbers or integers between −1 and 1. All the input data have to be normalized before being fed into the program. The output from one individual node can either be inputted into another node or be part of the NN's overall output. Each node performs its calculation and function independently from the rest of the nodes. The only association between the nodes is that the output from a node might be the input for another node. This type of architect is also known as a parallel structure, which allows for the exploration of numerous hypotheses. In addition, this parallel architect also permits the NN to make full use of conventional personal computers.

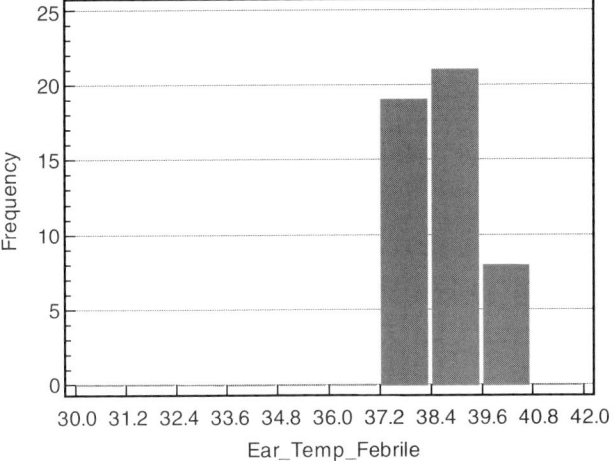

FIGURE 16.8 Distribution of ear temperature for febrile cases.

FIGURE 16.9 Distribution of maximum temperature at eye range for febrile cases.

The main advantage of ANN is that the tolerance of failure of an individual node or neuron is relatively high. This includes the weighted interconnection, because it might be erroneous too. The weights can be obtained by utilizing a trained algorithm and through iteration and adjustments. The eventual transfer function is obtained with regard to the desired output.

When given a set of inconsistent or incomplete data, ANN is able to give an approximate answer rather than a wrong answer. The performance of the NN will undergo a gradual degradation should there be any failures from individual nodes in the network. This is very useful in the medical arena as many a times, it is difficult to run a comprehensive test. The disadvantage of using ANN is that it does not have the capability to predict and forecast accurately beyond the range of previously trained data. In other words, the predicted outcome is based on the available set of data.

16.2.3 Radial Basis Function Network

Radial Basis Function Network is a kind of feed-forward and unsupervised learning paradigm. A simple RBFN consists of three separate layers—input layer, hidden layer and output layer as shown in Figure 16.12. The first part of the training cycles involves the clustering of input vectors. Mathematically, the clustering

FIGURE 16.10 Distribution of ear temperature for nonfebrile cases.

FIGURE 16.11 Distribution of maximum temperature at eye region for nonfebrile cases.

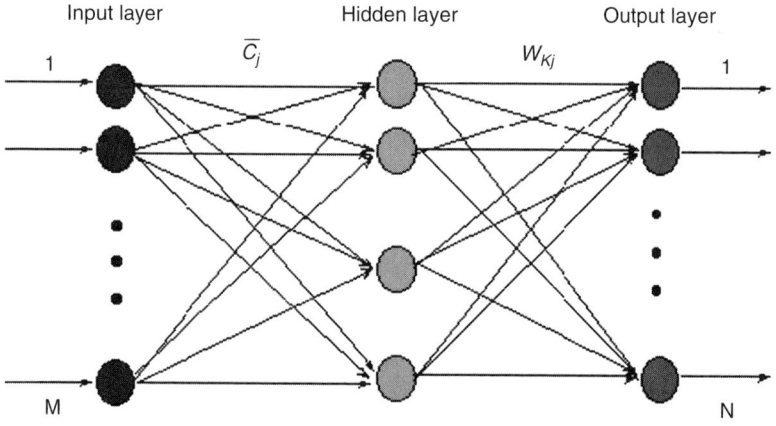

FIGURE 16.12 RBFN Architect [16,17].

is done using Dynamic K-Means algorithm [17]. At the end of the clustering process, the radius of the Gaussian functions at the middle of the clusters will be equivalent to the distance between the two nearest cluster centers [16].

During the training, the RBFN is required to fulfill two tasks. First, it is to determine the middle of each hypersphere (circle in 2-D and hypersphere in n-dimensional pattern space) and second, to obtain its radius. For the first task, it is done by allocating the weights of the processing elements. This can be done by using an unsupervised clustering algorithm. It is important to note that the output neuron in the prototypical layer of a RBFN is in a function of the Euclidean distance. This distance measures from the input vector to the weighted vector. The unsupervised learning phase in the hidden layer of RBFN is followed by another different supervised learning phase. This is the stage where the output neurons are trained to associate each individual cluster with their own distinct shapes and sizes. RBFN is selected for the current work since its training speed is faster than Back-Propagation network, able to detect data that are not within the norm and make better decision during classification problems.

The input and output neurons of RBFN and perceptron are alike [16]. The major difference lies in the hidden neuron. In most cases, it is governed by the Gaussian function. This is different from other processing neurons that produce an output based on the weighted sum of the inputs. On the contrary, the input neurons of the RBFN are not involved in the processing of information. Their sole function is to input the given data to the receiving nodes. Using a linear transfer function, these receiving nodes will decide the weights to be allocated to each processing element that follows. They are governed by the transfer functions:

$$y_i = f_r(r_i), \qquad r_i = \sqrt{\sum_{j=1}^{n}(x_j - w_{ij})^2}$$

where x_j is input vector, W_{ij} represents the amount of weights allocated to the inputs of the neuron i. f_r is a symmetrical function known as the radial basis function such as the Gaussian function, which is the preferred choice of most researchers.

$$f_r(r_i) = \exp\left(\frac{-r_i^2}{2\sigma_i^2}\right)$$

where σ_i is the standard deviation of the Gaussian distribution. Every neuron at each hidden layer will have its own unique σ_i value.

16.2.4 Bio-Statistical Methods

16.2.4.1 Regression Analysis

Regression (least squares) analysis is a statistical technique used to determine the unique curve or line that "best fits" all the data points (Figure 16.13). The underlying principle is to minimize the square of the distance of each data point to the line itself. In regression analysis, there are two variables—namely, dependent and independent. The former is the variable to be estimated or predicted.

The most important result obtained in the analysis is the R-squared, or coefficient of determination. R-squared is an indication of how tightly or sparsely clustered the data points are and it is a value that lies between 0 and 1. It is thus a measure of the correlation between the two variables. Correlation is the predictability of the change in the dependent variable given a change in the independent variable.

PR refers to using a parabolic curve to fit the data points. It is a simple yet effective way to obtain the correlation between the two variables. However, a few assumptions are made in using LR. First, a parabolic relationship is assumed between the two variables, which might not always be the case. Second, the dependent variable is assumed to be normally distributed with the same variance with its corresponding

FIGURE 16.13 A typical scattered plot.

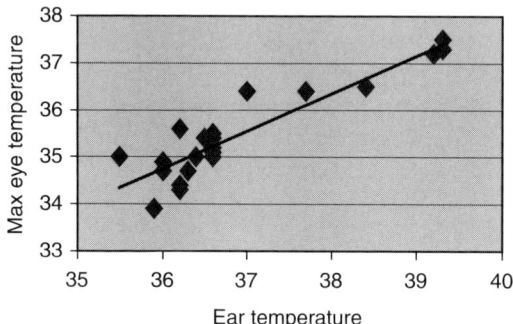

FIGURE 16.14 A regression line being fitted.

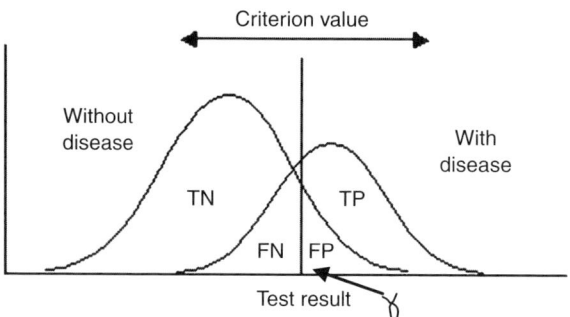

FIGURE 16.15 Discrimination curve.

value of independent variable. Mathematically, PR model is given by $Y = Ax^2 + Bx + C$ (Figure 16.14). PR usually offers a more realistic and better correlation between the two variables compared to LR.

16.2.4.2 ROC Curve

Receiver operating characteristics curves are used to assess the diagnostic performance of a medical test to discriminate unhealthy cases from healthy cases [21]. Very often a medical test, perfect separation between unhealthy and healthy cases is not possible if we were to discriminate them based on a threshold value. To illustrate this phenomenon, let us call the threshold value γ.

Figure 16.15 suggests that at the threshold value γ, the majority of those without the disease will be correctly diagnosed as healthy (TN). Similarly, the majority of those with the disease will be correctly diagnosed as unhealthy (TP). However, there will also be one group of diseased patients wrongly diagnosed

TABLE 16.1 Basic Mathematical Formulae for ROC Analysis

Test Result	Disease	Number	Disease	Number	Total
	Present	n	Absent	m	
Positive	True positive	a	False positive	c	$a + c$
Negative	False negative	b	True negative	d	$b + d$
Total		$a + b$		$c + d$	

TABLE 16.2 Important Terminology for ROC Analysis

Sensitivity	$a/(a+b)$
Specificity	$d/(c+d)$
Positive predictive value	Sensitivity/$(1 - $ specificity$)$
Negative predictive value	$(1 - $ sensitivity$)$/specificity

FIGURE 16.16 A typical ROC curve [21].

as healthy (FN) and one group of healthy patient wrongly diagnosed as unhealthy (FP). Table 16.1 summarizes all the possibilities—TN, TP, FN, and FP and their respective algebraic representation.

With that, four important criteria can be defined—sensitivity,* specificity,† positive predictive value (PPV),‡ and negative predictive value (NPV),§ and they are commonly used in ROC analysis to assess the credibility of the test. The mathematical formulas are summarized in Table 16.2.

In the ROC Curves analysis result (Figure 16.16), both sensitivity and specificity will be displayed for all criterions. This will allow the user to choose the optimum criterion, which ought to have a high value for both sensitivity and specificity. The value of sensitivity is inversely proportional to that of specificity. This can be easily illustrated by the threshold value γ. A low γ will ensure that those with the disease will be detected. But this will also cause those without the disease to be classified as diseased. On the

---

*Sensitivity—The probability that test is positive in the unhealthy population.
†Specificity—The probability that the test is negative in the healthy population.
‡PPV—Given a positive forecast, the probability that it is correct.
§NPV—Given a negative forecast, the probability that it is correct.

TABLE 16.3 Temperature Data of Forehead and Near Eye Regions

Forehead region	Near eye region
Minimum temperature	Minimum temperature
Maximum temperature	Maximum temperature
Average temperature	Average temperature

other hand, a high γ will allow correctly categorized the healthy group but will miss out on the diseased group.

An example of the ROC curves is presented in Figure 16.16. The vertical axis shows the sensitivity while the horizontal axis shows the (100 – specificity). This once again reinforces the fact that there is a trade-off between sensitivity and specificity.

The area under the ROC curve is important information obtained in the analysis. The value lies between 0.5 to 1. A value of 0.5 implies that the test cannot discriminate unhealthy from healthy group, whereas a value of 1 implies that the test can distinguish the two groups perfectly.

16.3 Designed Integrated Approach

16.3.1 Case 1: Advanced Integrated Technique (PR + ANN RBFN + ROC) for Febrile and Nonfebrile Cases

The proposed approach is a multipronged approach that comprises of PR, RBFN, and ROC analysis. It is a novel, integrative and powerful technique that can be used to analyze complicated and large numerical data.

16.3.1.1 Step 1: Parabolic Regression

Parabolic regression reflects the correlation between the variables and the actual health status (febrile or nonfebrile) of the subject, which is decided by means of a thermometer placed in the ear. The output is either 1 or 0, corresponding to febrile and nonfebrile cases respectively. The two input variables with the best correlation are chosen. The rational behind using PR over LR is it offers a more accurate and realistic approach in providing the correlation coefficient (LR results are also tabulated here for comparison purposes). Table 16.3 summarizes the temperature data from thermograms [6].

16.3.1.2 Step 2: ANN RBFN

On the basis of the various inputs fed into the network, RBFN is trained to produce the desired outcome, which are either positive (1) for febrile cases or negative (0) for nonfebrile cases. When this is done, the RBFN algorithm will possess the ability to predict the outcome when there are new input variables.

16.3.1.3 Step 3: ROC Analysis

Next, ROC is used to evaluate the accuracy, sensitivity, and specificity of the outcome of RBFN Test files (i.e., Is RBFN well built or not?).

Table 16.4 and Figure 16.17 reveal the software needed for the entire processes, including the steps prior to advanced integrated technique.

16.3.2 Case 2: Conventional Bio-Statistical Technique (LR + ROC) for Febrile and Nonfebrile Cases

The conventional bio-statistical technique comprises of LR and ROC to analyze the data collected from the thermal imager [3]. Similarly to the previous approach, regression is used to select the variable with

TABLE 16.4 Software Used of Advanced Integrated Technique for Febrile and Nonfebrile Thermograms

Purpose	Software
View thermograms from thermal imager and extract temperature data	Image J
Normalize raw temperature data Perform statistical analysis (e.g., mean, median, and standard deviation)	MS Excel Statistical Toolbox
Determine the correlation of each variable with the output (health status)	MedCal
Training and testing of data Building an algorithm for the data	NeuralWorks Pro II
To evaluate the effectiveness of the computed method	MedCal

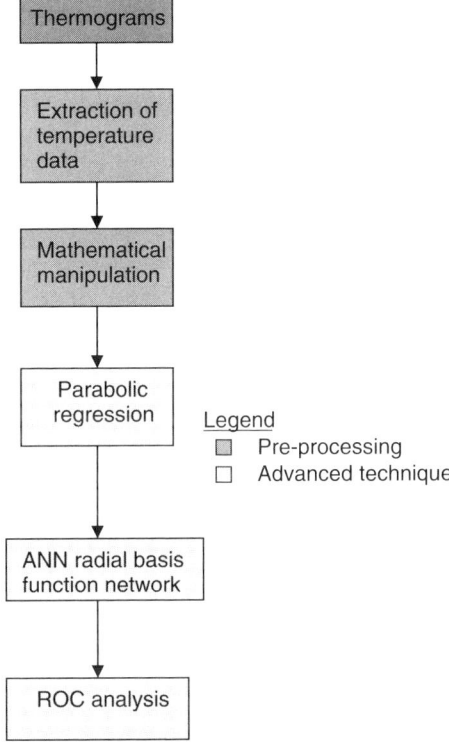

FIGURE 16.17 Flow chart for advanced integrated technique.

the strongest correlation with the outcome (health status of the patient). Subsequently, ROC is applied to obtain the optimal preset temperature based on the chosen variables. The temperature is dependent on the values of sensitivity and specificity from the ROC analysis results. The chosen threshold temperature must have high values of sensitivity and specificity. Also, the area under the ROC curve is to be high to determine whether or not a subject should be considered febrile (diseased) or nonfebrile (healthy). Table 16.5 and Figure 16.18 show the procedure of conventional technique used during the SARS-2003 outbreak [3–7].

TABLE 16.5 Software Used for Conventional Approach

Purpose	Software
View thermograms from thermal imager and extract temperature data	Image J
Normalize raw temperature data Perform statistical analysis (e.g., mean, median, and standard deviation)	MS Excel Statistical Toolbox
Determine correlation of each variable on the output (health status)	MedCal
Determine the optimal preset temperature Evaluate the effectiveness based on sensitivity and specifity	MedCal

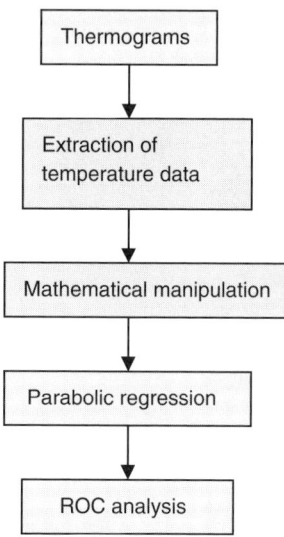

FIGURE 16.18 Flow chart for conventional approach.

16.4 Results and Discussion

16.4.1 Case 1: Advanced Integrated Technique (PR + ANN RBFN + ROC) for Febrile and Nonfebrile Cases

Table 16.6 tabulates results for PR, LR results are also included for comparison purposes. The PR coefficient of determination is always higher than that of LR. Thus, using simple LR with the present nonlinear data set are not always the best possible way to "fit the data," as it is frequently used.

When parabolic curve is used to generate the correlation coefficient, the *maximum temperature of near eye* and *maximum temperature of forehead regions* still remain to be the best correlated spots on the frontal face with regard to the core temperature. Hence, temperature data from these two regions are selected as input variables for the training of ANN. Although using parabolic function gives the better correlation coefficient, the outcome of the NN remains the same even if LR is used.

Table 16.7 gives the selected results for RBFN SLP with various combination of learn rule and transfer rate. The results for selected combination of learn rule & transfer rule (with various *options* tested) for RBFN SLP are included in Table 16.8.

Various combinations of learn rule, transfer rule and *options* were tested. With the inclusion of *options* (e.g., Connect Prior, Connect Bias), more NNs with an accuracy of 96% can be generated. The RBFN

TABLE 16.6 Summarized Results for Step 1 for Advanced Integrated Technique

Independent variable	Coefficient of determination	
	Linear	Parabolic
Maximum temperature at eye range	0.5507	0.6315
Minimum temperature at eye range	0.0672	0.1114
Standard deviation at eye range	0.0303	0.0588
Total average at eye range	0.4489	0.5721
Maximum temperature at forehead range	0.4973	0.6362
Minimum temperature at forehead range	0.1169	0.1798
Standard deviation at forehead range	0.0053	0.0053
Total average at forehead range	0.3759	0.5379

TABLE 16.7 Selected Results for RBFN SLP of Advanced Integrated Technique

Learn rule	Transfer rule	Score (%)
Delta Rule	Sigmoid	96
Delta Rule	DNNA	96
Norm-Cum-Delta	Linear	96
Norm-Cum-Delta	TanH	96
Norm-Cum-Delta	Sigmoid	96
Norm-Cum-Delta	Sine	96
Ext DBD	Linear	96

TABLE 16.8 Selected Results for RBFN SLP (with *Options* for Advanced Integrated Technique)

Learn rule	Transfer rule	Option	Score (%)
Delta Rule	Sigmoid	Connect Prior	96
Delta Rule	Sigmoid	Connect Bias	96
Delta Rule	Sigmoid	MinMax Table	96
Delta Rule	DNNA	Connect Prior	96
Delta Rule	DNNA	Linear O/P	96
Delta Rule	DNNA	Softmax O/P	96
Delta Rule	DNNA	Connect Bias	96
Delta Rule	DNNA	MinMax Table	96
Norm-Cum-Delta	TanH	Connect Prior	96
Norm-Cum-Delta	TanH	Linear O/P	96
Norm-Cum-Delta	TanH	Connect Bias	96
Norm-Cum-Delta	TanH	MinMax Table	96
Norm-Cum-Delta	Sigmoid	Connect Prior	96
Norm-Cum-Delta	Sigmoid	Linear O/P	96
Norm-Cum-Delta	Sigmoid	Connect Bias	96
Norm-Cum-Delta	Sigmoid	MinMax Table	96
Norm-Cum-Delta	Sine	Connect Prior	96
Norm-Cum-Delta	Sine	Linear O/P	96
Norm-Cum-Delta	Sine	Connect Bias	96
Norm-Cum-Delta	Sine	MinMax Table	96
Ext DBD	Linear	Connect Prior	96
Ext DBD	Linear	Linear O/P	96
Ext DBD	Linear	Connect Bias	96
Ext DBD	Linear	MinMax Table	96

TABLE 16.9 ROC Results for RBFN SLP with Various Combination of Learn Rule and Transfer Rule

No.	Learn rule	Transfer rule	Score (%)	Area under curve	Sensitivity	Specificity
1	Delta Rule	Sigmoid	96	0.972	100	84.1
2	Delta Rule	DNNA	96	0.971	91.7	94.3
3	Norm-Cum-Delta	Sigmoid	96	0.975	100	88.6

TABLE 16.10 ROC Results for RBFN SLP with Selected Combination of Learn Rule and Transfer Rule (with Various *Options* Tested)

No.	Learn rule	Transfer rule	Option	Score (%)	Area under curve	Sensitivity	Specificity
1	Delta Rule	Sigmoid	Connect Prior	96	0.972	100	84.1
2	Delta Rule	Sigmoid	MinMax Table	96	0.974	91.7	94.3
3	Delta Rule	DNNA	Connect Prior	96	0.971	91.7	94.3
4	Delta Rule	DNNA	Linear O/P	96	0.971	91.7	94.3
5	Delta Rule	DNNA	Softmax O/P	96	0.971	91.7	94.3
6	Delta Rule	DNNA	Connect Bias	96	0.970	91.7	94.3
7	Norm-Cum-Delta	TanH	Connect Bias	96	0.973	91.7	94.3
8	Norm-Cum-Delta	TanH	MinMax Table	96	0.978	100	87.5
9	Norm-Cum-Delta	Sigmoid	Connect Prior	96	0.975	100	88.6
10	Norm-Cum-Delta	Sigmoid	Linear O/P	96	0.975	100	88.6
11	Norm-Cum-Delta	Sigmoid	Connect Bias	96	0.970	100	85.2
12	Norm-Cum-Delta	Sigmoid	MinMax Table	96	0.981	100	94.3
13	Norm-Cum-Delta	Sine	Connect Bias	96	0.975	91.7	94.3
14	Norm-Cum-Delta	Sine	MinMax Table	96	0.975	91.7	94.3
15	Ext DBD	Linear	Connect Bias	96	0.980	100	93.2
16	Ext DBD	Linear	MinMax Table	96	0.984	100	94.3

is credible and has the ability to differentiate febrile from nonfebrile cases to a very large extent. There are always four input data which the model always predicts wrongly and accounts for the 4% error. This is due to inconsistencies between the patient's facial temperature (deduced from the thermograms) and his core temperature. For example, the Max Temp in the near eye region and Max Temp in the forehead region are very high and it indicates the fact that the person is having fever. Hence, ANN predicts that the person is having a fever. However, the core temperature taken by the thermometer suggests that the person is not having a fever. Thus, ANN's prediction is wrong. This is certainly not the ANN's fault because in these cases, the person's facial temperature has poor correlation with his core temperature. Without these exceptional cases, ANN should achieve an even higher accuracy rate. Tables 16.9 and 16.10 (with various *options* tested) summarize the selected results (of ROC Area >0.970) for ROC analysis.

The ROC area under curve for all the RBFNs shown in Tables 16.9 and 16.10 is larger than 0.97. These RBFNs also have high sensitivities (>90%) and high specificities (>80%). This suggests that the RBFN is well built and the overall diagnostic performance is reliable and can be used for mass screening of febrile subjects. The best performing RBFN is a Single Layered Perceptron with Ext DBD as the Learn Rule, Linear Function as the Transfer Rule and MinMax Table as the selected Option. The area under the ROC curve is 0.984 and its sensitivity and specificity are 100 and 94.3%, respectively.

16.4.2 Case 2: Conventional Bio-Statistical Technique (LR + ROC) for Febrile and Nonfebrile Cases

The LR analysis shows that the particular area on the skin surface that will produce the most consistent results with regard to the core temperature (taken using ear scanner) is the maximum temperature in

FIGURE 16.19 ROC curve for conventional technique (area of ROC = 0.972) [3,4,6].

TABLE 16.11 Summarized Results of LR for Conventional Approach

Independent variable	Coefficient of determination (linear)
Maximum temperature at eye range	0.5507
Minimum temperature at eye range	0.0672
Standard deviation at eye range	0.0303
Total average at eye range	0.4489
Maximum temperature at forehead range	0.4973
Minimum temperature at forehead range	0.1169
Standard deviation at forehead range	0.0053
Total average at forehead range	0.3759

TABLE 16.12 Selected Results of ROC Analysis for Conventional Bio-Statistical Technique [3,4,6]

Criterion	Sensitivity	Specificity
36.1	85.4	92.7
36.2	85.4	93.9
36.3*	85.4	95.0
36.4	83.3	96.2
36.5	75	96.9

*Selected criterion for preset temperature: 36.3°C.

the eye region with coefficient of correlation of 0.5507 (Table 16.11). The poorest correlated independent variable with the core temperature is the standard deviation for the forehead and eye regions (0.0053 and 0.0303) and the minimum temperature in the eye region (0.0672). Figure 16.19 shows the ROC plot in which the false positives are weighted the same as false negatives. Table 16.12 summarizes the sensitivity and specificity for various preset scanner temperature.

ROC curve analysis for the maximum eye region shows that the optimal preset (cut-off) temperature is 36.3°C. If a subject's maximum temperature in the eye region exceeds 36.3°C, it implies that he/she is having a fever. At this cut-off temperature, the sensitivity and specificity are 85.4 and 95.0%, respectively, with an accuracy rate of 93%.

16.4.3 Comparison Between the Advanced Integrated Technique and Conventional Bio-Statistical Technique

The advanced technique achieves 96% of accuracy rate whereas the conventional bio-statistical technique has 93% accuracy rate. Hence, there is a greater promise in using the advanced integrated technique for the thermogram analysis. In the conventional technique, after the "Max Temp in Eye region" is found to have the strongest correlation with the output, the rest of the variables (e.g., Max Temp in forehead region, Min Temp in forehead region, Min Temp in eye region, mode, median, etc.) are discarded. This implies that they will no longer be used in ANN. But in the advanced technique, it is possible and a common practice to use more than one input variable (besides Max Temp in eye region). For this study Max Temp in forehead region is used as the second input variable for ANN training and testing. These are two variables with the strongest correlation with the output. Further studies could be carried out to check if third, fourth, fifth … input variables would further improve the effectiveness of the advanced technique.

16.5 Conclusion and Future Work

The chapter focuses on the numerical analyses of the data, to the detriment of performing a scientifically rigorous test of the hypotheses that febrile patients can be detected using simple thermograms. Through the use of ANN and bio-statistical methods, progress is made in thermography application with regard to achieving a higher level of consistency. This is made possible with the introduction of the novel advanced integrated technique in thermogram analysis.

The advanced technique has a high level of accuracy rate in prediction based on the temperature data extracted from the thermograms. It improves the correlation and may prove more efficacious for mass fever screening. For elevated body temperature thermography, the advanced technique enables us to have in place a reliable system for mass screening of fever cases. The proposed approach (PR + ANN + ROC) has surpassed the conventional bio-statistical approach (LR + ROC), which was used for analytical purposes during the SARS-2003 pandemic. In other words, the advanced technique enables us to differentiate febrile from nonfebrile cases in as short time as possible. This is important in view of the SARS outbreak in 2003 and the potentially lethal Avian flu or malaria. Indonesia has recently reported the world's first laboratory-confirmed cluster of human-to-human transmission of bird flu, although scientists are as yet unsure of the significance for the multiple mutations in the H5N1 virus. In the event of such a virus being pandemic, we will be better prepared to set up thermography units in public places to mass screen populations for epidemic outbreaks. To sum it up, thermography application is like an unpolished gemstone, waiting for us to unleash its full potential.

The next focus in elevated body temperature thermography is testing other techniques like Adaptive Network-Based Fuzzy Inference System (ANFIS) to determine if the results can surpass ANN. Object Orientated Programming like Visual C++ can also be incorporated into ANN for coding purposes.

Acknowledgments

The first author would like to express his appreciation to members of the Technical Reference Committee on Thermal Imagers under Medical Technology Standards Division by SPRING, Dr. K.H. Pwee, Director of CSTA, Ministry of Health, Dr. G.J.L. Kaw, Consultant Radiologist, TTSH of National Health Group, Singapore for sharing of their views and interests on "Thermal Imagers for Fever Screening—Selection, Usage and Testing."

References

[1] Chan, L.S., Cheung, G.T.Y., Lauder, I.J., and Kumana, C.R. (2004). Screening for fever by remote-sensing infrared thermographic camera. *J Travel Med*, 11: 273–278.

[2] Hay, A.D., Peters, T.J., Wilson, A., and Fahey, T. (2004). The use of infrared thermometry for the detection of fever. *Br J Gen Pract*, 54: 448–450.

[3] Ng, E.Y.-K., Kaw, G.J.L., and Chang, W.M. (2004). Analysis of IR thermal imager for mass blind fever screening. *Microvasc Res*, 68: 104–109.

[4] Ng, E.Y.-K. (2005). Is thermal scanner losing its bite in mass screening of fever due to SARS? *Med Phys*, 32: 93–97.

[5] Ng, E.Y.-K., Chong, C., and Kaw, G.J.L. (2005). Classification of human facial and aural temperature using neural networks and IR fever scanner: a responsible second look. *J Mech Med Biol*, 5: 165–190.

[6] Ng, E.Y.-K. and Kaw, G.J.L. (March 2006). IR scanners as fever monitoring devices: physics, physiology and clinical Accuracy. In Nicholas Diakides (ed.) *Biomedical Engineering Handbook*, CRC Press, Boca Raton, FL, pp. 24–1 to 24–20.

[7] Ng, E.Y-K., Wiryani, M., and Wong, B.S. (2006). Study of facial skin and aural temperature using IR with and w/o TRS. *IEEE Eng Med Biol Mag*, 25: 68–74.

[8] Van Staaij, B.K., Rovers, M.M., Schilder, A.G., and Hoes, A.W. (2003). Accuracy and feasibility of daily infrared tympanic membrane temperature measurements in the identification of fever in children. *Intl J Pediatr Otorhinolaryngol*, 67: 1091–1097.

[9] Pettersson, M. and Strandell, A. (2000). Temperature measurements in health care: a question of quality assurance. *Lakartidningen*, 97: 4050.

[10] Ring, E.F. (1998). Progress in the measurement of human body temperature. *Eng Med Biol Mag*, 17: 19–24.

[11] Ng, E.Y.-K., Fok, S.C., Peh, Y.C., Ng, F.C., and Sim, L.S.J. (2002). Computerized detection of breast cancer with artificial intelligence and thermograms. *Intl J Med Eng Technol*, 26: 152–157.

[12] Ng, E.Y.-K. and Fok, S.C. (2003). A framework for early discovery of breast tumor using thermography with Artificial Neural Network. *Breast J*, 9: 341–343.

[13] Singapore Technologies Electronics Ltd: http://www.stee.st.com.sg/newsRm/2004/prt-09-02.htm (assessed September 8, 2005).

[14] WHO Bird Flu report: http://www.who.int/csr/disease/avian_influenza/country/cases_table_2006_05_29/en/index.html (assessed July 18, 2006).

[15] Essortment on Fever causes: http://ks.essortment.com/fevercauses_rker.htm (assessed June 8, 2005).

[16] Hopgood, A. (2000). Intelligent systems for engineers and scientists. Library of Congress Cataloging-in-Publication Data.

[17] Battelle: http://www.battelle.org/pipetechnology/(assessed June 10, 2005).

[18] FLIR Systems: http://www.flir.com (accessed July 17, 2006).

[19] Togawa, T. (1985). Body temperature measurement. *Clin Phys Physiol Meas*, 6: 83–108.

[20] Kaderavek, F. (1972). Clinical Thermometry (Czech). *Casopis Lekaru Ceskych*, 111: 1135–1138.

[21] Receiver Operating Characteristics (ROC): http://www.medcalc.be/ (accessed July 17, 2006).

17

Thermal Imaging in Diseases of the Skeletal and Neuromuscular Systems

17.1	Introduction..	17-1
17.2	Inflammation	17-2
17.3	Paget's Disease of Bone	17-3
17.4	Soft Tissue Rheumatism.................................	17-4
	Muscle Spasm and Injury • Sprains and Strains • Enthesopathies • Fibromyalgia	
17.5	Peripheral Nerves	17-6
	Nerve Entrapment • Peripheral Nerve Paresis	
17.6	Complex Regional Pain Syndrome	17-9
17.7	Thermal Imaging Technique...........................	17-11
	Room Temperature • Clinical Examination	
	References	17-11

Francis E. Ring
Glamorgan University

Kurt Ammer
Ludwig Boltzmann Research Institute for Physical Diagnostics and University of Glamorgan

17.1 Introduction

Clinical medicine has made considerable advances over the last century. The introduction of imaging modalities has widened the ability of physicians to locate and understand the extent and activity of a disease. Conventional radiography has dramatically improved, beyond the mere demonstration of bone and calcified tissue. Computed tomography ultrasound, positron emission tomography, and magnetic resonance imaging are now available for medical diagnostics.

Infrared imaging has also added to this range of imaging procedures. It is often misunderstood, or not been used due to lack of knowledge of thermal physiology and the relationship between temperature and disease.

In Rheumatology, disease assessment remains complex. There are a number of indices used, which testify to the absence of any single parameter for routine investigation. Most indices used are subjective.

Objective assessments are of special value, but may be more limited due to their invasive nature. Infrared imaging is noninvasive, and with modern technology has proved to be reliable and useful in rheumatology.

From early times physicians have used the cardinal signs of inflammation, that is, pain, swelling, heat, redness, and loss of function. When a joint is acutely inflamed, the increase in heat can be readily detected by touch. However, subtle changes in joint surface temperature occur and increase and decrease in temperature can have a direct expression of reduction or exacerbation of inflammation.

17.2 Inflammation

Inflammation is a complex phenomenon, which may be triggered by various forms of tissue injury. A series of cellular and chemical changes take place that are initially destructive to the surrounding tissue. Under normal circumstances the process terminates when healing takes place, and scar tissue may then be formed.

A classical series of events take place in the affected tissues. First, a brief arteriolar constriction occurs, followed by a prolonged dilatation of arterioles, capillaries, and venules. The initial increased blood flow caused by the blood vessel dilation becomes sluggish and leucocytes gather at the vascular endothelium. Increased permeability to plasma proteins causes exudates to form, which is slowly absorbed by the lymphatic system. Fibrinogen, left from the reabsorption partly polymerizes to fibrin. The increased permeability in inflammation is attributed to the action of a number of mediators, including histamines, kinins, and prostaglandins. The final process is manifest as swelling caused by the exudates, redness, and increased heat in the affected area resulting from the vasodilation, and increased blood flow. Loss of function and pain accompany these visible signs.

Increase in temperature and local vascularity can be demonstrated by some radionuclide procedures. In most cases, the isotope is administered intravenously and the resulting uptake is imaged or counted with a gamma camera. Superficial increases in blood flow can also be shown by laser Doppler imaging although the response time may be slow. Thermal imaging, based on infrared emission from the skin is both fast and noninvasive.

This means that it is a technique that is suitable for repeated assessment, and especially useful in clinical trials of treatment whether by drugs, physical therapy, or surgery.

Intra-articular injection, particularly to administer corticosteroids came into use in the middle of the last century. Horvath and Hollander in 1949 [1] used intra-articular thermocouples to monitor the reduction in joint inflammation and synovitis following treatment. This method of assessment while useful to provide objective evidence of anti-inflammatory treatment was not universally used for obvious ethical reasons.

The availability of noncontact temperature measurement for infrared radiometry was a logical progression. Studies in a number of centers were made throughout the 1960s to establish the best analogs of corticosteroids and their effective dose. Work by Collins and Cosh in 1970 [2] and Ring and Collins 1970 [3] showed that the surface temperature of an arthritic joint was related to the intra-articular joint, and to other biochemical markers of inflammation obtained from the exudates. In a series of experiments with different analogues of prednisolone (all corticosteroids), the temperature measured by thermal imaging in groups of patients can be used to determine the duration and degree of reduction in inflammation [4,5].

At this time, a thermal challenge test for inflamed knees was being used in Bath, based on the application of a standard ice pack to the joint. This form of treatment is still used, and results in a marked decrease of joint temperature, although the effect may be transient.

The speed of temperature recovery after an ice pack of 1 kg of crushed ice to the knee for 10 min, was shown to be directly related to the synovial blood flow and inflammatory state of the joint. The mean temperature of the anterior surface of the knee joint could be measured either by infrared radiometry or by quantitative thermal imaging [6].

A number of new nonsteroid anti-inflammatory agents were introduced into rheumatology in the 1970s and 1980s. Infrared imaging was shown to be a powerful tool for the clinical testing of these drugs, using temperature changes in the affected joints as an objective marker. The technique had been successfully used on animal models of inflammation, and effectively showed that optimal dose response curves could be obtained from temperature changes at the experimental animal joints. The process with human patients suffering from acute Rheumatoid Arthritis was adapted to include a washout period for previous medication. This should be capable of relieving pain but no direct anti-inflammatory action per se. The compound used by all the pharmaceutical companies was paracetamol. It was shown by Bacon et al. [7] that small joints such as fingers and metacarpal joints increased in temperature quite rapidly while paracetamol treatment was given, even if pain was still suppressed. Larger joints, such as knees and ankles required more than one week of active anti-inflammatory treatment to register the same effect. Nevertheless, the commonly accepted protocol was to switch to the new test anti-inflammatory treatment after one week of washout with the analgesic therapy. In every case if the dose was ineffective the joint temperature was not reduced. At an effective dose, a fall in temperature was observed, first in the small joints, then later in the larger joints. Statistical studies were able to show an objective decrease in joint temperature by infrared imaging as a result of a new and successful treatment. Not all the new compounds found their way into routine medicine; a few were withdrawn as a result of undesirable side effects. The model of infrared imaging to measure the effects of a new treatment for arthritis was accepted by all the pharmaceutical companies involved and the results were published in the standard peer reviewed medical journals. More recently attention has been focused on a range of new biological agents for reducing inflammation. These also are being tested in trials that incorporate quantitative thermal imaging.

To facilitate the use and understanding of joint temperature changes, Ring and Collins [3], Collins et al. [8] devised a system for quantitation. This was based on the distribution of isotherms from a standard region of interest. The Thermal Index was calculated as the mean temperature difference from a reference temperature. The latter was determined from a large study of 600 normal subjects where the average temperature threshold for ankles, knees, hands, elbows, and shoulder were calculated. Many of the clinical trials involved the monitoring of hands, elbows, knees, and ankle joints. Normal index figure obtained from controls under the conditions described was from 1 to 2.5 on this scale. In inflammatory arthritis this figure was increased to 4–5, while in osteoarthritic joints, the increase in temperature was usually less, 3–4. In gout and infection higher values around 6–7 on this scale were recorded.

However, to determine normal values of finger joints is a very difficult task. This difficulty arises partly from the fact, that cold fingers are not necessarily a pathological finding. Tender joints showed higher temperatures than nontender joints, but a wide overlap of readings from nonsymptomatic and symptomatic joints was observed [9]. Evaluation of finger temperatures from the reference database of normal thermograms [10] of the human body might ultimately solve the problem of being able to establish a normal range for finger joint temperatures in the near future.

17.3 Paget's Disease of Bone

The early descriptions of Osteitis Deformans by Czerny [11] and Paget [12] refer to "chronic inflammation of bone." An increased skin temperature over an active site of this disease has been a frequent observation and that the increase may be around 4°C. Others have shown an increase in peripheral blood flow in almost all areas examined. Increased periosteal vascularity has been found during the active stages of the disease. The vascular bed is thought to act as an arterio-venous shunt, which may lead to high output cardiac failure. A number of studies, initially to monitor the effects of calcitonin, and later bisphosphonate therapy have been made at Bath (UK). As with the clinical trials previously mentioned, a rigorous technique is required to obtain meaningful scientific data. It was shown that the fall in temperature during calcitonin treatment was also indicated more slowly, by a fall in alkaline phosphatase, the common biochemical marker. Relapse and the need for retreatment was clearly indicated by thermal imaging. Changes in the thermal index often preceded the onset of pain and other symptoms by 2 to 3 weeks. It was also shown that the level of increased temperature over the bone was related to the degree of bone pain. Those patients who had maximal temperatures recorded at the affected bone experienced severe bone pain. Moderate pain was found in those with raised temperature, and no pain in those patients with normal temperatures. The most dramatic temperature changes were observed at the tibia, where the bone is very close to the skin surface. In a mathematical model, Ring and Davies [13] showed that the increased temperature measured over the tibia was primarily derived from osseous blood flow and not from metabolic heat. This disease is often categorized as a metabolic bone disease.

17.4 Soft Tissue Rheumatism

17.4.1 Muscle Spasm and Injury

Muscle work is the most important source for metabolic heat. Therefore, contracting muscles contribute to the temperature distribution at the body's surface of athletes [14,15]. Pathological conditions such as muscle spasms or myofascial trigger points may become visible at regions of increased temperature [16]. An anatomic study from Israel proposes in the case of the levator scapulae muscle that the frequently seen hot spot on thermograms of the tender tendon insertion on the medial angle of the scapula might be caused by an inflamed bursae and not by a taut band of muscle fibers [17].

Acute muscle injuries may also be recognized by areas of increased temperature [18] due to inflammation in the early state of trauma. However, long lasting injuries and also scars appear at hypothermic areas caused by reduced muscle contraction and therefore reduced heat production. Similar areas of decreased temperature have been found adjacent to peripheral joints with reduced range of motion due to inflammation or pain [19]. Reduced skin temperatures have been related to osteoarthritis of the hip [20] or to frozen shoulders [21,22]. The impact of muscle weakness on hypothermia in patients suffering from paresis was discussed elsewhere [23].

17.4.2 Sprains and Strains

Ligamentous injuries of the ankle [24] and meniscal tears of the knee [25] can be diagnosed by infrared thermal imaging. Stress fractures of bone may become visible in thermal images prior to typical changes in x-rays [26]. Thermography provides the same diagnostic prediction as bone scans in this condition.

17.4.3 Enthesopathies

Muscle overuse or repetitive strain may lead to painful tendon insertions or where tendons are shielded by tendon sheaths or adjacent to bursae, to painful swellings. Tendovaginitis in the hand was successfully diagnosed by skin temperature measurement [27]. The acute bursitis at the tip of the elbow can be detected through an intensive hot spot adjacent to the olecranon [28]. Figure 17.1 shows an acute tendonitis of the Achilles tendon in a patient suffering from inflammatory spondylarthropathy.

17.4.3.1 Tennis Elbow

Painful muscle insertion of the extensor muscles at the elbow is associated with hot areas on a thermogram [29]. Thermal imaging can detect persistent tendon insertion problems of the elbow region in a similar way as isotope bone scanning [30]. Hot spots at the elbow have also been described as having a high association with a low threshold for pain on pressure [31]. Such hot areas have been successfully used as outcome measure for monitoring treatment [32,33]. In patients suffering from fibromyalgia, bilateral hot spots at the elbows is a common finding [34]. Figure 17.2 is the image of a patient suffering from tennis elbow with a typical hot spot in the region of tendon insertion.

17.4.3.2 Golfer Elbow

Pain due to altered tendon insertions of flexor muscles on the medial side of the elbow is usually named Golfer's elbow. Although nearly identical in pathogenesis as the tennis elbow, temperature symptoms in this condition were rarely found [35].

FIGURE 17.1 (**See color insert at the back of the book.**) Acute tendonitis of the right Achilles tendon in a patient suffering from inflammatory spondylarthropathy.

FIGURE 17.2 (**See color insert.**) Tennis elbow with a typical hot spot in the region of tendon insertion.

17.4.3.3 Periarthropathia of the Shoulder

The term periarthropathia includes a number of combined alterations of the periarticular tissue of the humero-scapular joint. The most frequent problems are pathologies at the insertion of the supraspinous and infraspinous muscles, often combined with impingement symptoms in the subacromial space. Long lasting insertion alteration can lead to typical changes seen on radiographs or ultrasound images, but

FIGURE 17.3 (**See color insert.**) Decreased temperature in patient with a frozen shoulder on the left-hand side.

unfortunately there are no typical temperature changes caused by the disease [22,36]. However, persistent loss in range of motion will result in hypothermia of the shoulder region [21,22,36,37]. Figure 17.3 gives an example of an area of decreased temperature over the left shoulder region in patient with restricted range of motion.

17.4.4 Fibromyalgia

The terms tender points (important for the diagnosis of fibromyalgia) and trigger points (main feature of the myofascial pain syndrome) must not be confused. Tender points and trigger points may give a similar image on the thermogram. If this is true, patients suffering from fibromyalgia may present with a high number of hot spots in typical regions of the body. A study from Italy could not find different patterns of heat distribution in patients suffering from fibromyalgia and patients with osteoarthritis of the spine [38]. However, they reported a correspondence of nonspecific hyperthermic patterns with painful muscle areas in both groups of patients. Our thermographic investigations in fibromyalgia revealed a diagnostic accuracy of 60% of hot spots for tender points [34]. The number of hot spot was greatest in fibromyalgia patients and the smallest in healthy subjects. More than 7 hot spots seem to be predictive for tenderness of more than 11 out of 18 specific sites [39]. Based on the count of hot spots, 74.2% of 252 subjects (161 fibromyalgia, 71 with widespread pain but less than 11 tender sites out of 18, and 20 healthy controls) have been correctly diagnosed. However, the intra- and inter-observer reproducibility of hot spot count is rather poor [40]. Software assisted identification of hot or cold spots based on the angular distribution around a thermal irregularity [41] might overcome that problem of poor repeatability.

17.5 Peripheral Nerves

17.5.1 Nerve Entrapment

Nerve entrapment syndromes are compression neuropathies at specific sites in human body. These sites are narrow anatomic passages where nerves are situated. The nerves are particularly prone to extrinsic or intrinsic pressure. This can result in paraesthesias such as tingling or numb feelings, pain, and ultimately in muscular weakness and atrophy.

Uematsu [42] has shown in patients with partial and full lesion of peripheral nerves that both conditions can be differentiated by their temperature reaction to the injury. The innervated area of partially lesioned nerve appears hypothermic caused by activation of sympathetic nerve fibers. Fully dissected nerves result in a total loss of sympathetic vascular control and therefore in hyperthermic skin areas.

The spinal nerves, the brachial nerve plexus, and the median nerve at the carpal tunnel are the most frequently affected nerves with compression neuropathy.

17.5.1.1 Radiculopathy

A slipped nucleus of an intervertebral disk may compress the adjacent spinal nerve or better the sensory and motor fibers of the dorsal root of the spinal nerve. This may or must not result in symptoms of compression neuropathy in the body area innervated by these fibers.

The diagnostic value of infrared thermal imaging in radiculopathies is still under debate. A review by Hoffman et al. [43] from 1991 concluded that thermal imaging should be used only for research and not in clinical routine. This statement was based on the evaluation of 28 papers selected from a total of 81 references.

The study of McCulloch et al. [44] planned and conducted at a high level of methodology, found thermography not valid. However, the applied method of recording and interpretation of thermal images was not sufficient. The chosen room temperature of 20 to 22°C might have been too low for the identification of hypothermic areas. Evaluation of thermal images was based on the criterion that at least 25% of a dermatome present with hypothermia of 1°C compared to the contralateral side. This way of interpretation might be feasible for contact thermography, but does not meet the requirements of quantitative infrared imaging.

The paper of Takahashi et al. [45] showed that the temperature deficit identified by infrared imaging is an additional sign in patients with radiculoapathy. Hypothermic areas did not correlate with sensory dermatomes and only slightly with the underlying muscles of the hypothermic area. The diagnostic sensitivity (22.9–36.1%) and the positive predictive value (25.2–37.0%) were low for both, muscular symptoms such as tenderness or weakness and for spontaneous pain and sensory loss. In contrast, high specificity (78.8–81.7%), high negative predictive values (68.5–86.2%), and a high diagnostic accuracy were obtained.

Only the papers by Kim and Cho [46] and Zhang et al. [47] found thermography of high value for the diagnosis of both lumbosacral and cervical radiculopathies. However, these studies have several methodological flaws. Although a high number of patients were reported, healthy control subjects were not mentioned in the study on lumbosacral radiculopathy. The clinical symptoms are not described and the reliability of the used thermographic diagnostic criteria remains questionable.

17.5.1.2 Thoracic Outlet Syndrome

Similar to fibromyalgia, the disease entity of the thoracic outlet syndrome (TOS) is under continuous debate [48]. Consensus exists, that various subforms related to the severity of symptoms must be differentiated. Recording thermal images during diagnostic body positions can reproducibly provoke typical temperature asymmetries in the hands of patients with suspected thoracic outlet syndrome [49,50]. Temperature readings from thermal images from patients passing that test can be reproduced by the same and by different readers with high precision [51]. The original protocol included a maneuver in which the fist was opened and closed 30 times before an image of the hand was recorded. As this test did not increase the temperature difference between index and little finger, the fist maneuver was removed from the protocol [52]. Thermal imaging can be regarded as the only technique that can objectively confirm the subjective symptoms of mild thoracic outlet syndrome. It was successfully used as outcome measure for the evaluation of treatment for this pain syndrome [53]. However, in a patient with several causes for the symptoms paraesthesias and coldness of the ulnar fingers, thermography could show only a marked cooling of the little finger, but could not identify all reasons for that temperature deficit [54]. It was also difficult to differentiate between subjects whether they suffer from TOS or carpal tunnel syndrome. Only

66.3% of patients were correctly allocated to three diagnostic groups, while none of the carpal tunnel syndromes have been identified [55].

17.5.1.3 Carpal Tunnel Syndrome

Entrapment of the median nerve at the carpal tunnel is the most common compression neuropathy. A study conducted in Sweden revealed a prevalence of 14.4%; for pain, numbness, and tingling in the median nerve distribution in the hands. Prevalence of clinically diagnosed carpal tunnel syndrome (CTS) was 3.8 and 4.9% for pathological results of nerve conduction of the median nerve. Clinically and electrophysiologically confirmed CTS showed a prevalence of 2.7% [56].

The typical distribution of symptoms leads to the clinical suspect of CTS [57], which must be confirmed by nerve conduction studies. The typical electroneurographic measurements in patients with CTS show a high intra- and inter-rater reproducibility [58]. The course of nerve conduction measures for a period of 13 years in patients with and without decompression surgery was investigated and it was shown that most of the operated patients presented with less pathological conduction studies within 12 months after operation [59]. Only 2 of 61 patients who underwent a simple nerve decompression by division of the carpal ligament as therapy for CTS had pathological findings in nerve conduction studies 2 to 3 years after surgery [60].

However, nerve conduction studies are unpleasant for the patient and alternative diagnostic procedures are welcome. Liquid crystal thermography was originally used for the assessment of patients with suspected CTS [61–64]. So et al. [65] used infrared imaging for the evaluation of entrapment syndromes of the median and ulnar nerves. Based on their definition of abnormal temperature difference to the contralateral side, they found thermography without any value for assisting diagnosis and inferior to electrodiagnostic testing. Tchou reported infrared thermography of high diagnostic sensitivity and specificity in patients with unilateral CTS. He has defined various regions of interest representing mainly the innervation area of the median nerve. Abnormality was defined if more than 25% of the measured area displayed a temperature increase of at least $1°C$ when compared with the asymptomatic hand [66].

Ammer has compared nerve conduction studies with thermal images in patients with suspected CTS. Maximum specificity for both nerve conduction and clinical symptoms was obtained for the temperature difference between the 3rd and 4th finger at a threshold of $1°C$. The best sensitivity of 69% was found if the temperature of the tip of the middle finger was by $1.2°C$ less than temperature of the metacarpus [67].

Hobbins [68] combined the thermal pattern with the time course of nerve injuries. He suggested the occurrence of a hypothermic dermatome in the early phase of nerve entrapment and hyperthermic dermatomes in the late phase of nerve compression. Ammer et al. [69] investigated how many patients with a distal latency of the median nerve greater than 6 msec present with a hyperthermic pattern. They reported a slight increase of the frequency of hyperthermic patterns in patients with severe CTS indicating that the entrapment of the median nerve is followed by a loss of the autonomic function in these patients.

Ammer [70] has also correlated the temperature of the index finger with the temperature of the sensory distribution of the median nerve on the dorsum of the hand and found nearly identical readings for both areas. A similar relationship was obtained for the ulnar nerve. The author concluded from these data that the temperature of the index or the little finger is highly representative for the temperature of the sensory area of the median or ulnar nerve, respectively.

Many studies on CTS have used a cold challenge to enhance the thermal contrast between affected fingers. A slow recovery rate after cold exposure is diagnostic for Raynaud's Phenomenon [71]. The coincidence of CTS and Raynaud's phenomenon was reported in the literature [72,73].

17.5.1.4 Other Entrapment Syndromes

No clear thermal pattern was reported for the entrapment of the ulnar nerve [65]. A pilot study for the comparison of hands from patients with TOS or entrapment of the ulnar nerve at the elbow found only 1 out of 7 patients with ulnar entrapment who presented with temperature asymmetry of the affected extremity [74]. All patients with TOS who performed provocation test during image recording showed at least in one thermogram an asymmetric temperature pattern.

17.5.2 Peripheral Nerve Paresis

Paresis is an impairment of the motor function of the nervous system. Loss of function of the sensory fibers may be associated with motor deficit, but sensory impairment is not included in the term paresis. Therefore, most of the temperature signs in paresis are related to impaired motor function.

17.5.2.1 Brachial Plexus Paresis

Injury of the brachial plexus is a severe consequence of traffic accidents and motor cyclers are most frequently affected. The loss of motor activity in the affected extremity results in paralysis, muscle atrophy, and decreased skin temperature. Nearly 0.5 to 0.9% of newborns acquire brachial plexus paresis during delivery [75]. Early recovery of the skin temperature in babies with plexus paresis precede the recovery of motor function as shown in a study from Japan [76].

17.5.2.2 Facial Nerve

The seventh cranial nerve supplies the mimic muscles of the face and an acquired deficit is often named Bell's palsy. This paresis has normally a good prognosis for full recovery. Thermal imaging was used as outcome measure in acupuncture trials for facial paresis [77,78]. Ammer et al. [79] found slight asymmetries in patients with facial paresis, in which hyperthermia of the affected side occurred more frequently than hypothermia. However, patients with apparent herpes zoster causing facial palsy presented with higher temperature differences to the contralateral side than patients with nonherpetic facial paresis [80].

17.5.2.3 Peroneal Nerve

The peroneal nerve may be affected by metabolic neuropathy in patients with metabolic disease or by compression neuropathy due to intensive pressure applied at the site of fibula head. This can result in "foot drop," an impairment in which the patient cannot raise his forefoot. The thermal image is characterized by decreased temperatures on the anterior lower leg, which might become more visible after the patient has performed some exercises [81].

17.6 Complex Regional Pain Syndrome

A temperature difference between the affected and the nonaffected limb equal or greater than 1°C is one of the diagnostic criteria of the complex regional pain syndrome (CRPS) [82]. Ammer conducted a study in patients after radius fracture treated conservatively with a plaster cast [83]. Within 2 h after plaster removal and 1 week later thermal images were recorded. After the second thermogram an x-ray image of both hands was taken. The mean temperature difference between the affected and unaffected hand was 0.6 after plaster removal and 0.63 one week later. In 21 out of 41 radiographs slight bone changes suspected of algodystropy have been found. Figure 17.4 summarizes the results with respect to the outcome of x-ray images. Figure 17.5 shows the time course of an individual patient.

It was also shown, that the temperature difference decrease during successful therapeutic intervention and temperature effect was paralleled by reduction of pain and swelling and resolution of radiologic changes [84].

Disturbance of vascular adaptation mechanism and delayed response to temperature stimuli was obtained in patients suffering from CRPS [85,86]. These alterations have been interpreted as being caused by abnormalities of the autonomic nerve system. It was suggested to use a cold challenge on the contralateral side of the injured limb for prediction and early diagnosis of CRPS. Gulevich et al. [87] confirmed the high diagnostic sensitivity and specificity of cold challenge for the CRPS. Wasner et al. [88] achieved similar results by whole body cooling or whole body warming. Most recently a Dutch study found that the asymmetry factor, which was based on histograms of temperatures from the affected and nonaffected

FIGURE 17.4 Diagram of temperatures obtained in patients with positive or negative x-ray images. (From Ammer, K. *Thermol. Österr.*, 1, 4, 1991. With permission.)

FIGURE 17.5 (**See color insert.**) Early CRPS after radius fracture. (a) Two hours after cast removal; (b) 1 week later.

hand had the highest diagnostic power for CRPS, while the difference of mean temperatures did not discriminate between disease and health [89].

17.7 Thermal Imaging Technique

The parameters for a reliable technique have been described in the past. Engel et al. [90] is a report published in 1978 by a European working group on Thermography in Locomotor Diseases. This paper discusses aspects of standardization including the need for adequate temperature control of the examination room and the importance of standard views used for image capture. More recently Ring and Ammer [91] described an outline of necessary considerations for good thermal imaging technique in clinical medicine. This outline has been subsequently expanded to encompass a revised set of standard views, and associated regions of interest for analysis. The latter is especially important for standardization, since the normal approach used is to select a region of interest subjectively. This means that without a defined set of reference points it is difficult for the investigator to reproduce the same region of interest on subsequent occasions. It is also even more difficult for another investigator to achieve the same, leading to unacceptable variables in the derived data. The aspects for standardization of the technique and the standard views and regions of interest recently defined are the product of a multicentered Anglo-Polish study who are pursuing the concept of a database of normal reference thermograms. The protocol can be found on a British University Research Group's website from University of Glamorgan [10].

17.7.1 Room Temperature

Room temperature is an important issue when investigating this group of diseases. Inflammatory conditions such as arthritis, are better revealed in a room temperature of 20°C, for the extremities, and may need to be at 18°C for examining the trunk. This presumes that the relative humidity will not exceed 45%, and a very low airspeed is required. At no time during preparatory cooling or during the examination should the patient be placed in a position where they can feel a draught from moving air. However in other clinical conditions where an effect from neuromuscular changes is being examined, a higher room temperature is needed to avoid forced vasoconstriction. This is usually performed at 22 to 24°C ambient. At higher temperatures, the subject may begin to sweat, and below 17°C shivering may be induced. Both of these thermoregulatory responses by the human body are undesirable for routine thermal imaging.

17.7.2 Clinical Examination

In this group of diseases, it can be particularly important that the patient receives a clinical examination in association with thermal imaging. Observations on medication, range of movement, experience of pain related to movement, or positioning may have a significant effect on the interpretation of the thermal images. Documentation of all such clinical findings should be kept on record with the images for future reference.

References

[1] Horvath, S.M. and Hollander, J.L. Intra-articular temperature as a measure of joint reaction. *J. Clin. Invest.*, 13, 615, 1949.
[2] Collins, A.J. and Cosh, J.A. Temperature and biochemical studies of joint inflammation. *Ann. Rheum. Dis.*, 29, 386, 1970.
[3] Ring, E.F.J. and Collins, A.J. Quantitative thermography. *Rheumatol. Phys. Med.*, 10, 337, 1970.
[4] Esselinckx, W. et al. Thermographic assessment of three intra-articular prednisolone analogues given in rheumatoid arthritis. *Br. J. Clin. Pharm.*, 5, 447, 1978.

[5] Bird, H.A., Ring, E.F.J., and Bacon, P.A. A thermographic and clinical comparison of three intra-articular steroid preparations in rheumatoid arthritis. *Ann. Rheum. Dis.*, 38, 36, 1979.
[6] Collins, A.J. and Ring, E.F.J. Measurement of inflammation in man and animals. *Br. J. Pharm.*, 44, 145, 1972.
[7] Bacon, P.A., Ring, E.F.J., and Collins, A.J. Thermography in the assessment of anti rheumatic agents, in *Rheumatoid Arthritis*. Gordon, J.L. and Hazleman, B.L., Eds., Elsevier/North Holland Biomedical Press, Amsterdam, 1977, p. 105.
[8] Collins, A.J. et al. Quantitation of thermography in arthritis using multi-isothermal analysis. I. The thermographic index. *Ann. Rheum. Dis.*, 33, 113, 1974.
[9] Ammer, K., Engelbert, B., and Kern, E. The determination of normal temperature values of finger joints. *Thermol. Int.*, 12, 23, 2002.
[10] Website address, Standard protocol for image capture and analysis, www.medimaging.org
[11] Czerny, V. Eine fokale Malazie des Unterschenkels. *Wien. Med. Wochenschr.*, 23, 895, 1873.
[12] Paget, J. On a form of chronic inflammation of bones. *Med. Chir. Transact.*, 60, 37, 1877.
[13] Ring, E.F.J. and Davies, J. Thermal monitoring of Paget's disease of bone. *Thermology*, 3, 167, 1990.
[14] Tauchmannova, H., Gabrhel, J., and Cibak, M. Thermographic findings in different sports, their value in the prevention of soft tissue injuries. *Thermol. Österr.* 3, 91–95, 1993.
[15] Smith, B.L, Bandler, M.K, and Goodman, P.H. Dominant forearm hyperthermia, a study of fifteen athletes. *Thermology*, 2, 25–28, 1986.
[16] Fischer, A.A. and Chang, C.H. Temperature and pressure threshold measurements in trigger points. *Thermology*, 1, 212, 1986.
[17] Menachem, A., Kaplan, O., and Dekel, S. Levator scapulae syndrome: an anatomic–clinical study. *Bull. Hosp. Jt. Dis.*, 53, 21, 1993.
[18] Schmitt, M. and Guillot, Y. Thermography and muscle injuries in sports medicine, in *Recent Advances in Medical Thermography*. Ring, E.F.J. and Philips, J., Eds., Plenum Press, London, 1984, p. 439.
[19] Ammer, K. Low muscular activity of the lower leg in patients with a painful ankle. *Thermol. Österr.*, 5, 103, 1995.
[20] Kanie, R. Thermographic evaluation of osteoarthritis of the hip. *Biomed. Thermol.*, 15, 72, 1995.
[21] Vecchio, P.C. et al. Thermography of frozen shoulder and rotator cuff tendinitis. *Clin. Rheumatol.*, 11, 382, 1992.
[22] Ammer, K. et al. Thermography of the painful shoulder. *Eur. J. Thermol.*, 8, 93, 1998.
[23] Hobbins, W.B. and Ammer, K. Controversy: why is a paretic limb cold, high activity of the sympathetic nerve system or weakness of the muscles? *Thermol. Österr.*, 6, 42, 1996.
[24] Ring, E.F.J. and Ammer, K. Thermal imaging in sports medicine. *Sports Med. Today*, 1, 108, 1998.
[25] Gabrhel, J. and Tauchmannova, H. Wärmebilder der Kniegelenke bei jugendlichen Sportlern. *Thermol. Österr.*, 5, 92, 1995.
[26] Devereaux, M.D. et al. The diagnosis of stress fractures in athletes. *JAMA*, 252, 531, 1984.
[27] Graber, J. Tendosynovitis detection in the hand. *Verh. Dtsch. Ges. Rheumatol.*, 6, 57, 1980.
[28] Mayr, H. Thermografische Befunde bei Schmerzen am Ellbogen. *Thermol. Österr.*, 7, 5–10, 1997.
[29] Binder, A.I. et al. Thermography of tennis elbow, in *Recent Advances in Medical Thermography*. Ring, E.F.J. and Philips, J., Eds., Plenum Press, London, 1984, p. 513.
[30] Thomas, D. and Savage, J.P. Persistent tennis elbow: evaluation by infrared thermography and nuclear medicine isotope scanning. *Thermology*, 3, 132; 1989.
[31] Ammer, K. Thermal evaluation of tennis elbow, in *The Thermal Image in Medicine and Biology*. Ammer, K. and Ring, E.F.J., Eds., Uhlen Verlag, Wien, 1995, p. 214.
[32] Devereaux, M.D., Hazleman, B.L., and Thomas, P.P. Chronic lateral humeral epicondylitis — a double-blind controlled assessment of pulsed electromagnetic field therapy. *Clin. Exp. Rheumatol.*, 3, 333, 1985.
[33] Ammer, K. et al. Thermographische und algometrische Kontrolle der physikalischen Therapie bei Patienten mit Epicondylopathia humeri radialis. *ThermoMed*, 11, 55–67, 1995.

[34] Ammer, K., Schartelmüller, T., and Melnizky, P. Thermography in fibromyalgia. *Biomed. Thermol.* 15, 77, 1995.
[35] Ammer, K. Only lateral, but not medial epicondylitis can be detected by thermography. *Thermol. Österr.*, 6, 105, 1996.
[36] Hirano, T. et al. Clinical study of shoulder surface temperature in patients with periarthritis scapulohumeralis (abstract). *Biomed. Thermol.*, 11, 303, 1991.
[37] Jeracitano, D. et al. Abnormal temperature control suggesting sympathetic dysfunction in the shoulder skin of patients with frozen shoulder. *Br. J. Rheumatol.*, 31, 539, 1992.
[38] Biasi, G. et al. The role computerized telethermography in the diagnosis of fibromyalgia syndrome. *Minerva Medica*, 85, 451, 1994.
[39] Ammer, K. Thermographic diagnosis of fibromyalgia. *Ann Rheum Dis. XIV European League Against Rheumatism Congress, Abstracts*, 135, 1999.
[40] Ammer, K., Engelbert, B., and Kern, E. Reproducibility of the hot spot count in patients with fibromyalgia, an intra- and inter-observer comparison. *Thermol. Int.*, 11, 143, 2001.
[41] Anbar, M. Recent technological developments in thermology and their impact on clinical applications. *Biomed. Thermol.*, 10, 270, 1990.
[42] Uematsu, S. Thermographic imaging of cutaneous sensory segment in patients with peripheral nerve injury. *J. Neurosurg.*, 62, 716–720, 1985.
[43] Hoffman, R.M., Kent, D.L., and. Deyo, R.A. Diagnostic accuracy and clinical utility of thermography for lumbar radiculopathy. A meta-analysis. *Spine*, 16, 623, 1991.
[44] McCulloch, J. et al. Thermography as a diagnostic aid in sciatica. *J. Spinal Disord.*, 6, 427, 1993.
[45] Takahashi, Y., Takahashi, K., and Moriya, H. Thermal deficit in lumbar radiculopathy. *Spine*, 19, 2443, 1994.
[46] Kim, Y.S. and Cho, Y.E. Pre- and postoperative thermographic imaging of lumbar disk herniations. *Biomed. Thermol.*, 13, 265, 1993.
[47] Zhang, H.Y., Kim, Y.S., and Cho, Y.E. Thermatomal changes in cervical disc herniations. *Yonsei Med. J.*, 40, 401, 1999.
[48] Cuetter, A.C. and Bartoszek, D.M. The thoracic outlet syndrome: controversies, overdiagnosism overtreatment and recommendations for management. *Muscle Nerve*, 12, 419, 1989.
[49] Schartelmüller, T. and Ammer, K. Thoracic outlet syndrome, in *The Thermal Image in Medicine and Biology*. Ammer, K. and Ring, E.F.J., Eds., Uhlen Verlag, Wien, 1995, p. 201.
[50] Schartelmüller, T. and Ammer, K. Infrared thermography for the diagnosis of thoracic outlet syndrome. *Thermol. Österr.*, 6, 130, 1996.
[51] Melnizky, P, Schartelmüller, T., and Ammer, K. Prüfung der intra-und interindividuellen Verläßlichkeit der Auswertung von Infrarot-Thermogrammen. *Eur. J. Thermol.*, 7, 224, 1997.
[52] Ammer, K. Thermographie der Finger nach mechanischem Provokationstest. *ThermoMed*, 17/18, 9, 2003.
[53] Schartelmüller, T., Melnizky, P., and Engelbert, B. Infrarotthermographie zur Evaluierung des Erfolges physikalischer Therapie bei Patenten mit klinischem Verdacht auf Thoracic Outlet Syndrome. *Thermol. Int.*, 9, 20, 1999.
[54] Schartelmüller, T. and Ammer, K. Zervikaler Diskusprolaps, Thoracic Outlet Syndrom oder periphere arterielle Verschlußkrankheit-ein Fallbericht. *Eur. J. Thermol.*, 7, 146, 1997.
[55] Ammer, K. Diagnosis of nerve entrapment syndromes by thermal imaging, in *Proceedings of The First Joint BMES/EMBS Conference. Serving Humanity, Advancing Technology*, October 13–16, 1999, Atlanta, GA, USA, p. 1117.
[56] Atroshi, I. et al. Prevalence of carpal tunnel syndrome in a general population. *JAMA*, 282, 153, 1999.
[57] Ammer, K., Mayr, H., and Thür, H. Self-administered diagram for diagnosing carpal tunnel syndrome. *Eur. J. Phys. Med. Rehab.*, 3, 43, 1993.

[58] Melnizky, P., Ammer, K., and Schartelmüller, T. Intra- und interindividuelle Verläßlichkeit der elektroneurographischen Untersuchung des Nervus medianus. *Österr. Z. Phys. Med. Rehab.*, 7, S83, 1996.

[59] Schartelmüller, T., Ammer, K., and Melnizky, P. Natürliche und postoperative Entwicklung elektroneurographischer Untersuchungsergebnisse des N. medianus von Patienten mit Carpaltunnelsyndrom (CTS). *Österr. Z. Phys. Med.*, 7, 183, 1997.

[60] Rosen, H.R. et al. Is surgical division of the carpal ligament sufficient in the treatment of carpal tunnel syndrome? *Chirurg*, 61, 130, 1990.

[61] Herrick, R.T. et al. Thermography as a diagnostic tool for carpal tunnel syndrome, in *Medical Thermology*, Abernathy, M. and Uematsu, S., Eds., American Academy of Thermology, 1986, p. 124.

[62] Herrick, R.T. and Herrick, S.K., Thermography in the detection of carpal tunnel syndrome and other compressive neuropathies. *J. Hand Surg.*, 12A, 943–949, 1987.

[63] Gateless, D., Gilroy, J., and Nefey, P. Thermographic evaluation of carpal tunnel syndrome during pregnancy. *Thermology*, 3, 21, 1988.

[64] Meyers, S. et al. Liquid crystal thermography, quantitative studies of abnormalities in carpal tunnel syndrome. *Neurology*, 39, 1465, 1989.

[65] So, Y.T., Olney, R.K., and Aminoff, M.J. Evaluation of thermography in the diagnosis of selected entrapment neuropathies. *Neurology*, 39, 1, 1989.

[66] Tchou, S. and Costich, J.F. Thermographic study of acute unilateral carpal tunnel syndromes. *Thermology*, 3, 249–252, 1991.

[67] Ammer, K. Thermographische Diagnose von peripheren Nervenkompressionssyndromen. *ThermoMed*, 7, 15, 1991.

[68] Hobbins, W.B. Autonomic vasomotor skin changes in pain states: significant or insignificant? *Thermol. Österr.*, 5, 5, 1995.

[69] Ammer, K. et al. The thermal image of patients suffering from carpal tunnel syndrome with a distal latency higher than 6.0 msec. *Thermol. Int.*, 9, 15, 1999.

[70] Ammer, K. and Melnizky, P. Determination of regions of interest on thermal images of the hands of patients suffering from carpal tunnel syndrome. *Thermol. Int.*, 9, 56, 1999.

[71] Ammer, K. Thermographic diagnosis of Raynaud's Phenomenon. *Skin Res. Technol.*, 2, 182, 1996.

[72] Neundörfer, B., Dietrich, B., and Braun, B. Raynaud–Phänomen beim Carpaltunnelsyndrom. *Wien. Klin. Wochenschr.*, 89, 131–133, 1977.

[73] Grassi, W. et al. Clinical diagnosis found in patients with Raynaud's phenomenon: a multicentre study. *Rheumatol. Int.*, 18, 17, 1998.

[74] Mayr, H. and Ammer, K. Thermographische Diagnose von Nervenkompressionssyndromen der oberen Extremität mit Ausnahme des Karpaltunnelsyndroms (abstract). *Thermol. Österr.*, 4, 82, 1994.

[75] Mumenthaler, M. and Schliack, H. *Läsionen periphere Nerven*. Georg Thieme Verlag, Stuttgart-New York, Auflage, 1982, p. 4.

[76] Ikegawa, S. et al. Use of thermography in the diagnosis of obstetric palsy (abstract). *Thermol. Österr.*, 7, 31, 1997.

[77] Zhang, D. et al. Preliminary observation of imaging of facial temperature along meridians. *Chen Tzu Yen Chiu*, 17, 71, 1992.

[78] Zhang, D. et al. Clinical observations on acupuncture treatment of peripheral facial paralysis aided by infra-red thermography — a preliminary report. *J. Tradit. Chin. Med.*, 11, 139, 1991.

[79] Ammer, K., Melnizky, P. and Schartelmüller, T. Thermographie bei Fazialisparese. *ThermoMed*, 13, 6–11, 1997.

[80] Schartelmüller, T., Melnizky, P., and Ammer, K. Gesichtsthermographie, Vergleich von Patienten mit Fazialisparese und akutem Herpes zoster ophthalmicus. *Eur. J. Thermol.*, 8, 65, 1998.

[81] Melnizky, P., Ammer, K., and Schartelmüller, T. Thermographische Überprüfung der Heilgymnastik bei Patienten mit Peroneusparese. *Thermol. Österr.*, 5, 97, 1995.

[82] Wilson, P.R. et al. Diagnostic algorithm for complex regional pain syndromes, in *Reflex Sympathetic Dystrophy, A Re-appraisal*. Jänig, W. and Stanton-Hicks, M., Eds., Seattle, IASP Press, 1996, p. 93.

[83] Ammer, K. Thermographie nach gipsfixierter Radiusfraktur. *Thermol. Österr.*, 1, 4, 1991.

[84] Ammer, K. Thermographische Therapieüberwachung bei M.Sudeck. *ThermoMed*, 7, 112–115, 1991.

[85] Cooke, E.D. et al. Reflex sympathetic dystrophy (algoneurodystrophy): temperature studies in the upper limb. *Br. J. Rheumatol.*, 8, 399, 1989.

[86] Herrick, A. et al. Abnormal thermoregulatory responses in patients with reflex sympathetic dystrophy syndrome. *J. Rheumatol.*, 21, 1319, 1994.

[87] Gulevich, S.J. et al. Stress infrared telethermography is useful in the diagnosis of complex regional pain syndrome, type I (formerly reflex sympathetic dystrophy). *Clin. J. Pain*, 13, 50, 1997.

[88] Wasner, G., Schattschneider, J., and Baron, R. Skin temperature side differences — a diagnostic tool for CRPS? *Pain*, 98, 19, 2002.

[89] Huygen, F.J.P.M. et al. Computer-assisted skin videothermography is a highly sensitive quality tool in the diagnosis and monitoring of complex regional pain syndrome type I. *Eur. J. Appl. Physiol.*, 91, 516, 2004.

[90] Engel, J.M. et al. Thermography in locomotor diseases, recommended procedure. Anglo-dutch thermographic society group report. *Eur. J. Rheumatol. Inflam.*, 2, 299–306, 1979.

[91] Ring, E.F.J. and Ammer, K. The technique of infra red imaging in medicine. *Thermol. Int.*, 10, 7, 2000.

18
Functional Infrared Imaging in the Evaluation of Complex Regional Pain Syndrome, Type I: Current Pathophysiological Concepts, Methodology, Case Studies, Clinical Implications

18.1 Introduction.. 18-2
    Overview, History, and Contemporary Issues • Ethics and the Imperatives for Evidence-Based Use of Functional Infrared (fIR) Imaging in Research and Practice • Detection, Discernment, and Diagnosis: The Bases for Effective Treatment

18.2 Pathophysiology of CRPS I............................ 18-4
    Sympathetic Neural Involvement • Neurogenic Inflammatory and Central Neural Interactions • Putative Genetic Factors

Timothy D. Conwell
Colorado Infrared Imaging Center

James Giordano
Georgetown University Medical Center

Steven J. Gulevich
Swedish Medical Center

18.3 Methodology—fIR Imaging 18-6
  Description • Brief Historical Context • Medical Infrared Equipment • Infrared Laboratory Environment • Patient Selection–Indication • Patient Preprocedure Protocol • Patient Protocol • Study Protocol for fIR Pain Studies • Methods for Obtaining the Three (3) Specific fIR Indices
18.4 Case Studies 18-9
  Integrating the Pathophysiology of CRPS I to Findings from fIR Case Studies • Interpretation of fIR Thermal Image Signatures • Normal fIR Thermal Signatures • Abnormal fIR Studies • Acute Trauma (Post-Traumatic Injury)—fIR Thermal Signatures • C-Fiber (Small Caliber Nociceptive Afferent Excitation) Mononeuropathy—fIR Thermal Signatures • Acute CRPS I Thermal Signatures • Acute CRPS I Thermal Signatures—Bilateral Presentation • Chronic CRPS I—Thermal Signatures • Clinical Implications and Potential
Dedication 18-21
Acknowledgments 18-21
References 18-21

18.1 Introduction

18.1.1 Overview, History, and Contemporary Issues

Complex regional pain syndrome, Type I (CRPS I) is a potentially disabling condition characterized by regional pain that is often disproportionate to or occurs in the absence of an identifiable inciting event. The condition is associated with hyperalgesia, allodynia, spontaneous pain, abnormal skin color, changes in skin temperature, abnormal sudomotor activity, edema, active and passive movement disorders, and trophic changes of nails and hair. CRPS I usually begins after minor or major trauma to soft tissue such as a strain, sprain, or surgery. Although rare, it can also occur following fracture, visceral trauma, or central nervous system insult (e.g., CVA). Although similar—if not identical—in presentation, a related syndrome, Type II (CRPS II), occurs following direct insult or injury to peripheral nerve. A complete address of CRPS- II is beyond the scope of this chapter [1, for review]. Epidemiologically, Sandroni et al. [2] report that CRPS I occurs more frequently than CRPS II (i.e., CRPS I incidence of 5.5/100,000 person years at risk vs. CRPS II incidence of 0.8/100,000 person years at risk) is more prevalent (21/100,000 vs. 4/100,000) and occurs more in females than males with reported ratios of 2:1 or greater [3].

Diagnosis of CRPS I is based on patient history and evaluation of presenting clinical signs and symptoms. Diagnosis can be complicated by the facts that (1) the severity of the symptoms is characteristically far greater than that of the instigating insult; (2) there is a tendency of the symptoms to spread proximally and in some cases to the contralateral limb, trunk, and face; and (3) although somewhat more rare, all four extremities may be involved [4,5]. In light of these diagnostic issues, a consensus workshop was convened in Orlando in 1993 to posit evaluative criteria and develop a more effective nomenclature for these disorders. From this work, the term CRPS was first introduced. Subsequently, the International Association for the Study of Pain (IASP) modified their taxonomy of pain to include these disorders, thus formalizing the use of CRPS I to identify and describe distinct syndromes [6–8]. Previously, CRPS I and II were known as reflex sympathetic dystrophy and causalgia, respectively, although both syndromes were rather arbitrarily referred to as algodystrophy, Sudeck's atrophy, sympathalgia, and sympathetically maintained pain (SMP). However, it should be noted that SMP remains in use as a diagnostic category for any pain syndrome that involves, and is perpetuated by autonomic hyper-reactivity, and thus may be considered a subtype of CRPS I that is identifiable by responsiveness to sympatholytic intervention (*vide infra*).

The IASP diagnostic criteria for CRPS I is based on nonstandardized signs and symptoms [9–12]. Rigorous discriminant function analyses (DFA) applied to these criteria have revealed problems in reliability and maintaining external validity. These studies have shown that there is significant potential for overdiagnosis due to low specificity [13–15], low interobserver reliability [16,17], and considerable variability in the recognition of relevant clinical signs. Such disparities promote inherent difficulties in the clinical management of CRPS I. The lack of coherence in detection, discernment, and diagnostic acumen arises first from a tendency to rely on sympathetic blockade as a diagnostic measure. Reiteratively, it is important to note that while some CRPS I patients will be responsive to sympatholytics (e.g., systemically administered adrenergic antagonists, interventional sympathetic blockade), such SMP does not occur in all CRPS I, and therefore is not an exclusory criterion. Second, given the heterogeneity of signs, symptoms, and overall presentations, there is a level of suspicion among nonsubspecialists regarding the validity of CRPS I as a diagnosis. Taken together, these lead to a tendency for either frank undertreatment or excessive utilization of therapeutic interventions that incur significant cost, time, and even health burdens for the patient. Thus, it can be seen that diagnosis is the pediment on which effective and sound treatment is built. Clearly, more reliable diagnostic capability is needed to advance our understanding and treatment of CRPS I.

18.1.2 Ethics and the Imperatives for Evidence-Based Use of Functional Infrared (fIR) Imaging in Research and Practice

Detection alone is not diagnosis. In formulating any diagnosis, the clinician must utilize distinct domains and types of knowledge to apprehend the subjective and objective features of a disorder as expressed in a particular patient. While this is important in the diagnosis of any malady, it is particularly critical to diagnosing (and treating) pain syndromes. Pain by its nature is subjective, and thus the clinician must utilize patient narrative and history, together with any/all objective findings to formulate a clinical impression [18]. The "goal" of this initial step of pain medicine is to detect what and how a disorder presents in a particular patient, differentiate these signs and symptoms from other possible disorders, discern the contextual basis of these features and establish a diagnosis, literally a "… seeing or a knowledge into the problem." This provides the basis for the scope, nature, and extent of subsequent care, and allows for prognosis (a knowledge of what could occur). It is clear that this process is not simply one of applied science, but takes on considerable ethical weight as it names the disorder (and by extension categorizes the patient), frames the patient within a larger community of others, and creates a foundation for the development and implementation of prudent care [19]. The diversity and individuality of signs and symptoms of CRPS I complicates this process. The ethical obligation to treat pain [19] compels research to determine those techniques and technologies that facilitate diagnoses and treatments that are safe and effective, and equally compels the utilization of these approaches in clinical practice [20–22].

By classical definition, medicine is dedicated to the ends of providing patient care that is technically correct and ethically sound, enacted through the clinical encounter [23]. Research facilitates these ends by affording knowledge that (1) enables the clinician to evaluate the relative value(s), benefits, and risks of particular diagnostic and therapeutic approaches, and ultimately resolve clinical equipoise and (2) empowers patients to be informed participants in clinical decisions relevant to care, thereby lessening their inherent vulnerability and decreasing the inequities of power and capacity [21]. The ethical obligations of research and practice are reciprocally sustaining. Findings from research inform practice, and evaluation of outcomes gained by employing various techniques in practice contributes to a progressive revision and expansion of an evidentiary base of knowledge to instigate and guide further study [22,24]. Thus, we argue that the investigational and clinical use of functional infrared (fIR) imaging is both ethically imperative and pragmatically valid (see also Giordano, this volume).

18.1.3 Detection, Discernment, and Diagnosis: The Bases for Effective Treatment

Functional infrared imaging effectively detects the thermal signature of vasomotor disturbances that are an important factor in establishing a diagnosis of CRPS I. Early detection of CRPS I is essential for successful treatment, yet detection of early-stage CRPS I is difficult because the signs and symptoms mimic other pathologies. Several studies have supported the utility of fIR in early detection [25–29]. Most studies have utilized quantitative homologous side-to-side temperature differences as the sole criterion in establishing the diagnosis. These temperature differences have ranged from 0.5 [25], 0.6 [30,31], 1 [28,32–34], 1.5 [35], and 2°C [29].

Bruehl et al. [30] evaluated thermal asymmetries in patients with CRPS I following equilibration in a 20°C examining room for 20 min, and demonstrated a sensitivity of 60% and specificity of 67% utilizing an asymmetry cutoff of 0.6°C in side-to-side computer-generated temperature differences. Gulevich et al. [34] demonstrated a 93% sensitivity and 89% specificity when three of the following four infrared image categories were present: (1) quantitative homologous side-to-side computer generated temperature differences of greater than 1.0°C in the region of interest (ROI); (2) the presence of abnormal, disrupted transverse distal thermal gradient lines visualized in the symptomatic extremity; (3) the presence of a "thermal marker" of the symptomatic extremity visualized in the isotherm view; and (4) abnormal warming of the symptomatic extremity secondary to functional cold-water autonomic stress testing of an asymptomatic limb. These contingencies are addressed elsewhere in this chapter (see Section 18.3). Similarly, Wasner et al. [36] showed a sensitivity of 76% and specificity of 93% when patients underwent controlled alteration of sympathetic activity by using thermoregulatory whole body cooling followed by computer-generated side-to-side temperature differences of homologous body regions.

The use of quantitative temperature differences alone lacks diagnostic specificity because other conditions can present with skin temperature asymmetry. For example, differences in skin temperature occur in focal inflammation and vascular disease. Moreover, thermal asymmetry can result from somatoautonomic vasoconstriction secondary to acute trauma, antidromic vasodilatation from small fiber distal neuropathy, and neuropathic pain with sympathetic activity. But fIR thermography does not merely measure limb temperature; the infrared thermogram yields a temperature map (thermal signature) of an extremity through which a trained examiner can differentiate the thermal patterns of CRPS I from trauma, inflammation, and vascular disease. There is literature to support that assessment of the thermal signature (vasomotor changes) is instrumental, if not mandatory for establishing an accurate diagnosis of CRPS I and II [37–39]. Furthermore, the information obtained from infrared thermographic studies is significantly enhanced when fIR is wed to the most current software that allows computer-generated side-to-side temperature differences to statistically evaluate the integrity (i.e., normality vs. abnormality) of distal thermal gradient lines and responses to cold-water autonomic functional stress testing [34].

An understanding of the capabilities and limitations of this technology are critical to establishing its significance in detecting physiologic changes that are relevant and meaningful to the diagnosis of CRPS I. Thus this chapter will present: (1) a brief overview of the pathophysiology of CRPS I, with particular emphasis on those autonomically mediated vasomotor effects that evoke clinically relevant changes in the radiant heat signature; (2) current fIR methodology that has been shown to be capable of effectively detecting such changes; (3) discussion of the current procedures and protocol methods for performing fIR studies of presumed CRPS I (and differentiating this from other pain syndromes); and (4) selected cases of acute trauma, neurogenic inflammation without sympathetic activity, small caliber fiber distal neuropathy, and acute and chronic CRPS I to illustrate clinical applications of this technology.

18.2 Pathophysiology of CRPS I

18.2.1 Sympathetic Neural Involvement

Any discussion of CRPS I (and other types of sympathetically maintained pain, as well) must address the role of autonomic dysfunction. Ordinarily, sympathetic efferents and sensory afferents are not conjoined [40,41]. However, functional and perhaps structural interaction between nociceptive C-fiber afferents and sympathetic efferent fibers in both the periphery and within the dorsal root ganglion has been elucidated in both animal models of sympathetically mediated pain [42] and in humans with CRPS I [43,44]. This interaction involves the de novo expression of alpha-2 adrenoceptor on C-fiber processes, with a resulting sensitivity to adrenergic stimulation [44,45]. It remains unclear whether structural synaptogenesis is involved in the periphery or the dorsal root, but clearly the functional properties of C-fiber afferents change, with alteration in excitation threshold(s), after-response duration and frequencies, and perhaps expansion of receptive fields [35,46]. However, while sympathetic contribution to C-fiber activity may be influential and can contribute to the loss of thermoregulatory function (via sensitized alpha-adrenoceptor response to norepinephrine that evokes C-fiber-mediated pain and a concomitant axon reflex vasodilatation [47–50]), such sympathetically mediated mechanisms are not uniform in all instances of CRPS I, and sympathetic dysregulation does not account for the entire constellation of neurologic features of the disorder. (Note that cold-water autonomic functional stress testing may be helpful in identifying those patients with a sympathetically mediated component who will respond to sympathetic nerve blocks. Those patients who have an empirically normal cold-water stress test response and who characteristically do not respond to sympathetic nerve blocks are considered to have the sympathetically independent pain (SIP) form of CRPS I.)

18.2.2 Neurogenic Inflammatory and Central Neural Interactions

Irrespective of sympathetic effects, a neurogenic inflammation appears to be perpetuated in CRPS I [51,52], thereby supporting the initial work of Sudeck et al. [53] over a century ago. This inflammatory response is initiated, at least in part by substance P, and involves a nitric oxide-mediated peripheral vasodilatation [54], with enhanced extravasation of serotonin 5-HT [55,56], as well as a variety of peptides [57] that restimulate C-fiber afferents (producing pain) and elevate local concentrations of proinflammatory cytokines [58–60]. The continued activation of C-fiber afferents, second-order neurons of the spinothalamic tract (STT), and higher supraspinal loci in the neuraxis can evoke plastic functional and structural changes in the CNS that (1) suppress endogenous pain modulatory mechanisms, (2) decrease pain thresholds, and (3) increase the duration and intensity of pain sensation and perception [20,61]. Such changes have been demonstrated in CRPS I, and may be responsible for "top-down" effects upon the sympathetic system that initiate and/or maintain increased activation of pronociceptive mechanisms [62,63], alter peripheral vaso- and sudo-motor control, and may affect the structural integrity of the innervated tissues (e.g., skin, hair, nails, bone).

18.2.3 Putative Genetic Factors

These plastic changes occur over a variable time course, and it is almost impossible to predict the rapidity of these effects. Thus, there is a considerable temporal and individual variation in the presentation of CRPS I. It is not known whether this variability reflects some genetic and/or endo-phenotypic diathesis, a circumstantial effect relative to the provocative insult, or a combination of both. Genetically, particular histocompatibilty complexes have been linked to (certain forms of) CRPS I; Van De Beek and colleagues [64] have shown that spontaneous-onset CRPS I is associated with a newly identified HLA I complex, and increased HLA-DQ1 and HLA-DR13 have been found in CRPS I patients [65,66]. To date, however, it is unclear whether the presence of these histocompatibility complexes are predictive, precipitative, or simply a copresentation of CRPS I. Still, these findings suggest that with further research, HLA testing may become a valuable contribution to the diagnosis of CRPS I. But while genetic testing may be useful to predict or correlate a predisposition to CRPS I, the strength of these findings remains dependent upon other objective measures that detect pathologic changes in support of patients' subjective reports (of pain, sensory and autonomic dysfunction, etc.) and thus reveal the disorder "in expression." It is in this light that we argue for the utility of fIR as a critical component in the evaluation of CRPS I.

18.3 Methodology—fIR Imaging

18.3.1 Description

Functional infrared thermography is a nonionizing pain-free physiologic assessment procedure that has no known adverse biological side effects, is completely safe for women who may become or are pregnant, patients with intractable pain, and patients who cannot tolerate painful invasive procedures. Functional IR imaging is not recommended for patients with casts, bandages or other technical factors (i.e., patients bound to a wheelchair) that preclude the ability to expose skin to temperature equilibration and imaging.

18.3.2 Brief Historical Context

Measuring human skin temperature as a means of medical assessment began in antiquity with practitioners and scholars who recognized that body temperature is altered during infection and disease. As early as 400 BC, Hippocrates applied thin layers of moistened clay to various body regions and measured drying times in order to show differences in body temperature, believing that "… *in whatever part of the body heat or cold is seated there is disease*" [67]. Some 2000 years later, Galileo Galilee invented the "thermoscope" to detect human body temperature. In the early eighteenth century, Gabriel Fahrenheit invented the mercury thermometer, a device that is strikingly similar to the contemporary thermometer. However, it was not until 1870 that the thermometer was used in medicine. In 1800, William Herschel discovered the infrared spectrum [68], and this ultimately provided the impetus for studies on thermal heat that culminated in the development of heat imaging of radiant emissions some 200 years later. The incipient use of infrared technology provided a rudimentary depiction of biological heat signatures, and it was not until the mid-1960s that these methods were directly employed as a potentially viable evaluative tool in medicine. In the early 1980s, highly sensitive infrared cameras were interfaced with computer software specifically designed for medical applications. The development of sophisticated computerized electronic infrared detectors that are coupled to state-of-the-art analytic software has overcome many of the technical and practical limitations of infrared thermography, and now allows accurate real-time, side-to-side homologous temperature differences of the extremities, as well as additional sophisticated computer-enhanced thermal images.

18.3.3 Medical Infrared Equipment

Medical infrared thermographic equipment is able to image and record the radiant infrared emission from skin surface radiation. The infrared radiant emission is focused through a germanium lens and detected (in most infrared cameras) by a mercury–cadmium–telluride (HgCdTe) element housed within the optics unit. This information is converted into an electronic signal that is processed by a computer and displayed on a color monitor in real time. Current infrared equipment can detect temperature differences as small as $0.02°C$, with high thermal sensitivity and resolution. This high-resolution infrared image is able to detect the subtle temperature differences that are required to evaluate patients with mild sensory and autonomic neuropathies. Advances in medical infrared imaging software allows for very accurate computer-generated side-to-side homologous temperature differences of the regions of interest to provide objective discrimination of thermal emissions. The thermal sensitivity range utilized by most clinicians with modern high-resolution IR equipment ranges from 0.2 to $1.0°C$. The thermal range is set according to the anatomic region being studied, as well as the discriminate information relative to the pathology studies. In addition, advanced software is capable of enhancing the thermal image to evaluate autonomic vasomotor tone and maintenance of the sympathetic vasoconstrictor reflex during cold-water autonomic functional stress testing.

18.3.4 Infrared Laboratory Environment

The infrared laboratory environment must be controlled to ensure obtaining accurate readings of the thermal emission that are free of artifact. The laboratory must be maintained at a constant temperature of $20 \pm 1°C$, and may require a 2 to 4°C reduction in temperature during the hot summer months in order to achieve the body cooling that is required before imaging. It is imperative that the subjects' autonomic thermoregulatory function is not affected by the ambient environment. Thus, the laboratory must be free of any ultraviolet rays that may cause aberrant heating of the surface skin temperature, and should be lit with fluorescent light bulbs. Similarly, all windows should be covered to eliminate solar radiation. The laboratory must maintain low humidity to ensure protection from aberrant cooling, and must be as draft-free as possible to prevent cold air from blowing on the patient. The laboratory must be carpeted to prevent an inadvertent cooling artifact of the plantar surface of the feet.

18.3.5 Patient Selection–Indication

Patients who are presumed or suspected to have CRPS I and II are common indicators for fIR studies (as are those patients with signs and symptoms of conditions that mimic CRPS I) [69,70]. Some of these conditions include small fiber distal mononeuropathies, acute trauma, localized inflammation, vascular pathology, peripheral neuropathy, and vasospastic disorders. Follow-up fIR studies may be helpful in determining the effectiveness of sympathetic blockade, sympathectomy, and/or spinal cord stimulator placement. Follow-up fIR studies may also be indicated when evaluating patients' response to treatment or evaluating progression of the underlying disease state.

18.3.6 Patient Preprocedure Protocol

Patients undergoing fIR testing must follow very specific preprocedural protocols [69,70]. These include discontinuing the use of nicotine and caffeine products 4 h before testing, discontinuing physical therapy and TENS unit the day before testing, and the avoidance of skin lotions, deodorants, moisturizers, liniments, topical OTC medications, skin powders, and makeup the day of testing. Patients are advised not to wear any tight fitting clothing on the day of the test, and to discontinue the use of braces, bandaging, or neoprene wraps for 24 h before evaluation. As well, patients must not have any form of invasive diagnostic procedures for 24 h before testing. Patients may be required to discontinue certain opioid and nonopioid analgesic, and sympatholytic medications up to 24 h before testing, as these may impact sympathetic function and alter surface skin temperature. All interventional (sympathetic, Bier and neurolytic) blocks must be discontinued for a minimum of 3 days before testing.

18.3.7 Patient Protocol

Before imaging, the patient is required to equilibrate body temperature in a $20 \pm 1°C$ environment for a minimum of 15 min in order to stimulate the thermoregulatory autonomic response. The equilibration time may be prolonged in patients who are carrying a heat load from a warm outside environment or who may have a high basal metabolic rate (BMR). A patient assessment should be performed before equilibration. This includes assessing the ability to tolerate the procedure, evaluation of any contraindications, taking an appropriate medical history, and conducting a physical examination. In addition, mental status, pain levels, symptoms/signs of allodynia, hyperalgesia, hyperpathia, vasomotor or sudomotor findings, and risk of vasomotor instability should be assessed. Documentation of the patient's current medications and therapies, results of any previous thermographic or vascular studies and results of any previous sympathetic or vascular interventions should also be acquired [69,70].

Before beginning equilibration, the patient is asked to disrobe and put on a loose fitting cotton gown that covers the breasts and genitalia. The patient is required to stand during the equilibration is period and, asked not to scratch, rub, or touch any area of the skin that is going to be imaged. During the equilibration period, the technician should ensure that the patient has followed all preprocedural protocols [69,70].

18.3.8 Study Protocol for fIR Pain Studies

Upper body fIR pain study (qualitative and quantitative images are of the same views):

Qualitative color IR images of
1. Posterior cervical region
2. Posterior thoracic region that includes posterior arms
3. Anterior thoracic region that includes anterior arms
4. Anterior forearms and palmar hands (preferably in one image)
5. Posterior forearms and dorsal hands (preferably in one image)
6. Radial forearms and hands (preferably in one image)
7. Ulnar forearms and hands (preferably in one image)

Quantitative side-to-side homologous computer-generated temperature measurements of
1. Anterior forearms and palmar hands (preferably in one image)
2. Posterior forearms and dorsal hands (preferably in one image)
3. Radial and ulnar forearms also

Black-white distal thermal gradient imaging of
1. Palmar hands (preferably in one image)
2. Dorsal hands (preferably in one image)

Cold-water autonomic functional stress testing of
1. Distal posterior forearms and dorsal hands (one image)

Lower body fIR pain study (qualitative and quantitative images are of the same views):

Qualitative color IR images of
1. Posterior lumbar and buttock region
2. Posterior thighs and legs (preferably in one image)
3. Anterior thighs and legs (preferably in one image)
4. Left lateral thigh and leg with medial right thigh and leg (one image)
5. Right lateral thigh and leg with medial left thigh and leg (one image)
6. Dorsal feet (preferably in one image)
7. Plantar feet (preferably in one image)

Quantitative side-to-side homologous computer-generated temperature measurements of
1. Anterior legs (preferably in one image)
2. Posterior legs (preferably in one image)
3. Dorsal feet (preferably in one image)
4. Plantar feet (preferably in one image)

Black–white distal thermal gradient imaging of
1. Dorsal feet (preferably in one image)
2. Plantar feet (preferably in one image)

Cold-water autonomic functional stress testing of
1. Distal anterior legs and dorsal feet (one image)

18.3.9 Methods for Obtaining the Three (3) Specific fIR Indices

1. Qualitative/Quantitative side-to-side homologous computer-generated temperature views. Both the quantitative and qualitative images are obtained by capturing baseline color qualitative thermal images 0 to 50°C, with 0.05-degree accuracy. The user can display the 12-bit data in color or gray scale with software-installed color maps. The images are displayed with an 85–100-color palette and 0.15°C thermal window. Once the qualitative thermal images are captured, the technician outlines the region of interest using the polygon drawing tool that is embedded in the medical software. In an upper body pain study, the technician draws a polygon around the anterior forearms, posterior forearms, palmar hands, and dorsal hands. In a lower body pain study, the technician draws a polygon around the anterior legs, posterior legs, dorsal feet, and plantar feet. The computer software calculates average temperature(s) within each polygon, allowing calculation of side-to-side homologous temperature differences. A side-to-side homologous temperature difference >1.0°C is generally considered indicative of an autonomic abnormality secondary to an underlying pathology. This 1.0°C temperature difference may range from 0.5 to 1.5°C depending on the laboratory bias.

2. Black–white distal thermal gradient imaging. The black–white distal transverse thermal gradient views are obtained by imaging the palmar and dorsal hand in an upper body pain study and the dorsal and plantar feet in a lower body pain study. The images are viewed in the black–white mode with a ten-color palette and 0.05°C thermal window.

3. Cold-water autonomic functional stress testing. The cold-water autonomic functional stress testing is best performed by utilizing real-time dynamic subtraction imaging that is available on most medical IR software programs. Real-time image subtraction is achieved by choosing a starting reference image, then choosing to view only the differences from the reference to the current image. If the individual pixel temperature rises, the difference will be shown in color; if the temperature drops, the image will be displayed in shades of gray. At any time during the imaging process the user can choose to view the reference, delta, or current image. All thermal data have a dynamic range of 12 bits, enabling the user to view 0.05-degree difference in a 0 to 50°C temperature range. This testing is performed by imaging the symptomatic and contralateral asymptomatic distal extremity for 5 min while an asymptomatic limb is placed in a 12 to 16°C cold-water bath. The immersion of a noninvolved limb activates autonomic thermoregulatory function. If autonomic function is intact, there is vasoconstriction in all four extremities due to the central vasoconstrictor reflex. If the autonomic vasoconstrictor reflex is inhibited or there is autonomic failure, then an axon vasodilatation reflex will occur. This reflex will be visualized by a warming of the symptomatic distal extremity, and on occasion the bilateral asymptomatic distal extremity, during the 5-min cold-water autonomic functional stress test.

18.4 Case Studies

18.4.1 Integrating the Pathophysiology of CRPS I to Findings from fIR Case Studies

Functional infrared imaging detects the thermal signature produced by changes in cutaneous blood flow regulated by central thermal and respiratory control that affects vasoconstrictor and sudomotor reflexes. This vaso- and sudomotor activity is predominantly, but not exclusively, dependent on hypothalamic mechanisms. Sympathetic preganglionic neurons project to the paravertebral ganglia and synapse with postganglionic neurons innervating target organs and cells. Postganglionic sympathetic neurons release norepinephrine and neuropeptide Y to regulate cutaneous blood flow. Studies suggest that the thermoregulatory dysfunction in CRPS I is due to central inhibition of the cutaneous sympathetic vasoconstrictor reflex [71].

In addition to inhibition of efferent sympathetic neurons, afferent neurons also regulate cutaneous blood flow. Sensitization of cutaneous, small caliber C fibers evokes orthodromic release of the tachykinin SP within the dorsal horn to engage the nociceptive neuraxis, and also causes antidromic release of SP, as well as calcitonin gene-related peptide (CGRP) to (1) elicit peripheral vasodilatation, causing extravasation of other pronociceptive and proinflammatory mediators (e.g., serotonin [5-HT], bradykinin, vasoactive intestinal peptide [VIP]), and (2) perpetuate a neurogenic inflammatory response [20,52–55,58,73–75]. This cutaneous vasodilatation is easily demonstrated with fIR imaging by visualizing the infrared hyperthermic radiation, and may be involved in the clinically observed vasomotor changes in patients with acute CRPS I.

18.4.2 Interpretation of fIR Thermal Image Signatures

Gulevich et al. [34] demonstrated 93% sensitivity and 89% specificity with fIR in diagnosing cases presumed to be CRPS I. These results were obtained by evaluating three separate and distinct infrared image indices:

1. Computer-generated side-to-side quantitative homologous temperature differences of the symptomatic and asymptomatic distal extremities obtained after the patient equilibrated in a controlled temperature environment of $\leq 20°C$ for 15 min (see Section 18.3).
2. Black-and-white distal transverse thermal gradient signatures evaluated for maintenance or presence of well-defined transverse gradient lines, which represent normal vasomotor presentation or disruption of the transverse gradient lines that represent an abnormal vasomotor presentation. The distal thermal gradient patterns are visualized in the hands or feet, paying particular attention to fingers and toes.
3. Responses to cold-water autonomic functional stress testing [34,76,77] of the symptomatic and asymptomatic distal extremity to evaluate for autonomic function with concomitant maintenance of the vasoconstrictor reflex. When autonomic function is intact, there is evidentiary cooling of the distal symptomatic extremity due to maintenance of the vasoconstrictor reflex. With autonomic dysfunction there is warming of the distal symptomatic extremity [34]. This warming may be due to inhibition/failure of the vasoconstrictor reflex [34,78–81] or adrenergic sensitization of nociceptors (viz, upregulation and/or hyperaffinity of alpha adrenergic receptors [82]) producing an axon reflex-mediated vasodilatation. This axon reflex-mediated vasodilatation is not suppressed by sympathetic activity due to central inhibition of the sympathetic efferent fiber.

18.4.3 Normal fIR Thermal Signatures (Table 18.1)

In an asymptomatic (i.e., healthy, normal control), patient population the three fIR image indices are entirely normal as demonstrated by: (1) symmetrical thermal emission; (2) normal well-defined transverse thermal gradient lines; and (3) normal response (i.e., cooling) to cold-water autonomic functional stress testing [34].

Image findings:

- Bilateral thermal symmetry in region of interest (ROI)
- Normal, well-defined and uniform, transverse distal thermal gradient lines
- Cooling of the symptomatic distal extremity during cold-water autonomic functional stress testing

Image indices description:

1. *Quantitative thermal emission (computer generated side-to-side temperature) image findings* Uematsu et al. [83] in a pioneer normative data study demonstrated that in a normal healthy asymptomatic patient population, the quantitative computer-generated side-to-side temperature differences of homologous body parts is in the range of 0.17 to 0.45°C, with a human surface temperature symmetry averaging $0.24 \pm 0.073°C$ between homologous sides [84]. The mean standard deviation for repetitive readings over time of computer-generated side-to-side temperature differences of homologous body parts was $30.8 \pm 0.032°C$ [85]. Uematsu's normative data have been confirmed by numerous authors [34,86,87].
2. *Distal thermal gradient image pattern findings* In normal, healthy asymptomatic patients, the distal transverse thermal gradient lines visualized in the distal extremities, particularly in the fingers and toes, are well maintained [34]. Normal distal thermal gradient patterns in the fingers and toes are represented by distinct uniform transverse lines that are closely aligned, forming an alternating black–white–black linear pattern. Normal distal thermal gradient lines may be a result of the normal rhythmic cycling of cutaneous blood flow that is seen in healthy asymptomatic individuals [88].

TABLE 18.1 Normal Study

Normal study	ROI delta $T°$	Distal thermal gradient lines	Cold-water autonomic functional stress test
Image findings: 1. Quantitative and qualitative thermal symmetry in the ROI	Image findings: 1. ROI symmetrical <1.0°C	Image findings: 1. Maintained distal gradient lines	Image findings: 1. Normal cooling of the symptomatic and asymptomatic distal extremity Putative Mechanism: 1. Normal ANS function with maintenance of the vasoconstrictor reflex
Upper body fIR study Thermal signature			
Lower body fIR study Thermal signature			

(See figures in color insert at the back of the book.)

3. *Cold-water autonomic functional stress test findings*   In normal, healthy asymptomatic patients with intact autonomic function there is cooling of the distal extremities when a noninvolved extremity is placed in a ≤15°C cold-water bath [34] or when subjected to whole-body cooling by perfusion of circulating water into a thermal suit [36,89]. Additional studies have shown that following the arousal stimuli and the cold pressor test, the vasoconstrictor response is observed in asymptomatic patients and is diminished or absent in patients with CRPS I [78–81]. The following fIR data and images of postcold-water autonomic functional stress testing were obtained by utilizing real-time dynamic subtraction imaging during the 5-min period [34].

18.4.4 Abnormal fIR Studies

18.4.4.1 Mimics of CRPS I

In symptomatic patients, numerous conditions "mimic" the IASP CRPS I criteria that make it difficult for the nonexpert to differentiate. We argue that they following three fIR image indices, with their specific thermal signatures, is beneficial in differentiating CRPS I from other pain syndromes.

18.4.5 Acute Trauma (Post-Traumatic Injury)—fIR Thermal Signatures (Table 18.2)

Following acute trauma, patients without strong clinical signs of sympathetic dysfunction or acute nerve injury may present with symptoms similar to CRPS I. This patient population presents with clinically relevant hypothermia in the symptomatic extremity that is likely due to maintenance of the vasoconstrictor reflex secondary to a peripheral pain generator [90].

Image findings:

- Unilateral **hypothermic** vascular disturbances in ROI
- Normal well-defined transverse distal thermal gradient lines
- Cooling of the symptomatic distal extremity during cold-water autonomic functional stress testing due to normal autonomic function with maintenance of the vasoconstrictor reflex

Image indices description:

1. *Quantitative thermal emission (computer-generated side-to-side temperature) findings*   In cases of acute trauma with an intact autonomic function, skin temperature cooling is a common finding of the affected symptomatic extremity when compared to the unaffected, contralateral extremity. Cooling in the symptomatic extremity is due to a somatoautonomic reflex secondary to a peripheral pain generator with a resultant increase in sympathetic vasoconstrictor activity. This normal somatoautonomic reflex vasoconstriction is due to excitation of sensory receptors or irritation of a sensory nerve that elicits increased sympathetic tone, resulting in skin cooling. This vasoconstriction is predominantly visualized in the territory in which the afferent stimulus originates [91].
2. *Distal thermal gradient lined patterns*   In post-traumatic states the distal thermal gradient lines are well-maintained. This is believed to be due to maintenance of normal sympathetic vasomotor tone.
3. *Cold-water autonomic functional stress test findings*   In post-traumatic states autonomic function is intact and elicits cooling of the symptomatic extremity during cold-water autonomic functional stress testing. Numerous researchers believe that maintenance of the sympathetic vasoconstrictor reflex may be a feature that allows differentiation of normal, post-traumatic states and CRPS I [75,81,92,93].

TABLE 18.2 Acute Trauma

Acute trauma	ROI delta T°	Distal thermal gradient Lines	Cold-water autonomic functional stress test
Image findings: 1. Quantitative and qualitative thermal asymmetry in the ROI Putative mechanism: 1. Increased sympathetic vasomotor tone secondary to a peripheral pain generator 2. No evidence of neurogenic inflammation–antidromic vasodilatation	Image findings: 1. ROI hypothermic $>1.0°C$	Image findings: 1. Maintained distal gradient lines	Image findings: 1. Normal cooling of the symptomatic and asymptomatic distal extremity Putative mechanism: 1. Normal ANS function with maintenance of the vasoconstrictor reflex
Upper body fIR study Thermal signature			
Lower body fIR study Thermal signature			

(See figures in color insert.)

18.4.6 C-Fiber (Small Caliber Nociceptive Afferent Excitation) Mononeuropathy—fIR Thermal Signatures (Table 18.3)

Excitation of peripheral sensory C-fiber nociceptive afferents produces both orthodromic and antidromic release of vasodilator substances from the involved nerve terminals. The vasodilatatory substances include SP and CGRP. The vasodilatatory effects induce a rise in surface temperature and increase in the resultant radiant heat signature. This hyperthermia is independent of sympathetic activity and is localized to the skin territory innervated by the particular C fiber [73,94,95].

Image findings:

- Unilateral **hyperthermic** vascular disturbances isolated to a specific nerve territory
- Disrupted transverse distal thermal gradient lines isolated to a specific nerve territory
- Normal cooling of the symptomatic distal extremity during cold-water autonomic functional stress testing due to normal autonomic function that suppresses vasodilatation induced by antidromic release of proinflammatory substances

Image indices description:

1. *Quantitative thermal emission (computer-generated side-to-side temperature) findings* In these cases there is skin temperature warming (hyperthermia) localized to the skin territory of the involved nerve that is independent of sympathetic activity. There is normal thermal symmetry of the asymptomatic extremity.
2. *Distal thermal gradient lined patterns* The distal thermal gradient lines are disrupted solely in the skin territory of the involved nerve with loss of the normal transverse lines.
3. *Cold-water autonomic functional stress test findings* Normal cooling of the symptomatic extremity is observed during cold-water autonomic functional stress testing because the observed vasodilatation is independent of sympathetic activity in this pathology. Therefore, the normal cooling is most likely due to intact autonomic function with maintenance of the vasoconstrictor reflex that suppresses the vasodilatation [90,94,96–98].

18.4.7 Acute CRPS I Thermal Signatures (Tables 18.4 and 18.5)

18.4.7.1 Abnormal fIR Signatures Visualized Solely in the Symptomatic Limb (Table 15.4)

The following fIR images are taken from case studies of patients who met both the IASP and Gulevich et al. [34] criteria for CRPS I, which taken together demonstrated a 93% sensitivity and 89% specificity in diagnosing patients with presumed CRPS I. These fIR cases show hyperthermia of the symptomatic distal extremity visualized by computer generated side-to-side homologous temperature differences $>1°C$. These cases also show evidence of inhibition of the vasoconstrictor reflex as revealed by abnormal hyperthermic response to cold-water autonomic functional stress testing. This fIR thermal presentation appears to be consistent with the hypothesized central inhibition of sympathetic activity that occurs in acute-stage CRPS I, producing decreased release of norepinephrine at the terminal sites and resulting in vasodilatation and increased cutaneous blood flow [72]. This central sympathetic inhibition results in abnormal warming during cold-water autonomic functional stress testing.

Image findings:

- Unilateral **hyperthermic** vascular disturbances in ROI
- Disrupted transverse distal thermal gradient lines in ROI
- Abnormal warming of the distal symptomatic extremity (generally seen in the fingers or toes of the involved extremity) during cold-water autonomic functional stress testing

Functional Infrared Imaging in Evaluation of Complex Regional Pain Syndrome

TABLE 18.3 Small Caliber Fiber Sensory Distal Mononeuropathy

Small caliber fiber sensory distal mononeuropathy	ROI delta $T°$	Distal thermal gradient lines	Cold-water autonomic functional stress testing
Image findings: 1. Vasodilatation (visualized hyperthermic emission) localized in specific skin territory of the involved nerve Putative mechanism: 1. Antidromic vasodilatation unrelated to sympathetic activity	Image findings: 1. ROI hypothermic >1.0°C localized to the specific skin territory of the involved nerve	Image findings: 1. Disrupted distal gradient lines localized to the skin territory of the sensitized peripheral nerve	Image findings: 1. Normal cooling of the symptomatic and asymptomatic distal limb Putative mechanism: 1. Normal ANS function that overrides the antidromic vasodilatation with maintenance of the vasoconstrictor reflex
Upper body fIR study Thermal signature			

(See figures in color insert.)

TABLE 18.4 Acute CRPS I

Acute CRPS I	ROI delta $T°$	Thermal gradient lines	Cold-water autonomic functional stress test
Image findings: 1. Vasodilatation (visualized hyperthermic emission) with global, nondermatomal skin warming in the affected distal extremity Putative mechanisms: 1. Neurogenic inflammation–afferent axon reflex vasodilatation 2. Central sympathetic inhibition	Image findings: 1. ROI hyperthermic $>1.0°C$	Image findings: 1. Disrupted distal gradient lines in a global, nondermatomal distribution in the symptomatic distal extremity and occasionally in the asymptomatic contralateral distal extremity	Image findings: 1. Abnormal warming of symptomatic distal extremity with occasional warming of the contralateral side Putative mechanisms: 1. Abnormal ANS function with impairment of the sympathetic vasoconstrictor reflex or sympathetic failure 2. Intense axon reflex vasodilatation secondary to C-fiber sensitivity to circulating NE
Upper body fIR study Thermal signature			
Lower body fIR study Thermal signature			

(See figures in color insert.)

TABLE 18.5 Acute CRPS I (Bilateral Thermal Findings)

Acute CRPS I Bilateral thermal findings	ROI delta T°	Distal thermal gradient lines	Cold-water autonomic functional stress test
Image findings: 1. Vasodilatation (visualized hyperthermic emission) with global, nondermatomal skin warming in the affected distal extremity Putative mechanisms: 1. Central sympathetic inhibition 2. Neurogenic inflammation–afferent axon reflex vasodilatation	Image findings: 1. ROI hypothermic >1.0°C	Image findings: 1. Bilateral disrupted distal thermal gradient lines (seen in the fingers or toes) visualized in a global nondermatomal distribution in the effected distal extremity and asymptomatic contralateral distal limb	Image findings: 1. Abnormal warming of symptomatic and asymptomatic distal extremity Putative mechanisms: 1. Abnormal ANS function with bilateral impairment of the sympathetic vasoconstrictor reflex or sympathetic failure 2. Bilateral axon reflex vasodilatation secondary to C-fiber sensitivity to circulating NE
Upper body fIR study Thermal signature			

(**See figures in color insert.**)

Image indices description:

1. *Quantitative thermal emission (computer-generated side-to-side temperature) findings* In the acute phase of CRPS I, the affected distal extremity shows abnormal vasodilatation with subsequent skin warming as compared to the contralateral asymptomatic extremity [71,81,97,99,100]. This vasodilatation is due, in part, to central inhibition of sympathetic activity and a decreased release of norepinephrine and neuropeptide Y at terminal sites of sympathetic neurons [101–103]. Decreased noradrenergic activity at the terminal sites results in an increased cutaneous blood flow, which produces the clinical picture of a warm, discolored extremity. Inhibition of neuronally mediated vasoconstrictor reflexes is not believed to be due to major damage to the peripheral nerve (as in CRPS II), but rather due to a central inhibition of the thermoregulatory function [36,97,100].
2. *Distal thermal gradient line patterns* In symptomatic patients with thermoregulatory dysfunction, the distal transverse thermal gradient lines visualized in the distal extremities (particularly in the fingers and toes) are disrupted [34]. The disrupted lines are represented by irregular black–white–black gradient lines that are highly irregular without evidence of the normal transverse well-maintained pattern alignment. The disrupted irregular patterns are felt to represent aberrations produced by abnormal sympathetic vasomotor tone.
3. *Cold-water autonomic functional stress test patterns* In the acute phase of CRPS I, the affected extremity abnormally warms during cold-water autonomic functional stress testing [34]. It is hypothesized that this abnormal warming is due to inhibition or complete failure of the vasoconstrictor reflex and concomitant axon reflex-mediated vasodilatation. The axon reflex vasodilatation prevails due to the absence or inhibition of vasoconstrictor reflexes that would normally suppress vasodilatation. This has been illustrated by a case presentation of a patient who developed complete failure of the tonic vasoconstrictor response to cooling within 2 weeks of CRPS I onset [97]. This has been further supported by literature showing diminished sympathetic vasoconstrictor reflexes in the affected limb during the early-acute phases of CRPS I [99,100]. This abnormal warming may be due to adrenergic sensitization of nociceptors [82].

18.4.8 Acute CRPS I Thermal Signatures—Bilateral Presentation (Table 18.5)

18.4.8.1 Abnormal fIR Signatures Visualized in Both the Symptomatic and Asymptomatic Limbs

There are reports in the literature of subclinical *contralateral* sympathetic involvement in CRPS I [78,79,88] that are associated with axon reflex vasodilatation (hyperthermia) in both the distal symptomatic and asymptomatic limbs [104]. The following fIR images are taken from case studies of patients who met IASP CRPS I criteria and the criteria of Gulevich et al. [34], which demonstrated 93% sensitivity and 89% specificity in diagnosing patients with presumed CRPS I who demonstrated bilateral vasomotor findings. These fIR cases show hyperthermia of both the symptomatic and asymptomatic distal extremity, evidenced by computer-generated side-to-side homologous temperature differences of a >1°C hyperthermia of the symptomatic distal extremity. These studies also show evidence of inhibition of the vasoconstrictor reflex subserved by an abnormal axon reflex vasodilatation during cold-water autonomic functional stress testing. The hypothermia is likely due to supersensitivity to circulating catecholamines evoking vasoconstriction [105]. These findings tend to support the notion that CRPS I may also involve central mediation via an increased activation of brainstem or hypothalamic–pituitary–adrenal mechanisms.

Image findings:

- Bilateral distal hyperthermic vascular disturbances with the symptomatic distal extremity (ROI) demonstrating a >1.0°C **hyperthermia** difference with the contralateral asymptomatic limb

- Bilateral disrupted transverse distal thermal gradient lines
- Bilateral abnormal warming of the distal extremities (generally seen in the fingers or toes) during cold-water autonomic functional stress testing

18.4.9 Chronic CRPS I—Thermal Signatures (Table 18.6)

The following fIR images are taken from case studies of patients who met the IASP criteria for chronic CRPS I as well as the Gulevich et al. [34] criteria. These fIR studies show hypothermia of the symptomatic distal extremity visualized by computer-generated side-to-side homologous temperature differences >1°C. These case studies also show evidence of inhibition of the vasoconstrictor reflex associated with an axon reflex vasodilatation that is readily visualized in the symptomatic distal extremity, and occasionally the asymptomatic distal extremity during the cold-water autonomic functional stress testing.

Image findings:

- Unilateral **hypothermic** vascular disturbances with the ROI being >1.0°C colder than the contralateral asymptomatic limb
- Unilateral or bilateral disrupted transverse distal thermal gradient lines
- Unilateral or bilateral (warming) abnormal response to cold-water autonomic functional stress testing

Image indices description:

1. *Quantitative thermal emission (computer-generated side-to-side temperature) findings* In the chronic phase of CRPS I, the affected distal extremity shows abnormal vasoconstriction with subsequent skin cooling of the involved distal limb as compared to the contralateral asymptomatic limb [33,34,36,105,106]. This vasoconstriction is felt to be due to supersensitivity to circulating catecholamines [107]. Numerous mechanisms are responsible for this adrenergic supersensitivity including, but not limited to, diminished neurotransmitter reuptake, enzyme degradation, increased alpha adrenoceptor binding affinity and/or density of receptor sites, increased expression of sodium channels and/or sodium–potassium pump inefficiency [108].
2. *Distal thermal gradient line patterns* The distal transverse thermal gradient lines in chronic CRPS I are disrupted with a loss of the normal well-defined transverse gradient lines [34]. It is hypothesized that this disruption is the result of vasomotor disturbances evoked by circulating catecholamines.
3. *Cold-water autonomic functional stress test findings* In the chronic phase of CRPS I, the affected extremity, and occasionally the contralateral unaffected extremity, shows abnormal warming during cold-water autonomic stress testing [34]. It is hypothesized that this abnormal warming is due to inhibition or complete loss of the vasoconstrictor reflex resulting in an axon reflex-induced vasodilatation.

18.4.10 Clinical Implications and Potential

These findings support our contention that fIR, when coupled to advanced computational software, can effectively detect thermal signatures that reflect particular vaso- and sudomotor disturbances that are important in establishing a differential diagnosis of CRPS I. Obviously, it is important to restate that these objective features cannot be taken in isolation, and thus we do not advocate that fIR be considered or utilized as a stand-alone diagnostic modality. However, it is equally important to recognize that the inherent ambiguities in the presentation of CRPS I (and a persistent reticence to acknowledge the validity of a diagnosis of CRPS I based upon lesser objective findings) fortify the utility of this technology as a part of the diagnostic workup. Functional IR testing, when administered and evaluated by a competently trained professional, can provide reliable data that can contribute to both the diagnosis of a particular patient, and to a progressive database that can be utilized to develop an objective standard for clinical discernment and diagnoses.

TABLE 18.6 Chronic CRPS I

Chronic CRPS I	ROI Delta T°	Distal thermal gradient lines	Cold-water autonomic functional stress test
Image findings: 1. Vasoconstriction (visualized hypothermic emission) with skin cooling in the affected distal extremity Putative mechanisms: 1. Supersensitivity to circulating catecholamines–adrenergic supersensitivity 2. Minimal or absent sympathetic inhibition	Image findings: 1. ROI hypothermic > 1.0°C	Image findings: 1. Bilateral disrupted distal thermal gradient lines (seen in the fingers or toes) visualized in a global nondermatomal distribution in the effected distal extremity and asymptomatic contralateral distal limb	Image findings: 1. Abnormal warming of the symptomatic distal extremity with occasional warming of the contralateral asymptomatic extremity Putative mechanisms: 1. Abnormal ANS function with bilateral impairment of the sympathetic vasoconstrictor reflex or sympathetic failure 2. Bilateral axon reflex vasodilatation secondary to C-fiber sensitivity to circulating NE

Upper body fIR study
Thermal signature

(**See figures in color insert.**)

Extant concerns and refutations of the plausibility of IR thermography reflected inadequacies of older technology, and were valid criticisms of the lack of specificity, inappropriate and/or inapt use by untrained personnel, and the entrepreneurial overuse of IR as a "diagnostic" test. However, these biases are no longer applicable as the enjoinment of current technology (based upon declassified military instrumentation) and advanced statistical software has rendered all prior iterations of thermographic detection almost obsolete and established a new benchmark for technical efficiency and accuracy.

This technology will only improve, and thus it is important to both study fIR further to develop new avenues for clinical use, and employ these methods in the detection of CRPS I and other diagnostically difficult syndromes.

Dedication

This chapter is dedicated to the memory of a gifted neurologist and friend, Neil Rosenberg M.D. During the early days of infrared thermography, Dr. Rosenberg recognized the potential for this technology through research. Dr. Rosenberg is internationally recognized for his groundbreaking work in evaluating and treating children with addiction from toxic chemical inhalation.

Acknowledgments

Contributions to this work were supported in part by Colorado Infrared Imaging Center, Denver Colorado. The fIR case studies were obtained from the center's patient files.

TC gratefully acknowledges Drs. L. Barton Goldman, Rick S. Schwettmann, Floyd O. Ring, Jr., and Richard L. Stieg for their intellectual and scientific pursuit in the advancement of this emerging technology.

Contributions to this work were also supported in part by Georgetown University Medical Center, Washington, DC and a grant from the Hunt-Travis Foundation (JG). JG gratefully acknowledges Sherry Loveless for assistance on preparation of this chapter, and Drs. Edmund Pellegrino and Pierre LeRoy for ongoing intellectual exchange.

We express our sincere thanks to Maurice Bales, founder and president, Bales Scientific, for his valuable and lifelong dedication to medical infrared imaging. The fIR images in this chapter were captured by a Bales Scientific Tip-50 infrared camera interfaced with sophisticated medical imaging software.

References

[1] Hendler, N., Complex regional pain syndrome types I and II, in *Weiner's Pain Management: A Practical Guide for Clinicians*, 7th ed., Boswell, M.V. and Cole, B.E., Eds., CRC Press, Boca Raton, FL, 2005.

[2] Sandroni, P. et al., Complex regional pain syndrome type I: incidence and prevalence in Olmsted County—a population based study, *Pain*, 103, 199, 2003.

[3] Allen, G., Galer, B.S., and Schwartz, L., Epidemiology of complex regional pain syndrome: a retrospective chart review of 134 patients, *Pain*, 80, 539, 1999.

[4] Harden, R.N., Baron, R., and Janig, W., *Complex Regional Pain Syndrome, Progress in Pain Research and Management*, IASP Press, Seattle, Vol. 22, 2001.

[5] Janig, W. and Levine, J.D., Autonomic–endocrine–immune interactions in acute and chronic pain, in *Wall and Melzack's Textbook of Pain*, 5th ed., McMahon, S.P. and Koltzenburg, M., Eds., Churchill Livingston, Edinburgh, 2005.

[6] Merskey, H. and Bogduk, N. *Classification of Chronic Pain: Descriptions of Chronic Pain Syndrome and Definitions of Pain Terms*, 2nd ed., IASP Press, Seattle, 1994.

[7] Stanton-Hicks, M. et al., Reflex sympathetic dystrophy: changing concepts and taxonomy, *Pain*, 63, 127, 1995.

[8] Janig, W. and Stanton-Hicks, M., Eds. *Reflex Sympathetic Dystrophy: A Reappraisal, Progress and Pain Research and Management*, IASP Press, Seattle, Vol. 6, 1996.

[9] Bonica, J.J., *The Management of Pain*, Lea and Febiger, Philadelphia, PA, 1953.

[10] Kozin, F. et al., Reflex sympathetic dystrophy (RSDS), III: scintigraphic studies, further evidence for the therapeutic efficacy of systemic corticosteroids and proposed diagnostic criteria, *Am. J. Med.*, 70, 23, 1981.

[11] Blumberg, H., A new clinical approach for diagnosing reflex sympathetic dystrophy, in *Proceedings of the VI World Congress on Pain*, Bond, M.R., Charlton, J E., and Woolf, C.J., Eds., Elsevier, New York, p. 399, 1991.

[12] Gibbons, J.J. and Wilson, P.R., RSD score: criteria for the diagnosis of reflex sympathetic dystrophy and causalgia, *Clin. J. Pain*, 8, 260, 1992.

[13] Harden, R.N. and Bruehl, S.P., Diagnostic criteria: the statistical deviation of the four criteria factors, in *CRPS: Current Diagnosis and Therapy*, Wilson, P.R., Stanton Hicks, M., and Harden, R.N., Eds., IASP Press, Seattle, Vol. 32, 2005.

[14] Galer, B.S., Bruehl, S., and Harden, R.N., IASP diagnostic criteria for complex regional pain syndrome: a preliminary comparable validation study, *Clin. J. Pain*, 14, 48, 1998.

[15] Bruehl, S. et al., External validation of IASP diagnostic criteria for complex regional pain syndrome and proposed research diagnostic criteria, *Pain*, 81, 147, 1999.

[16] Van de Beek, W.J. et al., Diagnostic criteria used in studies of reflex sympathetic dystrophy, *Neurology*, 8, 522, 2002.

[17] Van den Vusse, A.C. et al., Interobserver reliability of the diagnosis in patients with CRPS, *Eur. J. Pain*, 7, 259, 2003.

[18] Giordano, J., On knowing: domains of knowledge and intellectual virtue in practical pain management, *Prac. Pain Manage.*, 6, 71, 2006.

[19] Giordano, J., Toward a core philosophy and virtue-based ethics of pain medicine, *Pain Practitioner*, 15, 59, 2005.

[20] Giordano, J., The neuroscience of pain and analgesia, in *Weiner's Pain Management: A Practical Guide for Clinicians*, 7th ed., Boswell, M.V. and Cole, B.E., Eds., CRC Press, Boca Raton, FL, 2005.

[21] Giordano, J., Moral agency in pain medicine: philosophy, practice and virtue, *Pain Phys.*, 9, 71, 2006.

[22] Giordano, J., Good as gold? The randomized controlled trial—pragmatic and ethical issues in pain research, *Am. J. Pain Manage.*, 16, 68, 2006.

[23] Pellegrino, E.D., The healing relationship: the architectonics of clinical medicine, in *The Clinical Encounter: The Moral Fabric of the Patient–Physician Relationship*, Philosophy and Medicine Series 4, Shelp, E.E., Ed., Dordrecht, D., Reidel, 1983.

[24] Giordano, J., Pain research: can paradigmatic revision bridge the needs of medicine, scientific philosophy and ethics? *Pain Phys.*, 7, 459, 2004.

[25] Karstetter, K.W. and Sherman, R.A., Use of thermography in initial detection of early reflex sympathetic dystrophy, *J. Am. Pediatr. Med. Assoc.*, 81, 198, 1991.

[26] Perelman, R.B., Adler, D., and Humphries, M., Reflex sympathetic dystrophy: electronic thermography as an aid in diagnosis, *Orthop. Rev.*, 16, 561, 1987.

[27] Lightman, H.I. et al., Thermography in childhood reflex sympathetic dystrophy, *J. Pediatr.*, 111, 551, 1987.

[28] Lewis, R., Racz, G., and Fabian, G., Therapeutic approaches to reflex sympathetic dystrophy of the upper extremity, *Clin. Issues Reg. Anesth.*, 1, 1, 1985.

[29] Uematsu, S. et al., Thermography and electromyography in the differential diagnosis of chronic pain syndromes and reflex sympathetic dystrophy, *Electromyogr. Clin. Neurophysiol.*, 21, 165, 1981.

[30] Bruehl, S. et al., Validation of thermography in the diagnosis of reflex sympathetic dystrophy, *Clin. J. Pain*, 12, 316, 1996.

[31] Cooke, E.D. et al., Reflex sympathetic dystrophy (algoneurodystrophy): temperature studies in the upper limb, *Br. J. Rheumatol.*, 28, 399, 1989.

[32] McLeod, J.G. and Tuck, R.R., Disorders of the autonomic nervous system, *Ann. Neurol.*, 21, 419, 1987.

[33] Low, P.A. et al., Laboratory findings in reflex sympathetic dystrophy: a preliminary report, *Clin. J. Pain*, 10, 235, 1994.

[34] Gulevich, S.J. et al., Stress infrared telethermography is useful in the diagnosis of complex regional pain syndrome, type 1 (formally reflex sympathetic dystrophy), *Clin. J. Pain*, 13, 50, 1997.

[35] Birklein, F. et al., Neurological findings in complex regional pain syndrome-analysis of 145 cases, *Acta Neurol. Scand.*, 101, 262, 2000.

[36] Wasner, G., Schattschneider, J., and Baron, R., Skin temperature side differences: a diagnostic tool for CRPS? *Pain*, 98, 19, 2002.

[37] Rommel, O., Habler, H.J., and Schurmann, M., Laboratory tests for complex regional pain syndrome, in *CRPS: Current Diagnosis and Therapy*, Wilson, P.R., Stanton-Hicks, M., Harden, R.N., Eds., IASP Press, Seattle, Vol. 32, 2005.

[38] Hooshmand, H., *Chronic Pain: Reflex Sympathetic Dystrophy Prevention and Management*, CRC Press, Boca Raton, FL, 1993.

[39] Stanton-Hicks, M., Janig, W., and Boas, R.A., *Reflex Sympathetic Dystrophy*, Kluwer Academic Publications, Norwell, MA, 1990.

[40] Baron, R. and Maier C., Reflex sympathetic dystrophy: skin blood flow, sympathetic vasoconstrictor reflexes and pain before and after surgical sympathectomy, *Pain*, 67, 317, 1996.

[41] Wasner, G. et al., No effect of sympathetic sudomotor activity on capsaicin-evoked ongoing pain and hyperalgesia, *Pain*, 84, 331, 2000.

[42] McLachlan, E.M., et al., Peripheral nerve injury triggers noradrenergic sprouting within the dorsal root ganglia, *Nature*, 363, 543, 1993.

[43] Ali, Z., et al., Intradermal injection of norepinephrine evokes pain in patients with sympathetically maintained pain, *Pain*, 88, 161, 2000.

[44] Baron, R. et al., Relation between sympathetic vasoconstrictor activity and pain and hyperalgesia in complex regional pain syndromes: a case control study, *Lancet*, 359, 1655, 2002.

[45] Shi, T.S. et al., Distribution and regulation of alpha(2)—adrenoceptors in rat dorsal root ganglia, *Pain*, 84, 319, 2000.

[46] Sieweke, N. et al., Patterns of hyperalgesia in complex regional pain syndrome, *Pain*, 80, 171, 1999.

[47] Janig, W. and Habler, H.J., Organization of the autonomic nervous system: structure and function, in *Handbook of Clinical Neurology*, Appenzeller, O., Ed., Elsevier, Amsterdam, Vol. 74, p. 1, 1999.

[48] Janig, W. and Habler, H.J., Neurophysiological analysis of target-related sympathetic pathways from animal to human: similarities and differences, *Acta. Physiol. Scand.*, 177, 255, 2003.

[49] Janig, W. and MacLachlan, E.M., Neurobiology of the autonomic nervous system, in *Autonomic Failure: A Textbook of Clinical Disorders of the Autonomic Nervous System*, 4th ed., Mathias, C.J. and Bannister, R., Eds., Oxford University Press, Oxford, p. 3, 1999.

[50] Janig, W., The autonomic nervous system and its coordination by the brain, in *Handbook of Affective Sciences, Part II*, Davidson, R.J., Scherer, K.R., and Goldsmith, H.H., Eds., Oxford University Press, Oxford, p. 135, 2003.

[51] Oyen, W.J. et al., Reflex sympathetic dystrophy of the hand: an excessive inflammatory response? *Pain*, 55, 151, 1993.

[52] Weber, M. et al., Facilitated neurogenic inflammation in complex regional pain syndrome, *Pain*, 91, 251, 2001.

[53] Sudeck, P., Über die acute (trophoneurotische) Knochenatrophie nach Entzündugen und Traumen der Extremitüten. *Deutsche Medizinische Wochenschrift*, 28, 336, 1902.

[54] Hartrick, C.T., Increased production of nitric oxide stimulated by interferon-gamma from peripheral blood monocytes in patients with complex regional pain syndrome, *Neurosci. Lett.*, 323, 75, 2002.

[55] Giordano, J. and Dyche, J., Differential analgesic action of serotonin 5-HT3 receptor antagonists in three pain tests, *Neuropharmacology*, 28, 431, 1989.

[56] Giordano, J. and Schultea, T., Serotonin 5-HT3 receptor mediation of pain and anti-nociception, *Pain Phys.*, 7, 141, 2003.
[57] Kozin, F. et al., The reflex sympathetic dystrophy syndrome: I. Clinical and histologic studies: evidence for bilaterality, response to corticosteroids and articular involvement, *Am. J. Med.*, 60, 321, 1976.
[58] Sufka, K., Schomberg, F., and Giordano, J., Receptor mediation of 5-HT-induced inflammation and nociception in rats, *Pharmacol. Biochem. Behav.*, 41, 53, 1992.
[59] Giordano, J. and Sacks, S., Topical ondansetron attenuates capsaicin-induced inflammation and pain, *Eur. J. Pharmacol.*, 354, 13, 1998.
[60] Huygen, F.J., et al., Evidence for local inflammation in complex regional pain syndrome type 1, *Mediators Inflamm.*, 11, 47, 2002.
[61] Giordano, J., Neurobiology of nociceptive and anti-nociceptive systems, *Pain Phys.*, 8, 277, 2005.
[62] Apkarian, A.V. et al., Prefrontal cortical hyperactivity in patients with sympathetically mediated chronic pain, *Neurosci. Lett.*, 311, 193, 2001.
[63] Juttonen, K. et al., Altered central sensorimotor processing in patients with complex regional pain syndrome, *Pain*, 98, 315, 2002.
[64] Van de Beek, W.J. et al., Susceptibility loci for complex regional pain syndrome, *Pain*, 103, 93, 2003.
[65] Kemler, M.A. et al., HLA-DQ1 associated with reflex sympathetic dystrophy, *Neurology*, 53, 1350–1351, 1999.
[66] Van Hilten, J.J., Van de Beek, W.J., and Roep, B.O., Multifocal or generalized tonic dystonia of complex regional pain syndrome: A distinct clinical entity associated with HLA-DR13, *Ann. Neurol.*, 48, 113–116, 2000.
[67] Galen, *Hippocrates Writings*, Franklin Library, Franklin Center, PA, 1979.
[68] Clark, R.P., Human skin temperature and its relevance in physiology and clinical assessment, in *Recent Advances in Medical Thermology*, Ring, E.F.J. and Phillips, B., Eds. Plenum Press, New York, 5, 1984.
[69] American Chiropractic College of Infrared Imaging a College of the Council on Diagnostic Imaging, *Technical Protocols for High Resolution Infrared Imaging*, American Chiropractic Association, 1999.
[70] Schwartz, R.G., Chair, Practice guidelines committee, Guidelines for neuromusculoskeletal thermography, American Academy of Thermology, *Thermology International*, 5, 2006.
[71] Wasner, G. et al., Vascular abnormalities in reflex sympathetic dystrophy (CRPS I): mechanisms and diagnostic value, *Brain*, 124, 587, 2001.
[72] Giordano, J. and Gerstmann, H., Patterns of serotonin- and 2-methylserotonin-induced pain may reflect 5-HT3 receptor sensitization, *Eur. J. Pharmacol.*, 483, 267, 2004.
[73] Ochoa, J.L. et al., Intrafascicular nerve stimulation elicits regional skin warming that matches the projected field of evoked pain, in *Fine Afferent Nerve Fibers and Pain*, Schmidt, R.F., Schaible, H.G., and Vahle-Hinz, C., Eds., VCH Verlagsgesellschaft, Weinheim, Germany, 1987.
[74] Holzer, P., Peptidergic sensory neurons in the control of vascular functions: mechanisms and significance in the cutaneous and splanchnic vascular beds, *Rev. Physiol. Biochem. Pharmacol.*, 121, 49, 1992.
[75] Birklein, F., Kunzel, W., and Sieweke, N., Despite clinical similarities there are significant differences between acute limb trauma and complex regional pain syndrome I (CRPS I), *Pain*, 93, 165, 2001.
[76] Hobbins, W.B., Differential diagnosis of painful conditions and thermography, in *Contemporary Issues in Chronic Pain Management*, Norwell, M.A., Ed., Kluwer Academic Publishers, Paris 251, 1991.
[77] Edwards, B.E. and Hobbins, W.B., Pain management and thermography, in *Practical Management of Pain*, 2nd ed., Raj, P.P., Ed., Mosby-Year Book, St. Louis, p. 168, 1992.
[78] Rosen, L. et al., Skin microvascular circulation in the symptomatic dystrophy is evaluated by videophotometric capillaroscopy and laser Doppler fluxmetry, *Eur. J. Clin. Invest.*, 18, 305, 1998.

[79] Kurvers, H.J. et al., The spinal component to skin blood flow abnormalities in reflex sympathetic dystrophy, *Arch. Neurol.*, 53, 50, 1996.
[80] Schurmann, M., Grab, G., and Furst, H., A standardized bedside test for assessment of peripheral sympathetic nervous function using laser doppler flowmetry, *Microvasc. Res.*, 52, 157, 1996.
[81] Schurmann, M. et al., Assessment of peripheral sympathetic nervous function for diagnosing early post-traumatic complex regional pain syndrome type 1, *Pain*, 80, 149, 1999.
[82] Campbell, J.N., Maier, R.A., and Raja, S.N., Is nociceptor activation by alpha-1 adrenoceptors the culprit in sympathetically maintained pain? *APS J.*, 1, 3, 1992.
[83] Uematsu, S., Thermographic imaging of the sensory dermatomes, *Soc. Neurosci.*, abstract, 9, 324, 1983.
[84] Uematsu, S., Thermographic imaging of cutaneous sensory segments in patients with peripheral nerve injury, *J. Neurosurg.*, 62, 716, 1985.
[85] Uematsu, S. et al., Quantification of thermal asymmetry, Part 1: normal values and reproducibility, *J. Neurosurg.*, 69, 552, 1988.
[86] Feldman, F. and Nickoloff, E.L., Normal thermographic standards for the cervical spine and upper extremities, *Skeletal Radiol.*, 12, 235, 1984.
[87] Goodman, P.A., Computer-assisted thermography, in *Proceedings of the 14th Annual Meeting of the American Academy of Thermology*, abstract, 36, 1985.
[88] Bej, M.D. and Schwartzman, R.J., Abnormalities of cutaneous blood flow regulation in patients with reflex sympathetic dystrophy as measured by laser doppler fluxmetry, *Arch. Neurol.*, 48, 912, 1991.
[89] Bini, G. et al., Thermography and rhythm-generating mechanisms governing the sudomotor and vasoconstrictor outflow in human cutaneous nerves, *J. Physiol.* (London), 206, 537, 1980.
[90] Ochoa, J.L. et al., Interactions between sympathetic vasoconstrictor outflow and C-nociceptors-induced antidromic vasodilatation, *Pain*, 54, 191, 1993.
[91] Bennett, G.J. and Ochoa, L.J., Thermographic observations on rats with experimental neuropathic pain, *Pain*, 45, 61, 1991.
[92] Schurmann, M. et al., Peripheral sympathetic function as a predictor of complex regional pain syndrome type I (CRPS I) in patients with radial fracture, *Autonom. Neurosci.*, 86, 127, 2000.
[93] Rosenbaum, R.B. and Ochoa, J.L., Thermography, in *Carpal Tunnel Syndrome and Other Disorders of the Median Nerve*, Rosenbaum, R.B. and Ochoa, J.L., Eds., Butterworth-Heindmann, Boston, p. 185, 1993.
[94] Cline, M.A., Ochoa, J.L., and Torebjork, H.E., Chronic hyperalgesia and skin warming caused by sensitized C nociceptors, *Brain*, 112, 621, 1989.
[95] Ochoa, J.L., The newly recognize painful ABC syndrome: thermographic aspects, *Thermology*, 2, 65, 1986.
[96] Ochoa, J.L. et al., Antidromic vasodilatation overridden by somatosympathetic reflexes in man-intraneural stimulation and thermography (abstract), *Soc. Neurosci.*, 16, 1280, 1990.
[97] Wasner, G. et al., Vascular abnormalities in acute reflex sympathetic dystrophy (CRPS I): complete inhibition of sympathetic nerve activity with recovery, *Arch. Neurol.*, 56, 613, 1999.
[98] Hornyak, M.E. et al., Sympathetic activity influences the vascular axon reflex in the skin, *Acta. Physiol. Scand.*, 139, 77, 1990.
[99] Kurvers, H.J. et al., Reflex sympathetic dystrophy: evolution of microcirculatory disturbances in time, *Pain*, 60, 333, 1995.
[100] Birklein, F. et al., Sympathetic vasoconstrictor reflex pattern in patients with complex regional pain syndrome, *Pain*, 75, 93, 1998.
[101] Drummond, P.D., Finch, P.M., and Smythe, G.A., Reflex sympathetic dystrophy: the significance of differing plasma catecholamine concentrations in affected and unaffected limbs, *Brain*, 114, 2025, 1991.
[102] Drummond, P.A. et al., Plasma neuropeptide Y in the symptomatic limb of patients with causalgia pain, *Clin. J. Pain*, 12, 222, 1996.

[103] Harden, R.N. et al., Norepinephrine and epinephrine levels in affected versus unaffected limbs in sympathetically maintained pain, *Clin. J. Pain*, 10, 324, 1994.
[104] Leis, S. et al., Facilitated neurogenic inflammation in unaffected limbs of patients with complex regional pain syndrome, *Neurosci. Lett.*, 359, 163, 2004.
[105] Baron, R. and Maier, C., Reflex sympathetic dystrophy: skin blood flow, sympathetic vasoconstrictor reflexes and pain before and after surgical sympathectomy, *Pain*, 67, 317, 1996.
[106] Birklein, F. et al., Pattern of autonomic dysfunction in time course of complex regional pain syndrome, *Clin. Auto. Res.*, 8, 79, 1998.
[107] Cannon, W.B. and Rosenblueth, A., *The Supersensitivity of Denervation Structures: A Law of Denervation*, Macmillan, New York, 1949.
[108] Fleming, W.W. and Westphal, D.P., Adaptive supersensitivity, in *Catecholamines I, Handbook of Experimental Pharmacology*, Trendelenburg, U. and Weiner, N., Eds., New York, Springer, Vol. 9, p. 509, 1988.

19
Thermal Imaging in Surgery

19.1	Overview	19-1
19.2	Energized Systems	19-2
19.3	Thermal Imaging Systems	19-3
19.4	Calibration	19-3
19.5	Thermal Imaging during Energized Surgery	19-4
	RF Electrosurgery • Analysis of Collateral Damage	
19.6	Laser Applications in Dermatology	19-6
	Overview	
19.7	Laser–Tissue Interactions	19-8
19.8	Optimizing Laser Therapies	19-9
19.9	Thermographic Results of Laser Positioning	19-11
19.10	Computerized Laser Scanning	19-11
	Case Study 1: Port Wine Stain • Case Study 2: Laser Depilation	
19.11	Conclusions	19-15
References		19-17

Paul Campbell
Ninewells Hospital

Roderick Thomas
Swansea Institute of Technology

19.1 Overview

Advances in miniaturization and microelectronics, coupled with enhanced computing technologies, have combined to see modern infrared imaging systems develop rapidly over the past decade. As a result, the instrumentation has become considerably improved, not only in terms of its inherent resolution (spatial *and* temporal) and detector sensitivity (values ca. 25 mK are typical) but also in terms of its portability: the considerable reduction in bulk has resulted in light, camcorder (or smaller) sized devices. Importantly, cost has also been reduced so that entry to the field is no longer prohibitive. This attractive combination of factors has led to an ever increasing range of applicability across the medical spectrum. Whereas the mainstay application for medical thermography over the past 40 years has been with rheumatological and associated conditions, usually for the detection and diagnosis of peripheral vascular diseases such as Raynaud's phenomenon, the latest generations of thermal imaging systems have seen active service within new surgical realms such as orthopaedics, coronary by-pass operations, and also in urology. The focus of this chapter relates not to a specific area of surgery per se, but rather to a generic and pervasive aspect of all modern surgical approaches: the use of *energized* instrumentation during surgery. In particular, we will concern ourselves with the use of thermal imaging to accurately monitor temperature within the tissue locale surrounding an energy-activated instrument. The rationale behind this is that it facilitates optimization of operation specific protocols that may either relate to thermally based therapies, or else to reduce the extent of collateral damage that may be introduced when inappropriate power levels, or excessive pulse durations, are implemented during surgical procedures.

19.2 Energized Systems

Energy-based instrumentation can considerably expedite fundamental procedures such as vessel sealing and dissection. The instrumentation is most often based around ultrasonic, laser, or radio-frequency (RF)-current based technologies. Heating tissue into distinct temperature regimes is required in order to achieve the desired effect (e.g., vessel sealing, cauterization, or cutting). In the context of electrical current heating, the resultant effect of the current on tissue is dominated by two factors: the temperature attained by the tissue; and the duration of the heating phase, as encapsulated in the following equation:

$$T - T_0 = \frac{1}{\sigma \rho c} J^2 \delta t \tag{19.1}$$

where T and T_0 are the final and initial temperatures (in degrees Kelvin [K]) respectively, σ is the electrical conductivity (in S/m), ρ is the tissue density, c is the tissue specific heat capacity (J kg^{-1} K^{-1}), J is the current density (A/m^2), and δt is the duration of heat application. The resultant high temperatures are not limited solely to the tissue regions in which the electrical current flow is concentrated. Heat will flow away from hotter regions in a time dependence fashion given by the Fourier equation:

$$Q(r, t) = -k \nabla T(r, t) \tag{19.2}$$

where Q is the heat flux vector, the proportionality constant k is a scalar quantity of the material known as the thermal conductivity, and $\nabla T(r, t)$ is the temperature gradient vector. The overall spatio-temporal evolution of the temperature field is embodied within the differential equation of heat flow (alternatively known as the diffusion equation)

$$\frac{1}{\alpha} \frac{\partial T(r, t)}{\partial t} = \nabla^2 T(r, t) \tag{19.3}$$

where α is the thermal diffusivity of the medium defined in terms of the physical constants, k, ρ, and c thus:

$$\alpha = k/\rho c \tag{19.4}$$

and temperature T is a function of both the three dimensions of space (r) and also of time t. In other words, high temperatures are not limited to the region specifically targeted by the surgeon, and this is often the source of an added surgical complication caused by collateral or proximity injury. Electrosurgical damage, for example, is the most common cause of iatrogenic bowel injury during laparoscopic surgery and 60% of mishaps are missed, that is, the injury is not recognized during surgery and declares itself with peritonitis several days after surgery or even after discharge from hospital. This level of morbidity can have serious consequences, in terms of both the expense incurred by re-admission to hospital, or even the death of the patient. By undertaking *in vivo* thermal imaging during energized dissection it becomes possible to determine, in real time, the optimal power conditions for the successful accomplishment of specific tasks, and with minimal collateral damage. As an adjunct imaging modality, thermal imaging may also improve surgical practice by facilitating easier identification and localization of tissues such as arteries, especially by less experienced surgeons. Further, as tumors are more highly vascularized than normal tissue, thermal imaging may facilitate their localization and staging, that is, the identification of the tumor's stage in its growth cycle. Figure 19.1 shows a typical set-up for implementation of thermography during surgery.

FIGURE 19.1 Typical set-up for a thermal imaging in surgery. The camera is tripod mounted toward the foot of the operating table and aimed at the surgical access site (camera visible over the left shoulder of the nearmost surgeon).

19.3 Thermal Imaging Systems

As skin is a close approximation to an ideal black body (the emissivity, ε, of skin is 0.98, whereas that of an ideal black body has $\varepsilon = 1$), then we can feel reasonably confident in applying the relevant physics directly to the situation of thermography in surgery. One important consideration must be the waveband of detector chosen for thermal observations of the human body. It is known from the thermal physics of black bodies, that the wavelength at which the maximum emissive power occurs, λ_{max} (i.e., the peak in the Planck curve), is related to the body's temperature T through Wien's law:

$$\lambda_{max} T = 0.002898 \tag{19.5}$$

Thus for bodies at 310 K (normal human body temperature), the peak output is around 10 μm, and the majority of the emitted thermal radiation is limited to the range from 2 to 20 μm. The optimal detectors for passive thermal imaging of normal skin should thus have best sensitivity around the 10 μm range, and this is indeed the case with many of the leading thermal imagers manufactured today, which often rely on GaAs quantum well infrared photodetectors (QWIPs) with a typical waveband of 8–9 μm. A useful alternative to these longwave detectors involves the use of indium–antimonide (InSb) based detectors to detect radiation in the mid-wave infrared (3–5 μm). Both these materials have the benefit of enhanced temperature sensitivity (ca. 0.025 K), and are both wholly appropriate even for quantitative imaging of hotter surfaces, such as may occur in energized surgical instrumentation.

19.4 Calibration

Whilst the latest generation of thermal imaging systems are usually robust instruments exhibiting low drift over extended periods, it is sensible to recalibrate the systems at regular intervals in order to preserve the integrity of captured data. For some camera manufacturers, recalibration can be undertaken under a service agreement and this usually requires shipping of the instrument from the host laboratory. However for other systems, recalibration must be undertaken in-house, and on such occasions, a black body source (BBS) is required.

Most BBS are constructed in the form of a cavity at a known temperature, with an aperture to the cavity that acts as the black body, effectively absorbing all incident radiation upon it. The cavity temperature must be measured using a high accuracy thermometric device, such as a platinum resistance thermometer

(PRT), with performance characteristics traceable to a thermometry standard. Figure 19.2b shows one such system, as developed by the UK National Physical Laboratory at Teddington, and whose architecture relies on a heat-pipe design. The calibration procedure requires measurement of the aperture temperature at a range of temperature set-points that are simultaneously monitored by the PRT (e.g., at intervals of 5° between temperature range of 293 and 353 K). Direct comparison of the radiometric temperature measured by the thermal camera with the standard temperature monitored via the PRT allows a calibration table to be generated across the temperature range of interest. During each measurement, sufficient time must be allowed in order to let the programmed temperature set-point equilibrate, otherwise inaccuracies will result. Further, the calibration procedure should ideally be undertaken under similar ambient conditions to those under which usual imaging is undertaken. This may include aspects such as laminar, or even fan-assisted, flow around the camera body which will affect the heat transfer rate from the camera to the ambient and in turn may affect the performance of the detector (Figure 19.2b).

19.5 Thermal Imaging during Energized Surgery

Fully remote-controlled cameras may be ideally suited to overhead bracket mountings above the operating table so that a bird's eye view over the surgical site is afforded. However, without a robotized arm to fully control pitch and location, the view may be restrictive. Tripod mounting, as illustrated in Figure 19.1, and with a steep look-down angle from a distance of about 1 m to the target offers the most versatile viewing without compromising the surgeon's freedom of movement. However, this type of set-up demands that a camera operator be on hand continually in order to move the imaging system to those positions offering best viewing for the type of energized procedure being undertaken.

19.5.1 RF Electrosurgery

As mentioned earlier, the most common energized surgical instrumentation employ a physical system reliant on either (high frequency) electrical current, an ultrasonic mechanism, or else incident laser energy in order to induce tissue heating. Thermal imaging has been used to follow all three of these procedures. There are often similarities in approach between the alternative modalities. For example, vessel sealing often involves placement of elongated forcep-style electrodes across a target vessel followed by ratcheted compression, and then a pulse of either RF current, or alternatively ultrasonic activation of the forceps, is applied through the compressed tissue region. The latest generations of energized instrumentation may have active feedback control over the pulse to facilitate optimal sealing with minimal thermal spread (e.g., the Valleylab *Ligasure* instrument) however under certain circumstances, such as with calcified tissue or in excessively liquid environments the performance may be less predictable.

Figure 19.3 illustrates how thermal spread may be monitored during the instrument activation period of one such "intelligent" feedback device using RF current. The initial power level for each application is determined through a fast precursor voltage scan that determines the natural impedance of the compressed tissue. Then, by monitoring the temperature dependence of impedance (of the compressed tissue) during current activation, the microprocessor controlled feedback loop automatically maintains an appropriate power level until a target impedance is reached indicating that the seal is complete. This process typically takes between 1 and 6 sec, depending on the nature of the target tissue. Termination of the pulse is indicated by an audible tone burst from the power supply box. The performance of the system has been evaluated in preliminary studies involving gastric, colonic and small bowel resection [1]; hemorraoidectomy [2]; prostatectomy [3]; and cholecystectomy [4].

Perhaps most strikingly, the facility for real time thermographic monitoring, as illustrated in Figure 19.3, affords the surgeon immediate appreciation of the instrument temperature, providing a visual cue that automatically alerts to the potential for iatrogenic injury should a hot instrument come into close contact with vital structures. By the same token, the *in situ* thermal image also indicates when the tip of the instrument has cooled to ambient temperature. It should be noted that the amount by which the activated

Thermal Imaging in Surgery

FIGURE 19.2 Thermal cross-section (profile) through the black body calibration source together with equilibrated crushed ice, which acts as a convenient secondary temperature gauge *in situ*. (Insert [left] thermal view with linear region of interest highlighted, and [right] optical view of the black body cavity and beaker of [equilibrated] crushed ice to the lower right.) (b) Radiometric detector drift during start up under two different ambient conditions. The detector readout is centered on the black body cavity source shown in (a), which was itself maintained at a target temperature of 59.97°C throughout the measurements (solid circles). Without fan-assisted cooling of the camera exterior, the measured temperature drifted by 0.8°C over 2 h, hence the importance of calibration under typical operating conditions. With fan-assisted cooling, the camera "settles" within around 30 min of switching on. (Camera: Raytheon Galileo [Raytheon Systems].)

head's temperature rises is largely a function of device dimensions, materials, and the power levels applied together with the pulse duration.

19.5.2 Analysis of Collateral Damage

Whilst thermograms typical of Figure 19.3 offer a visually instructive account of the thermal scene and its temporal evolution, a quantitative analysis of the sequence is more readily achieved through the identification of a linear region of interest (LROI), as illustrated by the line bisecting the device head in Figure 19.4a. The data constituted by the LROI is effectively a snapshot thermal profile across those pixels lying on this designated line (Figure 19.4b). A graph can then be constructed to encapsulate the

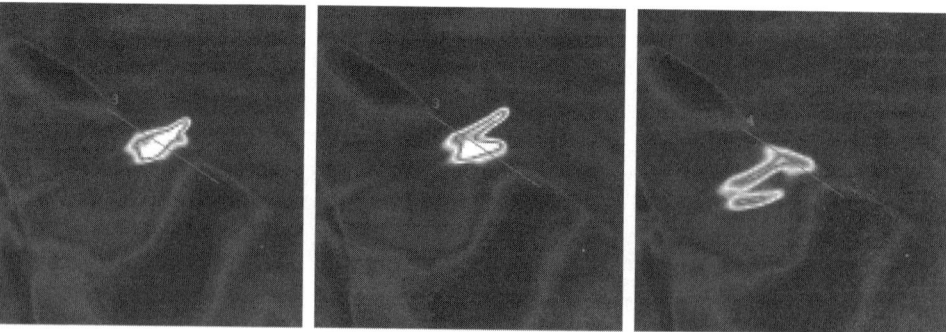

FIGURE 19.3 Thermographic sequence taken with the Dundee thermal imaging system and showing (19.1) energized forceps attached to bowel (white correlates with temperature), (19.2) detachment of the forceps revealing hot tissue beneath, (19.3) remnant hot-spot extending across the tissue and displaying collateral thermal damage covering 4.5 mm either side of the instrument jaws.

time dependent evolution of the LROI. This is displayed as a 3D surface (a function of spatial co-ordinate along the LROI, time, and temperature) upon which color-mapped contours are evoked to represent the different temperature domains across the LROI (Figure 19.4c). In order to facilitate measurement of the thermal spread, the 3D surface, as represented in matrix form, can then be interrogated with a mathematical programming package, or alternatively inspected manually, a process that is most easily undertaken after projecting the data to the 2D coordinate-time plane, as illustrated in Figure 19.4d. The critical temperature beyond which tangible heat damage can occur to tissue is assumed to be 45°C [5]. Thermal spread is then calculated by measuring the maximum distance between the 45°C contours on the planar projection, then subtracting the electrode "footprint" diameter from this to get the total spread. Simply dividing this result by two gives the thermal spread either side of the device electrodes.

The advanced technology used in some of the latest generations of vessel sealing instrumentation can lead to a much reduced thermal spread, compared with the earlier technologies. For example with the Ligasure LS1100 instrument, the heated peripheral region is spatially confined to less than 2 mm, even when used on thicker vessels/structures. A more advanced version of the device (LS1200 [*Precise*]) consistently produces even lower thermal spreads, typically around 1 mm (Figure 19.4). This performance is far superior to other commercially available energized devices.

For example, Kinoshita and co-workers [6] have observed (using infrared imaging) that the typical lateral spread of heat into adjacent tissue is sufficient to cause a temperature of over 60°C at radial distances of up to 10 mm from the active electrode when an ultrasonic scalpel is used. Further, when standard bipolar electro-coagulation instrumentation is used, the spread can be as large as 22 mm. Clearly, the potential for severe collateral and iatrogenic injury is high with such systems unless power levels are tailored to the specific procedure in hand and real time thermal imaging evidently represents a powerful adjunct technology to aid this undertaking.

Whilst the applications mentioned thusfar relate to "open" surgical procedures requiring a surgical incision to access the site of interest, thermal imaging can also be applied as a route to protocol optimization for other less invasive procedures also. Perhaps the most important surgical application in this regime involves laser therapy for various skin diseases/conditions. Application of the technique in this area is discussed below.

19.6 Laser Applications in Dermatology

19.6.1 Overview

Infrared thermographic monitoring (ITM) has been successfully used in medicine for a number of years and much of this has been documented by Prof. Francis Ring [http://www.medimaging.org/], who has

Thermal Imaging in Surgery

FIGURE 19.4 (a) Mid-infrared thermogram taken at the instant an energized forceps (Ligasure LS1200 "*Precise*") is removed from the surgical scene after having conducted a seal on the bile duct. The hot tips of the forceps are clearly evident in the infrared view (just left of center), as is the remnant hot-spot where the seal has occurred on the vessel. By generating a linear region of interest (LROI) through the hot-spot, as indicated by the highlighted line in the figure, it is possible to monitor the evolution of the hot-spot's temperature in a quantitative fashion. (b) Thermal profile corresponding to the LROI shown in (a). (c) By tracking the temporal evolution of the LROI, it is possible to generate a 3D plot of the thermal profile by simply stacking the individual profiles at each acquisition frame. In this instance the cooling behavior of the hot-spot is clearly identified. Manual estimation of the thermal spread is most easily achieved by resorting to the 2D contour plot of the thermal profile's temporal evolution, as shown in (d). In this instance, the maximal spread of the 45°C contours is measured as 4.28 mm. By subtracting the forcep "footprint" (2.5 mm for the device shown) and dividing the result by 2, we arrive at the thermal spread for the device. The average thermal spread (for 6 bile-duct sealing events) was 0.89 ± 0.35 mm.

established a database and archive within the Department of Computing at the University of Glamorgan, UK, spanning over 30 years of ITM applications. Examples include monitoring abnormalities such as malignancies, inflammation, and infection that cause localized increases in skin temperature, which show as hot spots or as asymmetrical patterns in an infrared thermogram.

A recent medical example that has benefited by the intervention of ITM is the treatment by laser of certain dermatological disorders. Advancements in laser technology have resulted in new portable laser therapies, examples of which include the removal of vascular lesions (in particular Port Wine Stains [PWS]), and also cosmetic enhancement approaches such as hair-(depilation) and wrinkle removal.

In these laser applications it is a common requirement to deliver laser energy uniformly without overlapping of the beam spot to a sub-dermal target region, such as a blood vessel, but with the minimum of collateral damage to the tissue locale. Temperature rise at the skin surface, and with this the threshold to burning/scarring is of critical importance for obvious reasons. Until recently, this type of therapy had not yet benefited significantly from thermographic evaluation. However, with the introduction of the latest generation thermal imaging systems, exhibiting the essential qualities of portability, high resolution, and high sensitivity, significant inroads to laser therapy are beginning to be made.

Historically, lasers have been used in dermatology for some 40 years [25]. In recent years there have been a number of significant developments particularly regarding the improved treatment of various skin disorders most notably the removal of vascular lesions using dye lasers [8,12,15,17,19] and depilation using ruby lasers [9,14,16]. Some of the general indicators as to why lasers are the preferred treatment of choice are summarized in Table 19.1.

19.7 Laser–Tissue Interactions

The mechanisms involved in the interaction between light and tissue depend on the characteristics of the impinging light and the targeted human tissue [24]. To appreciate these mechanisms the optical properties of tissue must be known. It is necessary to determine the tissue reflectance, absorption, and scattering properties as a function of wavelength. A simplified model of laser light interaction with the skin is illustrated in Figure 19.5.

Recent work has shown that laser radiation can penetrate through the epidermis and basal structure to be preferentially absorbed within the blood layers located in the lower dermis and subcutis. The process is termed selective photothermolysis, and is the specific absorption of laser light by a target tissue in order to eliminate that target without damaging surrounding tissue. For example, in the treatment of Port Wine

TABLE 19.1 Characteristics of Laser Therapy during and after Treatment

General indicators	Dye laser vascular lesions	Ruby laser depilation
During treatment	Varying output parameters Portable Manual and scanned Selective destruction of target chromophore (Haemoglobin)	Varying output parameters Portable Manual and scanned Selective destruction of target chromophore (melanin)
After treatment (desired effect)	Slight bruising (purpura)	Skin returns to normal coloring (no bruising)
	Skin retains its elasticity	Skin retains surface markings
	Skin initially needs to be protected from UV and scratching	Skin retains its ability to tan after exposure to ultraviolet light
	Hair follicles are removed	Hair removed

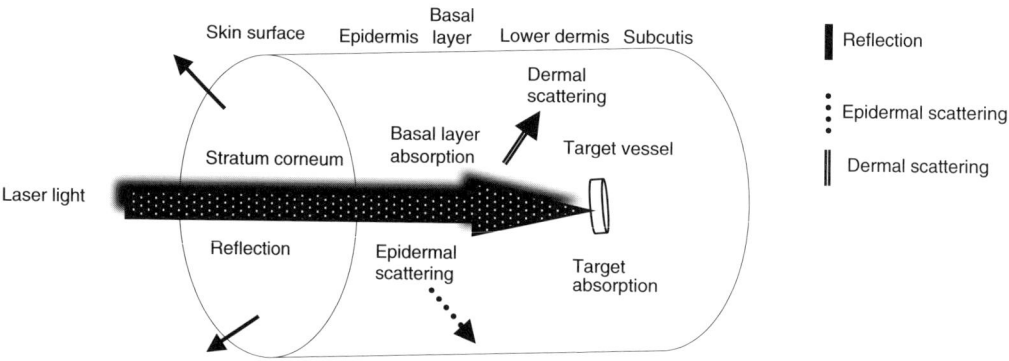

FIGURE 19.5 Passage of laser light within skin layers.

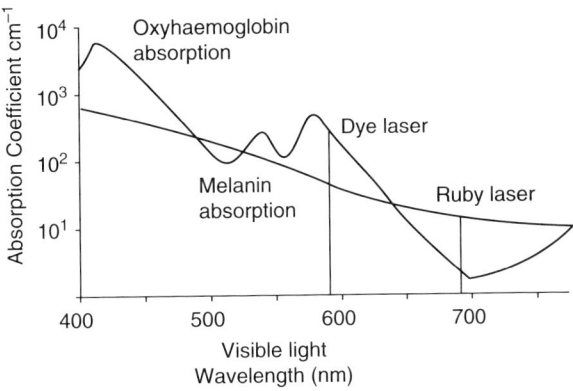

FIGURE 19.6 Spectral absorption curves for human blood and melanin.

TABLE 19.2 Interaction Effects of Laser Light and Tissue

Effect	Interaction
Photothermal	
Photohyperthermia	Reversible damage of normal tissue (37–42°C)
Photothermolysis	Loosening of membranes (odema), tissue welding (45–60°C)
Photocoagulation	Thermal-dynamic effects, micro-scale overheating
Photocarbonization	Coagulation, necrosis (60–100°C)
Photovaporization	Drying out, vaporization of water, carbonization (100–300°C)
	Pyrolysis, vaporization of solid tissue matrix (>300°C)
Photochemical	
Photochemotherapy	Photodynamic therapy, black light therapy
Photoinduction	Biostimulation
Photoionization	
Photoablation	Fast thermal explosion, optical breakdown, mechanical shockwave

Stains (PWS), a dye laser of wavelength 585 nm has been widely used [10] where the profusion of small blood vessels that comprise the PWS are preferentially targeted at this wavelength. The spectral absorption characteristics of light through human skin have been well established [7] and are replicated in Figure 19.6 for the two dominant factors: melanin and oxyhaemoglobin.

There are three types of laser–tissue interaction, namely: photothermal, photochemical, and protoionization (Table 19.2), and the use of lasers on tissue results in a number of differing interactions including photodisruption, photoablation, vaporization, and coagulation, as summarized in Figure 19.7.

The application of appropriate laser technology to medical problems depends on a number of laser operating parameters including matching the optimum laser wavelength for the desired treatment. Some typical applications and the desired wavelengths for usage are highlighted in Table 19.3.

19.8 Optimizing Laser Therapies

There are a number of challenges in optimizing laser therapy, mainly related to the laser parameters of wavelength, energy density, and spot size. Combined with these are difficulties associated with poor positioning of hand-held laser application that may result in uneven treatment [overlapping spots and/or uneven coverage (stippling) of spots], excessive treatment times, and pain. Therefore, for enhanced efficacy an improved understanding of the thermal effects of laser–tissue interaction benefits therapeutic

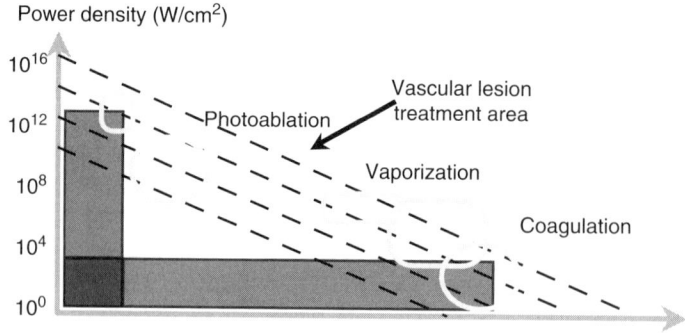

FIGURE 19.7 Physiological characteristics of laser therapy. (From Thomas et al., 2002, *Proceedings of SPIE*, 1–4 April, Orlando, USA. With permission.)

TABLE 19.3 Laser Application in Dermatology

Laser	Wavelength (nm)	Treatment
Flashlamp short-pulsed dye	510	Pigmented lesions, for example, freckles, tattoos
Flashlamp long-pulsed dye	585	PWS in children, warts, hypertrophic scars
Ruby single-pulse or Q-switched	694	Depilation of hair
Alexandrite Q-switched	755	Multicolored tattoos, viral warts, depilation
Diode variable	805	Multicolored tattoos, viral warts
Neodymium yitrium aluminum (Nd-YAG) Q-switched	1064	Pigmented lesions; adult port-wine stains, black/blue tattoos
Carbon dioxide continuous pulsed	10600	Tissue destruction, warts, tumors

approaches. Here, variables for consideration include:

1. Thermal effects of varying spot size
2. Improved control of hand-held laser minimising overlapping and stippling
3. Establishment of minimum gaps
4. Validation of laser computer scanning

Evaluation (Figure 19.8) was designed to elucidate whether or not measurements of the surface temperature of the skin are reproducible when illuminated by nominally identical laser pulses. In this case a 585 nm dye laser and a 694 nm ruby laser were used to place a number of pulses manually on tissue. The energy emitted by the laser is highly repeatable. Care must be taken to ensure that both the laser and radiometer position are kept constant and that the anatomical location used for the test had uniform tissue pigmentation.

Figure 19.8 shows the maximum temperature for each of twenty shots fired on the forearm of a representative Caucasian male with type 2 skin*. Maximum temperature varies between 48.90°C and 48.10°C representing a variance of 1°C (±0.45°C). This level of reproducibility is pleasing since it shows that, despite the complex scenario, the radiometer is capable of repeatedly and accurately measuring surface tissue temperatures. In practice the radiometer may be used to inform the operator when any accumulated temperature has subsided allowing further treatment without exceeding some damage threshold.

Energy density is also an important laser parameter and can be varied to match the demands of the application. It is normal in the discipline to measure energy density (fluence) in J/cm². In treating vascular lesions most utilize an energy density for therapy of 5 to 10 J/cm² [13]. The laser operator needs to be sure that the energy density is uniform and does not contain hot-spots that may take the temperature above the damage threshold inadvertently. Preliminary characterization of the spot with thermal imaging can

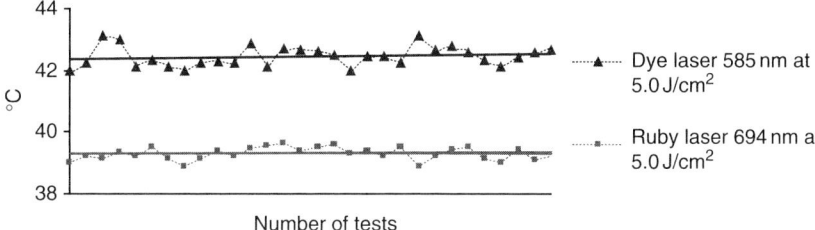

FIGURE 19.8 Repeatability of initial maximum skin temperatures (°C) of two lasers with similar energy density but different wavelengths.

then aid with fine tuning of the laser and reduce the possibility of excessive energy density and with that the possibility of collateral damage.

19.9 Thermographic Results of Laser Positioning

During laser therapy the skin is treated with a number of spots, applied manually depending on the anatomical location and required treatment. It has been found that spot size directly affects efficacy of treatment. The wider the spot size the higher the surface temperature [22]. The type and severity of lesion also determines the treatment required. Its color severity (dark to light) and its position on skin (raised to level). Therefore the necessary treatment may require a number of passes of the laser over the skin. It is therefore essential as part of the treatment that there is a physical separation between individual spots so that:

1. The area is not over treated with overlapping spots that could otherwise result in local heating effects from adjacent spots resulting in skin damage.
2. The area is not under treated leaving stippled skin.
3. The skin has cooled sufficiently before second or subsequent passes of the laser.

Figure 19.9 shows two laser shots placed next to each other some 4 mm apart. The time between the shots is 1 sec. There are no excessive temperatures evident and no apparent temperature build-up in the gap. This result, which concurs with Lanigan [18], suggests a minimum physical separation of 5 mm between all individual spot sizes.

The intention is to optimize the situation leading to a uniform therapeutic and aesthetic result without either striping or thermal build-up. This is achieved by initially determining the skin color (Chromotest) for optimum energy settings, followed by a patch test and subsequent treatment. Increasing the number of spots to 3 with the 4 mm separation reveals a continuing trend, as shown in Figure 19.10. The gap between the first two shots is now beginning to merge in the 2 sec period that has lapsed. The gap between shots 2 and 3 remains clear and distinct and there are clearly visible thermal bands across the skin surface of between 38–39 and 39–40°C. These experimental results supply valuable information to support the development of both free-hand treatment and computer-controlled techniques.

19.10 Computerized Laser Scanning

Having established the parameters relating to laser spot positioning, the possibility of achieving reproducible laser coverage of a lesion by automatic scanning becomes a reality. This has potential advantages, which include:

1. Accurate positioning of the spot with the correct spacing from the adjacent spots
2. Accurate timing allowing the placement at a certain location at the appropriate lapsed time

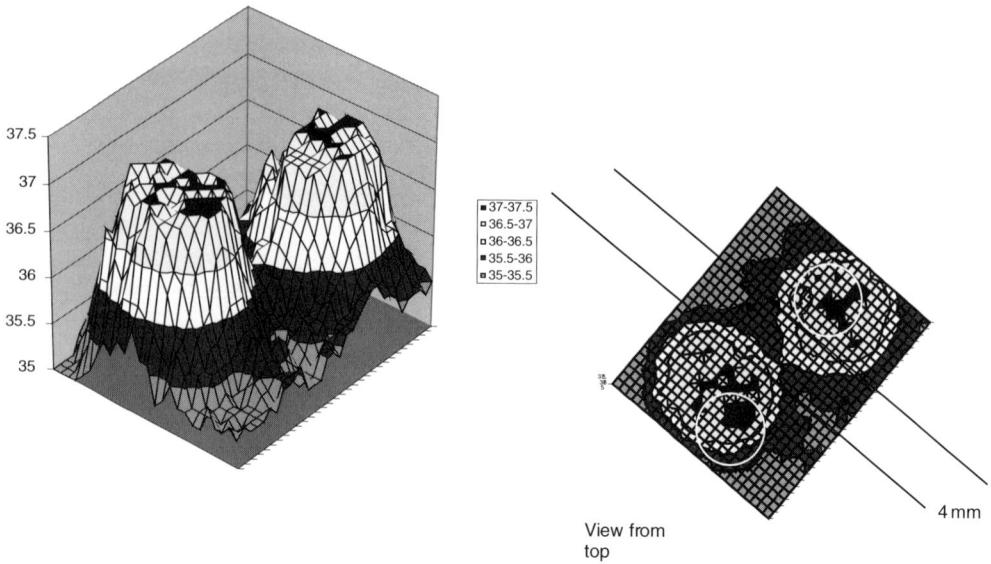

FIGURE 19.9 Two-dye laser spots with a minimum of 4 mm separation (585 nm at 4.5 J/cm^2, 5 mm spot).

FIGURE 19.10 Three-dye laser spots, 2 sec apart with a 5 mm separation (585 nm at 5 J/cm^2, 5 mm spot).

There are some disadvantages that include the need for additional equipment and regulatory approvals for certain market sectors.

A computerized scanning system has been developed [9] that illuminates the tissue in a pre-defined pattern. Sequential pulses are not placed adjacent to an immediately preceding pulse thereby ensuring the minimum of thermal build-up. Clement et al. [9] carried out a trial, illustrating treatment coverage using a hand-held system compared to a controlled computer scanning system. Two adjacent areas (lower arm) were selected and shaved. A marked hexagonal area was subjected to 19 shots using a hand-held system, and an adjacent area of skin was treated with a scanner whose computer control is designed to uniformly fill the area with exactly 19 shots. Such tests were repeated and the analyzed statistics showed that, on

FIGURE 19.11 Sample sequences during computer laser scanning.

average, only 60% of area is covered by laser spots. The use of thermography allowed the validation and optimization of this automated system in a way that was impossible without thermal imaging technology. The following sequence of thermal images, Figure 19.11, captures the various stages of laser scanning of the hand using a dye laser at 5.7 J/cm^2. Thermography confirms that the spot temperature from individual laser beams will merge and that both the positioning of spots and the time duration between spots dictate the efficacy of treatment.

19.10.1 Case Study 1: Port Wine Stain

Vascular naevi are common and are present at birth or develop soon after. Superficial lesions are due to capillary networks in the upper or mid dermis, but larger angiomas can be located in the lower dermis and subcutis. An example of vascular naevi is the Port-Wine Stain (PWS) often present at birth, is an irregular

TABLE 19.4 Vasculature Treatment Types

Treatment type	Process	Possible concerns
Camouflage	Applying skin colored pigments to the surface of the skin. Enhancement to this technique is to tattoo skin colored inks into the upper layer of the lesion	Only a temporary measure and is very time consuming. Efficacy dependant on flatter lesions
Cryosurgery	Involves applying super-cooled liquid nitrogen to the lesion to destroy abnormal vasculature	May require several treatments
Excision	Common place where the lesion is endangering vital body functions	Not considered appropriate for purely cosmetic reasons. Complex operation resulting in a scar. Therefore, only applicable to the proliferating haemangioma lesion
Radiation therapy	Bombarding the lesion with radiation to destroy vasculature	Induced number of skin cancer in a small number of cases
Drug therapy	Widely used administering steroids	Risk of secondary complications affecting bodily organs

red or purple macule which often affects one side of the face. Problems can arise if the naevus is located close to the eye and some cases where a PWS involves the trigeminal nerve's ophthalmic division may have an associated intracranial vascular malformation known as Sturge Weber Syndrome. The treatment of vascular naevi can be carried out a number of ways often dependent on the nature, type, anatomical and severity of lesion location, as highlighted in Table 19.4.

A laser wavelength of 585 nm is preferentially absorbed by haemoglobin within the blood, but there is partial absorption in the melanin rich basal layer in the epidermis. The objective is to thermally damage the blood vessel, by elevating its temperature, while ensuring that the skin surface temperature is kept low. For a typical blood vessel, the temperature–time graph appears similar to Figure 19.12. This suggests that it is possible to selectively destroy the PWS blood vessels, by elevating them to a temperature in excess of 100°C, causing disruption to the small blood vessels, whilst maintaining a safe skin surface temperature. This has been proven empirically via thermographic imaging with a laser pulsing protocol that was devised and optimized on the strength of Monte-Carlo based models [26] of the heat dissipation processes [11]. The two-dimensional Cartesian thermal transport equation is

$$\nabla T^2 + \frac{Q(x, y)}{k} = \frac{1}{\alpha} \frac{\partial T}{\partial t} \tag{19.6}$$

where temperature T has both an implied spatial and temporal dependence and the volumetric source term, $Q(x, y)$, is obtained from the solution of the Monte-Carlo radiation transport problem [27].

19.10.2 Case Study 2: Laser Depilation

The 694 nm wavelength laser radiation is preferentially absorbed by melanin, which occurs in the basal layer and particularly in the hair follicle base, which is the intended target using an oblique angle of laser beam (see Figure 19.13). A Monte-Carlo analysis was performed in a similar manner to *Case Study 1* above, where the target region in the dermis is the melanin rich base of the hair follicle. Figure 19.14a,b show the temperature–time profiles for 10 and 20 J cm^2 laser fluence [23]. These calculations suggest that it is possible to thermally damage the melanin-rich follicle base whilst restricting the skin surface temperature to values that cause no superficial damage. Preliminary clinical trials indicated that there is indeed a beneficial effect, but the choice of laser parameters still required optimizing.

Thermographic analysis has proved indispensable in this work. Detailed thermometric analysis is shown in Figure 19.15a. Analysis of this data shows that in this case, the surface temperature is raised to

Thermal Imaging in Surgery

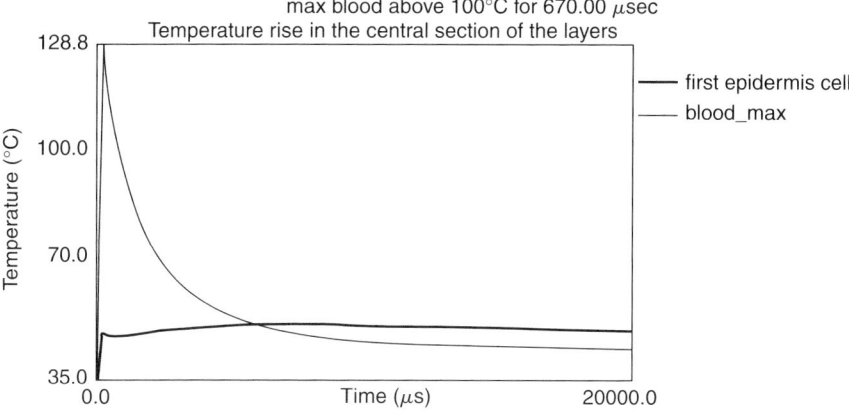

FIGURE 19.12 Typical temperatures for PWS problem, indicating thermal disruption of blood vessel, while skin surface temperature remains low.

FIGURE 19.13 Oblique laser illumination of hair follicle.

about 50°C. The thermogram also clearly shows the selective absorption in the melanin-dense hair. The temperature of the hair is raised to over 207°C. This thermogram illustrates direct evidence for selective wavelength absorption leading to cell necrosis. Further clinical trials have indicated a maximum fluence of 15 J cm^2 for type III caucasian skin. Figure 19.15b illustrates a typical thermographic image obtained during the real-time monitoring.

19.11 Conclusions

The establishment, development, and consequential success of medical infrared thermographic (MIT) intervention with laser therapy is primarily based on the understanding of the following, that are described in more detail below:

1. Problem/condition to be monitored
2. Set-up and correct operation of infrared system (appropriate and validated training)
3. Appropriate conditions during the monitoring process
4. Evaluation of activity and development of standards and protocol

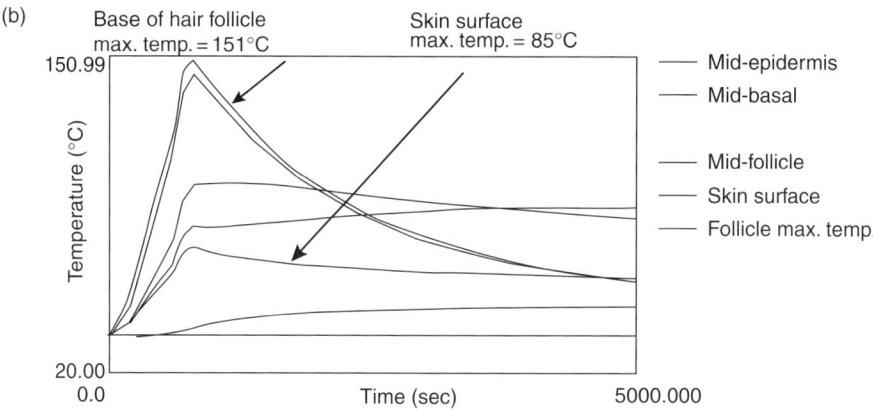

FIGURE 19.14 (a) Temperature–time profiles at 10 J cm^2 ruby (694 nm), 800 μsec laser pulse on caucasian skin type III. (b) Temperature–time profiles for 20 J cm^2 ruby (694 nm), 800 μsec laser pulse on Caucasian skin type III.

FIGURE 19.15 (a) Post-processed results of 5 mm. (b) Simplified thermogram diameter 694 nm 20 J cm^2 800 μsec ruby pulse of ruby laser pulse, with 5 mm spot at 20 J cm^2.

With reference to (1) above in the conclusions, the condition to be monitored, there needs to be a good knowledge as to the physiological aspects of the desired medical process; in laser therapy an understanding as to the mechanisms involved in laser–tissue interaction. A good reference source of current practice can be found in the Handbook of Optical Biomedical Diagnostics, published by The International Society for Optical Engineering (SPIE).

In this application fast data-capture (>50 Hz), good image quality (256 × 256 pixels), temperature sensitivity, and repeatability were considered important and an Inframetrics SC1000 Focal Plane Array Radiometer (3.4 to 5 μm, CMOS PtSi Cooled Detector) with a real-time data acquisition system (Dynamite) was used. There are currently very fast systems available with data acquisition speeds in terms of hundreds of Hertz with detectors that provide excellent image quality. In (2) the critical aspect is training [21]. Currently, infrared equipment manufacturers design systems with multiple applications in mind. This has resulted in many aspects of good practice and quality standards. This is one of the reasons why industrial infrared thermography is so successful. This has not necessarily been the case in medicine. However, it is worth noting that there are a number of good infrared training organizations throughout the world, particularly in the United States. The advantages of adopting training organizations such as these is that they have experience of training with reference to a very wide range and type of infrared thermographic systems, in a number of different applications. This will help in the identification of the optimum infrared technology. In (3) consideration as to the conditions surrounding the patient and the room environment are important for optimum results. In the United Kingdom, for example, Prof. Francis Ring, University of Glamorgan has led the way in the development and standardizations of clinical infrared practice [20]. Finally, (4) the evaluation of such practice is crucial if lessons are to be learnt and protocol and standards are to emerge.

Infrared thermal imaging provides an important tool for optimizing energized surgical interventions and facilitates validation of theoretical models of evolving temperature fields.

References

[1] Heniford, B.T., Matthews, B.D., Sing, R.F., Backus, C., Pratt, P., and Greene, F.L. (2001) Initial results with an electrothermal bipolar vessel sealer. *Surg. Endosc.* 15: 799–801.

[2] Palazzo, F.F., Francis, D.L., and Clifton, M.A. (2002) Randomised clinical trial of ligasure versus open haemorrhoidectomy. *Br. J. Surg.* 89: 154–157.

[3] Sengupta, S. and Webb, D.R. (2001) Use of a computer controlled bipolar diathermy system in radical prostatectomies and other open urological surgery. *ANZ J. Surg.* 71: 538–540.

[4] Schulze, S., Krztiansen, V.B., Fischer-Hansen, B., and Rosenberg, J. (2002) Sealing of the cystic duct with bipolar electrocoagulation. *Surg. Endosc.* 16: 342–344.

[5] Reidenbach, H.D. and Buess, G. (1992). Anciliary technology: electrocautery, thermoregulation and laser. In Cuschieri, A., Buess, G., and Perrisat, L. Eds., *Operative Manual of Endoscopic Surgery.* Springer-Verlag, Berlin-Heidelberg-New York, pp. 44–60.

[6] Kinoshita, T., Kanehira, E., Omura, K., Kawakami, K., and Watanabe, Y. (1999) Experimental study on heat production by a 23.5 kHz ultrasonically activated device for endoscopic surgery. *Surg. Endosc.* 13: 621–625.

[7] Andersen, R.R. and Parrish, J.A. (1981) Microvasculature can be selectively damaged using dye lasers. *Lasers Surg. Med.* 1: 263–270.

[8] Barlow, R.J., Walker, N.P.J., and Markey, A.C. (1996) Treatment of proliferative haemangiomas with 585nm pulsed dye laser. *Br. J. Dermatol.* 134: 700–704.

[9] Clement, R.M., Kiernan, M.N., Thomas, R.A., Donne, K.E., and Bjerring, P.J. (1999) The use of thermal imaging to optimise automated laser irradiation of tissue, *Skin Research and Technology.* Vol. 5, No. 2, *6th Congress of the International Society for Skin Imaging*, July 4–6, 1999, Royal Society London.

[10] Clement, R.M., Donne, K.D., Thomas, R.A., and Kiernan, M.N. (2000) Thermographic condition monitoring of human skin during laser therapy, *Quality Reliability Maintenance, 3rd International Conference*, St Edmund Hall, University of Oxford, 30–31 March 2000.

[11] Daniel, G. (2002) An investigation of thermal radiation and thermal transport in laser–tissue interaction, PhD Thesis, Swansea Institute.

[12] Garden, J.M., Polla, L.L., and Tan, O.T. (1988) Treatment of port wine stains by pulsed dye laser—analysis of pulse duration and long term therapy. *Arch. Dermatol.* 124: 889–896.

[13] Garden, J.M. and Bakus, W. (1996) Clinical efficacy of the pulsed dye laser in the treatment of vascular lesions. *J. Dermatol. Surg. Oncol.* 19: 321–326.

[14] Gault, D., Clement, R.M., Trow, R.B., and Kiernan, M.N. (1998) Removing unwanted hairs by laser. *Face* 6: 129–130.

[15] Glassberg, E., Lask, G., Rabinowitz, L.G., and Tunnessen, W.W. (1989) Capillary haemangiomas: case study of a novel laser treatment and a review of therapeutic options. *J. Dermatol. Surg. Oncol.* 15: 1214–1223.

[16] Grossman et al. (1997) Damage to hair follicle by normal mode ruby laser pulse. *J. Amer. Acad. Dermatol.* 889–894.

[17] Kiernan, M.N. (1997) An analysis of the optimal laser parameters necessary for the treatment of vascular lesions, PhD Thesis, The University of West of England.

[18] Lanigan, S.W. (1996) Port wine stains on the lower limb: response to pulsed dye laser therapy. *Clin. Exp. Dermatol.* 21: 88–92.

[19] Motley, R.J., Katugampola, G., and Lanigan, S.W. (1996) Microvascular abnormalities in port wine stains and response to 585 nm pulsed dye laser treatment. *Br. J. Dermatol.* 135: Suppl. 47: 13–14.

[20] Ring, E.F.J. (1995) History of thermography. In Ammer, K. and Ring, E.F.J., Eds., *The Thermal Image in Medicine and Biology*. Uhlen Verlag, Vienna, pp. 13–20.

[21] Thomas, R.A. (1999) *Thermography*. Coxmoor Publishers, Oxford, pp. 79–103.

[22] Thomas, R.A., Donne, K.E., Clement, R.M., and Kiernan, M. (2002) Optimised laser application in dermatology using infrared thermography, *Thermosense XXIV, Proceedings of SPIE*, April 1–4, Orlando, USA.

[23] Trow, R. (2001) The design and construction of a ruby laser for laser depilation, PhD Thesis, Swansea Institute.

[24] Welsh, A.J. and van Gemert, M.V.C. (1995) *Optical–Thermal Response of Laser-Irradiated Tissue*. Plenum Press, ISBN 0306449269.

[25] Wheeland, R.G. (1995) Clinical uses of lasers in dermatology. *Lasers Surg. Med.* 16: 2–23.

[26] Wilson, B.C. and Adam, G. (1983) A Monte Carlo model for the absorption and flux distributions of light in tissue. *Med. Phys. Biol.* 1.

[27] Donne, K.E. (1999) Two dimensional computer model of laser tissue interaction. Private communication.

20
Infrared Imaging Applied to Dentistry

20.1	The Importance of Temperature	20-1
20.2	The Skin and Skin-Surface Temperature Measurement	20-2
20.3	Two Common Types of Body Temperature Measurements	20-2
20.4	Diagnostic Applications of Thermography	20-3
20.5	The Normal Infrared Facial Thermography	20-3
20.6	Abnormal Facial Conditions Demonstrated with Infrared Facial Thermography	20-4
	Assessing Temporomandibular Joint (TMJ) Disorders with Infrared Thermography • Assessing Inferior Alveolar Nerve (IAN) Deficit with Infrared Thermography • Assessing Carotid Occlusal Disease with Infrared Thermography • Additional Applications of Infrared Thermography • Future Advances in Infrared Imaging	

Barton M. Gratt
University of Washington

	Acknowledgment	20-5
	References	20-5

20.1 The Importance of Temperature

Temperature is very important in all biological systems. Temperature influences the movement of atoms and molecules and their rates of biochemical activity. Active biological life is, in general, restricted to a temperature range of 0°C to 45°C [1]. Cold-blooded organisms are generally restricted to habitats in which the ambient temperature remains between 0°C and 40°C. However, a variety of temperatures well outside of this occurs on earth, and by developing the ability to maintain a constant body temperature, warm-blooded animals; for example, birds, mammals, including humans have gained access to a greater variety of habitats and environments [1].

With the application of common thermometers, elevation in the core temperature of the body became the primary indicator for the diagnosis of fever. Wunderlich introduced fever measurements as a routine procedure in Germany, in 1872. In 1930, Knaus inaugurated a method of basal temperature measurement, achieving full medical acceptance in 1952. Today, it is customary in hospitals throughout the world to take body temperature measurements on all patients [2].

The scientists of the first part of the twentieth century used simple thermometers to study body temperatures. Many of their findings have not been superseded, and are repeatedly confirmed by new investigators using new more advanced thermal measuring devices. In the last part of the twentieth century, a new discipline termed "thermology" emerged as the study of surface body temperature in both health and in disease [2].

20.2 The Skin and Skin-Surface Temperature Measurement

The skin is the outer covering of the body and contributes 10% of the body's weight. Over 30% of the body's temperature-receptive elements are located within the skin. Most of the heat produced within the body is dissipated by way of the skin, through radiation, evaporation, and conduction. The range of ambient temperature for thermal comfort is relatively broad (20°C to 25°C). Thermal comfort is dependent upon humidity, wind velocity, clothing, and radiant temperature. Under normal conditions there is a steady flow of heat from the inside of a human body to the outside environment. Skin temperature distribution within specific anatomic regions; for example, the head vs. the foot, are diverse, varying by as much as ±15°C. Heat transport by convection to the skin surface depends on the rate of blood flow through the skin, which is also variable. In the trunk region of the body, blood flow varies by a factor of 7; at the foot, blood flow varies by a factor of 30; while at the fingers, it can vary by a factor of 600 [3].

It appears that measurements of body (core) temperatures and skin (surface) temperature may well be strong physiologic markers indicating health or disease. In addition, skin (surface) temperature values appear to be unique for specific anatomic regions of the body.

20.3 Two Common Types of Body Temperature Measurements

There are two common types of body temperature measurements that are made and utilized as diagnostic indicators.

1. *The Measurement of Body Core Temperature.* The normal core temperature of the human body remains within a range of 36.0°C to 37.5°C [1]. The constancy of human core temperature is maintained by a large number of complex regulatory mechanisms [3]. Body core temperatures are easily measured orally (or anally) with contacting temperature devices including: manual or digital thermometers, thermistors, thermocouples, and even layers of liquid temperature sensitive crystals, etc. [4–6].
2. *The Measurement of Body Surface Temperature.* While body core temperature is very easy to measure, the body's skin surface temperature is very difficult to measure. Any device that is required to make contact with the skin cannot measure the body's skin surface temperature reliably. Since skin has a relatively low heat capacity and poor lateral heat conductance, skin temperature is likely to change on contact with a cooler or warmer object [2]. Therefore, an indirect method of obtaining skin surface temperature is required, a common thermometer on the skin, for example, will not work.

Probably the first research efforts that pointed out the diagnostic importance of the infrared emission of human skin and thus initiated the modern era of thermometry were the studies of Hardy in 1934 [7,8]. However, it took 30 years for modern thermometry to be applied in laboratories around the world. To conduct noncontact thermography of the human skin in a clinical setting, an advanced computerized infrared imaging system is required. Consequently, clinical thermography required the advent of microcomputers developed in the late 1960s and early 1970s. These sophisticated electronic systems employed advanced microtechnology, requiring large research and development costs.

Current clinical thermography units use single detector infrared cameras. These work as follows: infrared radiation emitted by the skin surface enters the lens of the camera, passes through a number of rapidly spinning prisms (or mirrors), which reflect the infrared radiation emitted from different parts of the field of view onto the infrared sensor. The sensor converts the reflected infrared radiation into electrical signals. An amplifier receives the electric signals from the sensor and boosts them to electric potential signals of a few volts that can be converted into digital values. These values are then fed into a computer. The computer uses this input, together with the timing information from the rotating mirrors, to reconstruct a digitized thermal image from the temperature values of each small area within the field of observation. These digitized images are easily viewed and can be analyzed using computer software and stored on a computer disk for later reference.

20.4 Diagnostic Applications of Thermography

In 1987, the *International Bibliography of Medical Thermology* was published and included more than 3000 cited publications on the medical use of thermography, including applications for anesthesiology, breast disease, cancer, dermatology, gastrointestinal disorders, gynecology, urology, headache, immunology, musculoskeletal disorders, neurology, neurosurgery, ophthalmology, otolaryngology, pediatrics, pharmacology, physiology, pulmonary disorders, rheumatology, sports medicine, general surgery, plastic and reconstructive surgery, thyroid, cardiovascular and cerebrovascular, vascular problems, and veterinary medicine [9]. In addition, changes in human skin temperature has been reported in conditions involving the orofacial complex, as related to dentistry, such as the temporomandibular joint [10–25], and nerve damage and repair following common oral surgery [25–27]. Thermography has been shown not to be useful in the assessment of periapical granuloma [28]. Reports of dedicated controlled facial skin temperature studies of the orofacial complex are limited, but follow findings consistent with other areas of the body [29,30].

20.5 The Normal Infrared Facial Thermography

The pattern of heat dissipation over the skin of the human body is normally symmetrical and this includes the human face. It has been shown that in normal subjects, the difference in skin temperature from side-to-side on the human body is small, about 0.2°C [31]. Heat emission is directly related to cutaneous vascular activity, yielding enhanced heat output on vasodilatation and reduced heat output on vasoconstriction. Infrared thermography of the face has promise, therefore, as a harmless, noninvasive, diagnostic technique that may help to differentiate selected diagnostic problems. The literature reports that during clinical studies of facial skin temperature a significant difference between the absolute facial skin temperatures of men vs. women was observed [32]. Men were found to have higher temperatures over all 25 anatomic areas measured on the face (e.g., the orbit, the upper lip, the lower lip, the chin, the cheek, the TMJ, etc.) than women. The basal metabolic rate for a normal 30-year-old male, 1.7 m tall (5 ft, 7 in.), weighing 64 kg (141 lbs), who has a surface area of approximately 1.6 m^2, is approximately 80 W; therefore, he dissipates about 50 W/m^2 of heat [33]. On the other hand, the basal metabolic rate of a 30-year-old female, 1.6 m tall (5 ft, 3 in.), weighing 54 kg (119 lbs), with a surface area of 1.4 m^2, is about 63 W, so that she dissipates about 41 W/m^2 of heat [33,34]. Assuming that there are no other relevant differences between males and females, women's skin is expected to be cooler, since less heat is lost per unit (per area of body surface). Body heat dissipation through the face follows this prediction. In addition to the effect of gender on facial temperature, there are indications that age and ethnicity may also affect facial temperature [32].

When observing patients undergoing facial thermography, there seems to be a direct correlation between vasoactivity and pain, which might be expected since both are neurogenic processes. Differences in facial skin temperature, for example, asymptomatic adult subjects (low temperatures differences) and adult patients with various facial pain syndromes (high temperature differences) may prove to be a useful criterion for the diagnosis of many conditions [35]. Right- vs. left-side temperature differences (termed: delta T or ΔT) between many specific facial regions in normal subjects were shown to be low ($<0.3°C$) [40], while similar ΔT values were found to be high ($>0.5°C$) in a variety of disorders related to dentistry [35].

20.6 Abnormal Facial Conditions Demonstrated with Infrared Facial Thermography

20.6.1 Assessing Temporomandibular Joint (TMJ) Disorders with Infrared Thermography

It has been shown that normal subjects have symmetrical thermal patterns over the TMJ regions of their face. Normal subjects had ΔT values of 0.1°C (±0.1°C) [32,36]. On the other hand, TMJ pain patients were found to have asymmetrical thermal patterns, with increased temperatures over the affected TMJ region, with ΔT values of +0.4°C (±0.2°C) [37]. Specifically, painful TMJ patients with internal derangement and painful TMJ osteoarthritis were both found to have asymmetrical thermal patterns and increased temperatures over the affected TMJ, with mean area TMJ ΔT of +0.4°C (±0.2°C) [22,24]. In other words, the correlation between TMJ pain and hyper perfusion of the region seems to be independent of the etiology of the TMJ disorder (osteoarthritis vs. internal derangement). In addition, a study of mild-to-moderate TMD (temporomandibular joint dysfunction) patients indicated that area ΔT values correlated with the level of the patient's pain symptoms [38]. And a more recent double-blinded clinical study compared active orthodontic patients vs. TMD patients vs. asymptomatic TMJ controls, and showed average ΔT values of +0.2, +0.4, and +0.1°C; for these three groups respectively. This study showed that thermography could distinguish between patients undergoing active orthodontic treatment and patients with TMD [39].

20.6.2 Assessing Inferior Alveolar Nerve (IAN) Deficit with Infrared Thermography

The thermal imaging of the chin has been shown to be an effective method for assessing inferior alveolar nerve deficit [40]. Whereas normal subjects (those without inferior alveolar nerve deficit) show a symmetrical thermal pattern (ΔT of +0.1°C [±0.1°C]); patients with inferior alveolar nerve deficit had elevated temperature in the mental region of their chin (ΔT of +0.5°C [±0.2°C]) on the affected side [41]. The observed vasodilatation seems to be due to blockage of the vascular neuronal vasoconstrictive messages, since the same effect on the thermological pattern could be invoked in normal subjects by temporary blockage of the inferior alveolar nerve, using a 2% lidocaine nerve block injection [42].

20.6.3 Assessing Carotid Occlusal Disease with Infrared Thermography

The thermal imaging of the face, especially around the orbits, has been shown to be an effective method for assessing carotid occlusal disease. Cerebrovascular accident (CVA), also called stroke, is well known as a major cause of death. The most common cause of stroke is atherosclerosotic plaques forming emboli, which travel within vascular blood channels, lodging in the brain, obstructing the brain's blood supply, resulting in a cerebral vascular accident (or stroke). The most common origin for emboli is located in the lateral region of the neck where the common carotid artery bifurcates into the internal and the external carotid arteries [43,44]. It has been well documented that intraluminal carotid plaques, which both restrict and reduce blood flow, result in decreased facial skin temperature [43–54]. Thermography has demonstrated the ability to detect a reduction of 30% (or more) of blood flow within the carotid arteries [55]. Thermography shows promise as an inexpensive painless screening test of asymptomatic elderly adults at risk for the possibility of stroke. However, more clinical studies are required before thermography may be accepted for routine application in screening toward preventing stroke [55,56].

20.6.4 Additional Applications of Infrared Thermography

Recent clinical studies assessed the application of thermography on patients with chronic facial pain (orofacial pain of greater than 4 month's duration). Thermography classified patients as being "normal" when selected anatomic ΔT values ranged from 0.0°C to ±0.25°C, and "hot" when ΔT values were >+0.35°C, and "cold" when area ΔT values were $<-0.35°C$. The study population consisted of 164 dental pain patients and 164 matched (control) subjects. This prospective, matched study determined that subjects classified with "hot" thermographs had the clinical diagnosis of (1) sympathetically maintained pain, (2) peripheral nerve-mediated pain, (3) TMJ arthropathy, or (4) acute maxillary sinusitis. Subjects classified with "cold" areas on their thermographs were found to have the clinical diagnosis of (1) peripheral nerve-mediated pain, or (2) sympathetically independent pain. Subjects classified with "normal" thermographs included patients with the clinical diagnosis of (1) cracked tooth syndrome, (2) trigeminal neuralgia, (3) pretrigeminal neuralgia, or (4) psychogenic facial pain. This new system of thermal classification resulted in 92% (301 or 328) agreement in classifying pain patients vs. their matched controls. In brief, ΔT has been shown to be within $\pm 0.4°C$ in normal subjects, while showing values greater than $+0.7°C$ and less than $-0.6°C$ in abnormal facial pain patients [10], making "ΔT" an important diagnostic parameter in the assessment of orofacial pain [35].

20.6.5 Future Advances in Infrared Imaging

Over the last 20 years there have been additional reports in the dental literature giving promise to new and varied applications of infrared thermography [57–63]. While, infrared thermography is promising, the future holds even greater potential for temperature measurement as a diagnostic tool, the most promising being termed dynamic area telethermometry (DAT) [64,65]. Newly developed DAT promises to become a new more advanced tool providing quantitative information on the thermoregulatory frequencies (TRFs) manifested in the modulation of skin temperature [66]. Whereas the static thermographic studies discussed above demonstrate local vasodilatation or vasoconstriction, DAT can identify the mechanism of thermoregulatory frequencies and thus it is expected, in the future, to significantly improve differential diagnosis [66].

In summary, the science of thermology, including static thermography, and soon to be followed by DAT, appears to have great promise as an important diagnostic tool in the assessment of orofacial health and disease.

Acknowledgment

This chapter is dedicated to Professor Michael Anbar, of Buffalo, New York: A brilliant scientist, my thermal science mentor, and "The Father of Dynamic Area Telethermography."

References

[1] Grobklaus, R. and Bergmann, K.E. Physiology and regulation of body temperature. In *Applied Thermology: Thermologic Methods*. J.-M. Engel, U. Fleresch, and G. Stuttgen, Eds., Federal Republic of Germany: VCH (1985), pp. 11–20.

[2] *Applied Thermology: Thermologic Methods*. J.-M. Engel, U. Fleresch, and G. Stuttgen, Eds., Federal Republic of Germany: VCH (1985), pp. 11–20.

[3] Kirsch, K.A. Physiology of skin-surface temperature. In *Applied Thermology: Thermologic Methods*. J.-M. Engel, U. Fleresch, and G. Stuttgen, Eds., Federal Republic of Germany: VCH (1985), pp. 1–9.

[4] Anbar, M., Gratt, B.M., and Hong, D. Thermology and facial telethermography: part I. History and technical review. *Dentomaxillofac. Radiol.* (1998) 27: 61–67.

[5] Anbar, M. and Gratt, B.M. Role of nitric oxide in the physiopathology of pain. *J. Musc. Skeletal Joint Pain* (1997) 14: 225–254.

[6] Rost, A. Comparative measurements with an infrared and contact thermometer for thermal stress reaction. In *Thermological Methods*. J.-M. Engel, U. Flesch, and G. Stuttgen, Eds., Weinheim: VCH Verlag (1985), pp. 169–170.

[7] Hardy, J.D. The radiation of heat from the human body: I–IV. *J. Clin. Invest.* (1934) 13: 593–620.

[8] Hardy, J.D. The radiation of heat from the human body: I–IV. *J. Clin. Invest.* (1934) 13: 817–883.

[9] Abernathy, M. and Abernathy, T.B. International bibliography of thermology. *Thermology* (1987) 2: 1–533.
[10] Berry, D.C. and Yemm, R. Variations in skin temperature of the face in normal subjects and in patients with mandibular dysfunction. *Br. J. Oral Maxillofac. Surg.* (1971) 8: 242–247.
[11] Berry, D.C. and Yemm, R. A further study of facial skin temperature in patients with mandibular dysfunction. *J. Oral Rehabil.* (1974) 1: 255–264.
[12] Kopp, S. and Haraldson, T. Normal variations in skin temperature of the face in normal subjects and in patients with mandibular dysfunction. *Br. J. Oral Maxillofac. Surg.* (1983) 8: 242–247.
[13] Johansson, A., Kopp, S., and Haraldson, T. Reproducibility and variation of skin surface temperature over the temporomandibular joint and masseter muscle in normal individuals. *Acta Odontol. Scand.* (1985) 43: 309–313.
[14] Tegelberg, A. and Kopp, S. Skin surface temperature over the temporo-mandibular and metacarpophalangeal joints in individuals with rheumatoid arthritis. *Odontol. Klin.*, Box 33070, 400 33 Goteborg, Sweden (1986) Report No. 31, pp. 1–31.
[15] Akerman, S. et al. Relationship between clinical, radiologic and thermometric findings of the temporomandibular joint in rheumatoid arthritis. *Odontol. Klin.*, Box 33070, 400 33 Goteborg, Sweden (1987) Report No. 41, pp. 1–30.
[16] Finney, J.W., Holt, C.R., and Pearce, K.B. Thermographic diagnosis of TMJ disease and associated neuromuscular disorders. *Special Report: Postgraduate Medicine* (March 1986), pp. 93–95.
[17] Weinstein, S.A. Temporomandibular joint pain syndrome—the whiplash of the 1980s, *Thermography and Personal Injury Litigation*, Ch. 7. S.D. Hodge, Jr., Ed., New York, USA: John Wiley & Sons (1987), pp. 157–164.
[18] Weinstein, S.A., Gelb, M., and Weinstein, E.L. Thermophysiologic anthropometry of the face in home sapiens. *J. Craniomand. Pract.* (1990) 8: 252–257.
[19] Pogrel, M.A., McNeill, C., and Kim, J.M. The assessment of trapezius muscle symptoms of patients with temporomandibular disorders by the use of liquid crystal thermography. *Oral Surg. Oral Med. Oral. Pathol. Oral Radiol. Endod.* (1996) 82: 145–151.
[20] Steed, P.A. The utilization of liquid crystal thermography in the evaluation of temporomandibular dysfunction. *J. Craniomand. Pract.* (1991) 9: 120–128.
[21] Gratt, B.M., Sickles, E.A., Graff-Radford, S.B., and Solberg, W.K. Electronic thermography in the diagnosis of atypical odontalgia: a pilot study. *Oral Surg. Oral Med. Oral Pathol. Oral Radiol. Endod.* (1989) 68: 472–481.
[22] Gratt, B.M. et al. Electronic thermography in the assessment of internal derangement of the TMJ. *J. Orofacial Pain* (1994) 8: 197–206.
[23] Gratt, B.M., Sickles, E.A., Ross, J.B., Wexler, C.E., and Gornbein, J.A. Thermographic assessment of craniomandibular disorders: diagnostic interpretation versus temperature measurement analysis. *J. Orofacial Pain* (1994) 8: 278–288.
[24] Gratt, B.M., Sickles, E.A., and Wexler, C.E. Thermographic characterization of osteoarthrosis of the temporomandibular joint. *J. Orofacial Pain* (1994) 7: 345–353.
[25] Progrell, M. A., Erbez, G., Taylor, R.C., and Dodson, T.B. Liquid crystal thermography as a diagnostic aid and objective monitor for TMJ dysfunction and myogenic facial pain. *J. Craniomand. Disord. Facial Oral Pain* (1989) 3: 65–70.
[26] Dmutpueva, B.C., and Alekceeva, A.H. Applications of thermography in the evaluation of the postoperative patient. *Stomatologiia* (1986) 12: 29–30 (Russian).
[27] Cambell, R.L., Shamaskin, R.G., and Harkins, S.W. Assessment of recovery from injury to inferior alveolar and mental nerves. *Oral Surg. Oral Med. Oral Pathol. Oral Radiol. Endod.* (1987) 64: 519–526.
[28] Crandall, C.E. and Hill, R.P. Thermography in dentistry: a pilot study. *Oral Surg. Oral Med. Oral Pathol. Oral Radiol. Endod.* (1966) 21: 316–320.
[29] Gratt, B.M., Pullinger, A., and Sickles, E.A. Electronic thermography of normal facial structures: A pilot study. *Oral Surg. Oral Med. Oral Pathol. Oral Radiol. Endod.* (1989) 68: 346–351.

[30] Weinstein, S.A., Gelb, M., and Weinstein, E.L. Thermophysiologic anthropometry of the face in homo sapiens. *J. Craniomand. Pract.* (1990) 8: 252–257.

[31] Uematsu, S. Symmetry of skin temperature comparing one side of the body to the other. *Thermology* (1985) 1: 4–7.

[32] Gratt, B.M. and Sickles, E.A. Electronic facial thermography: an analysis of asymptomatic adult subjects. *J. Orofacial Pain* (1995) 9: 222–265.

[33] Blaxter, K. Energy exchange by radiation, convection, conduction and evaporation. In *Energy Metabolism in Animals and Man.* New York: Cambridge University Press (1989), pp. 86–99.

[34] Blaxter, K. The minimal metabolism. In *Energy Metabolism in Animals and Man.* New York: Cambridge University Press (1989) 120–146.

[35] Gratt, B.M, Graff-Radford, S.B., Shetty, V., Solberg, W.K., and Sickles, E.A. A six-year clinical assessment of electronic facial thermography. *Dentomaxillofac. Radiol.* (1996) 25: 247–255.

[36] Gratt, B.M., and Sickles, E.A. Thermographic characterization of the asymptomatic TMJ. *J. Orofacial Pain* (1993) 7: 7–14.

[37] Gratt, B.M., Sickles, E.M., and Ross, J.B. Thermographic assessment of craniomandibular disorders: diagnostic interpretation versus temperature measurement analysis. *J. Orofacial Pain* (1994) 8: 278–288.

[38] Canavan, D. and Gratt, B.M. Electronic thermography for the assessment of mild and moderate TMJ dysfunction. *Oral Surg. Oral Med. Oral Pathol. Oral Radiol. Endod.* (1995) 79: 778–786.

[39] McBeth, S.A., and Gratt, B.M. A cross-sectional thermographic assessment of TMJ problems in orthodontic patients. *Am. J. Orthod. Dentofac. Orthop.* (1996) 109: 481–488.

[40] Gratt, B.M., Shetty, V., Saiar, M., and Sickles, E.A. Electronic thermography for the assessment of inferior alveolar nerve deficit. *Oral Surg. Oral Med. Oral Pathol. Oral Radiol. Endod.* (1995) 80: 153–160.

[41] Gratt, B.M., Sickles, E.A., and Shetty, V. Thermography for the clinical assessment of inferior alveolar nerve deficit: a pilot study. *J. Orofacial Pain* (1994) 80: 153–160.

[42] Shetty, V., Gratt, B.M., and Flack, V. Thermographic assessment of reversible inferior alveolar nerve deficit. *J. Orofacial Pain* (1994) 8: 375–383.

[43] Wood, E.H. Thermography in the diagnosis of cerebrovascular disease: preliminary report. *Radiology* (1964) 83: 540–546.

[44] Wood, E.H. Thermography in the diagnosis of cerebrovascular disease. *Radiology* (1965) 85: 207–215.

[45] Steinke, W., Kloetzsch, C., and Hennerici, M. Carotid artery disease assessed by color Doppler sonography and angiography. *AJR* (1990) 154: 1061–1067.

[46] Hu, H.-H. et al. Color Doppler imaging of orbital arteries for detection of carotid occlusive disease. *Stroke* (1993) 24: 1196–1202.

[47] Carroll, B.A., Graif, M., and Orron, D.E. Vascular ultrasound. In *Peripheral Vascular Imaging and Intervention.* D. Kim and D.E. Orron, Eds., St. Louis, MO, Mosby/Year Book (1992), pp. 211–225.

[48] Mawdsley, C., Samuel, E., Sumerling, M.D., and Young, G.B. Thermography in occlusive cerebrovascular diseases. *Br. Med. J.* (1968) 3: 521–524.

[49] Capistrant, T.D. and Gumnit, R.J. Thermography and extracranial cerebrovascular disease: a new method to predict the stroke-prone individual. *Minn. Med.* (1971) 54: 689–692.

[50] Karpman, H.L., Kalb, I.M., and Sheppard, J.J. The use of thermography in a health care system for stroke. *Geriatrics* (1972) 27: 96–105.

[51] Soria, E. and Paroski, M.W. Thermography as a predictor of the more involved side in bilateral carotid disease: case history. *Angiology* (1987) 38: 151–158.

[52] Capistrat, T.D. and Gumnit, R.J. Detecting carotid occlusive disease by thermography. *Stroke* (1973) 4: 57–65.

[53] Abernathy, M., Brandt, M.M., and Robinson, C. Noninvasive testing of the carotid system. *Am. Fam. Physic.* (1984) 29: 157–164.

[54] Dereymaeker, A., Kams-Cauwe, V., and Fobelets, P. Frontal dynamic thermography: improvement in diagnosis of carotid stenosis. *Eur. Neurol.* (1978) 17: 226–234.

[55] Gratt, B.M., Halse, A., and Hollender, L. A pilot study of facial infrared thermal imaging used as a screening test for detecting elderly individuals at risk for stroke. *Thermol. Int.* (2002) 12: 7–15.

[56] Friedlander A.H. and Gratt B.M. Panoramic dental radiography and thermography as an aid in detecting patients at risk for stroke. *J. Oral Maxillofac. Surg.* (1994) 52: 1257–1262.

[57] Graff-Radford, S.B., Ketalaer, M.-C., Gratt, B.M., and Solberg, W.K. Thermographic assessment of neuropathic facial pain: a pilot study. *J. Orofacial Pain* (1995) 9: 138–146.

[58] Pogrel, M.A., Erbez, G., Taylor, R.C., and Dodson, T.B. Liquid crystal thermography as a diagnostic aid and objective monitor for TMJ dysfunction and myogenic facial pain. *J. Craniobandib. Disord. Facial Oral Pain* (1989) 3: 65–70.

[59] Pogrel, M.A., Yen, C.K., and Taylor, R.C. Infrared thermography in oral and maxillo-facial surgery. *Oral Surg. Oral Med. Oral Pathol. Oral Radiol. Endod.* (1989) 67: 126–131.

[60] Graff-Radford, S.B., Ketalaer, M.C., Gratt, B.M., and Solberg, W.K. Thermographic assessment of neuropathic facial pain. *J. Orofacial Pain* (1995) 9: 138–146.

[61] Biagioni, P.A., Longmore, R.B., McGimpsey, J.G., and Lamey, P.J. Infrared thermography: its role in dental research with particular reference to craniomandibular disorders. *Dentomaxillofac. Radiol.* (1996) 25: 119–124.

[62] Biagioni, P.A., McGimpsey, J.G., and Lamey, P.J. Electronic infrared thermography as a dental research technique. *Br. Dent. J.* (1996) 180: 226–230.

[63] Benington, I.C., Biagioni, P.A., Crossey, P.J., Hussey, D.L., Sheridan, S., and Lamel, P.J. Temperature changes in bovine mandibular bone during implant site preparation: an assessment using infra-red thermography. *J. Dent.* (1996) 24: 263–267.

[64] Anbar, M. Clinical applications of dynamic area telethermography. In *Quantitative Dynamic Telthermography in Medical Diagnosis.* CRC Press: Boca Raton, FL (1994), pp. 147–180.

[65] Anbar, M. Dynamic area telethermography and its clinical applications. *SPIE Proc.* (1995) 2473: 3121–3323.

[66] Anbar M., Grenn, M.W., Marino, M.T., Milescu, L., and Zamani, K. Fast dynamic area telethermography (DAT) of the human forearm with a Ga/As quantum well infrared focal plane array camera. *Eur. J. Therol.* (1997) 7: 105–118.

21
Use of Infrared Imaging in Veterinary Medicine

Ram C. Purohit
Auburn University

Tracy A. Turner
Private Practice

David D. Pascoe
Auburn University

21.1	Historical Perspective...................................	**21-1**
21.2	Standards for Reliable Thermograms	**21-2**
21.3	Dermatome Patterns of Horses and Other Animal Species	**21-3**
21.4	Peripheral Neurovascular Thermography..............	**21-4**
	Horner's Syndrome • Neurectomies • Vascular Injuries	
21.5	Musculoskeletal Injuries................................	**21-5**
21.6	Thermography of the Testes and Scrotum in Mammalian Species	**21-6**
21.7	Conclusions	**21-6**
	References	**21-7**

21.1 Historical Perspective

In the mid-1960s and early 1970s, several studies were published indicating the value of IR (infrared) thermography in veterinary medicine [1–3]. In the 1965 research of Delahanty and George [2], the thermographic images required at least 6 min to produce a thermogram, a lengthy period of time during which the veterinarian had to keep the horse still while the scan was completed. This disadvantage was overcome by the development of high speed scanners using rotating IR prisms which then could produce instantaneous thermograms.

Stromberg [4–6] and Stromberg and Norberg [7] used thermography to diagnose inflammatory changes of the superficial digital flexor tendons in race horses. With thermography, they were able to document and detect early inflammation of the tendon, 1 to 2 weeks prior to the detection of lameness using clinical examination. They suggested that thermography could be used for early signs of pending lameness and it could be used for preventive measures to rest and treat race horses before severe lameness became obvious on physical examination.

In 1970, the Horse Protection Act was passed by the United States Congress to ban the use of chemical or mechanical means of "soring" horses. It was difficult to enforce this act because of the difficulty in obtaining measurable and recordable proof of violations. In 1975, Nelson and Osheim [8] documented that soring caused by chemical or mechanical means on the horse's digit could be diagnosed as having a definite abnormal characteristic IR emission pattern in the affected areas of the limb. Even though thermography at that time became the technique of choice for the detection of soring, normal thermography patterns in horses were not known. This prompted the USDA to fund research for the uses of thermography in veterinary medicine.

Purohit et al. [9] established a protocol for obtaining normal thermographic patterns of the horses' limbs and other parts of the body. This protocol was regularly used for early detection of acute and chronic inflammatory conditions in horses and other animal species. Studies at Auburn University vet school used an AGA 680 liquid cooled thermography system that had a black and white and an accessory color display units that allows the operator to assign the array of ten isotherms to temperature increments from $0.2°C$ to $10.0°C$. Images were captured within seconds rather than the 6 min required for earlier machines. In veterinary studies at Auburn University, the thermographic isotherms were imaged with nine colors and white assigned to each isotherm that varied in temperature between either $0.5°C$ or $1.0°C$.

In a subsequent study, Purohit and McCoy [10] established normal thermal patterns (temperature and gradients) of the horse, with special attention directed towards thoracic and pelvic limbs. Thermograms of various parts of the body were obtained 30 min before and after the exercise for each horse. Thermographic examination was also repeated for each horse on six different days. Thermal patterns and gradients were similar in all horses studied with a high degree of right to left symmetry in IR emission.

At the same time, Turner et al. [11] investigated the influence of the hair coat and hair clipping. This study demonstrated that the clipped leg was always warmer. After exercise, both clipped and unclipped legs had similar increases in temperature. The thermal patterns and gradients were not altered by clipping and/or exercise [10,11]. This indicated that clipping hair in horses with even hair coats was not necessary for thermographic evaluation. However, in some areas where the hair is long hair and not uniform, clipping may be required. Recently, concerns related to hair coat, thermographic imaging, and temperature regulation were investigated in llamas exposed to the hot humid conditions of the southeast [12]. While much of the veterinary research has focused on the thermographic imaging as a diagnostic tool, this study expanded its use into the problems of thermoregulation in various non endemic species.

Current camera technology has improved scanning capabilities that are combined with computer-assisted software programs. This new technology provides the practitioner with numerous options for image analysis, several hundred isotherms capable of capturing temperature differences in the hundredths of a degree Celsius, and better image quality. Miniaturized electronics have reduced the size of the units, allowing some systems to be housed in portable hand-held units. With lower cost of equipment, more thermographic equipment are being utilized in human and animal veterinary medicine and basic physiology studies.

It was obvious from initial studies by several authors that standards needed to be established for obtaining reliable thermograms in different animal species. The variations in core temperature and differences in the thermoregulatory mechanism responses between species emphasizes the importance of individually established norms for thermographic imagery.

A further challenge in veterinary medicine may occur when animal patient care may necessitate outdoor imaging.

21.2 Standards for Reliable Thermograms

Thermography provides an accurate, quantifiable, noncontact, noninvasive measure and map of skin surface temperatures. Skin surface temperatures are variable and change according to blood flow regulation to the skin surface. As such, IR thermography practitioner must be aware of the internal and external influences that alter this dynamic process of skin blood flow and temperature regulation. While imaging equipment can vary widely in price, these differences are often reflective of the wave-length capturing capability of the detectors and adjunct software that can aid in image analysis. The thermographer needs to understand the limitations of their IR system in order to make appropriate interpretations of their data. There have been some published studies that have not adhered to reliable standards and equipment prerequisites, thereby detracting from the acceptance of thermography as a valuable research and clinical technique. In some cases a simple cause–effect relationship was assumed to demonstrate the diagnosis of a disease or syndrome based on thermal responses as captured by thermographic images.

Internal and external factors have a significant effect on the skin surface temperature. Therefore, the use of thermography to evaluate skin surface thermal patterns and gradient requires an understanding of the dynamic changes which occur in blood flow at systemic, peripheral, regional, and local levels [9,10]. Thus, to enhance the diagnostic value of thermography, we recommend the following standards for veterinary medical imaging:

1. The environmental factors which interfere with the quality of thermography should be minimized. The room temperature should be maintained between 21°C and 26°C. Slight variations in some cases may be acceptable, but room temperature should always be cooler than the animal's body temperature and free from air drafts.
2. Thermograms obtained outdoors under conditions of direct air drafts, sunlight, and extreme variations in temperature may provide unreliable thermograms in which thermal patterns are altered. Such observations are meaningless as a diagnostic tool.
3. When an animal is brought into a temperature controlled room, it should be equilibrated at least 20 min or more, depending on the external temperature from which the animal was transported. Animals transported from extreme hot or cold environments may require up to 60 min of equilibration time. Equilibration time is adequate when the thermal temperatures and patterns are consistently maintained over several minutes.
4. Other factors affecting the quality of thermograms are exercise, sweating, body position and angle, body covering, systemic and topical medications, regional and local blocks, sedatives, tranquilizers, anesthetics, vasoactive drugs, skin lesions such as scars, surgically altered areas, etc. As stated prior, the hair coat may be an issue with uneven hair length or a thick coat.
5. It is recommended that the infrared imaging should be performed using an electronic non contact cooled system. The use of long wave detectors is preferable.

The value of thermography is demonstrated by the sensitivity to changes in heat on the skin surface and its ability to detect temporal and spatial changes in thermal skin responses that corresponds to temporal and spatial changes in blood flow. Therefore, it is important to have well documented normal thermal patterns and gradients in all species under controlled environments prior to making any claims or detecting pathological conditions.

21.3 Dermatome Patterns of Horses and Other Animal Species

Certain chronic and acute painful conditions associated with peripheral neurovascular and neuromuscular injuries are easy to confuse with spinal injuries associated with cervical, thoracic, and lumbar-sacral areas [13,14]. Similarly, inflammatory conditions such as osteoarthritis, tendonitis, and other associated conditions may also be confused with other neurovascular conditions. Thus, studies have been done over the last 25 years at Auburn University to map cutaneous and differentiate the sensory-sympathetic dermatome patterns of cervical, thoracic, and lumbosacral regions in horses [13,14]. Infrared thermography was used to map the sensory-sympathetic dermatome in horses. The dorsal or ventral spinal nerve(s) were blocked with 0.5% of mepevacine as a local anesthetic. The sensory sympathetic spinal nerve block produced two effects. First, blocking the sympathetic portion of the spinal nerve caused increased thermal patterns and produced sweating of the affected areas. Second, the areas of insensitivity produced by the sensory portion of the block were mapped and compared with the thermal patterns. The areas of insensitivity were found to correlate with the sympathetic innervations.

Thermography was used to provide thermal patterns of various dermatome areas from cervical areas to epidural areas in horses. Clinical cases of cervical area nerve compression provided cooler thermal patterns, away from the site of injuries. In cases of acute injuries, associated thermal patterns were warmer than normal cases at the site of the injury. Elucidation of dermatomal (thermatom) patterns provided location for spinal injuries for the diagnosis of back injuries in horses. Similarly, in a case of a dog where the neck injury (subluxation of atlanto-axis) the diagnosis was determined by abnormal thermal patterns and gradients.

21.4 Peripheral Neurovascular Thermography

When there are alterations in skin surface temperature, it may be difficult to distinguish and diagnose between nerve and vascular injuries. The cutaneous circulation is under sympathetic vasomotor control. Peripheral nerve injuries and nerve compression can result in skin surface vascular changes that can be detected thermographically. It is well known that inflammation and nerve irritation may result in vasoconstriction causing cooler thermograms in the afflicted areas. Transection of a nerve and/or nerve damage to the extent that there is a loss of nerve conduction results in a loss in sympathetic tone which causes vasodilation indicated by an increase in the thermogram temperature. Of course, this simple rationale is more complicated with different types of nerve injuries (neuropraxia, axonotomesis, and neurotmesis). Furthermore, lack of characterization of the extent and duration of injuries may make thermographic interpretation difficult.

Studies were done on horses and other animal species to show that if thermographic examination is performed properly under controlled conditions, it can provide an accurate diagnosis of neurovascular injuries. The rationale for a neurovascular clinical diagnosis is provided in the following Horner's Syndrome case.

21.4.1 Horner's Syndrome

In four horses, Horner's Syndrome was also induced by transaction of vagosympathetic trunk on either left or right side of the neck [15]. Facial thermograms of a case of Horner's Syndrome were done 15 min before and after the exercise. Sympathetic may cause the affected side to be warm by 2–3°C more than the non-transected side. This increased temperature after denervation is reflective of an increase in blood flow due to vasodilation in the denervated areas [15,16]. The increased thermal patterns on the affected side were present up to 6–12 weeks. In about 2–4 months, neurotraumatized side blood flow readjusted to the local demand of circulation. Thermography of both non-neuroectomized and neuroectomized sides looked similar and normal [16]. In some cases, this readjustment took place as early as five days and it was difficult to distinguish the affected side. The intravenous injection of 1 mg of epinephrine in a 1000 lb horse caused an increase in thermal patterns on the denervated side, the same as indicating the presence of Horner's Syndrome. Administration of I V acetyl promazine (30 mg/1000 lb horse) showed increased heat (thermal pattern) on the normal non-neuroectomized side, whereas acetylpromazine had no effect on the neurectomized side. Alpha-blocking drug acetylpromazine caused vasodilation and increased blood flow to normal non-neurectomized side, whereas no effect was seen in the affected neurectomized side due to the lack of sympathetic innervation [16–18].

21.4.2 Neurectomies

Thermographic evaluation of the thoracic (front) and pelvic (back) limbs were done before and after performing digital neurectomies in several horses. After posterior digital neurectomy there were significant increases in heat in the areas supplied by the nerves [17]. Within 3–6 weeks, readjustment of local blood flow occurred in the neurectomized areas, and it was difficult to differentiate between the non-neurectomized and the neurectomized areas. Ten minutes after administration of 0.06 mg/kg I V injection of acetylpromazine, a 2–3°C increase in heat was noted in normal non-neurectomized areas, whereas the neurectomized areas of the opposite limb were not affected.

21.4.3 Vascular Injuries

Thermography has been efficacious in the diagnosis of vascular diseases. It has been shown that the localized reduction of blood flow occurs in the horse with navicular disease [11]. This effect was more obvious on thermograms obtained after exercise than before exercise. Normally, 15–20 min of exercise will increase skin surface temperature by 2–2.5°C in horses [10,11]. In cases of arterial occlusion, the area distal to the occlusion in the horses' limb shows cooler thermograms. The effects of exercise or administration of alpha-blocking drugs like acetylpromazine causes increased blood flow to peripheral circulation in normal areas with intact vascular and sympathetic responses [17,18]. Thus, obtaining thermograms either after exercise or after administration of alpha-blocking drugs like acetylpromazine provides prognostic value for diagnosis of adequate collateral circulation. Therefore, the use of skin temperature as a measure of skin perfusion merits consideration for peripheral vascular flow, perfusion, despite some physical and physiological limitations, which are inherent in methodology [19].

Furthermore, interference with the peripheral vascular blood flow can result from neurogenic inhibition, vascular occlusion, and occlusion as a result of inflammatory vascular compression. Neurogenic inhibition can be diagnosed through the administration of alpha-blocking drugs which provide an increase in blood flow. Vascular impairment may also be associated with local injuries (inflammation, edema, swelling, etc.) which may provide localized cooler or hotter thermograms. Thus, evaluation using thermography should note the physical state and site of the injury.

21.5 Musculoskeletal Injuries

Thermography has been used in the clinical and subclinical cases of osteoarthritis, tendonitis, navicular disease, and other injuries such as sprains, stress fractures, and shin splints [10,11,20,21]. In some cases thermal abnormalities may be detected two weeks prior to the onset of clinical signs of lameness in horses, especially in the case of joint disease [21], tendonitis [10], and navicular problems [11,20].

Osteoarthritis is a severe joint disease in horses. Normally, diagnosis is made by clinical examination and radiographic evaluation. Radiography detects the problem after deterioration of the joint surface has taken place. Clinical evaluation is only done when horses show physical abnormalities in their gait due to pain. An early sign of osteoarthritis is inflammation, which can be detected by thermography prior to it becoming obvious on radiograms [21].

In studies of standard bred race horses, the effected tarsus joint can demonstrate abnormal thermal patterns indicating inflammation in the joint two to three weeks prior to radiographic diagnosis [21]. The abnormal thermograms obtained in this study were more distinct after exercise than before exercise. Thus, thermography provided a subclinical diagnosis of osteoarthritis in this study.

Thermography was used to evaluate the efficacy of corticosteroid therapy in amphotericine-B induced arthritis in ponies [22]. The intra-articular injection of 100 mg of methylprednisolone acetate was effective in alleviating the clinical signs of lameness and pain. It is important to note that when compared with clinical signs of non-treated arthritis, it was difficult to differentiate increased thermal patterns between corticosteroid treated vs. non-treated, arthritis-induced joints. However, corticosteroid therapy did not decrease the healing time of intercarpal arthritis, whereas corticosteroid therapy did decrease the time for return to normal thermographic patterns for tibiotarsal joints. In this study, thermography was useful in detecting inflammation in the absence of clinical signs of pain in corticosteroid treated joints and aiding the evaluation of the healing processes in amphotericin B-induced arthritis [22].

The chronic and acute pain associated with neuromuscular conditions can also be diagnosed by this technique. In cases where no definitive diagnosis can be made using physical examination and x-rays, thermography has been efficacious for early diagnosis of soft tissue injuries [10,23]. The conditions such as subsolar abscesses, laminitis, and other leg lameness can be easily differentiated using thermography [10,11]. We have used thermography for quantitative and qualitative evaluation of anti-inflammatory drugs such as phenylbutazone in the treatment of physical or chemically induced inflammation. The most useful application of thermography in veterinary medicine and surgery has been to aid early detection of an acute and chronic inflammatory process.

21.6 Thermography of the Testes and Scrotum in Mammalian Species

The testicular temperature of most mammalian species must be below body temperature for normal spermatogenesis. The testes of most domestic mammalian species migrates out of the abdomen and are retained in the scrotum, which provides the appropriate thermal environment for normal spermatogenesis [24,25]. The testicular arterial and venous structure is such that arterial coils are enmeshed in the pampiniform plexus of the testicular veins, which provides a counter current heating regulating mechanism by which arterial blood entering the testes is cooled by the venous blood leaving the testes [24,25]. In the ram, the temperature of the blood in the testicular artery decreases by 4°C from the external inguinal ring to the surface of the testes. Thus, to function effectively, the mammalian testes are maintained at a lower temperature.

Purohit [26,27] used thermography to establish normal thermal patterns and gradients of the scrotum in bulls, stallions, bucks, dogs, and llamas. The normal thermal patterns of the scrotum in all species studied is characterized by right to left symmetrical patterns, with a constant decrease in the thermal gradients from the base to the apex. In bulls, bucks, and stallions, a thermal gradient of 4–6°C from the base to apex with concentric hands signifies normal patterns. Inflammation of one testicle increased ipsilateral scrotal temperatures of 2.5–3°C [26,28] If both testes were inflamed, there was an overall increase of 2.5–3°C temperature and a reduction in temperature gradient was noted.

Testicular degeneration could be acute or chronic. In chronic testicular degeneration with fibrosis, there was a loss of temperature gradient, loss of concentric thermal patterns, and some areas were cooler than others with no consistent patterns [26]. Reversibility of degenerative changes depends upon the severity and duration of the trauma. The infrared thermal gradients and patterns in dogs [27] and llamas [27,29] are unique to their own species and the patterns are different from that of the bull and buck.

Thermography has also been used in humans, indicating a normal thermal pattern which is characterized by symmetric and constant temperatures between 32.5°C and 34.5°C [30–33]. Increased scrotal infrared emissions were associated with intrascrotal tumor, acute and chronic inflammation, and varicoceles [34,35]. Thermography has been efficacious for early diagnosis of acute and/or chronic testicular degeneration in humans and many animal species. The disruption of the normal thermal patterns of the scrotum is directly related to testicular degeneration. The testicular degeneration may cause transient or permanent infertility in the male. It is well established that increases in scrotal temperature above normal causes disruption of spermatogenesis, affects sperm maturation, and contributes toward subfertile or infertile semen quality. Early diagnosis of pending infertility has a significant impact on economy and reproduction in animals.

21.7 Conclusions

The value of thermography can only be realized if it is used properly. All species studied thus far have provided remarkable bilateral symmetrical patterns of infrared emission. The high degree of right-to-left symmetry provides a valuable asset in diagnosis of unilateral problems associated with various inflammatory disorders. On the other hand, bilateral problems can be diagnosed due to changes in thermal gradient and/or overall increase or decrease of temperature, away from the normal established thermal patterns in a given area of the body. Various areas of the body on the same side have normal patterns and gradients. This can be used to diagnose a change in gradient patterns. Alteration in normal thermal patterns and gradients indicates a thermal pathology. If thermal abnormalities are evaluated carefully, early diagnosis can be made, even prior to the appearance of clinical signs of joint disease, tendonitis, and various musculoskeletal problems in various animal species. Thermography can be used as a screening device for early detection of an impending problem, allowing veterinarian institute treatment before the problem becomes more serious. During the healing process post surgery, animals may appear physically sound. Thermography can be used as a diagnostic aid in assessing the healing processes. In equine sports medicine, thermography can be used on a regular basis for screening to prevent severe injuries to the horse. Early detection and treatment can prevent financial losses associated with delayed diagnosis and treatment.

The efficacy of non-contact electronic infrared thermography has been demonstrated in numerous clinical settings and research studies as a diagnostic tool for veterinary medicine. It has had a strong impact on veterinary medical practice and thermal physiology where accurate skin temperatures need to be assessed under normal conditions, disease pathologies, injuries, and thermal stress. The importance of infrared thermography as a research tool cannot be understated for improving the medical care of animals and for the contributions made through animal research models that improve our understanding of human structures and functions.

References

[1] Smith W.M. Application of thermography in veterinary medicine. *Ann. NY Acad. Sci.*, 121, 248, 1964.
[2] Delahanty D.D. and George J.R. Thermography in equine medicine. *J. Am. Vet. Med. Assoc.*, 147, 235, 1965.
[3] Clark J.A. and Cena K. The potential of infrared thermography in veterinary diagnosis. *Vet. Rec.*, 100, 404, 1977.
[4] Stromberg B. The normal and diseased flexor tendon in racehorses. *Acta Radiol.* [Suppl.] 305, 1, 1971.
[5] Stromberg B. Thermography of the superficial flexor tendon in race horses. *Acta Radiol.* [Suppl.] 319, 295, 1972.
[6] Stromberg B. The use of thermograph in equine orthopedics. *J. Am. Vet. Radiol. Soc.*, 15, 94, 1974.
[7] Stromberg B. and Norbert I. Infrared emission and Xe-disappearance rate studies in the horse. *Equine Vet. J.*, 1, 1–94, 1971.
[8] Nelson H.A. and Osheim D.L. Soring in Tennessee walking horses: detection by thermography. *USDA-APHIS, Veterinary Services Laboratories*, Ames, Iowa, pp. 1–14, 1975.
[9] Purohit R.C., Bergfeld II W.A. McCaoy M.D., Thompson W.M., and Sharman R.S. Value of clinical thermography in veterinary medicine. *Auburn Vet.*, 33, 140, 1977.
[10] Purohit R.C. and McCoy M.D. Thermography in the diagnosis of inflammatory processes in the horse. *Am. J. Vet. Res.*, 41, 1167, 1980.
[11] Turner T.A. et al. Thermographic evaluation of podotrochlosis in horses. *Am. J. Vet. Res.*, 44, 535, 1983.
[12] Heath A.M., Navarre C.B., Simpkins A.S., Purohit R.C., and Pugh D.G. A comparison of heat tolerance between sheared and non sheared alpacas (llama pacos). *Small Ruminant Res.*, 39, 19, 2001.
[13] Purohit R.C. and Franco B.D. Infrared thermography for the determination of cervical dermatome patterns in the horse. *Biomed. Thermol.*, 15, 213, 1995.
[14] Purohit R.C., Schumacher J, Molloy J.M., Smith, and Pascoe D.D. Elucidation of thoracic and lumbosacral dermatomal patterns in the horse. *Thermol. Int.*, 13, 79, 2003.
[15] Purohit R.C., McCoy M.D., and Bergfeld W.A. Thermographic diagnosis of Horner's syndrome in the horse. *Am. J. Vet. Res.*, 41, 1180, 1980.
[16] Purohit R.C. The diagnostic value of thermography in equine medicine. *Proc. Am. Assoc. Equine Pract.*, 26, 316–326, 1980.
[17] Purohit R.C. and Pascoe D.D. Thermographic evaluation of peripheral neurovascular systems in animal species. *Thermology*, 7, 83, 1997.

[18] Purohit R.C., Pascoe D.D., Schumacher J, Williams A., and Humburg J.H. Effects of medication on the normal thermal patterns in horses. *Thermol. Osterr.*, 6, 108, 1996.

[19] Purohit R.C. and Pascoe D.D. Peripheral neurovascular thermography in equine medicine. *Thermol. Osterr.*, 5, 161, 1995.

[20] Turner T.A., Purohit R.C., and Fessler J.F. Thermography: a review in equine medicine. *Comp. Cont. Education Pract. Vet.*, 8, 854, 1986.

[21] Vaden M.F., Purohit R.C. Mcoy, and Vaughan J.T. Thermography: a technique for subclinical diagnosis of osteoarthritis. *Am. J. Vet. Res.*, 41, 1175–1179, 1980.

[22] Bowman K.F., Purohit R.C., Ganjan, V.K., Peachman R.D., and Vaughan J.T. Thermographic evaluation of corticosteroids efficacy in amphotericin-B induced arthritis in ponies. *Am. J. Vet. Res.* 44, 51–56, 1983.

[23] Purohit R.C. Use of thermography in the diagnosis of lameness. *Auburn Vet.*, 43, 4, 1987.

[24] Waites G.M.H. and Setchell B.P. Physiology of testes, epididymis, and scrotum. In *Advances in Reproductive Physiology*. McLaren A., Ed., London, Logos, Vol. 4, pp. 1–21, 1969.

[25] Waites G.M.H. Temperature regulation and the testes. In *The Testis*, Johnson A.D., Grones W.R., and Vanderwork N.L., Eds., New York, Academy Press, Inc., Vol. 1, pp. 241–237, 1970.

[26] Purohit R.C., Hudson R.S., Riddell M.G., Carson R.L., Wolfe D.F., and Walker D.F. Thermography of bovine scrotum. *Am. J. Vet. Res.*, 46, 2388–2392, 1985.

[27] Purohit R.C., Pascoe D.D., Heath A.M. Pugh D.G., Carson R.L., Riddell M.G., and Wolfe D.F. Thermography: its role in functional evaluation of mammalian testes and scrotum. *Thermol. Int.*, 12, 125–130, 2002.

[28] Wolfe D.F., Hudson R.S., Carson R.L., and Purohit, R.C. Effect of unilateral orchiectomy on semen quality in bulls. *J. Am. Vet. Med. Assoc.*, 186, 1291, 1985.

[29] Heath A.M., Pugh D.G., Sartin E.A., Navarre B., and Purohit R.C. Evaluation of the safety and efficacy of testicular biopsies in llamas. *Theriogenology*, 58, 1125, 2002.

[30] Amiel J.P., Vignalou L., Tricoire J. et al. Thermography of the testicle: preliminary study. *J. Gynecol. Obstet. Biol. Reprod.*, 5, 917, 1976.

[31] Lazarus B.A. and Zorgiotti A.W. Thermo-regulation of the human testes. *Fertil. Steril.*, 26, 757, 1978.

[32] Lee J.T. and Gold R.H. Localization of occult testicular tumor with scrotal thermography. *J. Am. Med. Assoc.*, 1976, 236, 1976.

[33] Wegner G. and Weissbach Z. Application of palte thermography in the diagnosis of scrotal disease. *MMW*, 120, 61, 1978.

[34] Gold R.H., Ehrilich R.M., Samuels B. et al. Scrotal thermography. *Radiology*, 1221, 129, 1979.

[35] Coznhaire F., Monteyne R., and Hunnen M. The value of scrotal thermography as compared with selective retrograde venography of the internal spermatic vein for the diagnosis of subclinical varicoceles. *Fertil. Steril.*, 27, 694, 1976.

22
Standard Procedures for Infrared Imaging in Medicine

22.1	Introduction...	22-1
22.2	Definition of Thermal Imaging	22-2
	Accuracy • Precision • Responsiveness	
22.3	Sources of Variability of Thermal Images	22-3
	Object or Subject • Camera Systems, Standards, and Calibration • Patient Position and Image Capture • Information Protocols and Resources • Image Processing • Image Analysis • Image Exchange • Image Presentation	
References		22-9

Kurt Ammer
Ludwig Boltzmann Research Institute for Physical Diagnostics and University of Glamorgan

Francis E. Ring
Glamorgan University

22.1 Introduction

Infrared thermal imaging has been used in medicine since the early 1960s. Working groups within the European Thermographic Association (now European Association of Thermology) produced the first publications on standardization of thermal imaging in 1978 [1] and 1979 [2]. However, Collins and Ring established already in 1974 a quantitative thermal index [3], which was modified in Germany by J.-M. Engel in 1978 [4]. Both indices opened the field of quantitative evaluation of medical thermography.

Further recommendations for standardization appeared in 1983 [5] and 1984, the later related to essential techniques for the use of thermography in clinical drug trials [6]. J.-M. Engel published a booklet entitled "Standardized thermographic investigations in rheumatology and guideline for evaluation" in 1984 [7]. The author presented his ideas for standardization of image recording and assessment including some normal values for wrist, knee, and ankle joints. Engel's measurements of knee temperatures were first published in 1978 [4]. Normal temperature values of the lateral elbow, dorsal hands, anterior knee, lateral and medial malleolus and the 1st metatarsal joint were published by Collins in 1976 [8].

The American Academy of Thermology published technical guidelines in 1986 including some recommendations for thermographic examinations [9]. However, the American authors concentrated on determining the symmetry of temperature distribution rather than the normal temperature values of particular body regions. Uematsu in 1985 [10] and Goodman in 1986 [11] published the side to side variations of surface temperatures of the human body. These symmetry data were confirmed by E.F. Ring for the lower leg in 1986 [12].

In Japan, medical thermal imaging has been an accepted diagnostic procedure since 1981 [13]. Recommendations for the analysis of neuromuscular thermograms were published by Fujimasa et al. in 1986 [14]. Five years later more detailed proposals for the thermal image based analysis of physiological functions were published in *Biomedical Thermology* [15], the official journal of the Japanese Society of thermology. This paper was the result of a workshop on clinical thermography criteria.

Recently, the thermography societies in Korea have published a book, which summarizes in 270 pages general standards for imaging recording and interpretation of thermal images in various diseases [16].

As the relationship between skin blood flow and body surface temperature has been obvious from the initial use of thermal imaging in medicine, quantitative assessments were developed at an early stage. E.F. Ring developed a thermographic index for the assessment of ischemia in 1980, that was originally used for patients suffering from Raynauds' disease [17]. The European Association of Thermology published a statement in 1988 on the subject of Raynaud's Phenomenon [18]. Normal values for recovering after a cold challenge have been published since 1976 [19,20]. A range of temperatures were applied in this thermal challenge test, the technique was reviewed by E.F. Ring in 1997 [21].

An overview of recommendations gathered from, The Japanese Society of Biomedical Thermology and the European Association of Thermology was collated and published by Clark and Goff in 1997 [22]. This paper is based on the practical implications of the foregoing papers taken from the perspective of the modern thermal imaging systems available to medicine.

Finally, a project at the University of Glamorgan, aims to create an atlas of normal thermal images of healthy subjects [23]. This study, started in 2001, has generated a number of questions related to the influence of body positions on accuracy and precision of measurements from thermal images [24,25].

22.2 Definition of Thermal Imaging

Thermal imaging is regarded as a technique for temperature measurements based on the infrared radiation from objects. Unlike images created by x-rays or proton activation through magnetic resonance, thermal imaging is not related to morphology. The technique provides only a map of the distribution of temperatures on the surface of the object imaged.

Whenever infrared thermal imaging is considered as a method for measurement, the technique must meet all criteria of a measurement. The most basic features of measurement are accuracy (in the medical field also named validity) and precision (in medicine reliability). Anbar [26] has listed five other terms related to the precision of infrared based temperature measurements. When used as an outcome measure, responsiveness or sensitivity to change is an important characteristic.

22.2.1 Accuracy

Measurements are basic procedures of comparison namely to compare a standardized meter with an object to be measured. Any measurement is prone to error, thus a perfect measurement is impossible. However, the smaller the variation of a particular measurement from the standardized meter, the higher is the accuracy of the measurement or in other words, an accurate measurement is as close as possible to the true value of measurement. In medicine, accuracy is often named validity, mainly caused by the fact, that medical measurements are not often performed by the simple comparison of meter and object. For example, assessments from various features of a human being may be combined into a new construct, resulting in a innovative measurement of health.

22.2.2 Precision

A series of measurements can not achieve totally identical results. The smaller the variation between single results, the higher is the precision or repeatability (reliability) of the measurement. However, reliability without accuracy, is useless. For example, a sports archer who always hits the same peripheral sector of

TABLE 22.1 Conditions Affecting, Accuracy, Precision, and Responsiveness of Temperature Measures

Condition affecting	Accuracy	Precision	Responsiveness
Object or subject	X	X	X
Camera systems, standards, and calibration	X	X	X
Patient position and image capture		X	X
Information protocols and resources		X	X
Image analysis	X	X	X
Image exchange	X	X	X
Image presentation	X	X	X

the target, has very high reliability, but no validity, because such an athlete must find the centre of the target to be regarded as accurate.

22.2.3 Responsiveness

Both, accuracy and precision, have an impact on the sensitivity to change of outcome measures. Validity is needed to define correctly the symptom to be measured. Precision will affect the responsiveness also, because a change of the symptom can only be detected if this change is bigger than the variation of repeated measurements.

22.3 Sources of Variability of Thermal Images

Table 22.1 shows conditions in thermal imaging that may affect accuracy, precision, and responsiveness.

22.3.1 Object or Subject

As the emittance of infrared radiation is the source of remote temperature measurements, knowledge of the emissivity of the object is essential for the calculation of temperature related to the radiant heat. In non living objects emissivity is mainly a function of the texture of the surface.

Seventy years ago, Hardy [27] showed that the human skin acts like an almost perfect black body radiator with an emissivity of 0.98. Studies from Togawa in Japan have demonstrated that the emissivity of the skin is unevenly distributed [28]. In addition, infrared reflection from the environment and substances applied on the skin may also alter the emissivity [29–31]. Water is an efficient filter for infrared rays and can be bound to the superficial corneal layer of the skin during immersion for at least 15 min [32,33] or in the case of severe edema [34]. This can affect the emissivity of the skin.

The hair coat of animal may show a different emissivity than the skin after clipping the hair [35]. Variation in the distribution of the hairy coat will influence the emissivity of the animal's surface [36]. Variation in emissivity will influence the accuracy of temperature measurements.

Homeothermic beings, maintain their deep body (core) temperature through variation of the surface (shell) temperature, and show a circadian rhythm of both the core and shell temperature [37–40]. Repeated temperature registrations not performed at the same time of the day will therefore affect the precision of these measurements.

22.3.2 Camera Systems, Standards, and Calibration

22.3.2.1 The Imaging System

A new generation of infra red cameras have become available for medical imaging. The older systems normally single element detectors using an optical mechanical scanning process, were mostly cooled by the addition of liquid nitrogen [41–43]. However, adding nitrogen to the system, affects the stability of temperature measurements for a period up to 60 min [44]. Nitrogen cooled scanners had the effect of limiting the angle at which the camera could be used which restricted operation.

Electronic cooling systems were then introduced, which provided the use of image capturing without restrictions of the angle between the object and the camera. The latest generation of focal plane array cameras can be used without cooling, providing almost maintenance free technology [45]. However, repeated calibration procedures built inside the camera can affect the stability of temperature measurements [46].

The infrared wavelength, recorded by the camera, will not affect the temperature readings as long as the algoritm of calculation temperature from emitted radiation is correct. However, systems equipped with sensors sensitive in different bands of the infrared spectrum are capable to determine the emissivity of objects [47].

22.3.2.2 Temperature Reference

Earlier reports stipulate the requirement for a separate thermal reference source for calibration checks on the camera [9,48,49]. Many systems now include an internal reference temperature, with manufacturers claiming that external checks are not required. Unless frequent servicing is obtained, it is still advisable to use an external source, if only to check for drift in the temperature sensitivity of the camera. An external reference, which may be purchased or constructed, can be left switched on throughout the day. This allows the operator to make checks on the camera, and in particular provides a check on the hardware and software employed for processing. These constant temperature source checks may be the only satisfactory way of proving the reliability of temperature measurements made from the thermogram [48]. Linearity of temperature measurements which may be questionable in focal plane array equipment, can be checked with two ore more external temperature references. New low cost reference sources, based on the triple point of particular chemicals, are currently under construction in the United Kingdom [44].

22.3.2.3 Mounting the Imager

A camera stand which provides vertical height adjustment is very important for medical thermography. Photographic tripod stands are inconvenient for frequent adjustment and often result in tilting the camera at an undefined angle to the patient. This is difficult to reproduce, and unless the patient is positioned so that the surface scanned is aligned at 90° to the camera lens, distortion of the image is unavoidable. Undefined angles of the camera view affects the precision of measurements.

In the case of temperature measurements from a curved surface, the angle between the radiating object and the capturing device may be the critical source of false measurements [50–52]. At an angle of view beyond 30° small losses of capturing the full band of radiation start to occur, at an angel of 60° the loss of information becomes critically and is followed by false temperature readings. The determination of the temperature of the same forefoot in different views shows clearly, that consideration of the angel of the viewing is a significant task [53]. Unless corrected, thermal images of of evenly curved objects lack accuracy of temperature measurements [54].

Studio camera stands are ideal, they provide vertical height adjustment with counterbalance weight compensation. It should be noted that the type of lens used on the camera will affect the working distance and the field of view, a wide angle lens reduces distance between the camera and the subject in many cases, but may also increase peripheral distortion of the image [55].

22.3.2.4 Camera Initialization

Start up time with modern cameras are claimed to be very short, minutes or seconds. However, the speed with which the image becomes visible is not an indication of image stability. Checks on calibration will usually show that a much longer period from 10 min to several hours with an uncooled system are needed to achieve stable conditions for temperature readings from infrared images [5,46].

22.3.3 Patient Position and Image Capture

Standardized positions of the body for image capture and clearly defined fields of view can reduce systematic errors and increases both accuracy and precision of temperature readings from thermal images recorded in such a manner. In radiography, standardized positions of the body for image capture have been included in the protocol for quality assurance for a long time. Although thermal imaging does not provide much anatomical information compared to other imaging techniques, variation of body positions and the related fields of view affects the precision of temperature readings from thermograms. However, the intra- and inter-rater repeatability of temperature values from the same thermal image was found to be excellent [56].

22.3.3.1 Location for Thermal Imaging

The size of investigation room does not influence the quality of temperature measurements from thermal images, unless the least distance in one direction is not shorter than the distance between the camera and an object of 1.2 m height [57]. Such a condition will result in thermal images out of focus. Other important features of the examination room are thermal insulation and prevention of any direct or reflected infrared radiation sources. Following this proposal will result in an increase of accuracy and precisison of measurements.

22.3.3.2 Ambient Temperature Control

This is a primary requirement for most clinical applications of thermal imaging. A range of temperatures from 18 to 25°C should be attainable and held for at least 1 h to better than 1°C. Due to the nature of human thermoregulation, stability of the room temperature is a critical feature. It have been shown, that subjects acclimatized for 40–60 min to a room temperature of 22°C showed differences in surface temperature at various measuring sites of the face after lowering the ambient temperature by 2°C [58]. While the nose cooled on average by 4°C, the forehead and the meatus decreased the surface temperature by only by 0.4–0.45%. Similar changes may occur at other acral sites such as tips of fingers or toes, as both regions are highly involved in heat exchange for temperature regulation.

At lower temperatures, the subject is likely to shiver, and over 25°C room temperature will cause sweating, at least in most European countries. Variations may be expected in colder or warmer climates, in the latter case, room temperatures may need to be 1°C to 2°C higher [59].

Additonal techniques for cooling particular regions of the body have been developed [60,61]. Immersion of the hands in water at various tempeatures is a common challenge for the assessment of vasospastic disease [21].

Heat generated in the investigation room affects the room temperature. Possible heat sources are electronic equipment such as the scanner and its computer, but also human bodies. For this reason the air-conditioning unit should be capable of compensating for the maximum number of patients and staff likely to be in the room at any one time. These effects will be greater in a small room of 2×3 m or less.

Air convection is a very effective method of skin cooling and related to the wind speed. Therefore, air conditioning equipment should be located so that direct draughts are not directed at the patient, and that overall air speed is kept as low as possible. A suspended perforated ceiling with ducts diffusing the air distribution evenly over the room is ideal [62].

A cubicle or cubicles within the temperature controlled area is essential. These should provide privacy for disrobing and a suitable area for resting through the acclimatization period.

22.3.3.3 Pre-Imaging Equilibration

On arrival at the department, the patient should be informed of the examination procedure, instructed to remove appropriate clothing and jewellery, and asked to sit or rest in the preparation cubicle for a fixed time. The time required to achieve adequate stability in blood pressure and skin temperature is generally considered to be 15 min, with 10 min as a minimum [63–65]. After 30 min cooling, oszillations of the skin temperature can be detected, in different regions of the body with different amplitudes resulting in a temperature asymmetry between left and right sides [64].

Contact of body parts with the environment or with other body parts alters the surface temperature due to heat transfer by conduction. Therefore, during the preparation time the patient must avoid folding or crossing arms and legs, or placing bare feet on a cold surface. If the lower extremities are to be examined, a stool or leg rest should be provided to avoid direct contact with the floor [66]. If these requirements are not met, poor precision of measurements may result.

22.3.3.4 Positions for Imaging

As in anatomical imaging studies, it is preferable to standardize on a series of standard views for each body region. The EAT Locomotor Diseases Group recommendations include a triangular marker system to indicate anterior, posterior, lateral, and angled views [2,67]. However, reproduction of positions for angled views may be difficult, even when aids such as rotating platforms are used [68].

Modern image processing software provide comment boxes which can be used to encode the angle of view which will be stored with the image [69]. It should be noted that the position of the patient for scanning and in preparation must be constant. Standing, sitting, or lying down affect the surface area of the body exposed to the ambient, therefore an image recorded with the patient in a sitting position may not be comparable with one recorded on a separate occasion in a standing position. In addition, blood flow against the influence of gravity contributes to the skin temperature of fingers in various limb positions [70].

22.3.3.5 Field of View

Image size is dependent on the distance between the camera and the patient and the focal length of the infrared camera lens. The lens is generally fixed on most medical systems, so it is good practice to maintain a constant distance from the patient for each view, in order to acquire a reproducible field of view for the image. If in different thermograms different fields of the same subject are compared, the variable resolution can lead to false temperature readings [71]. However, maintaining the same distance between object and camera, cannot compensate for individual body dimensions, for example, big subjects will have big knees and therefore maintaining the same distance as for a tiny subjects knee is not applicable.

To overcome this problem, the field of view has been defined in the standard protocol at the University of Glamorgan in a twofold way, that is, body position and alignment of anatomical landmarks to the edge of the image [23]. These definitions enabled us to investigate the reproducibilty of body views using the distance in pixels between anatomical landmarks and the outline of the infrared images [24–72].

Figure 22.1 gives examples of the views, that have been investigated for the reproduciblity of body positions. Table 22.2 shows the mean value, standard deviation, and 95% confidence interval of the variation of body views of the upper and the lower part of the human body. Variations in views of the lower part of the body were bigger than in views of the upper part. The highest degree of variation was found in the view "Both Ankles Anterior," but the smallest variation in the view "Face."

22.3.4 Information Protocols and Resources

Human skin temperature is the product of heat dissipated from the vessels and organs within the body, and the effect of the environmental factors on heat loss or gain. There are a number of further influences which are controllable, such as cosmetics [29], alcohol intake [73–75], and smoking [76–78]. In general terms the patient attending for examination should be advised to avoid all topical applications such as ointments and cosmetics on the day of examination to all the relevant areas of the body [31,47,79,80]. Large meals and above average intake of tea or coffee should also be excluded, although studies supporting this recommendation are hard to find and the results are not conclusive [81,82].

Patients should be asked to avoid tight fitting clothing, and to keep physical exertion to a minimum. This particularly applies to methods of physiotherapy such as electrotherapy [83,85], ultrasound [86,87], heat treatment [88,90], cryotherapy [91–94], massage [95–97], and hydrotherapy [31,32,98,99], because thermal effects from such treatment can last for 4 to 6 h under certain conditions. Heat production by muscular exercise is a well documented phenomenon [65,100–103].

Standard Procedures for Infrared Imaging in Medicine

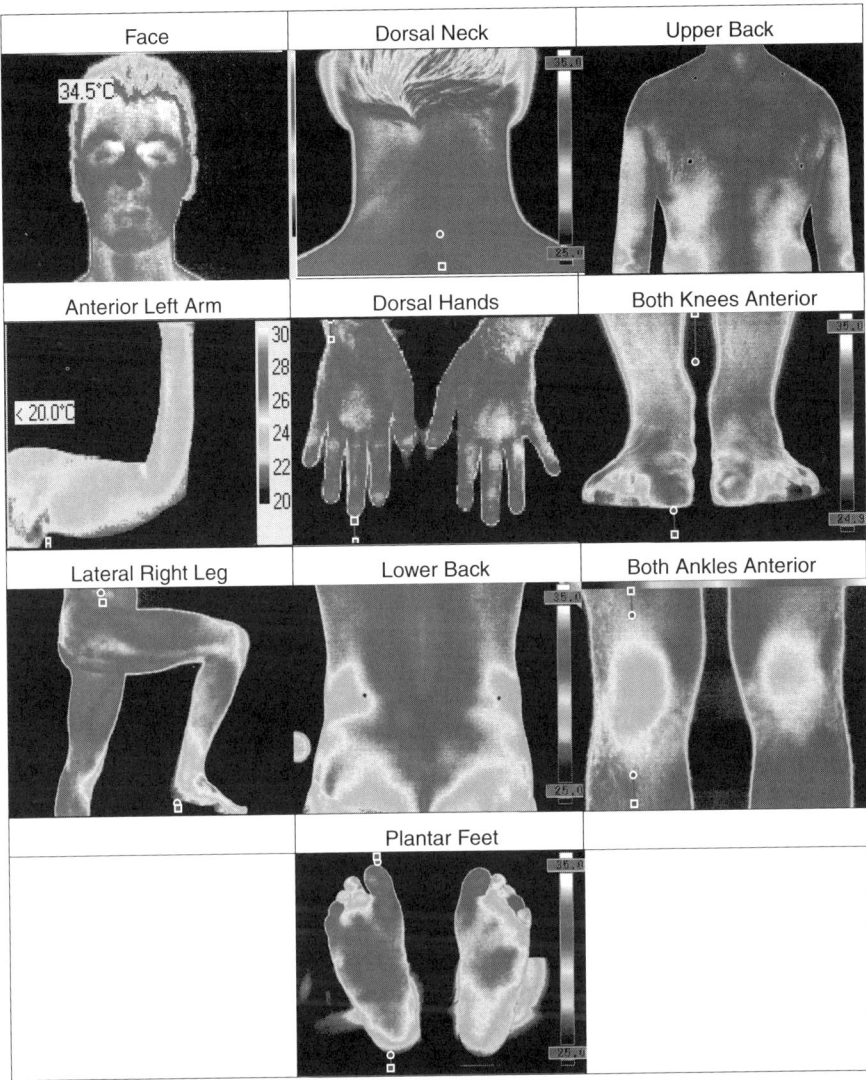

FIGURE 22.1 (See color insert at the back of the book.) Body views investigated.

TABLE 22.2 Variation of Positions of All the Investigated Views

View	Upper edge (pixel) mean ± SD (95% CI)	Lower edge (pixel) mean ± SD (95% CI)	Left side edge (pixel) mean ± SD (95% CI)
Face	0.5 ± 5.3 (−2.2 to 1.9)	4.0 ± 10.9 (−0.03 to 8.2)	
Dorsal neck	−8.4 ± 36.4 (−18.3 to 1.6)	122.6 ± 146.6 (82.6 to 162.6)	
Upper back	4.5 ± 9.9 (0.8 to 8.2)	28.1 ± 22.0 (19.9 to 36.4)	
Anterior left arm	22.4 ± 33.0 (8.7 to 36.0)	15.8 ± 15.4 (9.5 to 22.2)	12.5 ± 16.0 (5.9 to 19.1)
Dorsal hands	41.8 ± 17.8 (35.5 to 48.2)	33.2 ± 22.3 (25.3 to 41.5)	
Both knees anterior	80.7 ± 47.3 (60.7 to 100.7)	84.3 ± 37.0 (68.6 to 99.9)	
Lateral right leg	16.7 ± 21.0 (5.9 to 27.5)	17.2 ± 15.8 (9.0 to 25.3)	
Lower back	17.1 ± 4.2 (8.6 to 25.6)	16.3 ± 4.6 (16.3 to 34.9)	
Both ankles anterior	158.8 ± 12.2 (133.6 to 184.1)	54.9 ± 9.1 (36.1 to 37.8)	
Plantar feet	31.0 ± 24.1 (23.2 to 38.7)	25.7 ± 23.1 (18.3 to 33.1)	

Drug treatment can also affect the skin temperature. This phenomenon was used to evaluate the therapeutic effects of medicaments [6]. Drugs affecting the cardiovascular system must be reported to the thermographer, in order that the correct interpretation of thermal images will be given [104–107].

Omiting just one of the above mentioned conditions will result in reduced precision of temperature measurements.

22.3.5 Image Processing

Every image or block of images must carry the indication of temperature range, with color code/temperature scale. The color scale itself should be standardized. Industrial software frequently provides a grey-scale picture and one or more color scales. However, modern image processing software permits to squeeze the color scale in already recorded images in order to increase the image contrast. Such a procedure will affect the temperature readings from thermal images as temperatures outside of the compressed temperature scale will not be included in the statistics of selected regions of interest. This will result in erroneous temperature readings, affecting both accuracy and precision of measurements.

22.3.6 Image Analysis

Almost all systems now use image processing techniques and provide basic quantitation of the image [108–110]. In some cases this may be operated from a chip within the camera, of may be carried out through an on- or off-line computer. For older equipment like the AGA 680 series several hardware adaptations have been reported to achieve quantitation of the thermograms [111–113].

It has to be emphasized that false color coding of infrared images does not provide means for temperature measurement. If colors are separated by a temperature distance of $1°C$, the temperature difference between two points situated in adjacent colors may be between $0.1°C$ and $1.9°C$. It is obvious, that false colored images provide at its best an estimation of temperature, but not a measurement. The same is true for liquid crystal thermograms.

Nowadays, temperature measurements in thermal images are based on the definition of regions of interest (ROI). However, standards for shape, size and placement of these regions are not available or incomplete. Although a close correlation exists for ROI of different size in the same region [114], the precision of measurement is affected when ROIS of different size and location are used for repeated measurements.

The Glamorgan protocol [23] is the very first attempt to create a complete standard for the definition of regions of interest in thermal images based on anatomical limits. Furthermore, in the view "both knee anterior" the shape with the highest reproducibility was investigated. During one of the Medical Infrared Training-Courses at the University of Glamorgan, three newly trained investigators defined on the same thermal image of both anterior knees twice the region of interest in the shape of a box, an ellipsoid or as an hour-glass shape. Similar to the result of a pilot study that compared these shapes for repeateabilty, the highest reliability was found for temperature readings from the hour-glass shape, followed by readings from ellipsoids and boxes [53]. The repeatabilty of the regions on the view "Left Anterior Arm," "Both Ankles Anterior," "Dorsal Feet," and "Plantar Feet" were also investigated and resulted in reliabilty coefficients between 0.7 (right ankle) and 0.93 (forearm). The intraclass correlation coefficients ranged between 0.48 (upper arm) and 0.87 (forearm). Applying the Glamorgan protocol consequently, will result in precise temperature measurements from thermal images.

22.3.7 Image Exchange

Most of the modern infrared systems store the recorded thermal images in an own image format, which may not compatible with formats of thermal images from other manufacturers. However, most of this images can be transformed into established image formats such as TIF, JPEG, GIF, and others. As a thermal image is the pictographic representation of a temperature map, the sole image is not enough unless the related temperature information is not provided. Consequently, temperature measurements from standard computer images derived from thermograms is not possible.

Providing both temperature scale and a scale of grey shades, allows the exchange of thermal images over long distance and between different, but compatible image processing software [115]. The grey scale must be derived from the original grey shade thermal image. If it has been transformed from a false color image, the resulted black-and-white thermogram may not be representative for the original grey scale gradient as the grey scale of individual colors may deviate from the particular grey shade of the image. This can then result in false temperature readings.

22.3.8 Image Presentation

Image presentation does not influence the result of measurements from thermal images. However, if thermograms are read by eyes, their appearance will affect the credibility of the information in thermal images. This is for instance the case, when thermal images are use as evidence in legal trials [116].

It was stated, that for forensic acceptability of thermography standardization and repeatability of the technique are very important features [117]. This supports the necessity of quantitative evaluation of thermal images and standards strictly applied to the technique of infrared imaging will finally result in high accuracy and precision of this method of temperature measurement. At that stage it can be recommended as responsive outcome measure for clinical trials in rheumatology [6,8], angiopathies [107,118], neuromuscular disorders [119], surgery [120], and paedriatrics [121].

References

[1] Aarts, N.J.M. et al. Thermograp. terminology. *Acta Thermograp.*, 1978, Suppl. 2.
[2] Engel, J.M. et al. Thermography in locomotor diseases—recommended procedure. *Eur. J. Rheum. Inflamm.*, 2, 299, 1979.
[3] Collins, A.J. et al. Quantitation of thermography in arthritis using multi-isothermal analysis. *Ann. Rheum. Dis.*, 33, 113, 1974.
[4] Engel, J.-M. Quantitative Thermographie des Kniegelenks. *Z. Rheumatol.*, 37, 242, 1978.
[5] Ring, E.F.J. Standardisation of thermal imaging in medicine: physical and environmental factors, in *Thermal Assessment of Breast Health*, Gautherie, M., Albert, E., and Keith, L., Eds., MTP Press Ltd, Lancaster/Boston/The Hague, 1983, p. 29.
[6] Ring, E.F.J., Engel, J.M., and Page-Thomas, D.P. Thermologic methods in clinical pharmacology—skin temperature measurement in drug trials. *Int. J. Clin. Pharm. Ther. Tox.*, 22, 20, 1984.
[7] Engel, J.-M. and Saier, U. *Thermographische Standarduntersuchungen in der Rheumatologie und Richtlinien zu deren Befundung.* Luitpold, München, 1984.
[8] Collins, A.J. Anti-inflammatory drug assessment by the thermographic index. *Acta Thermograp.*, 1, 73, 1976.
[9] Pochaczevsky, R. et al. *Technical Guidelines*, 2nd ed. *Thermology*, 2, 108, 1986.
[10] Uematsu, S. Symmetry of skin temperatures comparing one side of the body to the other. *Thermology*, 1, 4, 1985.
[11] Goodman, P.H. et al. Normal temperature asymmetry of the back and extremities by computer-assisted infrared imaging. *Thermology*, 1, 195, 1986.
[12] Bliss, P. et al. Investigation of nerve root irritation by infrared thermography, in *Back Pain—Methods for Clinical Investigation and Assessment*, Hukins, D.W.L. and Mulholland, R.C., Eds., University Press, Manchester, 1986, p. 63.
[13] Atsumi, K. High technology applications of medical thermography in Japan. *Thermology*, 1, 79–80, 1985.
[14] Fujimasa, I. et al. A new computer image processing system for the analysis of neuromuscular thermograms: a feasibility study. *Thermology*, 1, 221, 1986.

[15] Fujimasa, I. A proposal for thermographic imaging diagnostic procedures for temperature related physiologic function analysis. *Biomed. Thermol.*, 11, 269, 1991.
[16] Lee, D.-I. (Ed.) *Practical Manual of Clinical Thermology*, ISBN 89-954013-04.
[17] Ring, E.F.J. A thermographic index for the assessment of ischemia. *Acta thermograp.*, 5, 35, 1980.
[18] Aarts, N. P. et al. Raynaud's phenomenon: assessment by thermography. *Thermology*, 3, 69, 1988.
[19] Acciarri, L., Carnevale, F., and Della Selva, A. Thermography in the hand angiopathy from vibrating tools. *Acta thermograp.*, 1, 18, 1976.
[20] Ring, E.F. and Bacon, P.A. Quantitative thermographic assessment of inositol nicotinate therapy in Raynaud's phenomena. *J. Int. Med. Res.*, 5, 217, 1977.
[21] Ring, E.F.J. Cold stress test for the hands, in *The Thermal Image in Medicine and Biology*, Ammer, K. and Ring, E.F.J., Eds., Uhlen-Verlag, Wien, 1995, p. 237.
[22] Clark, R.P. and de Calcina-Goff, M. Guidelines for standardisation in medical thermography draft international standard proposals. *Thermol. Osterr.*, 7, 47, 1997.
[23] Website address, Atlas of Normals, www.medimaging.org.
[24] Ammer, K. et al. Rationale for standardised capture and analysis of infrared thermal images, in *Proceedings Part II, EMBEC'02 2.European Medical & Biological Engineering Conference.* Hutten, H. and Krösel, P., Eds. IFMBE, Graz, 2002, p. 1608.
[25] Ring, E.F.J. et al. Errors and artefacts in thermal imaging, in *Proceedings Part II, EMBEC'02 2.European Medical & Biological Engineering Conference.* Hutten, H. and Krösel, P., Eds., IFMBE, Graz, 2002, p. 1620.
[26] Anbar, M. Recent technological developments in thermology and their impact on clinical applications. *Biomed. Thermol.*, 10, 270, 1990.
[27] Hardy, J.D. The radiation of heat from the human body. III. The human skin as a black body radiator. *J. Clin. Invest.*, 13, 615, 1934.
[28] Togawa, T. and Saito, H. Non-contact imaging of thermal properties of the skin. *Physiol. Meas.*, 15, 291, 1994.
[29] Engel, J.-M. Physical and physiological influence of medical ointments of infrared thermography, in *Recent Advances in Medical Thermology*, Ring, E.F.J. and Phillips, B., Eds., Plenum Press, New York, 1984, p. 177.
[30] Hejazi, S. and Anbar, M. Effects of topical skin treatment and of ambient light in infrared thermal images. *Biomed. Thermol.*, 12, 300, 1992.
[31] Ammer, K. The influence of antirheumatic creams and ointments on the infrared emission of the skin, in *Abstracts of the 10th International Conference on Thermogrammetry and Thermal Engineering in Budapest 18–20, June 1997*, Benkö, I. et al., Eds., MATE, Budapest, 1997, p. 177.
[32] Ammer, K. Einfluss von Badezusätzen auf die Wärmeabstrahlung der Haut. *ThermoMed*, 10, 71, 1994.
[33] Ammer, K. The influence of bathing on the infrared emission of the skin, in *Abstracts of the 9th International Conference on Thermogrammetry and Thermal Engineering in Budapest 14–16, June 1995*, Benkö, I., Lovak., and Kovacsics, I., Eds., MATE, Budapest, 1995, p. 115.
[34] Ammer, K. Thermographie in lymphedema, in *Advanced Techniques and Clinical Application in Biomedical Thermologie*, Mabuchi, K., Mizushina, S., and Harrison, B., Eds., Harwood Academic Publishers, Chur/Schweiz, 1994, p. 213.
[35] Heath, A.M. et al. A comparison of surface and rectal temperatures between sheared and non-sheared alpacas (*Lama pacos*). *Small Rumin. Res.*, 39, 19, 2001.
[36] Purohit, R.C. et al. Thermographic evaluation of animal skin surface temperature with and without haircoat. *Thermol. Int.*, 11, 83, 2001.
[37] Damm, F., Döring, G., and Hildebrandt, G. Untersuchungen über den Tagesgang von Hautdurchblutung und Hauttemperatur unter besonderer Berücksichtigung der physikalischen Temperaturregulation. *Z. Physik. Med. Rehabil.*, 15, 1, 1974.
[38] Reinberg, A. Circadian changes in the temperature of human beings. *Bibl. Radiol.*, 6, 128, 1975.

[39] Schmidt, K.-L., Mäurer, R., and Rusch, D. Zur Wirkung örtlicher Wärme und Kälteanwendungen auf die Hauttemperatur am Kniegelenk. *Z. Rheumatol.*, 38, 213, 1979.
[40] Kanamori, T. et al. Circadian rhythm of body temperature. *Biomed. Thermol.*, 11, 292, 1991.
[41] Friedrich, K.H. Assessment criteria for infrared thermography systems. *Acta thermograp.*, 5, 68, 1980.
[42] Alderson, J.K.A. and Ring, E.F.J. "Sprite" high resolution thermal imaging system. *Thermology*, 1, 110, 1985.
[43] Dibley, D.A.G. Opto-mechanical systems for thermal imaging, in *The Thermal Image in Medicine and Biology*, Ammer, K., and Ring, E.F.J., Eds., Uhlen-Verlag, Wien, 1995, p. 33.
[44] Plassmann, P. Advances in image processing for thermology, *Presented at Int. Cong. of Thermology*, Seoul, June 5–6, 2004, p. 3.
[45] Kutas, M. Staring focal plane array for medical thermal imaging, in *The Thermal Image in Medicine and Biology*, Ammer, K., and Ring, E.F.J., Eds., Uhlen-Verlag, Wien, 1995, p. 40.
[46] Ring, E.F.J., Minchinton, M., and Elvins, D.M. A focal plane array system for clinical infrared imaging. *IEEE/EMBS Proceedings*, Atlanta 1999, p. 1120.
[47] Hejazi, S. and Spangler, R.A. A multi-wavelength thermal imaging system, in *Proc. 11th Annual Int. Conf. IEEE Engineering in Medicine and Biology Society*, II, 1989, p. 1153.
[48] Ring, E.F.J. Quality control in infrared thermography, in *Recent Advances in Medical Thermology*, Ring, E.F.J. and Phillips, B., Eds., Plenum Press, New York, 1984, p. 185.
[49] Clark, R.P. et al. Thermography and pedobarography in the assessment of tissue damage in neuropathicand atherosclerotic feet. *Thermology*, 3, 15, 1988.
[50] Clark, J.A. Effects of surface emissivity and viewing angle errors in thermography. *Acta thermograp.*, 1, 138, 1976.
[51] Steketee, J. Physical aspects of infrared thermography, in *Recent Advances in Medical Thermology*, Ring, E.F.J. and Phillips, B., Eds., Plenum Press, New York, 1984, p. 167.
[52] Wiecek, B., Jung, A., and Zuber, J. Emissivity-Bottleneck and Challenge for thermography. *Thermol. Int.*, 10, 15, 2000.
[53] Ammer K. Need for standardisation of measurements, in *Thermal Imaging in Thermography and Lasers in Medicine*, Wiecek, B., Ed., Akademickie Centrum Graficzno-Marketigowe Lodart S.A, Lodz, 2003, p. 13.
[54] Anbar, M. Potential artifacts in infrared thermographic measurements. *Thermology*, 3, 273, 1991.
[55] Ring, E.F.J. and Dicks, J.M. Spatial resolution of new thermal imaging systems, *Thermol. Int.*, 9, 7, 1999.
[56] Melnizky, P., Schartelmüller, T., and Ammer, K. Prüfung der intra-und interindividuellen Verlässlichkeit der Auswertung von Infrarot-Thermogrammen. *Eur. J. Thermol.*, 7, 224, 1997.
[57] Ring, E.F.J. and Ammer, K. The technique of thermal imaging in medicine. *Thermol. Int.*, 10, 7, 2000.
[58] Khallaf, A. et al. Thermographic study of heat loss from the face. *Thermol. Österr.*, 4, 49, 1994.
[59] Ishigaki, T. et al. Forehead–back thermal ratio for the interpretation of infrared imaging of spinal cord lesions and other neurological disorders. *Thermology*, 3, 101, 1989.
[60] Schuber, T.R. et al. Directed dynamic cooling,a methodic contribution in telethermography. *Acta thermograp.*, 1, 94, 1977.
[61] Di Carlo, A. Thermography in patients with systemic sclerosis. *Thermol. Österr.*, 4, 18, 1994.
[62] Love, T.J. Heat transfer considerations in the design of a thermology clinic. *Thermology*, 1, 88, 1985.
[63] Ring, E.F.J. Computerized thermography for osteo-articular diseases. *Acta thermograp.*, 1, 166, 1976.
[64] Roberts, D.L. and Goodman, P.H. Dynamic thermoregulation of back and upper extremity by computer-aided infrared imaging. *Thermology*, 2, 573, 1987.

[65] Mabuchi, K. et al. Development of a data processing system for a high-speed thermographic camera and its use in analyses of dynamic thermal phenomena of the living body, in *The Thermal Image in Medicine and Biology*, Ammer, K., and Ring, E.F.J., Eds., Uhlen-Verlag, Wien, 1995, p. 56.

[66] Cena, K. Environmental heat loss, in *Recent Advances in Medical Thermology*, Ring, E.F.J. and Phillips, B., Eds., Plenum Press, New York, 1984, p. 81.

[67] Engel, J.-M. Kennzeichnung von Thermogrammen, in *Thermologische Messmethodik*, Engel, J.-M., Flesch, U., and Stüttgen, G., Eds., Notamed, Baden–Baden, 1983, p. 176.

[68] Park, J.-Y. Current development of medical infrared imaging technology, *Presented at Int. Congr. of Thermology*, Seoul, June 5–6, 2004, p. 9.

[69] Plassmann, P. and Ring, E.F.J. An open system for the acquisition and evaluation of medical thermological images. *Eur. J. Thermol.* 7, 216, 1997.

[70] Abramson, D.I. et al. Effect of altering limb position on blood flow, O_2 uptake and skin temperature. *J. Appl. Physiol.*, 17, 191, 1962.

[71] Schartelmüller, T. and Ammer, K. Räumliche Auflösung von Infrarotkameras. *Thermol. Österr.*, 5, 28, 1995.

[72] Ammer, K. Update in standardization and temperature measurement from thermal images, *Presented at Int. Cong. of Thermology*, Seoul, June 5–6, 2004, p. 7.

[73] Mannara, G., Salvatori, G.C., and Pizzuti, G.P. Ethyl alcohol induced skin temperature changes evaluated by thermography. Preliminary results. *Boll. Soc. Ital. Biol. Sper.*, 69, 587, 1993.

[74] Melnizky, P. and Ammer, K. Einfluss von Alkohol und Rauchen auf die Hauttemperatur des Gesichts, der Hände und der Kniegelenke. *Thermol. Int.*, 10, 191, 2000.

[75] Ammer, K., Melnizky, P., and Rathkolb, O. Skin temperature after intake of sparkling wine, still wine or sparkling water. *Thermol. Int.*, 13, 99, 2003.

[76] Gershon-Cohen, J., Borden, A.G., and Hermel, M.B. Thermography of extremities after smoking. *Br. J. Radiol.*, 42, 189, 1969.

[77] Usuki, K. et al. Effects of nicotine on peripheral cutaneous blood flow and skin temperature. *J. Dermatol. Sci.*, 16, 173, 1998.

[78] Di Carlo, A. and Ippolito, F. Early effects of cigarette smoking in hypertensive and normotensive subjects. An ambulatory blood pressure and thermographic study. *Minerva Cardioangiol.*, 51, 387, 2003.

[79] Collins, A.J. et al. Some observations on the pharmacology of "deep-heat," a topical rubifacient. *Ann. Rheum. Dis.*, 43, 411, 1984.

[80] Ring, E.F. Cooling effects of Deep Freeze Cold gel applied to the skin, with and without rubbing, to the lumbar region of the back. *Thermol. Int.*, 14, 64, 2004.

[81] Federspil, G. et al. Study of diet-induced thermogenesis using telethermography in normal and obese subjects. *Recent Prog. Med.*, 80, 455, 1989.

[82] Shlygin, G.K. et al. Radiothermometric research of tissues during the initial reflex period of the specific dynamic action of food. *Med. Radiol. (Mosk)*, 36, 10, 1991.

[83] Danz, J. and Callies, R. Infrarothermometrie bei differenzierten Methoden der Niederfrequenztherapie. *Z. Physiother.*, 31, 35, 1979.

[84] Rusch, F., Neeck, G., and Schmidt, K.L. Über die Hemmung von Erythemen durch Capsaicin. 3.Objektivierung des Capsaicin-Erythems mittels statischer und dynamischer Thermographie, *Z. Phys. Med. Baln. Med. Klim.*, 17, 18, 1988.

[85] Mayr, H., Thür, H., and Ammer, K. Electrical stimulation of the stellate ganglia, in *The Thermal Image in Medicine and Biology*, Ammer, K., and Ring, E.F.J., Eds., Uhlen-Verlag, Wien, 1995, p. 206.

[86] Danz, J. and Callies R. Thermometrische Untersuchungen bei unterschiedlichen Ultraschallintensitäten. *Z. Physiother.*, 30, 235, 1978.

[87] Demmink, J.H., Helders, P.J., Hobaek, H., and Enwemeka, C. The variation of heating depth with therapeutic ultrasound frequency in physiotherapy. *Ultrasound Med. Biol.*, 29, 113–118, 2003.

[88] Rathkolb, O. and Ammer, K. Skin temperature of the fingers after different methods of heating using a wax bath. *Thermol Österr.*, 6, 125, 1996.

[89] Ammer, K. and Schartelmüller, T. Hauttemperatur nach der Anwendung von Wärmepackungen und nach Infrarot-A-Bestrahlung. *Thermol. Österr.*, 3, 51, 1993.

[90] Goodman, P.H., Foote, J.E., and Smith, R.P. Detection of intentionally produced thermal artifacts by repeated thermographic imaging. *Thermology*, 3, 253, 1991.

[91] Dachs, E., Schartelmüller, T., and Ammer, K. Temperatur zur Kryotherapie und Veränderungen der Hauttemperatur am Kniegelenk nach Kaltluftbehandlung. *Thermol. Österr.*, 1, 9, 1991.

[92] Rathkolb, O. et al. Hauttemperatur der Lendenregion nach Anwendung von Kältepackungen unterschiedlicher Größe und Applikationsdauer. *Thermol. Österr.*, 1, 15, 1991.

[93] Ammer, K. Occurrence of hyperthermia after ice massage. *Thermol. Österr.*, 6, 17, 1996.

[94] Cholewka, A. et al. Temperature effects of whole body cryotherapy determined by thermography. *Thermol. Int.*, 14, 57, 2004.

[95] Danz, J., Callies, R., and Hrdina, A. Einfluss einer abgestuften Vakuumsaugmassage auf die Hauttemperatur. *Z. Physiother.*, 33, 85, 1981.

[96] Eisenschenk, A. and Stoboy, H. Thermographische Kontrolle physikalisch-therapeutischer Methoden. *Krankengymnastik*, 37, 294, 1985.

[97] Kainz, A. Quantitative Überprüfung der Massagewirkung mit Hilfe der IR-Thermographie. *Thermol. Österr.*, 3, 79, 1993.

[98] Rusch, D. and Kisselbach, G. Comparative thermographic assessment of lower leg baths in medicinal mineral waters (Nauheim Springs), in *Recent Advances in Medical Thermology*, Ring, E.F.J. and Phillips, B., Eds., Plenum Press, New York, 1984, p. 535.

[99] Ring, E,F.J., Barker, J.R., and Harrison, R.A. Thermal effects of pool therapy on the lower limbs. *Thermology*, 3, 127, 1989.

[100] Konermann, H. and Koob, E. Infrarotthermographische Kontrolle der Effektivität krankengymnastischer Behandlungsmaßnahmen. *Krankengymnastik*, 27, 39, 1975.

[101] Smith, B.L., Bandler, M.K., and Goodman, P.H. Dominant forearm hyperthermia: a study of fifteen athletes. *Thermology*, 2, 25, 1986.

[102] Melnizky, P., Ammer, K., and Schartelmüller, T. Thermographische Überprüfung der Heilgymnastik bei Patienten mit Peroneusparese. *Thermol. Österr.*, 5, 97, 1995.

[103] Ammer, K. Low muscular acitivity of the lower leg in patients with a painful ankle. *Thermol. Österr.*, 5, 103, 1995.

[104] Ring, E.F., Porto, L.O., and Bacon, P.A. Quantitative thermal imaging to assess inositol nicotinate treatment for Raynaud's syndrome. *J. Int. Med. Res.*, 9, 393, 1981.

[105] Lecerof, et al. Acute effects of doxazosin and atenolol on smoking-induced peripheral vasoconstriction in hypertensive habitual smokers. *J. Hypertens.*, 8, S29, 1990.

[106] Tham, T.C., Silke, B., and Taylor, S.H. Comparison of central and peripheral haemodynamic effects of dilevalol and atenolol in essential hypertension. *J. Hum. Hypertens.*, 4, S77, 1990.

[107] Natsuda, H. et al. Nitroglycerin tape for Raynaud's phenomenon of rheumatic disease patients—an evaluation of skin temperature by thermography. *Ryumachi*, 34, 849, 1994.

[108] Engel, J.M. Thermotom- ein Softwarepaket für die thermographische Bildanalyse in der Rheumatologie, in *Thermologische Messmethodik*, Engel, J.-M., Flesch, U., and Stüttgen, G., Eds., Notamed, Baden–Baden, 1983, p. 110.

[109] Bösiger, P. and Scaroni, F. Mikroprozessor-unterstütztes Thermographie-System zur quantitativewn on-line Analyse von statischen und dynamischen Thermogrammen, in *Thermologische Messmethodik*, Engel, J.-M., Flesch, U., and Stüttgen, G., Eds., Notamed, Baden–Baden, 1983, p. 125.

[110] Brandes, P. PIC-Win-Iris Bildverarbeitungssoftware. *Thermol. Österr.*, 4, 33, 1994.

[111] Ring, E.F.J. Quantitative thermography in arthritis using the AGA integrator. *Acta thermograp.*, 2, 172, 1977.

[112] Parr, G. et al. Microcomputer standardization of the AGA 680 M system, in *Recent Advances in Medical Thermology*, Ring, E.F.J. and Phillips, B., Eds., Plenum Press, New York, 1984, pp. 211–214.

[113] Van Hamme, H., De Geest, G., and Cornelis, J. An acquisition and scan conversion unit for the AGA THV680 medical infrared camera. *Thermology*, 3, 205, 1990.

[114] Mayr, H. Korrelation durchschnittlicher und maximaler Temperatur am Kniegelenk bei Auswertung unterschiedlicher Messareale. *Thermol. Österr.*, 5, 89, 1995.

[115] Plassmann, P. On-line Communication for Thermography in Europe, *Presented at Int. Cong. of Thermology*, Seoul, June 5–6, 2004, p. 50.

[116] Ring, E.F.J. Thermal imaging in medico-legal claims. *Thermol. Int.*, 10, 97, 2000.

[117] Sella, G.E. Forensic criteria of acceptability of thermography. *Eur. J. Thermol.*, 7, 205, 1997.

[118] Hirschl, M. et al. Double-blind, randomised, placebo controlled low level laser therapy study in patients with primary Raynaud's phenomenon. *Vasa*, 31, 91, 2002.

[119] Schartelmüller, T., Melnizky, P., and Engelbert, B. Infrarotthermographie zur Evaluierung des Erfolges physikalischer Therapie bei Patienten mit klinischem Verdacht auf Thoracic Outlet Syndrome. *Thermol. Int.*, 9, 20, 1999.

[120] Kim, Y.S. and Cho, Y.E. Pre- and postoperative thermographic imaging in lumbar disc herniations, in *The Thermal Image in Medicine and Biology*, Ammer, K., and Ring, E.F.J., Eds., Uhlen-Verlag, Wien, 1995, p. 168.

[121] Siniewicz, K, et al. Thermal imaging before and after physial exercises in children with orthostatic disorders of the cardiovascular system. *Thermol. Int.*, 12, 139, 2002.

23

Storage and Retrieval of Medical Thermograms

23.1	Introduction	23-1
23.2	The Need for a Standardized Thermogram Format	23-2
23.3	Compression of Thermograms	23-3
	Image Dataset • Compression Algorithms • Compression Results	
23.4	Retrieval of Thermograms	23-6
	Content-Based Retrieval • Browsing of Thermal Image Database	
23.5	Conclusions	23-13
	Acknowledgments	23-14
	References	23-14

Gerald Schaefer
Aston University

Thermal medical images are recorded and saved in digital form. Yet often little thought is given on the format the data is stored. In this chapter we stress the need for a standardized format for storing medical infrared images. We then evaluate several algorithms that allow thermograms to be stored in compressed form, resulting in reduced utilization of resources such as disk space or bandwidth. While storage is usually solely done for archival and legal reasons we further introduce an approach that retrieves thermograms that are similar to a given image and that are hence also likely to be medically relevant. Finally, we introduce a system that allows to visually browse a whole database of thermal medical images.

23.1 Introduction

Advances in camera technologies and reduced equipment costs have led to an increased interest in the application of thermal imaging in the medical fields [6]. Thermograms are typically recorded and stored in digital form, and computerized image processing techniques have been used in acquiring and evaluating medical thermal images [12,24] and have proved to be important tools for clinical diagnostics. Yet these tools rely on the digital images to be in a certain format. Unfortunately, manufacturers of medical infrared cameras all have their own proprietary format, with little or no possibility of data interchange between suppliers. There is therefore a need to develop a standardized format for storing and processing thermograms. In the first part of this chapter we will argue that the Digital Imaging and Communications in Medicine (DICOM) medical imaging standard [11] can be adopted for this purpose.

Obviously, the more images are captured the more attention has to be put on necessary resources such as storage space and bandwidth. For example, the images for one person captured according to Reference 13, which suggests 27 standard views, requires, assuming a 12-bit thermal camera with 680×512 resolution, more than 13 MB of disk space. The application of compression methods is therefore often a necessary step to reduce these storage requirements. For images there are two kinds of compression methods: lossless compression, which preserves all of the original information, and lossy compression, which sacrifices some of the visual quality to gain in terms of compression rate. While approaches for lossy compression of medical infrared images have been presented [17,18] clinicians often prefer lossless algorithms to ensure no information is lost. Also, in some countries it is forbidden by law to lossy compress images used for medical diagnosis.

In the second part of the chapter we evaluate several "standard" lossless image compression algorithms for compressing medical infrared images. Lossless JPEG [9], JPEG-LS [4], JPEG2000 [5], PNG [26], and CALIC [25] are compared on an image set comprising more than 380 thermal images organized into 20 groups according to Reference 13.

Thermograms are typically stored for archival and legal purposes only and are not being retrieved again once a successful diagnosis has been made. In the final part of this chapter we show how these images of past cases can be used to aid in the diagnosis of new ones. Our approach is based on the concept of content-based image retrieval (CBIR) that has been an active research area in the image-processing areas for more than a decade [21]. The principal aim is to retrieve digital images based not on textual annotations but on features derived directly from image data. These features are then stored alongside the image and serve as an index. Retrieval is often performed in a query by example fashion where a query image is provided by the user. The retrieval system is then searching through all images in order to find those with the most similar indices that are returned as the candidates most alike to the query.

We consider the application of CBIR for thermal medical images as a generic approach for the analysis and interpretation of medical infrared images. CBIR allows the retrieval of visually similar and hence usually relevant images based on a predefined similarity measure between image features derived directly from the image data. In terms of medical infrared imaging, images that are visually similar to a given sample will also be likely to have medical relevance. These known cases together with their medical reports should then provide a valuable asset for diagnostic purposes.

Finally, we also introduce an approach that allows the browsing of whole databases of thermograms, again based on visual features. Utilizing a feature-dimension reduction method, all thermal images are shown on the computer screen so that images that are close by are also visually similar; this provides an alternative method of navigating through these image collections as opposed to standard methods that are restricted to searching by patient name or similar attributes.

The rest of this chapter is organized as follows. Section 23.2 stresses the need for a standard format for thermograms. Section 23.3 evaluates the performance of several compression algorithms on thermograms, both in terms of compression speed and in terms of compression ratio. Section 23.4 details our methods of applying CBIR techniques to the domain of thermal medical images and introduces a system of visually navigating collections of thermograms. Section 23.5 concludes the chapter.

23.2 The Need for a Standardized Thermogram Format

Various camera suppliers are competing for their share in the market of medical infrared imaging. Unfortunately, each of these also store the captured images in their own, proprietary file format. This fact makes it hard to impossible to share thermograms between users of different systems, despite the urgent need for this facility in the light of increase of telemedicine and other emerging technologies. Thermal imaging packages such as CTHERM [12] allow the capture from various types of cameras and store images in a simple common format, yet this approach is only a step toward a suitable solution.

What is needed is a recognized standard for storage and interchange of thermograms. Clearly this standard needs to be supported by suppliers of both cameras and software packages. Most importantly, such a standard must support the preservation of the original radiometric information. What this also means is that it must support a variety of spatial and radiometric resolutions, both of which vary from camera model to camera model. Apart from the storage of the actual image information in digital form, a useful standard format will provide various other properties. Patient identification and the addition of patient information as well as attaching information on the clinicians and treatments should be supported and so should the addition of other information items deemed useful for interpreting the thermogram.

Looking at other medical fields that deal with storage and exchange of digital images, DICOM [11] has emerged as the major standard here and is in common use for many imaging modalities such as magnetic resonance image (MRI) or computed tomography (CT) scans. We therefore want to briefly investigate whether the DICOM standard can be adopted for use of thermograms.

DICOM supports arbitrary image resolutions and various bit depths of data. Saving the radiological information of thermograms accurately will therefore be ensured though the exact format will need to be specified. Storage of patient and medical information is also provided by default as is the possibility to provide annotations and extra information in form of tags. This feature can be employed to save information on which part of the anatomy is captured and the storage of region of interest information as suggested in Reference 13 and can hence be used to integrate the efforts of standardization there into a common file format. Furthermore, DICOM supports not only storage of the original image data but also compression thereof, which will be investigated in further detail in the next section of this chapter. Overall, DICOM supports the main requirements of a standard for storage and communication of medical thermograms while its application and enforcement will have a major positive impact on the community of users providing them with an effective and efficient way of sharing and interpreting medical infrared images.

23.3 Compression of Thermograms

23.3.1 Image Dataset

In order to provide a useful comparison of the performance of compression algorithms one requires an image set that reflects the diversity of types of thermal images that are typically captured. We have therefore compiled such a data set that follows the standard views introduced in Reference 13. There, 27 standard poses are defined that are designed to capture every view possible necessary for composing an atlas based on infrared imaging. Of these 27 views we omitted 7 poses that are very similar to some of the other ones owing to symmetry reasons (either left/right or anterior/dorsal). For each of the remaining 20 image groups, about 20 images were collected using CTHERM [12]; details regarding each group are given in Table 23.1. With a few exceptions all images are of size 680×512, and the image bit depth is 7 bits.

23.3.2 Compression Algorithms

We evaluated five popular compression algorithms of which four have also been adapted as international imaging standards. Below, we briefly characterize the algorithms and implementations we used:

1. Lossless JPEG—former JPEG committee standard for lossless image compression [9]. The standard describes predictive image compression algorithm with Huffman or arithmetic entropy coder. JPEG is supported by the DICOM standard. We used the Cornell University implementation (version 1.0, ftp://ftp.cs.cornell.edu/pub/multimed/ljpg.tar.Z) that applies Huffman coding. The results are reported for the predictor function SV2, which resulted in the best average compression ratio for the dataset.
2. JPEG-LS—standard of the JPEG committee for lossless and near-lossless compression of still images [4]. The standard describes low-complexity predictive image compression algorithm with entropy coding using modified Golomb-Rice family. The algorithm is based on the LOCO-I

TABLE 23.1 Image Groups in the Dataset

Abbreviation	Description	No. of images
ABD	Abdomen, anterior view	19
BAA	Both ankles, anterior view	21
BHD	Both hands, dorsal view	16
BKA	Both knees, anterior view	18
CA	Chest, anterior view	22
DF	Dorsal feet	15
FA	Face	23
LAD	Left arm, dorsal view	15
LB	Lower back, dorsal view	17
LLA	Lower legs, anterior view	20
LLD	Lower legs, dorsal view	19
LRL	Right leg, lateral view	19
ND	Neck, dorsal view	23
PF	Plantar feet	23
TA	Thighs, anterior view	20
TBA	Total body, anterior view	19
TBD	Total body, dorsal view	16
TBR	Total body, right view	17
TD	Thighs, dorsal view	18
UB	Upper body, dorsal view	22
Total		382

algorithm [23]. JPEG-LS is supported by the DICOM standard. We used the University of British Columbia implementation (version 2.2, ftp://ftp.netbsd.org/pub/NetBSD/packages/distfiles/jpeg_ls_v2.2.tar.gz).

3. JPEG2000—a recent JPEG committee standard describing an algorithm based on wavelet transform image decomposition and arithmetic coding [5]. Apart from lossy and lossless compressing and decompressing of whole images it delivers many interesting features (progressive transmission, region of interest coding, etc.) [1]. JPEG2000 is supported by the DICOM standard. We used the JasPer implementation by Adams (version 1.700.0, http://www.ece.uvic.ca/ mdadams/jasper/).

4. PNG—standard of the WWW Consortium for lossless image compression [26]. PNG is a predictive image compression algorithm using the LZ77 [27] algorithm and Huffman coding. We used the `pnmtopng` implementation (version 2.37.6, part of the NetPBM 10.25 toolkit, http://netpbm.sourceforge.net/) compiled with libraries `libpng` (version 1.2.8, http://libpng.sourceforge.net/) and `zlib` (version 1.2.2, http://www.gzip.org/zlib/). The results are reported for the "sub" predictor function (filter), which resulted in the best average compression ratio for the dataset.

5. CALIC—a relatively complex predictive image compression algorithm using arithmetic entropy coder, which because of its usually high compression ratios is commonly used as a reference for other image compression algorithms [25]. We used the implementation by Wu and Memon (ftp://ftp.csd.uwo.ca/pub/from_wu/).

23.3.3 Compression Results

Before detailing the experimental procedure it should be stressed that, although all evaluated algorithms are lossless, they are only able to preserve the data that is originally presented and which therefore has to be ensured to be radiometrically sound.

Experimental results were obtained on an HP Proliant ML350G3 computer equipped with two Intel Xeon 3.06 GHz (512 kB cache memory) processors and Windows 2003 operating system. Single-threaded

TABLE 23.2 Compression Speeds (Given in MB/s)

Images	Lossless JPEG	JPEG-LS	JPEG2000	PNG	CALIC
ABD	11.9	17.7	3.8	3.3	4.1
BAA	11.8	18.2	4.0	3.4	4.3
BHD	11.8	17.9	3.8	3.2	4.3
BKA	11.7	14.5	3.5	2.8	3.7
CA	11.6	14.2	3.4	2.6	3.8
DF	11.8	17.6	3.9	3.3	4.2
FA	12.0	20.2	4.1	3.8	4.7
LAD	12.1	22.4	4.3	4.0	5.0
LB	11.6	13.7	3.4	2.6	3.6
LLA	12.2	23.6	4.4	4.3	4.9
LLD	12.0	21.6	4.4	4.0	4.6
LRL	11.9	20.3	4.0	3.8	4.8
ND	11.6	15.3	3.6	2.9	3.8
PF	11.7	17.7	3.9	3.2	4.4
TA	11.8	19.0	4.0	3.7	4.4
TBA	12.4	29.7	4.7	4.9	5.7
TBD	12.5	28.8	4.6	4.9	5.5
TBR	12.5	30.2	4.8	4.8	5.7
TD	12.0	19.6	4.1	3.6	4.5
UB	11.7	14.6	3.5	2.7	3.7
All	11.9	19.6	4.0	3.6	4.5

applications of algorithms used for comparisons were compiled using Intel C++ 8.1 compiler. To minimize effects of the system load and the input–output subsystem the compressors were run several times. The time of the first run was ignored while the collective time of other runs (executed for at least 1 s, and at least 5 times) was measured and then averaged. The time measured is hence the sum of time spent by the processor in application code and in kernel functions called by the application, as reported by the operating system after application execution.

In Tables 23.2 and 23.3 we show the results obtained by the compression algorithms introduced in Section 23.3.2 for the image dataset described in Section 23.3.1. Results are given in terms of compression speed, expressed in megabytes per second [MB/s], where 1 MB = 2^{20} bytes (Table 23.2) and compression ratio defined as O/C, where O is the filesize of the original image and C that of the compressed file (Table 23.3). The numbers are calculated as an average for all images contained in the group; since not all groups contain the same number of images, the average results for all images may be slightly different from the average of all groups.

Among the tested algorithms, the JPEG-LS is clearly the best when we consider the compression speeds listed in Table 23.2. All other algorithms are noticeably slower—from 39 (Lossless JPEG) to 82% (PNG). Our aim in this study was to analyze popular "standard" image compression algorithms; however we note that there exist other methods with compression speeds over two times higher than JPEG-LS [2,22]. The speeds of JPEG2000, PNG, and CALIC are similar (CALIC is faster than the remaining two algorithms by 11 and 20%, respectively). Both CALIC and JPEG2000 use an arithmetic entropy coder in contrast to PNG, which is based on faster techniques (LZ77 and the Huffman coding). On the basis of this we expected PNG to obtain compression speeds close to Lossless JPEG with Huffman coding. Therefore, the low speed of PNG is probably due to the implementation used. Looking at the results on a group-by-group basis, the best compression speeds were obtained for groups TBA, TBD, and TBR i.e., all three groups where the total body is captured. The worst compression speeds were achieved for groups BKA, CA, LB, and UB.

Considering the compression ratios from Table 23.3 we see that the ratios for JPEG-LS and CALIC are higher than those for JPEG2000, which in turn performs better than PNG and Lossless JPEG. While for various continuous tone grayscale images JPEG2000 has been reported as close to or little worse than

TABLE 23.3 Compression Ratios

Images	Lossless JPEG	JPEG-LS	JPEG2000	PNG	CALIC
ABD	2.83	3.86	3.48	3.06	3.76
BAA	3.03	4.12	3.73	3.28	4.04
BHD	2.86	3.81	3.41	3.05	3.75
BKA	2.50	3.11	2.85	2.52	3.10
CA	2.41	3.06	2.78	2.55	3.01
DF	3.03	4.04	3.68	3.20	3.99
FA	3.18	4.73	4.23	3.70	4.57
LAD	3.48	5.23	4.68	4.12	4.98
LB	2.36	2.92	2.65	2.41	2.88
LLA	3.75	5.71	5.09	4.27	5.52
LLD	3.64	5.34	4.79	4.06	5.18
LRL	3.24	4.71	4.19	3.66	4.56
ND	2.55	3.33	3.04	2.78	3.28
PF	2.94	3.96	3.59	3.27	3.89
TA	3.14	4.40	3.98	3.44	4.28
TBA	4.21	7.35	6.36	5.42	6.96
TBD	4.20	7.19	6.22	5.36	6.84
TBR	4.26	7.36	6.39	5.64	6.92
TD	3.21	4.49	4.08	3.46	4.36
UB	2.53	3.24	2.95	2.65	3.20
All	3.04	4.21	3.79	3.35	4.11

JPEG-LS [15], our results indicate that for medical infrared images JPEG2000 is significantly worse than JPEG-LS, which is the best performing algorithm. CALIC performs slightly worse than JPEG-LS but is also computationally much more complex. Looking at the results for each image group, the highest compression ratios are achieved for the three body groups TBA, TBD, and TBR while images of groups BKA, CA, LB, and UB are least compressible. Correlating this with the compression speeds from Table 23.2 we see that there is a direct link between efficiency and efficacy.

Overall it is clear that JPEG-LS is the best performing algorithm for lossless compression of medical infrared images. Not only does it provide the highest compression ratios but it is also the fastest of the tested methods. Furthermore, JPEG-LS is already included in the DICOM standard and can hence be readily employed.

23.4 Retrieval of Thermograms

23.4.1 Content-Based Retrieval

23.4.1.1 Moment Invariant Features

In CBIR techniques, each image is characterized by a set of features that serve as an index into the database. The features we propose to store as indices for thermal images are invariant combinations of moments of an image. Two-dimensional geometric moments m_{pq} of order $p+q$ of a density distribution function $f(x,y)$ are defined as

$$m_{pq} = \int_{-\infty}^{\infty} \int_{-\infty}^{\infty} x^p y^q f(x,y) \, dx dy \qquad (23.1)$$

In terms of a digital image $g(x,y)$ of size $N \times M$ the calculation of m_{pq} becomes discretized and the integrals are hence replaced by sums leading to

$$m_{pq} = \sum_{y=0}^{M-1} \sum_{x=0}^{N-1} x^p y^q g(x,y) \qquad (23.2)$$

Rather than m_{pq} often central moments

$$\mu_{pq} = \sum_{y=0}^{M-1} \sum_{x=0}^{N-1} (x - \bar{x})^p (y - \bar{y})^q g(x, y) \tag{23.3}$$

with

$$\bar{x} = \frac{m_{10}}{m_{00}}, \quad \bar{y} = \frac{m_{01}}{m_{00}}$$

are used, that is, moments where the centre of gravity has been moved to the origin (i.e., $\mu_{10} = \mu_{01} = 0$). Central moments have the advantage of being invariant to translation.

It is well known that a small number of moments can characterize an image fairly well; it is equally known that moments can be used to reconstruct the original image [3]. In order to achieve invariance to common factors and operations such as scale, rotation, and contrast, rather than using the moments themselves algebraic combinations thereof known as moment invariants are used that are independent of these transformations. It is a set of such moment invariants that we use for the retrieval of thermal medical images. In particular, the descriptors we use are based on Hu's original moment invariants [3].

$$\begin{aligned}
M_1 &= \mu_{20} + \mu_{02} \\
M_2 &= (\mu_{20} - \mu_{02})^2 + 4\mu_{11}^2 \\
M_3 &= (\mu_{30} - 3\mu_{12})^2 + 3(\mu_{21} + \mu_{03})^2 \\
M_4 &= (\mu_{30} + \mu_{12})^2 + (\mu_{21} + \mu_{03})^2 \\
M_5 &= (\mu_{30} - 3\mu_{12})(\mu_{30} + \mu_{12})[(\mu_{30} + \mu_{12})^2 - 3(\mu_{21} + \mu_{03})^2] \\
&\quad + (3\mu_{21} - \mu_{03})(\mu_{21} + \mu_{03})[3(\mu_{30} + \mu_{12})^2 - (\mu_{21} + \mu_{03})^2] \\
M_6 &= (\mu_{20} - \mu_{02})[(\mu_{30} + \mu_{12})^2 - (\mu_{21} + \mu_{03})^2] + 4\mu_{11}(\mu_{30} + \mu_{12})(\mu_{21} + \mu_{03}) \\
M_7 &= (3\mu_{21} - \mu_{03})(\mu_{30} + \mu_{12})[(\mu_{30} + \mu_{12})^2 - 3(\mu_{21} + \mu_{03})^2] \\
&\quad + (\mu_{30} - 3\mu_{12})(\mu_{21} + \mu_{03})[3(\mu_{30} + \mu_{12})^2 - (\mu_{21} + \mu_{03})^2]
\end{aligned} \tag{23.4}$$

Combinations of Hu's invariants can be found to achieve invariance not only in translation and rotation but also in scale and contrast [10]:

$$\begin{aligned}
\beta_1 &= \frac{\sqrt{M_2}}{M_1} \\
\beta_2 &= \frac{M_3 \mu_{00}}{M_1 M_2} \\
\beta_3 &= \frac{M_4}{M_3} \\
\beta_4 &= \frac{\sqrt{M_5}}{M_4} \\
\beta_5 &= \frac{M_6}{M_1 M_4} \\
\beta_6 &= \frac{M_7}{M_5}
\end{aligned} \tag{23.5}$$

23.4.1.2 Similarity Metric

Each thermal image is characterized by the six-moment invariants from Equation 23.5 that form a vector $\Phi = \{\beta_i, i = 1, \ldots, 6\}$. It should be noted that in the context of the DICOM standard, these features can be integrated into the thermogram through a set of annotations and can hence be shared by different users.

As similarity metric or distance measure between two thermograms, we use the Mahalanobis norm that takes into account different magnitudes of different components in Φ. The Mahalanobis distance between two invariant vectors $\Phi(I_1)$ and $\Phi(I_2)$ computed from two thermal images I_1 and I_2 is defined as

$$d(I_1, I_2) = \sqrt{(\Phi_1 - \Phi_2)^T C^{-1}(\Phi_1 - \Phi_2)}, \qquad (23.6)$$

where C is the covariance matrix of the distribution of Φ.

23.4.1.3 Retrieval through Query by Example

One main advantage of using the concept of CBIR is that it represents a generic approach to the automatic processing of images. Rather than employing specialized techniques that will capture only one type of image or pose (or one kind of disease or defect), image retrieval, when supported by a sufficiently large medical image database, will provide those cases that are most similar to a given one. The Query by example (QBE) method, whereby an image is provided to the system and corresponding images from the database are retrieved and returned in order of decreasing similarity, is perfectly suited for this task. Typically, it is sufficient to restrict the attention to the top 20 retrieved images.

The moment invariant descriptors described in Section 23.4.1.1 were used to index an image database of 350 thermal medical images provided by the University of Glamorgan [7]. An example of an image of an arm was used to perform QBE retrieval on the whole dataset. The result of this query is given in Figure 23.1, which shows those 20 images that were found to be closest to the query (sorted according to descending similarity from left to right, top to bottom). As can be seen all 13 other arm images present in the database were retrieved in the top 20 by our retrieval algorithm. Figure 23.2 shows another QBE retrieval example based on a thermogram of the neck. Again the top 20 retrieval images are returned. The ten images retrieved as the most similar ones are all neck images as was the given query. The QBE method can hence be effectively employed to retrieve similar thermograms from an existing medical image repository. If coupled with patient data and related medical records, a powerful information retrieval process supporting clinical diagnosis can be initiated.

23.4.1.4 Comparison with Database of Normals

The QBE paradigm is well suited for checking an existing database of thermal images for similar cases, for example, cases of the same disease or similar manifestations of a disease. Based on a sufficiently comprehensive database is available it will hence provide a useful aid for medical diagnosis. However, in many cases this prerequisite on the database is not realistic. In such instances an alternative approach based on dissimilarities rather than similarities can be taken. On the basis of the assumption that a dysfunction will show on the taken thermogram, it can be compared, on the basis of the features and similarity measure described above, to a dataset of healthy subjects captured in the same pose (such a database is described in Reference 13). If the average distance to the healthy subjects is much larger than the intercluster distances within this group of normals, then this provides an indication of a certain dysfunction that needs further investigation by the clinician.

Figure 23.3 shows three infrared images of hands. Two of the images depict healthy subjects. However, the third one shows a clear inflammation on one of the fingers and generally cooler hands. Following the strategy laid out in this section, all hand images in the database were taken and their inter-cluster distance, that is, the average distance (again, based on the moment invariant features) between any two hand images, was calculated. This was then compared with average distance of the third image to all "healthy" hand thermograms. While the average distance between two images of healthy individuals was 3.53, the distance of the image with the inflammation was 15.78. The difference between the thermogram showing an inflammation and images of healthy subjects is hence calculated as about four times the

Storage and Retrieval of Medical Thermograms

FIGURE 23.1 (See color insert at the back of the book.) Example of retrieving thermal images based on a query of an *arm* image. The query image is the one on the top left; the other images are those most similar to the query ordered in decreasing similarity (from left to right, top to bottom).

average difference among the images of normals. The presented image indexing techniques can therefore also be employed when no comprehensive database of pathologic cases is present. Thermal images falling outside the range of thermograms recorded from healthy subjects can so automatically be detected and should give a clear indication to the clinician to instigate further investigation.

23.4.2 Browsing of Thermal Image Database

When storing thermograms (or other medical images), often little thought is given to the actual organization and management of these image collections. While in typical medical image databases data records are accessed by patients' names or other similar attributes, here we propose a method that allows access to and navigation through the database based on visual cues. All images in the collection are projected onto a two-dimensional (2D) space in such a way that images that are similar to each other are located close to one another in this configuration. The result is then displayed on screen and provides a picture of the complete dataset. That visually similar images are located close to each other (i.e., clustered) is fundamental to this approach as it provides an intuitive and easy to understand interface for the user.

23.4.2.1 Features and Similarity Measure

Since the browsing approach taken in this chapter is again based on visual similarity between images, we make use of the features and the similarity metric we introduced and described in Sections 23.4.1.1 and 23.4.1.4 (i.e. moment invariants and Mahalanobis distance). Doing so allows the same features to be used for both retrieval and browsing without any additional overhead.

FIGURE 23.2 (**See color insert.**) Example of retrieving thermal images based on a query of a *neck* image. The result is laid out in the same structure as that of Figure 23.1.

FIGURE 23.3 (**See color insert.**) Thermal hand images of healthy subjects (a) and (b) together with a thermogram showing an inflammation (c).

23.4.2.2 Multidimensional Scaling

Multidimensional scaling (MDS) [8] expresses the similarities between different objects in a small number of dimensions, allowing for a complex set of interrelationships to be summarized in a single figure. MDS can be used to analyze any kind of distance or similarity/dissimilarity matrix created from a particular dataset.

There are two types of MDS methods: metric and non-metric MDS. In metric MDS the distances between the data items are given and a configuration of points that would give rise to the distances is sought. This perfect reproduction of distances is not always possible in which case nonmetric MDS can be applied. In nonmetric MDS the calculations between rank orders of similarity Euclidean distances and rank orders in the original space are computed to produce a set of metric co-ordinates that most closely approximate their nonmetric distances.

In this chapter we follow ideas from Reference 14 and apply MDS for thermal medical image database display and navigation. By applying MDS based on the distances between moment invariant vectors of thermal images we produce a way of visualizing the retrieved images not only in terms of decreasing similarities but also according to their common similarities. All images are implanted (based on their similarities) in a 2D Euclidean space where the original distances are preserved as closely as possible.

In detail, first a distance matrix that contains all pairwise distances between the medical images in the databases needs to be obtained. As mentioned above we define as the distance d between two images the Mahalanobis distance between their moment invariant vectors. Euclidean distances $\hat{d}_{i,j}$ are calculated and initially compared using Kruskals' stress formula [8]:

$$\text{Stress} = \frac{\sum_{i,j}(\hat{d}_{i,j} - d_{i,j})}{\sum_{i,j} d_{i,j}^2} \qquad (23.7)$$

which expresses the difference between the distances d and the Euclidean values $\hat{d}$ between all images. The aim of nonmetric MDS is to assign locations to the input data so that the overall stress is minimal.

Typically an initial configuration is found through principal components analysis (PCA). While the degree of goodness-of-fit after this is in general fairly high, it is not optimal. To move toward a better solution the locations of the points are updated in such a way as to reduce the overall stress. If, for instance, the distance between two specific samples has been overestimated it will be reduced to correct this deviation. It is clear that this modification will have implications for all other distances calculated. Therefore, the updating of the coordinates and the recalculation of the stress is being performed in an iterative way, where during each iteration the positions are slightly changed until the whole configuration is stable and the algorithm has converged into a minimum where the distances between the projected samples correspond accurately to the original distances. Several termination conditions can be applied, such as an acceptable degree of goodness-of-fit, a predefined maximal number of iterations, or a threshold for the overall changes in the configuration. Once the calculation is terminated the images can then be plotted at the calculated coordinates on the screen.

23.4.2.3 Browsing

Navigation through the image database starts typically with a global display of the entire dataset with images positioned in relation to how similar they are to all others. From here the user has the ability to zoom into certain regions of interest to enlarge for further querying. For each localized visualization occurrence, the images selected in the area have their distance matrix recalculated and projected back into 2D format. This accommodates for the enlargement so as to occupy the entire screen when displayed.

The same image database as employed for the retrieval experiments has been used to test our browsing method. The triangular distance matrix between all invariant vectors was obtained using the Mahalanobis distance from Equation 23.6. On the basis of this distance matrix, MDS was applied as explained in Section 23.4.2.2. The resulting global view is shown in Figure 23.4 where all images are projected (although some are occluded by others) onto the visualization plane, which is then displayed on screen. It can be seen that similar images are indeed placed close to each other and that clusters or groups are formed. Typically the user will then zoom into one of the clusters or areas of interest to narrow down the search, as was done to produce Figure 23.5, which displays a zoomed-in area showing mainly *legs* and *upper body* images. As mentioned in Section 23.4.2.2, MDS is reapplied to the images in the localized area to provide a less cluttered view. Also shown in Figure 23.5 is the possibility to retrieve further information on a certain image, which is displayed in a pop-up window. Clearly, additional medical information such as the patient's medical history, medication, or current diagnosis information can be added to this view, which hence provides an intuitive interface.

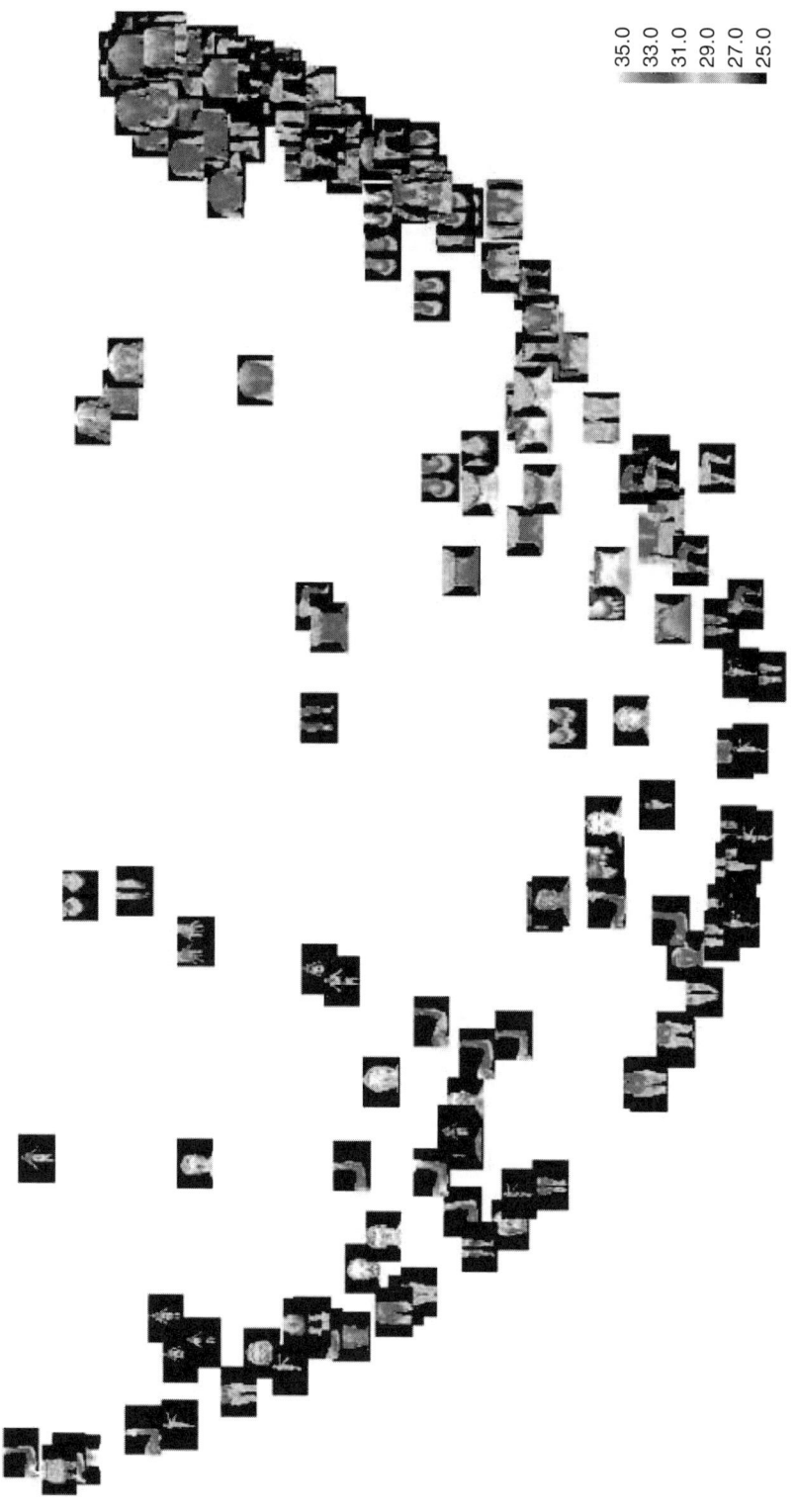

FIGURE 23.4 (See color insert.) Global visualization view of complete thermal image database.

FIGURE 23.5 (**See color insert.**) Zoomed-in area showing leg and upper body images.

23.5 Conclusions

In this chapter we have looked at issues regarding the storage and retrieval of medical thermograms. First, we stressed the need of a standard format for storage and communication of thermograms and suggested the adoption of the DICOM standard for this purpose.

A number of lossless compression algorithms were then evaluated on a large database of thermal medical images. It was shown that, depending on the type of image, compression ratios of up to 1:4 are possible. Furthermore, it was shown that JPEG-LS seems the most suitable algorithm to employ, as it provides both the best compression performance and is also the fastest of the tested algorithms. As JPEG-LS is also certified as an international standard and is further integrated into the DICOM standard for the exchange of medical imagery, it could be recommended as a standard for storing and exchanging thermal medical images.

We have also proposed the application of CBIR to the domain of thermal medical images. Each image is characterized by a set of moment invariants that are independent to translation, scale, rotation, and contrast. Retrieval is performed by returning those images whose moments are most similar to the ones of a given query image. In addition to retrieval, the same features can be used to provide an intuitive interface for browsing a collection of thermograms. Using MDS, all images are projected onto a visualization plane so that images that are visually similar are also located close to each other. Experimental results for both techniques have been presented and have demonstrated the usefulness of the proposed techniques.

Acknowledgments

This chapter is based on the work published in References 16, 19, and 20. The author would like to thank Roman Starosolski (Silesian Technical University), Shao Ying Zhu and Brian Jones (University of Derby), and Simon Ruszala (Nottingham Trent University) for their contributions, as well as the Medical Computing Research Group of the University of Glamorgan for providing the test image dataset. Comments from Nicholas Diakides, the editor of this book, on an earlier draft of this chapter were also greatly appreciated.

References

[1] C. Christopoulos, A. Skodras, and T. Ebrahimi. The JPEG2000 still image coding system: An overview. *IEEE Transaction on Consumer Electronics*, 46:1103–1127, 2000.

[2] Consultative Committee for Space Data Systems. Lossless data compression. *CCSDS Recommendation for Space System Data Standards, CCSDS 121.0-B-1, Blue Book*, 1997.

[3] M.K. Hu. Visual pattern recognition by moment invariants. *IRE Transactions on Information Theory*, 8:179–187, February 1962.

[4] ISO. Lossless and near-lossless compression of continuous-tone images (JPEG-LS). *ISO Working Document ISO/IEC JTC1/SC29/WG1 N522*, 1997.

[5] ISO. JPEG2000 image coding system. *ISO/IEC FCD 15444-1 JPEG2000 Part I Final Committee Draft Version 1.0*, 2000.

[6] B.F. Jones. A reappraisal of infrared thermal image analysis for medicine. *IEEE Transaction on Medical Imaging*, 17:1019–1027, 1998.

[7] B.F. Jones. EPSRC Grant GR/R50134/01 Report, 2001.

[8] J.B. Kruskal and M. Wish. *Multidimensional Scaling*. Sage Publications, 1978.

[9] G. Langdon, A. Gulati, and E. Seiler. On the JPEG model for lossless image compression. In *2nd Data Compression Conference*, pp. 172–180, 1992.

[10] S. Maitra. Moment invariants. *Proceedings of the IEEE*, 67:697–699, 1979.

[11] National Electrical Manufacturers Association. Digital Imaging and Communications in Medicine (DICOM). *Standards Publication PS 3.1-2004*, 2004.

[12] P. Plassmann and E.F.J. Ring. An open system for the acquisition and evaluation of medical thermological images. *European Journal of Thermology*, 7:216–220, October 1997.

[13] E.F.J. Ring, K. Ammer, A. Jung, P. Murawski, B. Wiecek, J. Zuber, S. Zwolenik, P. Plassmann, C. Jones, and B.F. Jones. Standardization of infrared imaging. In *26th IEEE International Conference on Engineering in Medicine and Biology*, pp. 1183–1185, 2004.

[14] Y. Rubner, L. Guibas, and C. Tomasi. The earth mover's distance, multi-dimensional scaling, and color-based image retrieval. In *Image Understanding Workshop*, pp. 661–668, 1997.

[15] D. Santa-Cruz and T. Ebrahimi. A study of JPEG2000 still image coding versus other standards. In *10th European Signal Processing Conference*, pp. 673–676, 2000.

[16] G. Schaefer, R. Starosolski, and S.Y. Zhu. An evaluation of lossless compression algorithms for medical infrared images. In *27th IEEE International Conference Engineering in Medicine and Biology*, pp. 1125–1128, 2005.

[17] G. Schaefer and S.Y. Zhu. Compressing thermal medical images. *Thermology International*, 14(4):147, 2004.

[18] G. Schaefer and S.Y. Zhu. Lossy compression of medical infrared images. In *3rd European Medical and Biological Engineering Conference*, pp. 3118–3121, 2005.

[19] G. Schaefer, S.Y. Zhu, and B. Jones. Retrieving thermal medical images. In *International Conference on Computer Vision and Graphics*, Computational Imaging and Vision. Springer, 2006.

[20] G. Schaefer, S.Y. Zhu, and S. Ruszala. Visualisation of medical infrared image databases. In *27th IEEE International Conference Engineering in Medicine and Biology*, pp. 1139–1142, 2005.

[21] A.W.M. Smeulders, M. Worring, S. Santini, A. Gupta, and R.C. Jain. Content-based image retrieval at the end of the early years. *IEEE Transaction on Pattern Analysis and Machine Intelligence*, 22:1349–1380, December 2000.

[22] R. Starosolski. Simple fast and adaptive lossless image compression algorithm. Software—Practice and Experience, 37(1):65–91, 2007.

[23] M.J. Weinberger, G. Seroussi, and G. Sapiro. The LOCO-I lossless image compression algorithm: Principles and standardization into JPEG-LS. *IEEE Transaction on Image Processing*, 9:1309–1324, 1996.

[24] B. Wiecek, S. Zwolenik, A. Jung, and J. Zuber. Advanced thermal, visual and radiological image processing for clinical diagnostics. In *21st IEEE International Conference on Engineering in Medicine and Biology*, 1999.

[25] X. Wu and N. Memon. Context-based adaptive lossless image codec. *IEEE Transactions on Communications*, 45:437–444, 1997.

[26] WWW Consortium. PNG (Portable Network Graphics) specification. *Version 1.0*, 1996.

[27] J. Ziv and A. Lempel. A universal algorithm for sequential data compression. *IEEE Transactions of Information Theory*, 32:337–343, 1977.

24

Ethical Obligations in Infrared Imaging Research and Practice

James Giordano
Center for Clinical Bioethics, and Division of Palliative Medicine, Georgetown University Medical Center

24.1	Introduction..	24-1
	A Perspective on Ethical Issues in the Use of Infrared Technology in Medicine • On the Need for Continuing and Progressive Research	
24.2	Domains of Knowledge in Clinical Medicine..........	24-3
24.3	The Contribution of fIR Detection to Diagnostic Value(s)	24-5
	Ethical Obligations for Education and Training • The Role of Policy	
	Acknowledgment...	24-6
	References	24-7

24.1 Introduction

24.1.1 A Perspective on Ethical Issues in the Use of Infrared Technology in Medicine

Over the past two decades, technological advancement has led to increased capability, and efficacy of functional infrared imaging (fIR). Developments in computerized image acquisition, data processing, and interpretation derived and directly incorporated from formerly classified military applications have increased and solidified the medical utility of fIR. Previous and residual concerns and criticisms of IR as being inadequate to effectively detect thermal signatures that are important to establishing particular differential diagnoses have been assuaged and refuted by the functional sophistication produced through the merging of advanced image acquisition and computerized analytic systems. There is recurrent contention surrounding the inapt use of fIR by untrained personnel, and the overuse of IR as an improperly administered or interpreted "diagnostic" test. I believe that the aforementioned progress in (the technological domains) of the field has deepened concerns over the ethical use of fIR, and compels a need for increased stringency in the education, training, and certification of professionally qualified, competent clinicians, and technicians to be the sole providers of this technology.

In this chapter, I address the ethical obligations that compel and sustain the use of fIR in medical research and practice. I base this discussion on the premise that medicine is not merely applied science, but rather is a profession that mandates the use of scientific (i.e., theoretical) information in ways that sustain and are resonant to the humanitarian essence of the interaction between clinician and patient (Dell'Oro, 2005). To be sure, there are areas of medicine (e.g., basic science research, epidemiology/public health, etc.) that are not explicitly focused upon the clinical encounter. Yet, their relevance to the clinician–patient relationship, while indirect, implicitly reinforces the scope, tenor, and basis of patient care. This is perhaps most evident in basic sciences' research; while the proximate goal of the basic sciences is the contribution of theoretical knowledge (i.e., "knowledge for knowledge's sake"), this theoretical information contributes to a larger body of epistemic capitol that is applied within the context of clinical practice as a fundamental domain of relevant knowledge (Feinstein, 1967). It is in this light that I discuss the imperative to conduct and advance research that is aimed at elucidating the capacities, enhancing the efficacy, and evaluating the outcomes of IR technology as a component of clinical paradigms of detection, discernment, and ultimately diagnosis.

But how this knowledge is utilized is as important as what this knowledge entails, and thus I provide a brief overview of the domains of knowledge that maintain the intellectual virtues important for clinical medicine. For if the information gained from basic sciences' studies of IR is to be the bedrock on which its use in medical practice is to be built, then we must recognize the moral obligations to utilize such knowledge and technical acumen in prudent ways that support the humanitarian dimensions that define medicine as an interpersonal act. This is particularly true when regarding IR technology as a viable method of detection to facilitate diagnosis, as the values in and of diagnosis ultimately establish the subsequent construct(s), content, and context of care.

Thus, I argue that the use of IR (or any technique or technology) in the medical milieu must be explicitly relevant to and consistent with (if not wholly supportive of) the moral obligations and ethical integrity of clinical encounter between patient and clinician. The clinical encounter is, in essence, a nexus for (1) the multidimensional aspects of medicine as a science, engaging research findings within the context of a complex practice and (2) the enactment of medicine as a humanitarian endeavor, in which the enjoinment of participatory agents who maintain the expectation that the ends, or *telos*, of technically right and morally good care is enabled and provided (Pellegrino, 1983). Therefore, the capacities and limitations of IR must be recognized and explicated, so as to insure (technically and ethically) appropriate use within the medical fiduciary.

24.1.2 On the Need for Continuing and Progressive Research

Research facilitates the defined *telos* of medicine by affording knowledge that (1) enables the clinician to evaluate the relative value(s), benefits, and risks of particular diagnostic and therapeutic approaches, and ultimately resolve equipoise and (2) empowers patients to be informed participants in clinical decisions relevant to care, thereby lessening their inherent vulnerability and decreasing the inequalities of power and capacity (Freedman, 1987; Giordano, 2006a). Of course, such research must be methodologically rigorous and ethically sound (Fried, 1974; see Levine, 1986 for review). The relationship of research and practice is reciprocal. Findings from research inform practice, and evaluation of outcomes gained by employing various techniques in practice contributes to a progressive revision and expansion of an evidentiary base of knowledge to instigate and guide further study (Giordano, 2004, 2006b).

In both cases, the imperative for developing, implementing, and promoting ongoing research to assess and evaluate the capabilities and clinical application(s) of fIR is grounded upon the moral obligation of beneficence (Frankena, 1982). Irrespective of the ethical system that is utilized to guide medical research or care (e.g., employment of *prima facie* principles, casuistic approaches, ethic of care, virtue ethics, etc.), the primacy of patient benefit is a critical, if not fundamental to morally sound conduct of clinical research and practice (Giordano, 2006a). Pellegrino and Thomasma (1988) have defined beneficence in the clinical encounter as fourfold, encompassing the biomedical (i.e., technical) good, the good as relevant to the choices of the patient, the good for the patient as a (*n* autonomous) person, and the existential good, in context. Obviously, research is instrumental in determining the technical or practical "good" of a particular technique or technology, such as fIR. But even at this level, application as a meaningful biomedical "good" requires translational studies that evaluate the broader implications of use-in-practice to determine viability in real-world medical settings. In recognizing and achieving the biomedical good the somewhat more passive maxim of nonharm can be concomitantly realized. By understanding the actions, effects and capabilities of fIR, we can also recognize, weigh, and may be able to compensate for (1) inherent limitations of the technology in various applications; (2) potential risks of use or nonuse; and (3) possible burdens incurred to the patient, as well as the medical system.

This knowledge serves to illustrate the potential viability of fIR as a tool within the armamentarium of evaluative techniques that contribute to accurate diagnosis. When coupled to an understanding of the mechanisms of particular pathologies, such knowledge allows the clinician to address whether fIR can, and indeed should, be employed in specific determinative clinical situations. If properly employed, fIR can fortify the informational base necessary toward the resolution of equipoise, and thus allow treatment that is appropriate to the pathologic state, as well as the choices and overall integrity of a particular patient. Ultimately, this process, together with the prudent, practical wisdom of the clinician (i.e., *phronesis*) distinguishes what care *should* be rendered, from what care *can* be rendered (Davis, 1997).

Information fuels this decisional process, and as this volume well illustrates, the technical sophistication of current iterations of fIR enable its utility as a tool in detecting thermal changes that reflect pathologic processes of several disorders (e.g., complex regional pain syndrome, certain vasculopathies, tumorigenesis, etc.). Still, there is equivocal discussion that questions the salience and necessity of continuing fIR research. The majority of contention is focused on the incapability of fIR to accurately detect thermal variation with sufficient sensitivity to be relevant to the clinical discernment of particular pathophysiological states. From this assumption would arise the issue that fIR research is impractical, or worse, that time and effort spent pursuing clinical application of fIR are pragmatically, temporally, and economically wasteful and therefore constitute an unethical exploitation of research resources or patient trust and expectation. I do not feel that these criticisms are valid based on the following grounds: first, to reiterate, the wedding of advanced image acquisition systems to state-of-the-art computerized systems using complex statistical data analyses, has allowed for increased image clarity and specificity of signal-to-noise discrimination (Kakuta et al., 2002). The technical advancement of current fIR has rendered previous iterations of this technology obsolete (Irvine, 2002). Second, it must be borne to mind that the applied goals of basic (and clinical) research are to address, identify, and develop methods of overcoming problematic issues that affect or impede medical care (Goodman, 2003). But research is not merely a means to these ends, rather it is an end unto itself, being a moral enterprise that must sustain the moral obligations to patients (as research subjects) and society as a public good (Giordano, 2006c; Pedroni, 2006). As a public good it should be (1) effective in achieving goals consistent with stated ends (in this case, of medicine); (2) not be burdensome to individual patient subjects or society (May, 2003); and (3) be relatively self-advancing — that is, maintain a reciprocally translational focus that contributes to the knowledge base that infuses and advances the benefits of patient care (see also Giordano, 2004). Contemporary fIR research satisfies each of these requirements, and thus I argue that contentions against ongoing research in this area are ill informed, improperly directed and hence, unjustified.

But if the knowledge acquired through well-designed and rigorously conducted research studies is to be of any meaningful value, it must be appropriately and effectively used within the clinical encounter. How such knowledge gained from research is to be incorporated within the larger fabric of clinically relevant information is important to both its practical and ethical use, and reflects the intellectual skills necessary to the act of medicine (Pellegrino and Thomasma, 1993; Toulmin, 1975).

24.2 Domains of Knowledge in Clinical Medicine

Arguably, medicine as a science relies on theoretical knowledge that affords understanding of mechanisms of physiological process(es), disease, and diagnostic and therapeutic interventions. Such knowledge is based not only in part on *a priori* understanding of the workings of the world as natural phenomena that are logically consistent, but also on the acquisition of new knowledge that modifies our basic concepts and, as such, provides a somewhat changing epistemological capitol of "truth(s)" (Fuller, 2003; Kuhn, 1962).

Philosophically, this reflects the essence of science as being self-critical and self-revising as new information is acquired and incorporated into the accepted fund of knowledge (Nagel, 1961). Theoretical knowledge is gained through research, both as an observational and experimental undertaking; this criticality of epistemic knowledge supports the importance of research to science and medicine, in general, and in the present case, undergirds the importance of progressive research to advance an understanding and the capabilities of fIR.

Given my position that medicine is not just applied science, I believe that its practice involves far more than a theoretical knowledge of physiological systems, pathologies, and the mechanics of particular tests, tools, and interventions. I hold that knowing "what should be done" mandates understanding of "how", "when", and "why" something is done (Giordano, 2006b,c). Specifically, knowing whether fIR represents an appropriate detective protocol for a particular clinical case requires understanding not only of the technology (and its capacities and limitations) but also the suspected pathology, the physiological changes it incurs, the viability of fIR to detect such changes, as well as how the technology (of both image acquisition conditions and data analyses) should be employed to meet the particular circumstances. This necessitates experience in differing situations and across time. Experiential knowledge can be gained through an expanding body of research findings, and may be acquired through training and direct activity (Davis, 1997; Giordano, 2006b,c). The necessity of experiential knowledge in clinical contexts further endorses the need for continued research in mechanisms and applications of fIR, and additionally supports the continued utilization of fIR in practice so as to contribute to a growing database of clinically relevant applications and possibilities. Ultimately, theoretical and experiential knowledge work synergistically when relating current cases to paradigmatic examples (i.e., the casuistic approach), and in this way theory and experience are conjoined to determine if, how and why fIR can and should be utilized as a step in the process of diagnosing particular pathology in a specific patient.

In this situation, contextual knowledge allows the clinician to

1. Utilize technical and experiential knowledge of fIR as a tool in detecting the thermal signatures of certain pathophysiological states
2. Use this theory and experience to determine whether fIR represents an appropriate evaluative method
3. Utilize theoretical and experiential understanding to formulate and implement the right conditions for use and interpretation of fIR in a given case

Taken together, contextual knowledge fuses research to practice (Giordano, 2006c), and allows the clinician to avoid a simplistic "one-size-fits-all" approach to assessment of those pathologies for which fIR has been shown to be a valid and effective evaluative tool.

Experiential and contextual knowledge rely on a theoretical foundation, and both require and infuse skill. However, it is important to note that there is an abstract dimension to medicine. Indeed, medicine has been described as both skill and art (i.e., *tekne*) that establishes the distinction between simply applied science and the finesse that empowers its subjective, hermeneutic character (Edelstein, 1967; Owens, 1977; Svenaeus, 2000). The critical intellectual, practical, and moral step in medical practice occurs as description, detection, and differentiation coalesce into the process of diagnosis (Wulff, 1976). It is from this point of determining "what is wrong" with a particular patient that the possibilities for and selection of subsequent treatment can be ascertained (Pellegrino, 1979). Indeed, this is the point at which individual and clinical equipoise are reconciled and resolved on grounds that provide the best choice(s) for ethically good patient care. This process of using theoretical, experiential, and contextual knowledge, together with any and all tools and methods that are nonburdensome, manifest low risk and which effectively produce reliable data to generate an evidence-based approach is essential to clinical decision making. I have argued that *phronesis*, the intellectual virtue of practical wisdom, is imperative to determine (1) which tools, tests, and approaches best contribute to the diagnostic process; (2) the meaning and relative value(s) of findings; and (3) how these findings facilitate diagnosis (Giordano, 2005, 2006a,b; see also Davis, 1997). As well, *phronesis* allows the clinician to intuit the nature and power in and of diagnosis as an act of naming the disorder, claiming particular "truths" about the disorder and its care, and framing the patient within a population of those with this disorder and establishing the trajectory of subsequent clinical interaction(s) (Giordano, 2006b). The power of this step is exceptional, and as such the inherent responsibilities must be borne by individuals who are capable of integrating multidimensional knowledge, weighing the complex choices arising from diverse circumstances, prudently determining the reasons to guide right action(s), and recognizing and accepting consequences of those actions (Pellegrino, 1979). For fIR to be accurately, effectively, and thus ethically employed, it must be administered and interpreted by individuals who are not simply repeating a task by rote (even if safely, and efficiently), but rather by individuals who exercise practical wisdom in the professional responsibilities of the diagnostic process (i.e., by one who utilizes and embodies *phronesis* by virtue of character — a *phronimos*). By Aristotelian definition, a *phronimos* is concerned not just with knowing the right things, but in using that knowledge in the right ways to achieve the good(s) intrinsic to the practice (Aristotle, 1999; Edelstein, 1967).

24.3 The Contribution of fIR Detection to Diagnostic Value(s)

Yet, detection and discernment are not diagnosis; fIR cannot and should not be considered or utilized as a singular method of detection or explicitly diagnostic technique. However, the use of IR evaluation by a competently trained professional, acting prudently to weigh the value of information gained, can serve as an important diagnostic asset. The word diagnosis is derived from the Greek *diagignoskein*, meaning "… to distinguish." This distinguishing quality reflects the abilities of the clinician to utilize the aforementioned domains of knowledge to apprehend the features of a disorder as expressed in a particular patient, differentiate these signs and symptoms from other possible disorders, discern the contextual basis of these features and in so doing establish diagnosis, literally as a "… seeing or a knowledge into the problem" (Mainetti, 1992). Any and all contributory acts and methods of diagnosis should be oriented toward (1) simplification, (2) ongoing re-evaluation and interpretation, (3) synergizing theoretical and contextual understanding and moral intention, and (4) the primacy of the patients' best interest(s) (Sadler, 2004, 2005). Each of these criteria can be met by fIR, for as this volume illustrates, the technical advances that have been made in the past 20 years have allowed fIR to be used to (1) facilitate detection and thus simplify particular diagnoses, (2) afford the ability for (re-)evaluation and interpretation of pathologic advancement or effects of therapeutic intervention, and (3) incur low/minimal risk and thus be nonburdensome to the best interest(s) of the patient (*vide infra*). In this latter regard, it should be noted that as part of a more expansive diagnostic protocol, fIR may lessen the risks and burdens of medical care through earlier detection of particular pathologies, to prompt better diagnosis and care that ultimately could reduce the extent, duration as well as negative (personal and financial) impact of subsequent intervention(s). It is clear that this process takes on considerable ethical weight as it provides the basis for prognosis (a knowledge of what could occur), and creates a foundation for the development and implementation of prudent care (Giordano, 2005a). Thus, diagnosis also relies, at least in part on *phronesis*, as its technical rectitude and moral gravity must be oriented to and consistent with the *telos* of medicine. I argue that these telic obligations compel both research to determine those techniques and technologies that enhance diagnoses, as well as the utilization of these approaches in clinical practice (Giordano, 2005b, 2006b,c).

24.3.1 Ethical Obligations for Education and Training

If research is to inform practice, and the actions of morally sound practice are reliant on the phronetic integration of distinct types and domains of knowledge, then how can this relationship be fortified to ensure that fIR is aptly utilized? It is notable that the more befouling criticisms of fIR have centered around its use by poorly trained "technicians" or nonprofessionals, and on unethical claims for financial reimbursement for improper characterization and employment as a "diagnostic" technique. Both of these denunciations reflect inadequacies or improprieties in education and training. Thus, I argue that the clinical understanding of fIR technology, use and applications must be provided by stringent programs of didactic pedagogy, practical training, and evaluation that reflect the complexity and advancement of the field, acknowledge the technical and ethical power of this technology in medical diagnosis and care, and uphold a high standard of professionalism. I impugn those approaches and programs that claim to "certify" individuals as fIR "technicians" or experts after a course of brief home study, weekend seminar and/or superficial "examination." Such programs are wholly iniquitous, depreciate the field and threaten patient care and the integrity of the medical fiduciary. Rather, I propose that fIR be incorporated into extant training programs of medical imaging, either as an additional curricular focus, or as a specialized program of study. Similarly, I propose that fIR training be provided to licensed medical professionals (i.e., physicians, veterinarians) through continuing education and postgraduate programs that 1) afford thorough information on the technology, conditions and constraints of use, limitations and delimiting factors in clinical application, and 2) mandate practical training and experience in fIR use and methods of data analysis and outcomes evaluation. Progress in technological development should not be ethically undermined by capricious, unprofessional utilization engendered through improper education, training, and certification.

To be sure, these insurances are demanding, and require revision and ongoing monitoring of research, education, training, and application(s) in practice. Yet, as technology progresses, so too do the responsibilities to utilize and apply such technology in ways that are consistent with an expanding epistemology and are adherent to moral obligations and ethical affirmations for good and nonharm (Jonas, 1975).

24.3.2 The Role of Policy

But while these incentives may affect change on a grass-roots level, meaningful change in the "culture" of medicine (and the economic strata that support it) cannot be fully actualized without "top-down" implementation. This is the role of policy. If positive change is to occur, it must reflect the technological progress in the field, identify and be consonant with the purpose of those individuals who embrace and utilize these developments for identifiably good ends, and enact a process that engages each of the tiers affected (i.e., research, education, training, and application; Light, 2000). The voices of the research, clinical and patient communities must reflect valuation of fIR as a meaningful clinical tool that requires further study, development, and application, thus necessitating policy that provides enablement and economic support of these endeavors. In this way "bottom-up" values and interests will encourage "top-down" enactment of public policy programs for subsidizing these enterprises. How could this be realistically achieved? First, it is important to recognize that learning must precede change—the vectors for change agency can only be empowered when the potential and possibilities that change incurs are generally appreciated as positive and nonthreatening to some real or perceived status quo. By demonstrating the progress in fIR and pragmatically addressing the potential, possibilities, and implications that such progress may afford to healthcare, a pediment to learning can, and hopefully has been achieved. This is critical for dispelling prior and extant misconceptions, and engendering favorable reappraisal. But "bottom-up" efforts must also reflect a "house cleaning" of sorts, to fortify the field from within, ensuring professionalism that adheres to, and reflects strict ethical standards, as previously described. Without such, any viability of fIR as a technology and technique will be overshadowed by ethical improbity in application, and the value of policy to support further research and clinical use will be abrogated.

The fusion of "bottom-up" and "top-down" change to advance the medical use of fIR requires a multipartite effort of (1) integrating research into formalized education and training, (2) instilling and ensuring high ethical standards for the use of fIR by competent professionals, and (3) public policy to assure ongoing administrative and economic support. The work described by this volume certainly serves both as a cornerstone to such efforts and a catalyst for progress in the ethical use of this technology.

Acknowledgment

This work was supported, in part, by the Center of Clinical Bioethics, Georgetown University Medical Center, Washington, DC, and by the Manchikanti Distinguished Lectureship in Pain Medicine and Ethics of the American Society of Interventional Pain Physicians.

References

Aristotle. *The Nicomachean Ethics* (T. Irwin, trans.), Hackett Publishing, Indianapolis, 1999.
Davis FD. Phronesis, reasoning and Pellegrino's philosophy of medicine. *Theoret. Med.*, 1997; 18: 173–198.
Dell'Oro R. Interpreting clinical judgment: epistemological notes on the praxis of medicine. In: Viafora C (ed.) *Clinical Bioethics—A Search for Foundations*. Springer, Dordrecht, 2005.
Edelstein L. The professional ethics of the Greek physician. In: Temkin, O and Temkin, CL (eds.) *Ancient Medicine: The Selected Papers of Ludwig Edelstein*. Johns Hopkins Press, Baltimore, MD, 1967.
Feinstein AR. *Clinical Judgment*. Williams and Wilkins, Baltimore, MD, 1967.
Frankena W. Beneficence in an ethics of virtue. In: Shelp, E (ed.) *Beneficence and Health Care*. D. Reidel, Dordrecht, 1982.
Freedman B. Equipoise and the ethics of clinical research. *N. Engl. J. Med.*, 1987; 317: 141–145.
Fried C. *Medical Experimentation: Personal Integrity and Social Policy*. North-Holland, Amsterdam, 1974.
Fuller S. *Kuhn vs. Popper: The Struggle for the Soul of Science*. Columbia University Press, New York, 2003.
Giordano J. Pain research: Can paradigmatic revision bridge the needs of medicine, scientific philosophy and ethics? *Pain Phys.*, 2004; 7: 459–463.
Giordano J. Toward a core philosophy and virtue-based ethics of pain medicine. *Pain Pract.*, 2005; 15: 59–66.
Giordano J. Good as gold? The randomized controlled trial—paradigmatic revision and ethical responsibility in pain research. *Am. J. Pain Mangt.*, 2006a; 16: 68–71.
Giordano J. On knowing: Domains of knowledge and intellectual virtue in practical pain management. *Pract. Pain Mangt.*, 2006b; 6: 65–67.
Giordano J. Moral agency in pain medicine: Philosophy, practice and virtue. *Pain Phys.*, 2006c; 9: 71–76.
Goodman KW. *Ethics and Evidence-Based Medicine: Fallibility and Responsibility in Clinical Science*. Cambridge University Press, Cambridge, 2003.
Irvine JM. Targeting breast cancer detection with military technology; applicability of automated target recognition technology to early screening for breast cancer. *Eng. Biol. Med.*, 2002; 21: 36–40.
Jonas H. Technology and responsibility. *Social Res.*, 1973; 40: 31–54.
Kakuta N, Yokoyama S, and Mabuchi K. Human thermal models for evaluating infrared images: comparing infrared images under various thermal environmental conditions through normalization of skin surface temperature. *Eng. Biol. Med.*, 2002; 21: 65–72.
Kuhn T. *The Structure of Scientific Revolutions*. University of Chicago Press, Chicago, IL, 1962.
Levine RJ. *Ethics and Regulation of Clinical Research*. 2nd ed. Yale University Press, New Haven, CT, 1986.
Light DW. The sociological character of health care. In: Albrecht, GL, Fitzpatrick, R, and Scrimshaw, SC (eds.) *Healthcare Markets, Handbook of Social Studies in Health*. Sage Publications, London, 2000.
Mainetti JA. Embodiment, pathology, diagnosis. In: Peset JL and Gracia D (eds.) *The Ethics of Diagnosis*. Philosophy and Medicine Series, Vol. 40, Kluwer, Boston, MD, 1992.
May WF. Contending images of the healer in an era of turnstile medicine. In: Walter JK and Klein EP (eds.) *The Story of Bioethics: From Seminal Works to Contemporary Explorations*. Georgetown University Press, Washington, DC, 2003.
Nagel E. *The Structure of Science: Problems in the Logic of Scientific Explanation*. Harcourt, Brace and World, New York, 1961.
Owens J. Aristotelian ethics, medicine and the changing nature of man. In: Spicker S and Engelhardt HT (eds.) *Philosophical Medical Ethics—Its Nature and Significance*, vol. 3. D. Reidel, Dordrecht, 1977.
Pedroni J. Going off the gold standard—pain research beyond the randomized controlled trial. *Am. J. Pain Mangt.*, 2006; 16: 61–65.
Pellegrino ED. The anatomy of clinical judgments: some notes on right reason and right action. In: Engelhardt HT, Spicker S and Towers B (eds.) *Clinical Judgment: A Critical Appraisal*. D. Reidel, Dordrecht, 1979.
Pellegrino ED. The healing relationship: architectonics of clinical medicine. In: Shelp E (ed.) *The Clinical Encounter: The Moral Fabric of the Patient–Physician Relationship*. Philosophy and Medicine Series, vol. 4, D. Reidel, Dordrecht, 1983.

Pellegrino ED and Thomasma DC. *For the Patient's Good: The Restoration of Beneficence in Health Care.* Oxford University Press, New York, 1988.

Pellegrino ED and Thomasma DC. *The Virtues in Medical Practice.* Oxford University Press, New York, 1993.

Sadler JZ. Diagnosis/antidiagnosis. In: Radden J (ed.) *The Philosophy of Psychiatry: A Companion.* Oxford University Press, New York, 2004.

Sadler JZ. *Values and Psychiatric Diagnosis.* Oxford University Press, New York, 2005.

Svenaeus F. *The Hermeneutics of Medicine and the Phenomenology of Health: Steps Toward a Philosophy of Medical Practice.* Kluwer, Dordrecht, 2000.

Toulmin S. Concepts of function and mechanism in medicine and medical science (Hommage a Claude Bernard). In: Engelhardt HT and Spicker S (eds.) *Evaluation and Explanation in the Biomedical Sceinces.* Philosophy and Medicine Series, Vol. 1. D. Reidel, Dordrecht, 1975.

Wulff HR. *Rational Diagnosis and Treatment.* Blackwell, Oxford, 1976.

Index

A

Abnormal facial conditions demonstrated with infrared facial thermography, **20**-4–**20**-5
  carotid occlusal disease, assessing, **20**-4
  inferior alveolar nerve (IAN) deficit, assessing, **20**-4
  temporomandibular joint (TMJ) disorders, assessing, **20**-4
Active dynamic thermal IR-imaging (ADT IR-imaging), **7**-2–**7**-4, **7**-12, **7**-14
Advanced breast cancer
  digital high-resolution functional infrared imaging to monitor, **10**-14–**10**-20
Advanced thermal image processing, **12**-1–**12**-13
  classification, **12**-9–**12**-12
  histogram-based first order thermal signatures, **12**-3–**12**-5
  second order statistical parameters, **12**-5–**12**-7
  wavelet transformation, **12**-8–**12**-9
Allologous transplantation, **6**-15
Anabolism, **11**-3
Angiogenesis, **10**-7, **11**-3
Anisotropic scattering, **14**-3
Arteriovenous anastamoses (AVA), **6**-3
Artificial Neural Network (ANN), **12**-3, **12**-9, **16**-2
  advantage of, **16**-7
  as a screening tool, for infectious diseases outbreak, **16**-6–**16**-7
Asymmetry analysis
  breast cancer detection from thermal IR images by, **11**-1–**11**-14
  early detection of breast cancer, **11**-4
  human body and cancer cells, metabolic activity of, **11**-2–**11**-3; *see also* under Metabolism
  human body temperature measurement, **11**-2
Autologous transplantation, **6**-15
Automatic segmentation, **11**-4–**11**-8
  edge-based techniques, **11**-4
  experimental results, **11**-6–**11**-8
  Hough transform for edge linking, **11**-5–**11**-6
  region-based techniques, **11**-4
  segmentation based on feature boundaries, **11**-6
  threshold-based techniques, **11**-4
Automatic target recognition (ATR), **1**-6, **1**-7, **3**-24, **9**-17
Average correlation coefficients (ACC), **12**-3

B

Barnes thermograph, **10**-2
Bayes' theorem, **13**-4
  Bayesian segmentation of face, **13**-5
Beer's Lambert Law, **14**-3
Biologic heat flow equation, **7**-7
Biological tissue
  optical properties, **14**-3–**14**-5
  thermal properties of, **7**-3–**7**-6
Biomedical applications of fIR, **15**-1–**15**-20
  τ image technique
  quantifying the relevance and stage of disease with, **15**-7–**15**-11
  Raynaud's phenomenon and scleroderma, **15**-4–**15**-7
  skin temperature and metabolism during exercise, **15**-11–**15**-17
  varicocele, diagnosis and follow-up of the treatment, **15**-2–**15**-4
Biomedical dynamic thermal assessment, **8**-2–**8**-7
  cellular DTI methodology
  cancer effect on perfusion, **8**-5–**8**-6
  clinical applications, **8**-4
  early history, **8**-2–**8**-3
  'quantitative dynamic area telethermometry in medical diagnosis and management', **8**-3–**8**-6
Bio-statistical methods
  as a screening tool, for infectious diseases outbreak, **16**-9–**16**-12
  regression analysis, **16**-9–**16**-10
  ROC curve, **16**-10–**16**-12
Blackbody radiation, **5**-2
Blackbody source (BBS), **19**-3
Bolometer operation, **3**-6
Brachial plexus paresis, **17**-9

Breast, fIR imaging of,
10-1–**10**-30
  breast cancer detection
      demonstration projects
      (BCDDP) era,
      10-3–**10**-5
  mammography, **10**-4
  future considerations,
      10-24–**10**-28
  historical perspectives,
      10-2–**10**-7
  post-breast cancer detection
      demonstration projects
      era, **10**-5–**10**-7
  pre-breast cancer detection
      demonstration projects
      era, **10**-2–**10**-3
  Isard's work, **10**-2–**10**-3
  Ville Marie multi-disciplinary
      breast center
      experience, **10**-7–**10**-24
Breast, IR imaging of, **9**-1–**9**-22
  actual process of imaging, **9**-4
  breast cancer detection and
      demonstration project
      (BCDDP), **9**-13–**9**-15;
      see also under Breast
      cancer
  breast cancer detection,
      current status of,
      9-16–**9**-17
  in cancer detection, **9**-9–**9**-11
  fundamentals and standards
      in, **9**-2–**9**-9
    equipment considerations,
      9-3
    image interpretation,
      9-7–**9**-8
    laboratory and patient
      preparation
      protocols, **9**-3–**9**-4
    physics, **9**-2
    special tests, **9**-6–**9**-7
  future advancements in, **9**-17
  mammography and infrared
      imaging, **9**-15–**9**-16
  pathology and infrared
      imaging, correlation
      between, **9**-8–**9**-9
  positioning of the patient prior
      to imaging, **9**-4–**9**-6
  as a prognostic indicator,
      9-12–**9**-13
  as a risk indicator, **9**-11–**9**-12
Breast cancer
  breast cancer detection and
      demonstration project
      (BCDDP), **9**-13–**9**-15,
      10-3–**10**-5
    critical areas, **9**-15
    study design, **9**-14
    untrained personnel and
      protocol violations,
      9-14–**9**-15

  detection, from thermal
      infrared images by
      asymmetry analysis,
      11-1–**11**-14; *see also*
      under Asymmetry
      analysis
  early detection of, **10**-7–**10**-14
Breast cancer, IR technique for,
      1-3, **1**-5–**1**-7
  detection modalities approved
      by FDA, **1**-5
  early breast cancer detection
      method, **1**-5
  ideal characteristics for, **1**-5
  image processing and medical
      applications, **1**-6
  in United States, **1**-5–**1**-6
  website and database, **1**-6
    sensor technology, **1**-6
Bruce's scheme, **15**-12

C

CALIC, compression algorithm,
      23-4
Camera characterization,
      infrared, **4**-1–**4**-10
  cooled scanning systems, **4**-1
  cooled staring systems, **4**-1
  dimensional noise, **4**-3–**4**-5;
      see also 3D noise model
  dynamic range, **4**-6–**4**-8
  defined by linearity, **4**-7
  minimum resolvable
      temperature, **4**-8–**4**-9
  modulation transfer function
      (MTF), **4**-8–**4**-9
  noise equivalent temperature
      difference (NETD),
      4-5–**4**-6
  scanning and staring system
      designs, **4**-1
  spatial resolution, **4**-9
    pixel size, **4**-9
    of thermal imaging systems,
      1-11
  uncooled staring systems, **4**-1
Cancer research
  IR technique for, **1**-3
Cardiac surgery, **7**-22–**7**-25
  in vivo experiments on pigs,
      7-22–**7**-25
    thermal conductivity
      distribution in burn
      fields, **7**-23
    thermal transients of, **7**-23
Carotid occlusal disease,
      assessing, **20**-4
Carpal tunnel syndrome (CTS),
      6-4, **8**-15, **17**-8
Cascade image tube, **2**-3
Catabolism, **11**-3
Celsius scale, **2**-1

Chalcogenide glasses, **5**-13
Clinical thermometer, **2**-1
Complex regional pain syndrome
      (CRPS) evaluation,
      fIR in, **17**-9–**17**-11,
      18-1–**18**-26
  abnormal fIR studies, **18**-12
  acute CRPS I thermal
      signatures,
      18-14–**18**-18
  acute trauma (post-traumatic
      injury), **18**-12–**18**-13
  case studies, **18**-9–**18**-21
  C-fiber (small caliber
      nociceptive afferent
      excitation)
      mononeuropathy,
      18-14, **18**-15
  clinical implications and
      potential, **18**-19–**18**-21
  CRPS I, **18**-2
  detection, discernment, and
      diagnosis, **18**-3–**18**-4
  ethics and imperatives for
      evidence-based use of,
      18-3
  fIR thermal image signatures,
      interpretation of,
      18-10
  methodology, **18**-6–**18**-9
    description, **18**-6
    equipment, **18**-6
    historical context, **18**-6
    laboratory environment,
      18-7
    patient preprocedure
      protocol, **18**-7
    patient protocol, **18**-7
    patient selection–indication,
      18-7
    study protocol for fIR pain
      studies, **18**-8
  normal fIR thermal signatures,
      18-10–**18**-12
    cold-water autonomic
      functional stress test
      findings, **18**-12
    distal thermal gradient
      image pattern
      findings, **18**-10
    quantitative thermal
      emission, **18**-10
  overview, history, and
      contemporary issues,
      18-2–**18**-3
  three (3) specific fIR indices,
      methods for obtaining,
      18-8–**18**-9
    black–white distal thermal
      gradient imaging,
      18-9
    cold-water autonomic
      functional stress
      testing, **18**-9

Index

qualitative/quantitative side-to-side homologous computer-generated temperature views, **18**-8
Computerized laser scanning, **19**-11–**19**-15
   advantages, **19**-11
   disadvantages, **19**-12
   sequences during, **19**-13
Continuous wave (CW), **14**-5
Co-occurrence matrix, **12**-5–**12**-6
CRPS I, **18**-2
   acute CRPS I thermal signatures, **18**-14–**18**-18
   bilateral presentation, **18**-18–**18**-19
   in symptomatic limb, **18**-14–**18**-18
   chronic CRPS I, thermal signatures, **18**-19, **18**-20
   diagnosis, **18**-2
   pathophysiology of, **18**-4–**18**-5
     neurogenic inflammatory and central neural interactions, **18**-5
     putative genetic factors, **18**-5
     sympathetic neural involvement, **18**-4
Cutaneous circulation measurement techniques, **6**-5–**6**-7
Cutaneous temperature (Tc), **15**-11
CW techniques, **14**-5

D

Database thermal image, browsing of, **23**-9–**23**-13
   browsing, **23**-11–**23**-13
   features and similarity measure, **23**-9–**23**-10
   multidimensional scaling (MDS), **23**-10–**23**-11
Deep inferior epigastric perforator (DIEP), **6**-15
Dentistry, infrared imaging applied to, **20**-1–**20**-8
   abnormal facial conditions, **20**-4–**20**-5
   body temperature measurements, types, **20**-2–**20**-3
   normal infrared facial thermography, **20**-3
   skin and skin-surface temperature measurement, **20**-2

temperature, importance of, **20**-1–**20**-2
thermography, diagnostic applications of, **20**-3
Dermatology
   dermatome patterns of horses and other animal species, **21**-3–**21**-4
   laser applications in, **19**-6–**19**-8
Detector materials, **3**-7–**3**-12
   $Hg_{1-x}Cd_xTe$ alloys, **3**-7–**3**-8
   InSb, **3**-7
     crystals of InSb, **3**-7
     photovoltaic InSb, **3**-7
   quantum well infrared photodetectors (QWIPs), **3**-7–**3**-8
   uncooled bolometers, **3**-7
Detector readouts, **3**-12–**3**-14
   hybrid detector array structure, **3**-12
   for photon detectors, **3**-12–**3**-13
   readout evolution, **3**-13–**3**-14
   rolling frame mode, **3**-13
   snapshot mode, **3**-13
   thermal detector readouts, **3**-13
Digital high-resolution functional infrared imaging to monitor advanced breast cancer, **10**-14–**10**-20
Digital Imaging and Communications in Medicine (DICOM), **23**-2–**23**-3
Digital mammography, **10**-25
   Digital Mammographic Imaging Screening Trial (DMIST), **9**-15
Direct problems, **7**-7
Disease processes, functional monitoring of
   infrared thermal monitoring, **14**-16–**14**-28
     clinical study, **14**-19–**14**-23
     emissivity corrected temperature, **14**-16–**14**-17
     temperature calibration, **14**-17–**14**-19
   IR imaging for, **14**-1–**14**-28
   NIR quantitative imaging, **14**-2–**14**-15
Doppler measurement, **6**-6
DTA experimentation (1997–2001), **8**-7–**8**-11
   early DTA experimentation, **8**-7
   preliminary DTA findings on melanoma and diabetes, **8**-10–**8**-11

research at Millard Fillmore hospital at Buffalo, **8**-7–**8**-10
   limitations, **8**-9–**8**-10
   methodology of assessment, **8**-8–**8**-9
   physiological considerations and their implications, **8**-10
   statistical analysis and findings, **8**-9
DTA studies (2000–2005), **8**-11–**8**-16
   brain function and brain malignancies study, **8**-12–**8**-13
   on complex regional pain syndrome, **8**-15
   in diabetes mellitus study, **8**-15
   to diagnose upper extremity musculoskeletal disorders, **8**-15
   intraoperative DTI in surgical procedures, **8**-13–**8**-14
   cardiac and transplant surgery, **8**-14
   reconstructive and vascular surgery, **8**-14
   malignancy, detection of and treatment of, **8**-11–**8**-12
   to monitor reperfusion of tissues, **8**-15
   in ophthalmology, **8**-15
DuBois formula, **6**-6
Dyes, **6**-5
Dynamic infrared imaging (DIRI), **8**-1–**8**-2
Dynamic range, of thermal imaging systems, **1**-8–**1**-9
Dynamic thermal assessment (DTA), **8**-1–**8**-23
   biomedical dynamic thermal assessment, **8**-2–**8**-7
   DTA experimentation (1997–2001), **8**-7–**8**-11
   recent DTA studies (2000–2005), **8**-11–**8**-16; see also under DTA studies
Dynamic thermography, **6**-14

E

Edge-based techniques, **11**-4–**11**-5
Edges, **11**-5
Education and training, ethical obligations for, **24**-5–**24**-6
Electronic cooling systems, **22**-4
Emissivity corrected temperature, **14**-16–**14**-17

Energized systems, **19**-2–**19**-3
Enthesopathies, thermal imaging, **17**-4–**17**-6
   fibromyalgia, **17**-6
   Golfer elbow, **17**-4–**17**-5
   periarthropathia of the shoulder, **17**-5–**17**-6
   tennis elbow, **17**-4
Entropy, **12**-4, **12**-7
Ethical obligations in IR imaging research and practice, **24**-1–**24**-8
   clinical medicine, domains of knowledge in, **24**-3–**24**-5
   need for continuing and progressive research, **24**-2–**24**-3
   education and training, ethical obligations for, **24**-5–**24**-6
   fIR contribution to diagnostic value(s) detection, **24**-5–**24**-6
   perspective on, **24**-1–**24**-2
   role of policy, **24**-6
Evans Blue Dye to, **6**-5

F

Face recognition in the thermal infrared spectrum, **13**-1–**13**-16
   architecture of, **13**-1
   experimental results, **13**-11–**13**-14
      frontal pose and arbitrary pose experiments, **13**-12–**13**-14
      low permanence problem, **13**-12
   facial skin region, segmentation, **13**-6
   feature extraction, **13**-3–**13**-9
      algorithm, architecture, **13**-3
      extraction of TMPs, **13**-8–**13**-9; see also under Thermal Minutia Points
   face segmentation, **13**-3–**13**-6
   goal of, **13**-1
   matching, **13**-9–**13**-11
      facial pose, estimation, **13**-9–**13**-10
   phases of, **13**-1
      off-line phase, **13**-2
      on-line phase, **13**-2–**13**-3
   superficial blood vessels, **13**-3
      segmentation of, **13**-7–**13**-8

      vascular network extraction, **13**-8
   Feature extraction, **13**-3–**13**-9; see also under Face recognition
      on segmented images, **11**-11
      entropy, **11**-11
      joint entropy, **11**-11
      moments of the intensity image, **11**-11
      peak pixel intensity of the correlated image, **11**-11
Febrile thermogram, **16**-4–**16**-8
Fibromyalgia, thermal imaging, **17**-6
'First cluster ratio' (FCR), **8**-9
Florescin, **6**-5
Fluorescence, **14**-4
f/number, **5**-9
Focal plane array (FPA), **4**-3, **5**-3
Forward Looking InfraRed (FLIR) systems, **2**-3
Functional infrared imaging (fIR)
   biomedical applications of, **15**-1–**15**-20; see also under Biomedical applications
   of the breast, **10**-1–**10**-30; see also under Breast
   in complex regional pain syndrome evaluation, **18**-1–**18**-26; see also under Complex regional pain syndrome
Functional monitoring of disease processes
   IR imaging for, **14**-1–**14**-28; see also under Disease processes

G

Gain detector, **5**-6–**5**-9
   gain calculation
      high temperature, **5**-8
      low temperature, **5**-8
      processed using computed gain, **5**-8
      processed using uniform gain, **5**-8
   nonuniformity calibration, **5**-6–**5**-7
   operational considerations, **5**-7–**5**-8
Galileo's experiments, **2**-1
Germanium, **5**-13
Golfer elbow, thermal imaging, **17**-4–**17**-5

H

Heat transfer
   modeling equations for microcirculation, **6**-4–**6**-5
   by radiation, **2**-2
Homeostasis, **2**-2
Horner's syndrome, **21**-4
Hough transform for edge linking, **11**-5–**11**-6
Human body
   asymmetry identification; see also Feature extraction
      using supervised learning based on feature extraction, **11**-11–**11**-12
      by unsupervised learning, **11**-8–**11**-11
   in breast cancer detection, **11**-4–**11**-12
      automatic segmentation, **11**-4–**11**-8
   and cancer cells, metabolic activity of, **11**-2–**11**-3; see also under Metabolism
   temperature measurement, **11**-2
Human-in-the-loop (HITL) performance, **4**-2
Hyperfocal distance (HFD), **5**-11

I

τ Image technique
   quantifying the relevance and stage of disease with, **15**-7–**15**-11
   reliability and value of, **15**-9
Indocyanine green (ICG), **6**-5
Infectious diseases outbreak, fever mass screening tool for, **16**-1–**16**-19
   designed integrated approach, **16**-12–**16**-14
      advanced integrated technique (PR+ANN RBFN+ROC), **16**-12, **16**-14–**16**-16
      conventional bio-statistical technique (LR+ROC), **16**-12–**16**-14, **16**-16–**16**-18
   for febrile and nonfebrile thermograms, **16**-13
   methodology, **16**-3–**16**-12
      bio-statistical methods, **16**-9–**16**-12
      data acquisition, **16**-3–**16**-6

Index

radial basis function network, **16**-7–**16**-9
thermal images, processing, **16**-6
Inferior alveolar nerve (IAN) deficit, assessing, **20**-4
Inflammation, **17**-2–**17**-3
Infrared camera and optics for medical applications, **5**-1–**5**-14
  gain detector, **5**-6–**5**-9
  infrared imaging, major components, **5**-3
    background, **5**-3: major challenges accompanying, **5**-3
    object of interest, **5**-3
  infrared optical considerations, **5**-8–**5**-9
    f/number, **5**-9
    resolution, **5**-8–**5**-9
  infrared sensor calibration, **5**-4–**5**-5
  optical materials for
    chalcogenide glasses, **5**-13
    coatings, **5**-13
    germanium, **5**-13
    reflective optics, **5**-13–**5**-14
    selecting, **5**-11–**5**-14
    silicon, **5**-13
    special considerations, **5**-12–**5**-13
    ZnS, **5**-13
  spectral requirement, **5**-10–**5**-11
    depth of field (DOF), **5**-10–**5**-11
    first order parameters resolution, **5**-10
Infrared detectors and detector arrays, **3**-1–**3**-26
  detector materials, **3**-7–**3**-12
  detector readouts, **3**-12–**3**-14
  photon (or quantum) detectors, **3**-1
  technical challenges for, **3**-14–**3**-24
    cost challenges, **3**-19
    detector readout challenges, **3**-17
    electronics challenges, **3**-16–**3**-17
    optics challenges, **3**-17–**3**-18
    performance challenges, **3**-21–**3**-24
    sensor format and packaging issues, **3**-19–**3**-20
    temperature cycling fatigue, **3**-20–**3**-21
    third-generation cooled imagers, challenges for, **3**-18–**3**-24

    uncooled infrared detector challenges, **3**-14–**3**-16
  thermal detectors, **3**-1
Infrared (IR) imaging
  applied to dentistry, **20**-1–**20**-8; *see also* under Dentistry
  breast imaging, **9**-1–**9**-22; *see also* under Breast
  in medicine, *see* Medical infrared imaging
  in veterinary medicine, **21**-1–**21**-8; *see also* Veterinary medicine
Infrared-nondestructive testing (IR-NDT), **7**-2
Infrared sensor calibration, **5**-4–**5**-5
Injury, sports medicine injury, **6**-15–**6**-16
Instantaneous field of view (IFOV), **5**-8
Integrated artificial intelligence with bio-statistical approach
  in thermogram analysis, **16**-1–**16**-19; *see also* under Infectious diseases outbreak
Isotropic scattering, **14**-4

J

Javelin cooler coefficient, **3**-24
Jet Propulsion Laboratory (JPL), **8**-7
Johnson noise term, **3**-2, **3**-4
Jones, **3**-3
JPEG2000, compression algorithm, **23**-4
JPEG-LS, compression algorithm, **23**-3

K

Kaposi sarcoma, **1**-4
  infrared thermal monitoring of, **14**-19–**14**-23
Karhunen-Loeve transform, **12**-1
k-means algorithm, **11**-8, **16**-9
Kronecker delta, **12**-3
Kruskals' stress formula, **23**-11
Kurtosis, **11**-11, **12**-4

L

Laser tissue interactions, **19**-8–**19**-9
  laser light passage within skin layers, **19**-8

  laser therapy during and after treatment, characteristics of, **19**-8
'Lie detection', **8**-3
Linear discriminant analysis (LDA), **12**-3
Linear region of interest (LROI), **19**-5–**19**-7
Linear regression (LR), **16**-2
Liquid crystal sensors for temperature, **2**-2
Liquid crystal thermography (LCT), **9**-8
locally advanced breast cancer (LABC), **10**-14
Long wavelength infrared (LWIR) imaging, **1**-10, **3**-7, **4**-2
Lossless JPEG, compression algorithm, **23**-3

M

Mahalanobis distance, **23**-11
Malignancy
  detection of and treatment of, **8**-11–**8**-12
Mammography
  in cancer detection, **10**-4
  and infrared imaging, **9**-15–**9**-16
  versus IR imaging in early breast cancer detection, **11**-4
Matching, in face recognition, **13**-9–**13**-11
Maxwell's equations, **14**-3
Mean, **11**-11
Medical infrared imaging
  advances in, **1**-1–**1**-13
  applications and methods, **1**-2
  for breast screening, **1**-3; *see also* under Breast cancer
  important issues, **1**-1
  standard procedures, **22**-1–**22**-14
  thermal imaging, **22**-2–**22**-3
  thermal imaging systems, **1**-7–**1**-12
  worldwide use of, **1**-2–**1**-5
    Austria, **1**-4
    Canada, **1**-2
    China, **1**-3
    Germany, **1**-4
    Italy, **1**-5
    Japan, **1**-4
    Korea, **1**-4
    Poland, **1**-4
    United Kingdom, **1**-4
    United States of America, **1**-2

Medical thermograms
  compression of, **23**-3–**23**-6
    compression algorithms, **23**-3–**23**-4
    compression results, **23**-4–**23**-6
    image dataset, **23**-3
  storage and retrieval of, **23**-1–**23**-15; *see also* under Storage and retrieval
Medium wavelength infrared (MWIR) imaging, **1**-10, **3**-7
Mercury–cadmium–telluride (HgCdTe) element, **18**-6
Metabolism
  of human body and cancer cells, **11**-2–**11**-3
    anabolism, **11**-3
    catabolism, **11**-3
Microencapsulation, **2**-2
Microvascular density (MVD), **9**-8
Mie scattering, **14**-3, **14**-22
Minimum detectable temperature difference (MDTD), **4**-8
Minimum resolvable temperature difference (MRTD), **4**-2, **4**-8
Modulation transfer function (MTF), **4**-2, **4**-8–**4**-9, **5**-13–**5**-14
Multidimensional scaling (MDS), **23**-10–**23**-11
  metric MDS, **23**-10
  nonmetric MDS, **23**-10
Muscle spasm and injury, thermal imaging, **17**-4
Muscle tissue, thermal properties of, **7**-5
Musculoskeletal injuries, **21**-5–**21**-6
  osteoarthritis, **21**-5

N

Nearest neighbor classification (NNC), **12**-3
Near-infrared imaging (NIR), **14**-1–**14**-15; *see also* under NIR quantitative imaging
Nerve entrapment, **17**-6–**17**-9
Neural network (NN), **16**-2
Neurectomies, **21**-4
NIR quantitative imaging of deep tissue structure, **14**-2–**14**-15
  measurable quantities and experimental techniques, **14**-5–**14**-6
  optical properties of biological tissue, **14**-3–**14**-5; *see also* under Optical properties
  photon migration in tissue, models, **14**-6–**14**-9
  quantitative fluorescence imaging and spectroscopy, **14**-12–**14**-15
Nitris oxide (NO)
  in cancer biology, **8**-5
  as chemical messenger, **8**-4–**8**-5
  in infrared breast imaging, **9**-8
  NO–fat hypothesis, **8**-10
Noise equivalent temperature difference (NETD), **3**-14, **4**-2, **4**-5–**4**-6, **5**-3
3D noise model, **4**-3
  data cube for, **4**-4
  3D noise components, **4**-4–**4**-5
Nonfebrile thermogram, **16**-4–**16**-8
Normal infrared facial thermography, **20**-3

O

Objective thermography, **6**-7–**6**-18
  dynamic IR-thermography to highlight perforating vessels, **6**-14–**6**-15
  heat transport in the skin of hand, **6**-8
  infrared-thermography and laser Doppler mapping of skin blood flow, **6**-12–**6**-14
  median nerve block in the hand, **6**-11–**6**-12
  reduced blood flow, effect of, **6**-8–**6**-11
  sports medicine injury, **6**-15–**6**-16
  transplanted tissue, reperfusion of, **6**-15
Optical properties of biological tissue, **14**-3–**14**-5
  light propagation, **14**-3
  light–tissue interactions, **14**-3
  of tumor and background breast tissue, **14**-12
  wave propagation, **14**-3
Osteoarthritis, **21**-5

P

Paget's disease of bone, thermal imaging, **17**-3–**17**-4
Palomo's technique, **15**-4
Parabolic Regression (PR), **16**-2
Pathology and infrared imaging, correlation between, **9**-8–**9**-9
Pennes model, **6**-4
Performance challenges, of infrared detectors, **3**-21–**3**-24
  dynamic range and sensitivity constraints, **3**-21–**3**-23
  higher operating temperature, **3**-24
  high frame rate operation, **3**-23–**3**-24
  Javelin cooler coefficient of performance vs. temperature, **3**-24
Periarthropathia of the shoulder, thermal imaging, **17**-5–**17**-6
Peripheral nerves, thermal imaging, **17**-6–**17**-9
  nerve entrapment, **17**-6–**17**-9
    brachial plexus paresis, **17**-9
    carpal tunnel syndrome, **17**-8
    facial nerve, **17**-9
    peripheral nerve paresis, **17**-9
    peroneal nerve, **17**-9
    radiculopathy, **17**-7
    thoracic outlet syndrome, **17**-7–**17**-8
Peripheral neurovascular thermography, **21**-4–**21**-5
  Horner's syndrome, **21**-4
  neurectomies, **21**-4
  vascular injuries, **21**-5
Peroneal nerve, **17**-9
Photon detectors, **3**-1–**3**-5
  energy of photons, **3**-1
  photoconductive detector geometry, **3**-2
    current–voltage characteristics of, **3**-2
  photoconductive detectors, **3**-2
    noise in, **3**-2
    response of, **3**-2
  photovoltaic detectors, **3**-2–**3**-5
    current–voltage characteristics of, **3**-4
    mechanism of, **3**-3
    noise in, **3**-4
    structure, **3**-3
Photon generation-recombination term, **3**-2, **3**-4
Photon migration in tissue, models, **14**-6–**14**-9; *see also* Random Walk Theory (RWT)
  transport equation, **14**-6
Phronesis, **24**-4–**24**-5
Pixel count, **1**-9
Pixel size, **4**-9

Planck's blackbody law, **5**-1–**5**-2, **9**-3
Plethysmography, **6**-5–**6**-6
   venous occlusion plethysmography (VOP), **6**-5–**6**-6
PNG, compression algorithm, **23**-4
Polaroid photography, **2**-2
Pontamine Sky Blue dyes, **6**-5
Pre-operative chemohormonotherapy-induced changes, monitoring, **10**-14–**10**-20
Pre-operative or neo-adjuvant chemotherapy (PCT), **10**-15–**10**-16
Principal component analysis (PCA), **12**-1, **13**-9, **23**-11
Pulsed thermography (PT), **7**-12
   hot spots and cold spots images, **7**-13
   maximal thermal contrast index, **7**-13
   normalized differential PT index (NDPTI), **7**-13
Pulse phase thermography (PPT), **7**-12, **7**-14
   calculation of synthetic pictures in, **7**-16
'Pyroscan', **2**-2

Q

Quantitative active dynamic thermal IR-imaging and thermal tomography
   biological tissues, thermal properties of, **7**-3–**7**-6; *see also* Thermal tissue properties
   data and image processing, procedures of, **7**-12–**7**-17
   experiments and applications, **7**-17–**7**-25
      cardiac surgery, **7**-22–**7**-25
      in vivo experiments on animals, **7**-18
      location of experimental burns, **7**-18
      organization of experiments, **7**-17–**7**-19
      skin burns, **7**-19–**7**-22; *see also* under Skin
   measurement equipment, **7**-11–**7**-12
      fast data acquisition system, **7**-11
      IR-camera, **7**-11
      set of excitation sources with a synchronized driving unit, **7**-11
   measurement procedures, **7**-8–**7**-10
      ADT and TT instrumentation, **7**-9
      data acquisition system (DAS), **7**-9
      nondestructive evaluation of defects, **7**-10
      registration process in, **7**-9–**7**-10
   in medical diagnostics, **7**-1–**7**-29
   thermal models and equivalent/synthetic parameters, **7**-7–**7**-8
   thermal tomography (TT), **7**-2–**7**-3
Quantitative fluorescence imaging and spectroscopy, **14**-12–**14**-15
Quantum well infrared photodetectors (QWIPs), **3**-7–**3**-9, **8**-7, **19**-3
   representative spectral response of, **3**-10
Query by example (QBE) method, **23**-8

R

Radial Basis Function Network (RBFN), **16**-2, **16**-7–**16**-9
   hidden layer, **16**-7
   input layer, **16**-7
   output layer, **16**-7
Radiculopathy, **17**-7
Random Walk Theory (RWT), **14**-7–**14**-9
   applied to quantitative spectroscopy of the breast, **14**-9–**14**-12
Rayleigh limit, **5**-11
Raynaud's phenomenon, **15**-4–**15**-7
Readout integrated circuit (ROIC), **4**-2
Readouts, detector, *see* Detector readouts
Receiver Operating Characteristics (ROC), **16**-2
'Reflex sympathetic dystrophy', **8**-3
Region-based techniques, **11**-4–**11**-5
Regression analysis, **16**-9–**16**-10
Research and practice, in IR imaging, **24**-1–**24**-8; *see also* under Ethical obligations
Resolution, **5**-8–**5**-9

and sensitivity, of thermal imaging systems, **1**-9
Retrieval of thermograms, **23**-6–**23**-13
   content-based retrieval, **23**-6–**23**-9
   comparison with database of normals, **23**-8
   moment invariant features, **23**-6–**23**-7
   retrieval through query by example, **23**-8
   similarity metric, **23**-8
   thermal image database, browsing of, **23**-9–**23**-13; *see also* under Data base
RF electrosurgery, **19**-4–**19**-5
ROC curve, **16**-10–**16**-12
   basic mathematical formulae for, **16**-11
   important terminology for, **16**-11
Rudimentary hand-held thermopile, **10**-2

S

Scleroderma, **15**-4–**15**-7
Segmentation, *see* Automatic segmentation
Sensitivity, **4**-5
Sensor technology for medical applications, **1**-6
Severe acute respiratory syndrome (SARS), **16**-2
Signal PRocessing In The Element (Sprite) detector, **2**-4
Silicon, **5**-13
Single band imagers, of thermal imaging systems, **1**-10
Sjøgren's Syndrome (SS), **14**-12
Skeletal and neuromuscular diseases, thermal imaging in, **17**-1–**17**-15
   complex regional pain syndrome (CRPS), **17**-9–**17**-11
   inflammation, **17**-2–**17**-3
   Paget's disease of bone, **17**-3–**17**-4
   peripheral nerves, **17**-6–**17**-9
   soft tissue rheumatism, **17**-4–**17**-6
   technique, **17**-11
      clinical examination, **17**-11
      room temperature, **17**-11
Skewness, **11**-11, **12**-4
Skin
   anatomy, **7**-19
   equivalent thermo-electric model, **7**-19

Skin (continued)
    three-layer structural model, 7-19
    blood flow, **6**-2
    skin blood flow for heat transfers, regulation, 6-3–**6**-4
    skin burns, 7-19–**7**-22
        in vivo experiments on pigs, 7-19–**7**-22
        relative thickness of, 7-20
    and skin-surface temperature measurement, **20**-2
    skin temperature and metabolism during exercise, **15**-11–**15**-17
        A/τ during incremental load and recovery phases, 15-14
        Tav variation, **15**-14–**15**-16
    skin tissue, nutritive needs of, **6**-2
    thermal properties in response to stress, **6**-2–**6**-3
Soft tissue rheumatism, **17**-4–**17**-6
    enthesopathies, **17**-4–**17**-6
    muscle spasm and injury, **17**-4
    sprains and strains, **17**-4
Spatial resolution, **4**-9
Sports medicine injury, **6**-15–**6**-16
Sprains and strains, thermal imaging, **17**-4
Stains, **6**-5
Static infrared (IR) thermal imaging, **7**-1
Static thermal imaging, **8**-1
Stefan–Boltzmann Law, **9**-2
Stimulated Raman scattering, **14**-6
Storage and retrieval of medical thermograms, **23**-1–**23**-15
    retrieval of thermograms, **23**-6–**23**-13
    standardized thermogram format, need for, **23**-2–**23**-3
Support Vector Machine (SVM), **13**-9
Surgery, thermal imaging in, **19**-1–**19**-18
    calibration, **19**-3–**19**-4
    computerized laser scanning, **19**-11–**19**-15
    dermatology, laser applications in, **19**-6–**19**-8
    during energized surgery, **19**-4–**19**-6
        collateral damage, analysis, **19**-5–**19**-6
        RF electrosurgery, **19**-4–**19**-5

    energized systems, **19**-2–**19**-3
    laser tissue interactions, **19**-8–**19**-9
    optimizing laser therapies, **19**-9–**19**-11
    thermographic results of laser positioning, **19**-11
System intensity transfer function (SITF), **4**-5

T

Talytherm, **2**-4
Temperature
    body temperature measurements, types, **20**-2–**20**-3
    body core temperature, **20**-2
    body surface temperature, **20**-2
    importance of, **20**-1–**20**-2
    skin and skin-surface temperature measurement, **20**-2
Temporal Point Spread Function (TPSF), **14**-6
Temporomandibular joint (TMJ) disorders, assessing, **20**-4
Tendovaginitis, **17**-4
Tennis elbow, thermal imaging, **17**-4
Testes and scrotum in mammalian species, **21**-6
'Therapeutic window', **14**-3
Thermal detectors, **3**-1, **3**-6–**3**-7
    sensitivity of, **3**-6
    thermal detector readouts, **3**-13
Thermal diffusivity, **7**-4
Thermal generation-recombination term, **3**-2, **3**-4
Thermal imaging, in medicine/medical applications, **1**-7–**1**-12; *see also* Medical Thermograms
    accuracy, **22**-2
    applications and image formats, **1**-8
    background, **1**-8
    calibration, **1**-9–**1**-10
        external calibration, **1**-10
        internal calibration, **1**-10
    camera technology, **1**-11
        beginning, **1**-11–**1**-12
    definition of, **22**-2–**22**-3
    dynamic range, **1**-8–**1**-9
    for medical R&D, **1**-8
    precision, **22**-2–**22**-3
    resolution and sensitivity, **1**-9
        good sensitivity, **1**-9
        modest sensitivity, **1**-9

    spatial resolution, **1**-9
    responsiveness, **22**-3
    single band imagers, **1**-10
    in skeletal and neuromuscular diseases, **17**-1–**17**-15; *see also* under Skeletal and neuromuscular diseases
    sources of variability of, **22**-3–**22**-9
        camera initialization, **22**-4
        camera systems, standards, and calibration, **22**-3–**22**-4
        image analysis, **22**-8
        image exchange, **22**-8
        image presentation, **22**-9
        image processing, **22**-8
        imaging system, **22**-3–**22**-4
        information protocols and resources, **22**-6–**22**-8
        mounting the imager, **22**-4
        object or subject, **22**-3
        patient position and image capture, **22**-4–**22**-6
        temperature reference, **22**-4
    in surgery, **19**-1–**19**-18; *see also* under Surgery
    thermal image processing; *see also* Advanced thermal image processing
Thermal infrared spectrum
    face recognition in, **13**-1–**13**-16; *see also* under Face recognition
Thermal Minutia Points (TMPs)
    extraction of, **13**-8–**13**-9
    matching of, **13**-10–**13**-11
        global minutiae matching algorithms, **13**-10
        local minutiae matching algorithms, **13**-10
Thermal models and equivalent/synthetic parameters, **7**-7–**7**-8
    explicit method, **7**-8
    implicit method, **7**-8
Thermal signals, physiology of, **6**-1–**6**-20
    cutaneous circulation measurement techniques, **6**-5–**6**-7
    clearance measurement, **6**-6
    Doppler measurement, **6**-6
    dyes and stains, **6**-5
    measurement techniques, **6**-7
    plethysmography, **6**-5–**6**-6
    procedures and techniques, **6**-5
    thermal skin measurement, **6**-6–**6**-7

Index

objective thermography, **6**-7–**6**-18
heat transfer modeling equations for microcirculation, **6**-4–**6**-5
skin thermal properties in response to stress, **6**-2–**6**-3; *see also* under Skin
Thermal skin measurement, **6**-6–**6**-7
Thermal time constant, **3**-15
Thermal tissue properties
   for the equivalent three-component model, **7**-6
   taken *in vitro*, mean values of, **7**-6
   temperature dependence of, **7**-5
Thermal tomography (TT), **7**-2–**7**-4, **7**-14–**7**-17
   3-parameter model, **7**-15
   5-parameter model, **7**-15
Thermistor, **6**-7
Thermograms, **2**-2; *see also* Medical thermograms
   analysis
      integrated artificial intelligence with bio-statistical approach in, **16**-1–**16**-19; *see also* under Infectious diseases outbreak
   diagnostic applications of, **20**-3
   John Herschel's thermogram, **2**-2
Thermometry and thermal imaging; *see also* Thermograms
   computer technology in, **2**-3

   historical development of, **2**-1–**2**-5
   thermal index, **2**-4
   uncooled bolometer arrays, **2**-4
Thoracic outlet syndrome (TOS), **17**-7–**17**-8
Three-dimensional (3D) noise model, **4**-2
Threshold-based techniques, **11**-4–**11**-5
   hysteresis thresholding, **11**-5
Time-domain techniques, **14**-5
Time-of-flight (TOF), **14**-5, **14**-10
Tomography, **7**-2–**7**-3
Transport equation, **14**-6
Tricore method, **9**-7

U

Uncooled bolometers, **3**-7
Uncooled infrared detector challenges, **3**-14–**3**-16

V

Variance, **11**-11
Varicocele, diagnosis and follow-up of the treatment, **15**-2–**15**-4
Vascular injuries, **21**-5
Vascularization, **11**-3
Vasodilator system, **6**-3–**6**-4
Veterinary medicine, IR imaging in, **21**-1–**21**-8
   dermatome patterns of horses and other animal species, **21**-3–**21**-4
   historical perspective, **21**-1–**21**-2
   musculoskeletal injuries, **21**-5–**21**-6

   peripheral neurovascular thermography, **21**-4–**21**-5
   standards for reliable thermograms, **21**-2–**21**-3
   testes and scrotum in mammalian species, **21**-6
Ville Marie multi-disciplinary breast center
   breast cancer detection and monitoring, with high-resolution digital infrared imaging for, **10**-7–**10**-24
   early detection of breast cancer, **10**-7–**10**-14
   clinical and multi-imaging breast cancer detection strategy, **10**-8
   Ville Marie IR grading scale, **10**-10
   modified, **10**-20

W

Wavefront coding, **5**-11
Wavelet transformation, **12**-8–**12**-9
Wein's Law, **5**-2, **9**-3, **19**-3

X

X-ray mammography, in early breast cancer detection, **11**-4

Z

ZnS, **5**-13

FIGURE 1.1 An application of IR technique for breast screening: (a) healthy and (b) pathological breast. (Courtesy: Prof. Reinhold Berz, MD. Informatics Germany.)

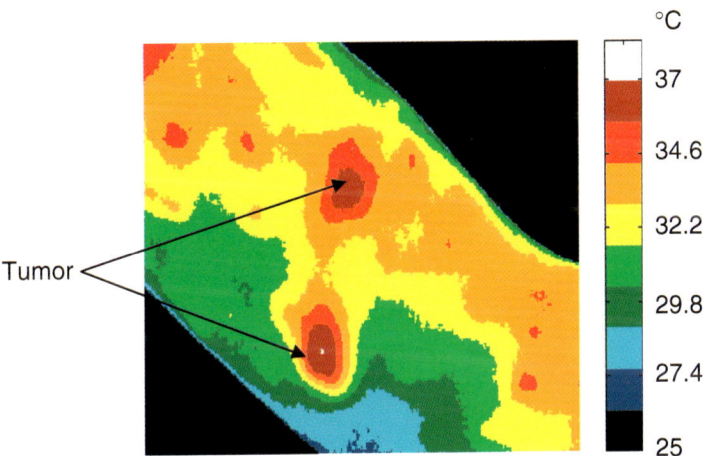

FIGURE 1.2 An application of IR technique for cancer research. (From Hassan, M., et al., 2004. *Technology in Cancer Research and Treatment*, 3, 451–457. With permission.)

FIGURE 6.1 (a) A Thermogram of a healthy 52-year-old male subject in a cold environment (ca. 15°C; left panel) and in a warm environment (ca. 25°C; right panel). In the cold environment arteriovenous anastomoses in the nose and the auricle region of the ears are closed, resulting in low skin temperatures at these sites. Also note reduced blood flow in the cheeks but not on the forehead, where the blood vessels in the skin are unable to vasoconstrict. (b) Efficiency of skin blood flow as a heat transporter. The photograph in the upper left panel shows a rubber mat being heated with a water-filtered infrared-A irradiator at high intensity (400 mW/cm^2) for a period of 20 min. In the lower panel the time course of surface temperature of the mat at five selected spots as measured by an IR-camera is given. During the last 10 min of the 20-min heating period, the left hand of a healthy 54-year-old male subject was placed on the mat. Note that skin surface temperature of the hand remains below 39°C.

(a)

30 min equilibration in cool environment (20°C, 30% rh)

30 min equilibration in warm environment (41°C, 30% rh)

Range of temperature (°C) within regions at two climatic conditions.

	Anterior torso	Posterior torso	Anterior arms	Posterior arms	Palmer hands	Dorsal hands
Cool 20°C	5.0	5.1	6.3	4.5	5.2	4.0
Warm 41°C	3.0	3.2	3.2	3.6	4.0	3.5

(b)

FIGURE 6.2 (a) A thermoregulatory response of the torso when exposed to a cool or warm environment. Note the heterogeneous temperature distribution in the cool environment as opposed to the more homogeneous temperature distribution in the warm environment. Different colors represent different temperatures. One might recognize the difficulty related to choosing one point (thermocouple data) as the reference value in a region. (b) Skin heating with and without intact circulation in a 65-year-old healthy male subject. The two panels on the right show the time course of 6 selected measuring sites (4 spot measurements and 2 area measurements) of skin temperatures as determined by IR-thermography before, during, and after a period in which the skin surface on the back of the left hand was heated with a water-filtered infrared-A irradiator at high intensity (400 mW/cm^2) in two separate experiments. The results shown in the upper right panel were performed under a situation with a normal intact blood circulation, while the results shown in the lower left panel were made during total occlusion of circulation in the right arm by means of an inflated pressure cuff placed around the upper arm. The time of occlusion is indicated. The IR-thermogram on the left was taken just prior to the end of the heating period in the experiment described in the upper panel. The location of the temperature measurement sites on the hand (4 spot measurements [Spot 1 to Spot 4] and the average temperature within a circle [Areas 5 and 6]) are indicated on the thermogram.

FIGURE 6.3 (a) The distribution of cutaneous nerves to the hand. (b) IR-thermogram of a 40-year-old female patient following a successful nerve block of the left median nerve. (c) and (d) IR-thermograms of the hands of a 36-year-old female patient whose left wrist (middle of the red circle) was punctured with a sharp object resulting in partial nerve damage (motor and sensory loss). The strong vasodilatory response resulting from partially severed nerves can be easily seen.

FIGURE 6.4 IR-thermograms, temperature profiles, scanning laser doppler (SLD) scans, and blood flow profiles (perfusion units PU) of the abdominal area of a 44-year-old healthy female subject before (a), immediately after (b), and 5 min (c), 10 min (d) and 20 min (e) after a 20 min heating of the right side of the abdomen with a water-filtered infrared-A irradiation lamp. The blue horizontal lines in the IR-thermograms indicate the position of the temperature profiles. The red horizontal lines in the SLD scans indicate the position of the blood flow profiles. In IR-thermogram (b) the white color indicates skin temperatures greater than 36°C.

FIGURE 6.5 Abdominal cooling in a 32-year-old female patient prior to breast reconstruction surgery. In this procedure skin and fat tissue from the abdominal area was used to reconstruct a new breast. The localization of suitable perforating vessels for reconnection to the mammary artery is an important part of the surgical procedure. In this sequence of thermograms the patient was first subjected to a mild cooling of the abdominal skin (2 min fan cooling). IR-thermograms of the skin over the entire abdominal area were taken prior to, immediately after, and at various time intervals during the recovery period following the cooling period. To help highlight the perforating vessels, an outline function has been employed in which all skin areas having a temperature greater than 32.5°C are enclosed in solid lines.

FIGURE 6.6 Infrared thermal images of an abdominal skin flap during breast reconstruction surgery. The sequence of IR-thermal images demonstrates the return of heat to the excised skin flap following reestablishing its blood supply (anastomizing of a mammary artery and vein to a single branch of the deep inferior epigastric artery and a concomitant vein). Prior to this procedure the excised skin flap had been without a blood supply for about 50 min and consequently cooled down. The photograph in the upper left panel shows the skin flap in position on the chest wall prior to being shaped into a new breast.

FIGURE 6.7 An American football player who suffered a helmet impact to the right shoulder (left side of image). The athlete was unable to flex his arm above shoulder level. Note the asymmetrical torso pattern in the posterior torso.

FIGURE 7.13 Classical thermogram (a) and PT normalized differential thermography index pictures of burns (b) and (c).

FIGURE 7.16 Thermal transients of burn fields of degree: I, IIa, IIb, IIb.

FIGURE 7.18 Pig's heart after heart infarct evoked by the indicated clamp (a), the cross section of the heart with visible area of the stroke (the necrosis of the left ventricle wall—under the finger—is evidenced by darker shadow) (b) and the micro-histopathologic picture showing the cell necrosis (c).

FIGURE 7.19 Thermograms of the heart: before (a) and after the evoked infarct (b). The change of the PT/ADT pictures in time (indicated in the subscript of the thermogram) 0.5 h after the LAD clamping (the tissue is still alive) (c), and 3 h later (the necrosis is evidenced by the change of thermal properties of the tissue) (d).

FIGURE 7.21 ADT picture of clinical intervention—before the CABG (a) and after the operation (b). Important is more uniform temperature distribution after the operation proving that intervention was fully successful.

FIGURE 9.1 Bilateral frontal.

FIGURE 9.2 Right oblique.

FIGURE 9.3 Left oblique.

FIGURE 9.4 Right close-up.

FIGURE 9.5 Left close-up.

FIGURE 9.6 TH1 (normal uniform nonvascular).

FIGURE 9.7 Right TH5 (severely abnormal).

FIGURE 10.2 (a) Tumor angiogenesis. (b) High nuclear grade ductal carcinoma *in situ* with numerous blood vessels (angiogenesis) (Tabar). (c) Invasive ductal carcinoma with central necrosis and angiogenesis (Tabar).

FIGURE 10.4 (a) A 46-year-old patient: Lump in the upper central area of the right breast. *Infrared imaging* (A): Significant vascular asymmetry (SVA) in the upper central area of the right breast (IR-3). *Mammography* (B): Corresponding speculated opacity. *Surgical histology*: 2 cm infiltrating ductal carcinoma with negative sentinel nodes. (b) A 44-year-old patient: *Infrared imaging* (A): Revealed a significant vascular asymmetry in the upper central and inner quadrants of the right breast with a ΔT of 1.8°C (IR-4.8). *Corresponding mammography* (B): Reveals a spiculated lesion in the upper central portion of the right breast. *Surgical histology*: 0.7 cm infiltrating ductal carcinoma. Patient underwent adjuvant brachytherapy. (c) A 52-year-old patient: Presented with a mild fullness in the lower outer quadrant of the right breast. *Infrared imaging* (A): Left breast (B): right breast reveals extensive significant vascular asymmetry with a ΔT of 1.35°C (IR-5.3). A 2 cm cancer was found in the lower outer area of the right breast. (d) A 37-year-old patient: *Infrared image* (A): Significant vascular asymmetry in the upper inner quadrant of the left breast with a ΔT of 1.75°C (IR-4) (mod IR-4.75). *Mammography* (B): Corresponding spiculated lesion. *Ultrasound* (C): 6 mm lesion. *Surgical histology*: 0.7 cm infiltrating ductal carcinoma.

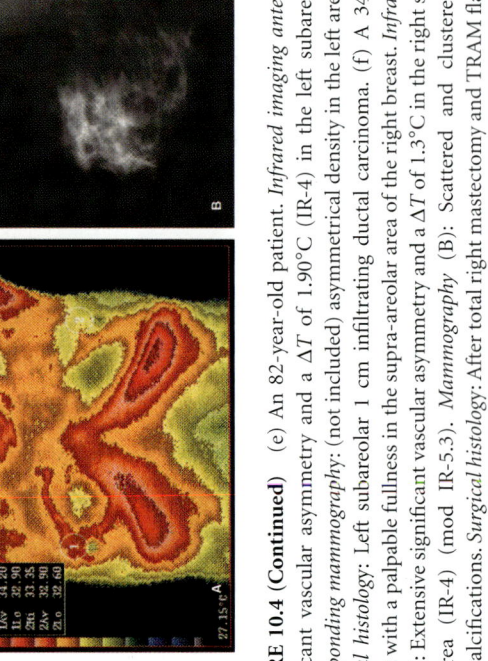

FIGURE 10.4 (Continued) (e) An 82-year-old patient. *Infrared imaging anterior view:* Significant vascular asymmetry and a ΔT of 1.90°C (IR-4) in the left subareolar area. *Corresponding mammography:* (not included) asymmetrical density in the left areolar area. *Surgical histology:* Left subareolar 1 cm infiltrating ductal carcinoma. (f) A 34-year-old patient with a palpable fullness in the supra-areolar area of the right breast. *Infrared imaging* (A): Extensive significant vascular asymmetry and a ΔT of 1.3°C in the right supra areolar area (IR-4) (mod IR-5.3). *Mammography* (B): Scattered and clustered central microcalcifications. *Surgical histology:* After total right mastectomy and TRAM flap: multifocal DCIS and infiltrating ductal CA centered over a 3 cm area of the supra areolar area.

FIGURE 10.5 (a) A 48-year-old patient *Infrared imaging* (A): Significant vascular asymmetry and a ΔT of 0.8°C (IR-3) in the lower inner quadrant of the left breast. *Corresponding mammography* (B): A nonspecific density. *Surgical histology:* 1.6 cm left lower inner quadrant infiltrating ductal carcinoma. (b) A 40-year-old patient. *Infrared imaging* (A): left breast (B) right breast: focal hot spot in the right subareolar area on a background of increased vascular activity with a ΔT of 1.1°C (IR-4). *Corresponding mammography* (C): Reveals dense tissue bilaterally. *Surgical histology:* reveals a 1 cm right infiltrating ductal carcinoma and positive lymph nodes.

FIGURE 10.5 (Continued) (c) A 51-year-old patient. *Infrared imaging* (A): Significant vascular asymmetry and a ΔT of 2.2°C (IR-5) in the upper central area of the left breast. *Corresponding mammography* (B): Mild scattered densities. *Surgical histology*: 2.5 cm infiltrating ductal carcinoma in the upper central area of the left breast. (d) A 44-year-old patient. *Infrared imaging* (A): Significant vascular asymmetry and a ΔT of 1.58°C (IR-4) in the upper inner quadrant of the left breast. *Corresponding mammography* (B): A nonspecific corresponding density. *Surgical histology*: A 0.9 cm left upper inner quadrant infiltrating ductal carcinoma. (e) A 45-year-old patient with a nodule in central area of left breast. *Infrared imaging* (A): Extensive significant vascular asymmetry (SVA) in the central inner area of the left breast with a ΔT of 0.75°C (IR-3) (mod IR-4.75). *Mammography* (B): Non-contributory. *Surgical histology*: 1.5 cm infiltrating ductal carcinoma with necrosis in the central inner area and 3 + axillary nodes. (f) A 51-year-old patient. *Infrared imaging* (A): Extensive significant vascular asymmetry and a ΔT of 2.2° (IR-5) in the upper central area of the left breast. *Corresponding mammography* (B) scattered densities. *Surgical histology*: 2.5 cm infiltrating ductal carcinoma in the upper central area of the left breast.

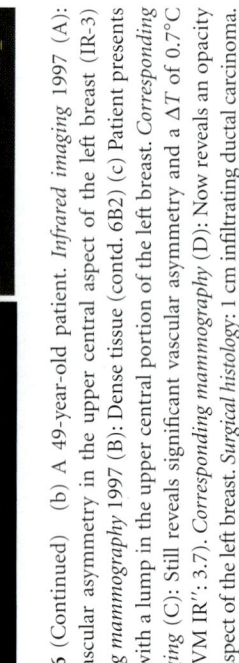

FIGURE 10.5 (Continued) (g) A 74-year-old patient. *Infrared imaging* (A): significant vascular asymmetry in the upper central portion of the right breast with a ΔT of 2.8°C (IR-5) (Mod VM IR: 6.8). *Corresponding mammography* (B): Bilateral extensive density. *Surgical histology*: 1 cm right central quadrant infiltrating ductal carcinoma.

FIGURE 10.5 (Continued) (b) A 49-year-old patient. *Infrared imaging* 1997 (A): Significant vascular asymmetry in the upper central aspect of the left breast (IR-3) *Corresponding mammography* 1997 (B): Dense tissue (contd. 6B2) (c) Patient presents 2 years later with a lump in the upper central portion of the left breast. *Corresponding infrared imaging* (C): Still reveals significant vascular asymmetry and a ΔT of 0.7°C (IR-3) (Mod VM IR'': 3.7). *Corresponding mammography* (D): Now reveals an opacity in the upper aspect of the left breast. *Surgical histology*: 1 cm infiltrating ductal carcinoma.

FIGURE 10.6 (a) A 66-year-old patient. Initially seen 2 years prior to diagnosis of left breast cancer for probable fibrocystic disorder (FCD) and scattered cysts, mostly on the left side. *Initial infrared imaging* (A): Extensive significant vascular asymmetry left breast and a near global ΔT of 1.4°C (IR-4) (Mod IR: 5.4). *Initial mammography* (B): Scattered opacities and ultrasound and cytologies were consistent with FCD. Two years later a 1.7 cm cancer was found in the central portion of the left breast.

FIGURE 10.7 (a) A 52-year-old patient. *Infrared imaging* (A): Extensive vascular asymmetry (SVA) in the right breast with a ΔT of 1.2°C (IR-5.2). The patient was started on pre-operative chemotherapy (PCT). *Post-PCT infrared imaging* (B): Resolution of previously noted SVA (IR-2). *Surgical histology*: no residual carcinoma in the resected right breast specimen. (b) A 32-year-old patient. *Infrared imaging* (A): Extensive significant vascular asymmetry and tortuous vascular pattern and a ΔT of 1.3°C (IR-5.3) in the right breast. *Corresponding mammography* (B): Scattered densities. Patient was started on pre-operative chemotherapy (PCT). *Post-PCT infrared image* (C —left breast; D — right breast): Notable resolution of SVA, with a whole breast ΔT of 0.7°C (IR-2). *Surgical histology*: No residual right carcinoma and chemotherapy induced changes. (c) A 47-year-old patient. *Infrared imaging* (A): Extensive significant vascular asymmetry in the inner half of the left breast with a ΔT of 2°C (IR-6.0). The patient was started on pre-operative chemotherapy (PCT). *Post-PCT infrared imaging* (B): no residual asymmetry (IR-1). *Surgical histology*: No viable residual carcinoma, with chemotherapy induced dense fibrosis surrounding nonviable tumor cells. (d) A 56-year-old patient. *Pre-chemotherapy infrared imaging* (A): Significant vascular asymmetry overlying the central portion of the left breast with a ΔT of 1.35°C (IR-4.35). The patient was given pre-operative chemotherapy (PCT). *Post-PCT infrared* (C): mild bilateral vascular symmetry (IR-). *Surgical histology*: no residual tumor. (e) A 54-year-old patient. *Infrared image* (A): extensive significant vascular asymmetry right breast with a rT of 2.8°C (IR-6.8). Received pre-operative chemotherapy (PCT). *Post-PCT infrared* (B): Mild local residual vascular asymmetry with a rT of 1.65°C (IR-3.65). *Surgical pathology*: No residual viable carcinoma.

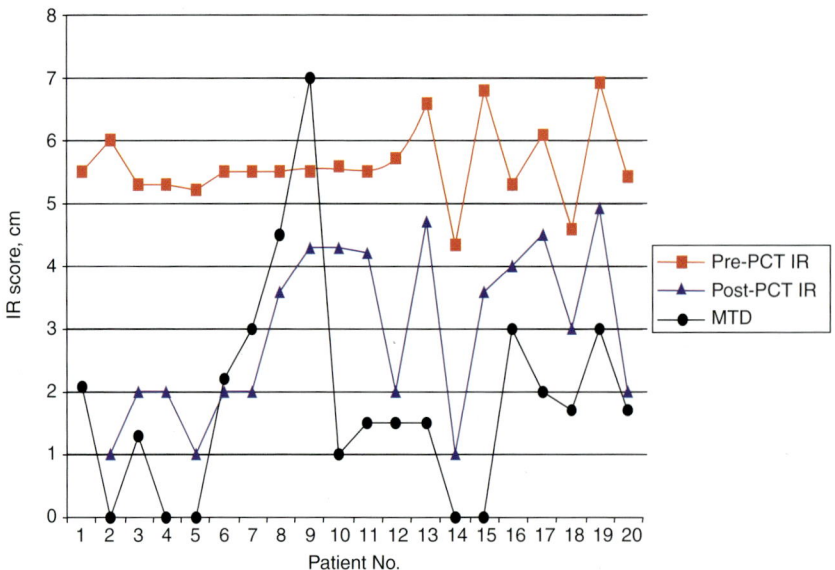

FIGURE 10.8 Pre- and Post-PCT IR Score and histological maximum tumor dimension (MTD).

FIGURE 10.9 (a) A stable vascular distribution in the lower inner quadrant of the left breast over a 12-month period. *Infrared imaging* of the breast usually remains remarkably stable in the absence of any on going developing significant pathology. It is important in grading these images to determine if the findings are to be considered evolving and important or stable and possibly relating to the patient's vascular anatomy. (b) An identical vascular distribution of the left breast over a 12-month period. (c) A stable vascular distribution in both breasts over a 12-month period.

FIGURE 10.10 (a) A 50-year-old patient. *Infrared imaging* (A): Significant vascular asymmetry and a ΔT of 3.4°C (IR-5) in the right breast. *Corresponding mammography* (B): Increased density and microcalcifications in the right breast. *Surgical histology*: extensive right multi-focal infiltrating ductal carcinoma requiring a total mastectomy. (b) A 50-year-old patient. *Infrared imaging* (A): Significant vascular asymmetry with a near global ΔT of 2.35°C in the left breast (IR-5). *Mammography* (not available) diffuse density. *Surgical histology*: Left multi-focal infiltrating ductal carcinoma requiring a total mastectomy.

FIGURE 10.11 (a) Four years post right partial mastectomy, the patient is recurrence free. Current *Infrared imaging* (A): shows no activity and *Mammography* (B): shows scar tissue. (b) *Infrared image*, 5 years following a left partial mastectomy and radiotherapy for carcinoma revealing slight asymmetry of volume, but no abnormal vascular abnormality and resolution of radiation-induced changes. The patient is disease free.

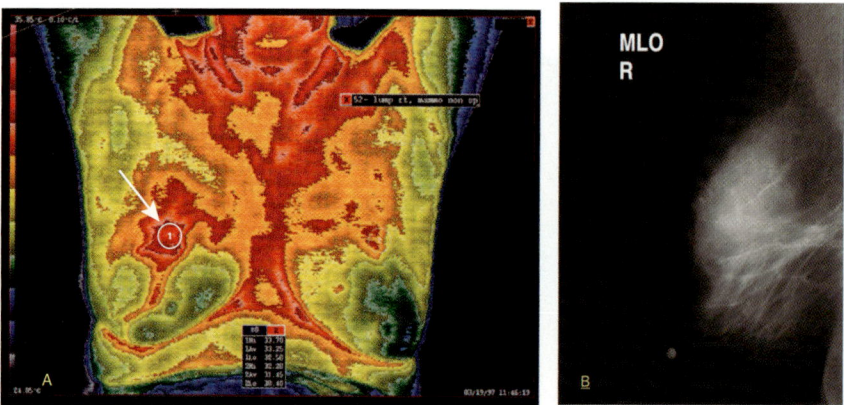

FIGURE 10.12 A 52-year-old patient, 5 years following right partial mastectomy, radiation, and chemotherapy for right breast cancer. Recent follow-up Infrared Imaging (A) now reveals significant vascular asymmetry (SVA) in the right breast with a ΔT of 1.5°C in the area of the previous surgery (IR-4). *Corresponding mammography* (B): Density and scar issue vs. possible recurrence. *Surgical histology*: 4 cm, recurrent right carcinoma in the area of the previous resection.

FIGURE 10.13 (a) A 45-year-old patient with small nodular process just inferior and medial to the left nipple areolar complex. *Infrared imaging* (A), without digital enhancement, was carried out and circles were placed on the nipple area rather than just below and medial to it. The nonenhanced IR-image was thus initially misinterpreted as normal with a ΔT of 0.25°C. The same image was recalled and *repeated* (B), now with appropriate digital enhancement and once again, documented the presence of increased vascular activity just inferior and medial to the left nipple areolar complex with a ΔT of 1.15°C (IR-4.15). A 1.5 cm. cancer was found just below the left nipple. (b) A 37-year-old patient with lump in the upper inner quadrant of the left breast. Mammography confirms spiculated mass. *Infrared imaging* (A): Reported as "normal." Infrared imaging was repeated after appropriate *digital adjustment* (B): Now reveals obvious significant vascular asymmetry in the same area and a ΔT of 1.75°C (Ir-4) (mod IR-4.75). Using a different IR-camera on the *same patient* (C) confirms same finding. *Surgical histology*: 1.5 cm infiltrating ductal CA.

FIGURE 12.1 ROI of thermal image and its histogram.

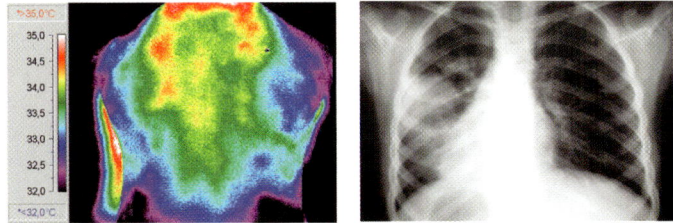

FIGURE 12.2 Nonsymmetrical temperature distribution for pneumonia with corresponding x-ray image.

FIGURE 12.3 Thermal image of the healthy breast.

FIGURE 12.4 Thermal image of the breast with malignant tumor (left side).

FIGURE 12.12 Example of thermal image with the tumor.

FIGURE 13.1 Architecture of our face recognition system.

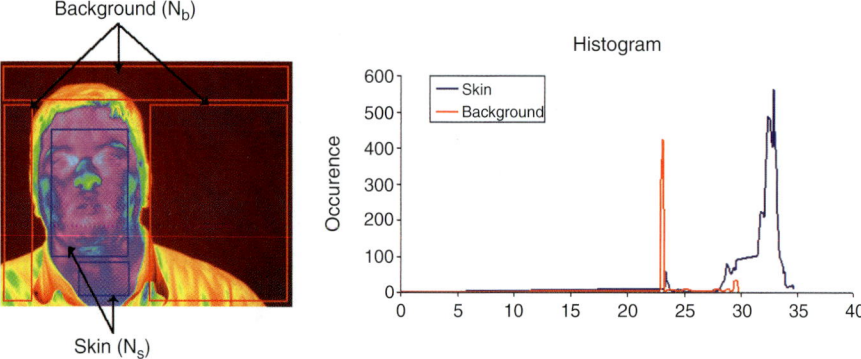

FIGURE 13.4 Skin and background: (a) selection of samples for EM algorithm and (b) corresponding bimodal temperature distributions.

FIGURE 13.5 Segmentation of facial skin region: (a) original thermal facial image and (b) result of Bayesian segmentation.

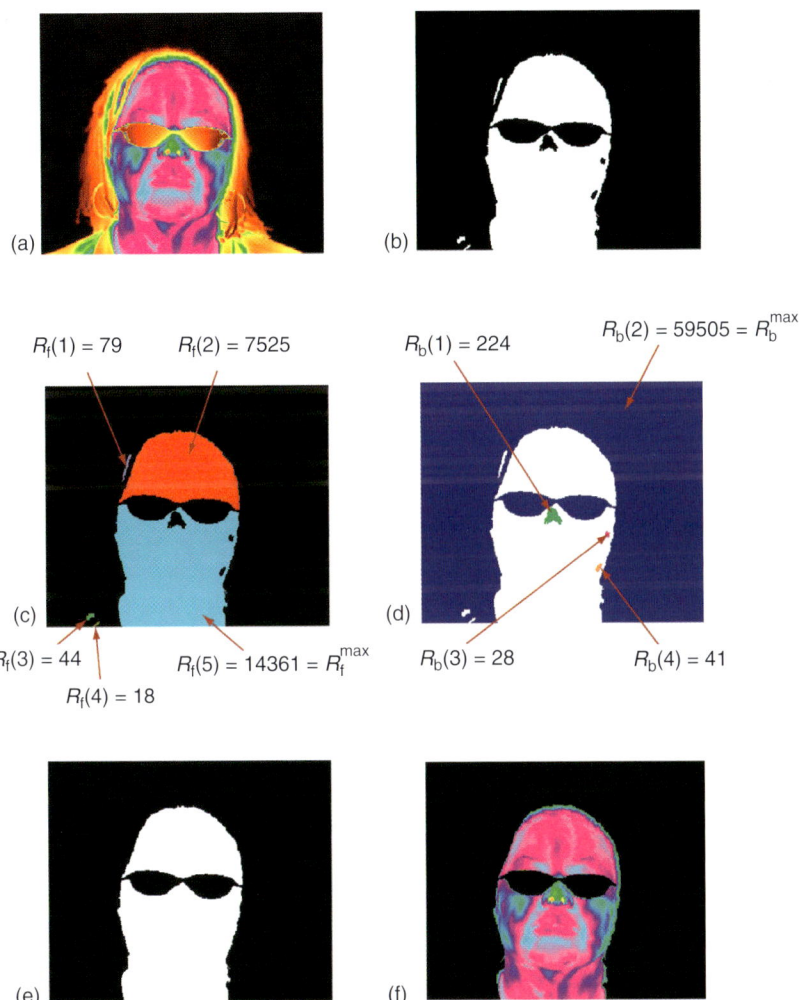

FIGURE 13.6 Segmentation of facial skin region: (a) original thermal facial image; (b) binary segmented image; (c) foreground regions each represented in different color; (d) background regions each represented in different color; (e) binary mask after foreground and background corrections; and (f) final segmentation result after postprocessing.

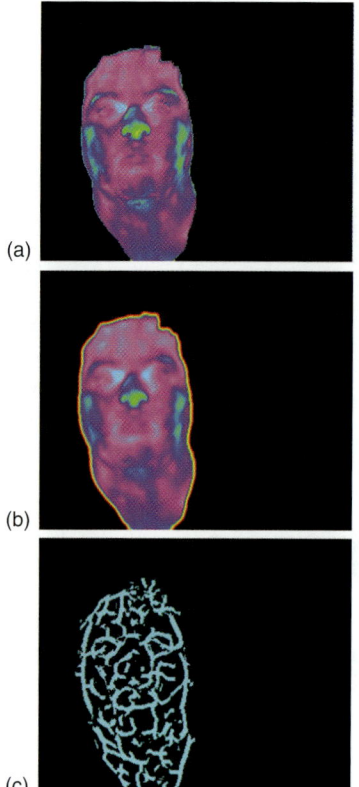

FIGURE 13.7 Vascular network extraction: (a) original segmented image; (b) anisotropically diffused image; and (c) blood vessels extracted using white top-hat segmentation.

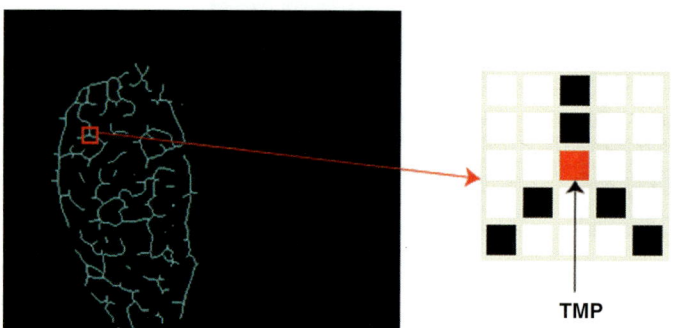

FIGURE 13.8 TMP extracted from the thinned vascular network.

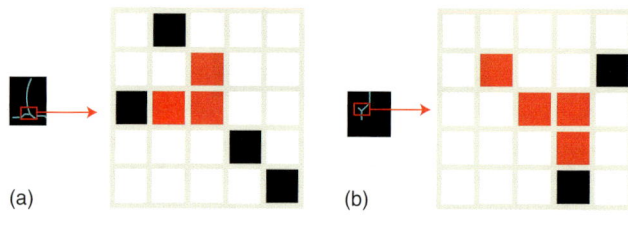

FIGURE 13.9 Spurious TMPs: (a) clustered TMPs and (b) spike formed due to a trivially short branch.

FIGURE 13.10 Visualization of the various stages of the vascular feature extraction algorithm: (a) a typical thermal facial image; (b) facial tissue delineated from the background; (c) network of vascular contours extracted from the thermal facial image; (d) skeletonized vessel map; (e) extracted TMPs from branching points; and (f) cleaned TMP set.

FIGURE 13.11 Samples from our training set featuring five (5) different poses per subject. From left to right the views depicted are left profile, mid-left profile, center, mid-right profile, and right profile.

FIGURE 13.12 (a) Thermal facial image of a subject acquired on October 17, 2003; (b) corresponding vascular network; (c) thermal facial image of the same subject acquired on April 29, 2004; and (d) corresponding vascular network.

FIGURE 13.13 (a) Test image and (b) corresponding vascular network. (c) Mid-left profile image picked from training database by pose estimation and (d) corresponding vascular network.

FIGURE 14.1 Absorption spectra of the three major components of tissue in the NIR region; oxy- and deoxy-hemoglobin, and water.

FIGURE 14.2 Functional imaging of rat cranium during changes in inhaled oxygen concentration. (a) MRI image; (b) creation of the mesh to distinguish different compartments in the brain; (c) map of hemoglobin concentration and oxygen saturation of the rat brain without structural constraints from MRI; and (d) same as (c) with structural constraints including tissue heterogeneity. In (c) and (d) the rows from top correspond to 13, 8, and 0% (after death) oxygen inhaled. (Courtesy of Dartmouth College.)

FIGURE 14.8 An example of images obtained from the forearm of a normal healthy male subject. (a) Original thermogram; (b) emissivity image; and (c) thermogram corrected by emissivity.

FIGURE 14.10 Typical multimodality images obtained from a patient with KS lesion. The number '1' and '5' in the visual image were written on the skin to identify the lesions for tumor measurement. The solid line in the thermal and LDI demarks the border of the visible KS lesion. Shown is a representative patient from the study reported in Reference 95.

FIGURE 14.12 Typical example of lesion obtained from a subject with KS (a) before, and (b) after the treatment. Improvement after the treatment can be assessed by the thermal or LDI images after 18 weeks. Shown is a patient from the clinical trial reported in Reference 95.

FIGURE 14.13 Set of comparative images of a KS patient. (a) Visual, (b) thermal, (c) laser Doppler, (d) HbO$_2$ fraction, and (e) tissue blood volume fraction images are provided [110].

FIGURE 15.1 (a) Second grade right varicocele. The temperature distribution all over the scrotum clearly highlights significant differences between affected and unaffected testicles. (b) The same scrotum after varicocelectomy. The surgical treatment reduced the increased temperature on the affected hemiscrotum and restored the symmetry in the scrotal temperature distribution. (c) Third-grade left varicocele. (d) The same scrotum after varicocelectomy. The treatment was unsuccessful in repairing the venous reflux, as documented by the persisting asymmetric scrotal distribution.

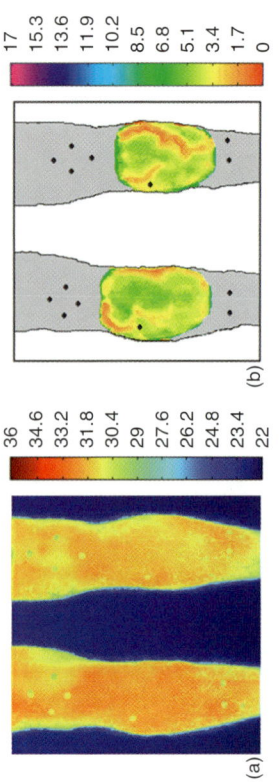

FIGURE 15.6 Second-class muscular lesion on the left leg abductor—medial view. (a) Static thermography image. The color bar shows the pixel temperature color mapping. The light gray spots indicate the presence of the trauma. (b) Time constant τ image after mild cold stress. The color bar illustrates the recovery time, in minutes, for each pixel. The black spots are the markers used as position references. (From Merla, A., et al., Quantifying the relevance and stage of disease with Tau imaging technique. *IEEE Eng. Biol. Meg.*, 21, 86, 2002, by permission of the editor.)

FIGURE 15.7 Raynaud's Phenomenon Secondary to Scleroderma. (a) Static thermography image. The color bar shows the pixel temperature mapping. (b) Time constant τ image after mild cold stress. The color bar illustrates the recovery time, in minutes, for each pixel. The regions associated with longer recovery times identify the main damaged finger regions. (From Merla, A., et al., Quantifying the relevance and stage of disease with Tau imaging technique. *IEEE Eng. Biol. Meg.*, 21, 86, 2002, by permission of the editor.)

FIGURE 15.8 Bi-lateral vein thrombosis. (a) Static thermography image. The color bar shows the pixel temperature color mapping. (b) Time constant τ image after mild cold stress. The color bar illustrates the recovery time, in minutes, for each pixel. The areas associated with shorter recovery times identify the regions interested by the thrombosis. (From Merla, A., et al., Quantifying the relevance and stage of disease with Tau imaging technique. *IEEE Eng. Biol. Meg.*, 21, 86, 2002, by permission of the editor.)

FIGURE 15.9 Total body Tc changes during incremental load exercise for a trained subject. (a) baseline Tc distribution; (b) Tc distribution immediately before reaching the age-predicted maximal HR value; (c) Tc distribution at the start of the recovery period (treadmill speed set at stage 1 value); (d) Tc distribution during postexercise period. The color bar reports the pseudo-colors associated the values of Tc.

FIGURE 17.1 Acute tendonitis of the right Achilles tendon in a patient suffering from inflammatory spondylarthropathy.

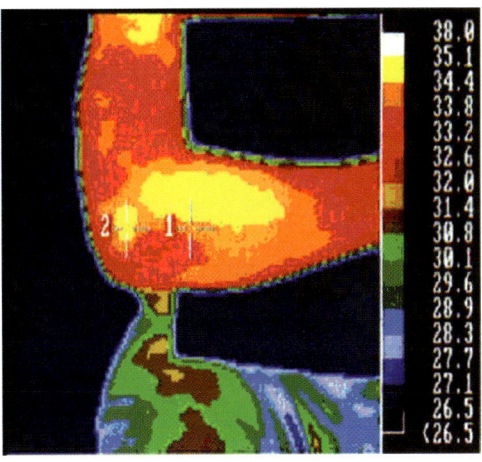

FIGURE 17.2 Tennis elbow with a typical hot spot in the region of tendon insertion.

FIGURE 17.3 Decreased temperature in patient with a frozen shoulder on the left-hand side.

FIGURE 17.5 Early CRPS after radius fracture. (a) 2 h after cast removal; (b) 1 week later.

TABLE 18.1 Normal study. Upper body fIR study (thermal signature).

TABLE 18.1 Normal study. Lower body fIR study (thermal signature).

TABLE 18.2 Acute trauma. Upper body fIR study (thermal signature).

TABLE 18.2 Acute trauma. Lower body fIR study (thermal signature).

TABLE 18.3 Small caliber fiber sensory distal mononeuropathy. Upper body fIR study (thermal signature).

TABLE 18.4 Acute CRPS I. Upper body fIR study (thermal signature).

TABLE 18.4 Acute CRPS I. Lower body fIR study (thermal signature).

TABLE 18.5 Acute CRPS I (bilateral thermal findings). Upper body fIR study (thermal signature).

TABLE 18.6 Chronic CRPS I. Upper body fIR study (thermal signature).

FIGURE 22.1 Body views investigated.

FIGURE 23.1 Example of retrieving thermal images based on a query of an *arm* image. The query image is the one on the top left; the other images are those most similar to the query ordered in decreasing similarity (from left to right, top to bottom).

FIGURE 23.2 Example of retrieving thermal images based on a query of a *neck* image. The result is laid out in the same structure as that of Figure 23.1.

FIGURE 23.3 Thermal hand images of healthy subject (a) and (b) together with a thermogram showing an in ammation (c).

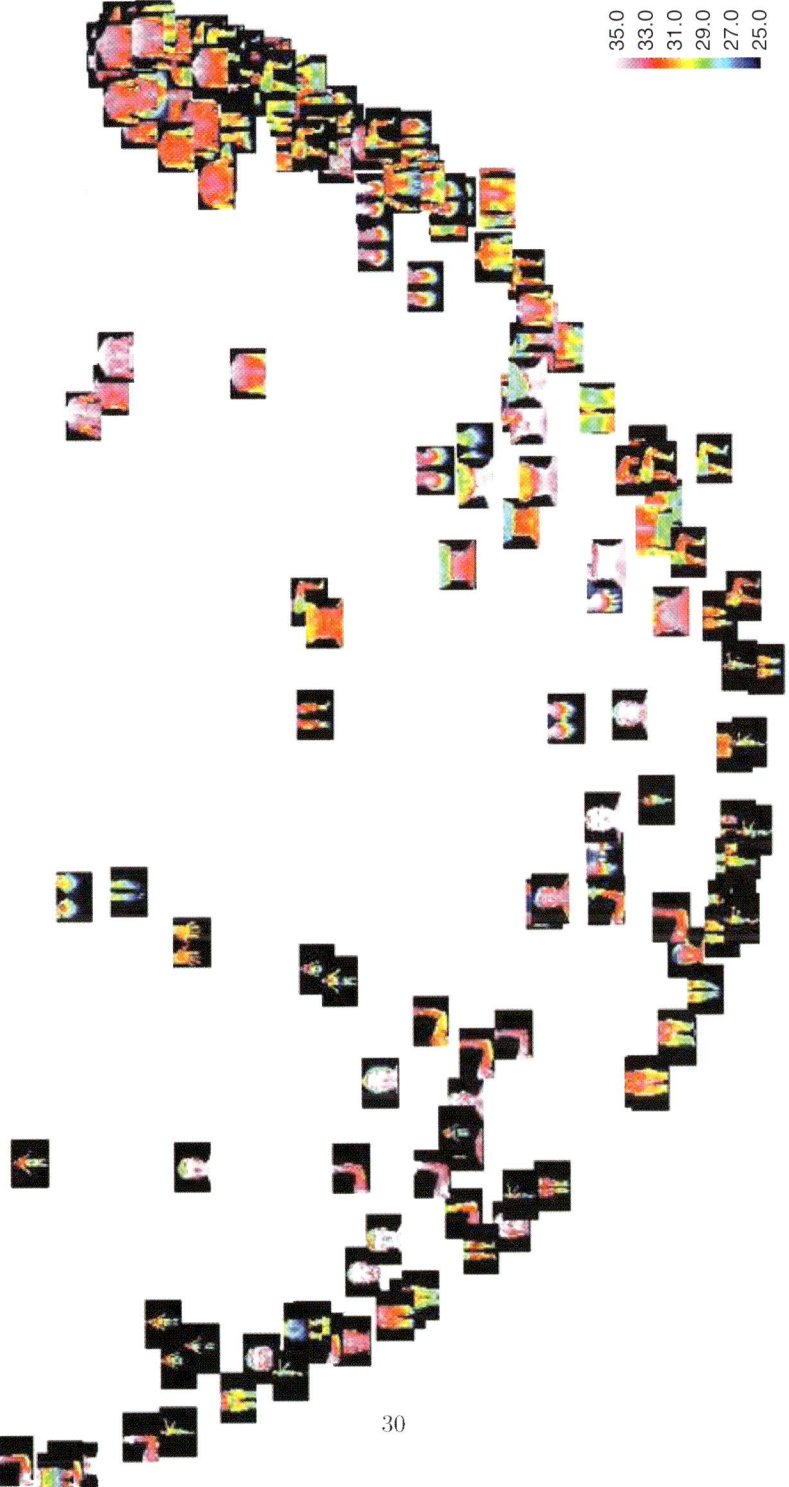

FIGURE 23.4 Global visualisation view of complete thermal image database.

FIGURE 23.5 Zoomed-in area showing leg and upper body images.